PHARMACOLOGY

for the PREHOSPITAL PROFESSIONAL

Second Edition

Jeffrey S. Guy

JONES & BARTLETT
LEARNING

World Headquarters
Jones & Bartlett Learning
5 Wall Street
Burlington, MA 01803
978-443-5000
info@jblearning.com
www.jblearning.com
www.psglearning.com

Jones & Bartlett Learning books and products are available through most bookstores and online booksellers. To contact the Jones & Bartlett Learning Public Safety Group directly, call 800-832-0034, fax 978-443-8000, or visit our website, www.psglearning.com.

Substantial discounts on bulk quantities of Jones & Bartlett Learning publications are available to corporations, professional associations, and other qualified organizations. For details and specific discount information, contact the special sales department at Jones & Bartlett Learning via the above contact information or send an email to specialsales@jblearning.com.

04146-0

Production Credits

General Manager and Executive Publisher: Kimberly Brophy
VP, Product Development: Christine Emerton
Senior Managing Editor: Donna Gridley
Product Manager: Tiffany Sliter
Associate Development Editor: Ashley Procum
VP, Sales, Public Safety Group: Matthew Maniscalco
Project Manager: Kristen Rogers
Project Specialist: John Fuller
Digital Products Manager: Jordan McKenzie
Digital Project Specialist: Angela Dooley
Director of Marketing Operations: Brian Rooney
Marketing Manager: Jessica Carmichael
Associate Marketing Manager: Hayley Lorge

Production Services Manager: Colleen Lamy
VP, Manufacturing and Inventory Control: Therese Connell
Composition: S4Carlisle Publishing Services
Project Management: S4Carlisle Publishing Services
Cover Design: Matthew Oliva
Text Design: Kristin E. Parker
Senior Media Development Editor: Shannon Sheehan
Media Development Editor: Troy Liston
Rights & Media Specialist: John Rusk
Cover Image (Title Page, Part Opener, Chapter Opener):
  © Andrew Brookes/Getty Images
Printing and Binding: LSC Communications
Cover Printing: LSC Communications

Library of Congress Cataloging-in-Publication Data
Names: Guy, Jeffrey S., author.
Title: Pharmacology for the prehospital professional / Jeffrey S. Guy.
Description: Second edition. | Burlington, MA : Jones & Bartlett Learning,
  [2020] | Includes bibliographical references and index.
Identifiers: LCCN 2019011665 | ISBN 9781284041460 (paperback : alk. paper)
Subjects: | MESH: Pharmacological Phenomena | Pharmaceutical
  Preparations--administration & dosage | Pharmacokinetics | Drug
  Therapy--methods | Emergency Medical Services--methods
Classification: LCC RM300 | NLM QV 4 | DDC 615/.1--dc23 LC record available at https://lccn.loc.gov/2019011665

6048

Printed in the United States of America
23 22 21 20 19   10 9 8 7 6 5 4 3 2 1

To my wife, Deanna, and my children,
Danielle, Christian, Madeline, Spencer, and Layne.
I love all of you and I am blessed.

Brief Contents

Contents

Preface

▶ Second Edition

Finally, a textbook that makes pharmacology for prehospital providers easy and understandable! This text puts EMS pharmacology in perspective and presents information the way you learn it and use it—case by case and step by step.

To safely and effectively administer drugs to your patients, you must understand what is happening in their bodies when they are sick or injured, and you must understand how the right drug works to improve these processes. Further, you will need to know how to calculate the correct dosage for a specific patient in a specific situation and will need to ensure that your actions are legal and ethical. This textbook introduces these concepts, then applies them to the prehospital scenarios that you will encounter. Along the way, it walks you through important drug administration procedures and real-world case studies.

Pharmacology for the Prehospital Professional, Second Edition contains over 90 profiles of drugs commonly used in the prehospital setting. Each drug profile includes detailed information about drug administration, including classification, action, indication, adverse effects, contraindications, dosage, and special considerations. Product photographs and illustrations will help you identify the drugs discussed. A thorough review of special considerations, such as critical care transport and special patient populations, will help prepare you to work in a challenging and dynamic environment. Finally, Appendices A and B reframe the information provided in the chapters, and Appendices C and D familiarize you with common herbal supplements and over-the-counter medications that must not be overlooked when considering the big picture of your patient's care.

▶ About the Author

Dr. Jeffrey S. Guy, a former paramedic, is the director of the Vanderbilt Burn Center. He is board certified by the American Board of Surgery in General Surgery and Surgical Critical Care. Additionally, Dr. Guy is fellowship trained in trauma surgery as well as pediatric and adult burn surgery. He is the medical director for the paramedic training program at Columbia State Community College and the medical director for Tennessee State Parks. He previously served on the PHTLS Executive Council. He has a particular interest in emergency medical services.

Acknowledgments

The author and publisher wish to acknowledge and thank the many reviewers and editors of this book who devoted countless hours to intensive review. Their commitments were invaluable in helping develop and fine-tune the manuscript. A special thank you goes out to Andrew Bartkus and Mike Boblitt for their work in developing this second edition.

▶ Reviewers

Peter Connick, NREMT, EMT I/C
Emergency Medical Teaching Services, Inc.
Pembroke, Massachusetts
Fire Chief
Chatham Fire Department
Chatham, Massachusetts

Kevin Curry, NRP, CCEMTP
Augusta Fire Rescue
Augusta, Maine

Fidel O. Garcia, Paramedic
Professional EMS Education
Grand Junction, Colorado

Jamie O. Gray, BS, AAS, NRP
Alabama Department of Public Health
Office of EMS
Montgomery, Alabama

Jason D. Haag, CCEMT-P, CIC
Finger Lakes Ambulance
Clifton Springs, New York
Wayne County Advanced Life Support Services
Marion, New York
Finger Lakes Regional Emergency Medical Services
    Council
Geneva, New York

Anthony S. Harbour, MEd, BSN, RN, NRP
Director
Southern Virginia Emergency Medical Services
Roanoke, Virginia

Chad S. Kim, MBA, NRP
Albuquerque Fire Department
Albuquerque, New Mexico
University of New Mexico
Albuquerque, New Mexico

Nicholas J. Montelauro, BS, NRP, FP-C, NCEE, CHSE
Indiana University Health Emergency Response
    Training Institute
Indianapolis, Indiana

Keito Ortiz, Paramedic
Paramedic Training Coordinator
Jamaica Hospital Medical Center
Jamaica, New York

Deb Petty, BS, EMT-P
Captain Training Officer
St. Charles County Ambulance District
St. Charles, Missouri

Scott Vanderkooi, MEd, BS, NRP
Blue Ridge Community College
Weyers Cave, Virginia

▶ First-Edition Reviewers

David K. Anderson, BS, EMT-P
Director, Paramedic Education Program
Northwest Regional Training Center
Vancouver, Washington

Jeffrey K. Benes, BS, NREMT-P
Owner/Consultant/Educator
Jeff Benes Company
Antioch, Illinois

Chip Boehm, RN, EMT-P/FF
EMS Educator
Portland Fire Department
Portland, Maine

Robert P. Breese, EMT-P, FP-C
Monroe Community College
Rochester, New York

Rob Brouhard, AA, EMT-P
Modesto, California

Anthony J. Brunello, BS, RN, PHRN, TNS, EMS-LI
Provena St. Mary's Hospital
Kankakee, Illinois

JoAnn Cobble, EdD, NREMT-P, RN
Dean, Division of Health Professions
Oklahoma City Community College
Oklahoma City, Oklahoma

Peter Connick, NREMT, EMT I/C
Emergency Medical Teaching Services, Inc.
Pembroke, Massachusetts
Fire Chief
Chatham Fire Department
Chatham, Massachusetts

Ken Davis, NREMT-P, CCEMT-P, FP-C
Paramedic Coordinator
Eastern New Mexico University
Roswell, New Mexico

Daryl D. DePestel, PharmD
Clinical Assistant Professor
University of Michigan College of Pharmacology
Ann Arbor, Michigan

Dennis Edgerly, EMT-P
EMS Instructor
HealthONE EMS
Englewood, Colorado

John F. Elder, CCEMT-P, EMT-P
Director of Education
CareFlight
Fort Worth, Texas

Sloan B. Fleming, PharmD
Vanderbilt University Medical Center
Nashville, Tennessee

Fidel O. Garcia, Paramedic
Professional EMS Education
Grand Junction, Colorado

Danna S. Hatley, PharmD
East Alabama Medical Center
Opelika, Alabama

Chad S. Kim, MBA, NRP
Albuquerque Fire Department
Albuquerque, New Mexico
University of New Mexico
Albuquerque, New Mexico

Michael W. Lynch, AS, CCEMT-P, NREMT-P
Administrative Director
Crozer Chester Medical Center
Media, Pennsylvania

Dean Martin, AAS, EMT-P
Division Chief
Fire Marshal/Training/EMS Division
Columbia Fire Department
Columbia, Missouri

Denise Martin, MS
Oakland Community College
Auburn Hills, Michigan

Joanne McCall, MA, BAS, RN, CEN, CFN, SANE-A
Providence Park Hospital
Novi, Michigan

Christine C. McEachin, BSN, RN, CEN, Paramedic/IC
Clinical Nurse Specialist—Emergency Services
William Beaumont Hospital—Troy
Troy, Michigan

Greg Mullen, MS, BS, NREMT-P
Education Coordinator
National EMS Academy
Lafayette, Louisiana

Joshua J. Neumiller, Pharm D, CDE, CGP, FASCP
Assistant Professor of Pharmacology
Washington State University
Spokane, Washington

Deb Petty, BS, EMT-P
Captain Training Officer
St. Charles County Ambulance District
St. Charles, Missouri

Lynn Pierzchalski-Goldstein, PharmD
Clinical Coordinator Pharmacy
Penrose St. Francis Health System
Colorado Springs, Colorado

Gregg D. Ramirez, BS, EMT-P
Student Services Director
Army Medical Department, Northwest Regional
Training Center
Vancouver, Washington

Ken Reardon, Flight Paramedic
LifeNet New York
Valhalla, New York

Judith A. Ruple, PhD, RN, NREMT-P
The Ruple Group/Education Consultants
The Villages, Florida
Professor (Retired)
University of Toledo
Toledo, Ohio

Janet L. Schulte, BS, AS, NR-CCEMT-P
Director of Continuing Education
IHM Health Studies Center
St. Louis, Missouri

Stephen M. Setter, PharmD, CDE, CGP, DVM
Associate Professor of Pharmacotherapy
Washington State University—Spokane
Elder Services, Visiting Nurses Association
Spokane, Washington

Douglas R. Smith, MAT, EMT-P, I/C
Educational Consultant
Platinum Educational Group, LLC
Jenison, Michigan

David L. Sullivan, PhD(c), NREMT-P
St. Petersburg College EMS/CE
Pinellas Park, Florida

Anthony Tedesco, RN, NREMT-P
St. Petersburg College
Pinellas Park, Florida

Donna G. Tidwell, BS, RN, EMT-P
Director of EMS Personnel Licensure and Education
Tennessee Department of Health Division of EMS
Nashville, Tennessee

▶ Second-Edition Contributor

Andrew Bartkus, JD, MSN, RN, CEN, CCRN, CFRN, NREMT-P, FP-C
Emergency Department Director
Sandoval Regional Medical Center
Rio Rancho, New Mexico

▶ First-Edition Contributors

Deanna L. Aftab Guy, MD
Assistant Professor of Pediatrics, Division of Pediatric
    Endocrinology
Vanderbilt University Medical Center
Nashville, Tennessee
Vanderbilt Children's Hospital
Nashville, Tennessee

Angela Allen, MSN, RN, ACNP-BC, CCRN, NREMT-B
Nurse Educator
Vanderbilt University Medical Center Burn Center
Nashville, Tennessee

Will Chapleau, EMT-P, RN, TNS
Manager, ATLS Program
American College of Surgeons
Chicago, Illinois

Gregory J. Chapman, BS, RRT, REMT-P
Program Director
Institute of Prehospital Emergency Medicine
Hudson Valley Community College
Troy, New York

Brenna Michelle Farmer, MD
Emergency Medicine Resident Physician
Vanderbilt University Department of Emergency
    Medicine
Vanderbilt University Medical Center
Nashville, Tennessee

William W. Goldsmith, DO
Assistant Professor of Clinical Anesthesiology
Vanderbilt University Medical Center
Nashville, Tennessee
Staff Anesthesiologist
Sacred Heart Hospital
Pensacola, Florida

Kirby R. Gross, MD, FACS
Commander
772nd Forward Surgical Team
Fort Campbell, Kentucky

Michelle M. McLean, MD, NREMT-P
Emergency Physician
Emergency Care Center
Covenant Hospital
Saginaw, Michigan

Leanna R. Miller, MN, RN, CCRN, CEN, NP
Assistant in Surgery
Vanderbilt University Medical School
Nashville, Tennessee
Educator: Trauma, Burn, Life Flight
Vanderbilt University Medical Center
Nashville, Tennessee

Deanna Moore, MSN, RN, ACNP-BC, CCRN, NREMT-P, FP-C
Acute Care Nurse Practitioner
Neurocare ICU
Vanderbilt University Hospital
Nashville, Tennessee

Mary Jane Pavlick, BA, AAS, RN, CEN, EMT-P, EMS-I
Guest Instructor
School of EMS, Cleveland Clinic Health System,
  Eastern Region
Euclid, Ohio
Human Resources Development
Hillcrest Hospital
Mayfield Heights, Ohio
Program Manager, Emergency Management
Hillcrest Hospital
Mayfield Heights, Ohio

Corey M. Slovis, MD, FACP, FACEP
Professor of Emergency Medicine
Chairman, Department of Emergency Medicine
Vanderbilt University School of Medicine
Nashville, Tennessee
Medical Director
Nashville Fire Department
Nashville, Tennessee

Steven J. White, MD, FACEP, FAAP
Assistant Professor of Emergency Medicine and
  Pediatrics
Vanderbilt University School of Medicine
Nashville, Tennessee
Emergency Department Attending Physician
Vanderbilt University Medical Center
Monroe Carrell Jr. Children's Hospital
Nashville, Tennessee

Stephen R. Wirth, Esq, MS, EMT-P
Partner
Page, Wolfberg & Wirth, LLC
Mechanicsburg, Pennsylvania
Adjunct Professor
University of Pittsburgh EMS Program
Pittsburgh, Pennsylvania
Adjunct Professor
George Washington University EMS Program
Washington, District of Columbia

Douglas M. Wolfberg, JD, BS, EMT-A
Partner
Page, Wolfberg & Wirth, LLC
Mechanicsburg, Pennsylvania
Adjunct Professor
Widener University School of Law
Harrisburg, Pennsylvania
Adjunct Professor
University of Pittsburgh EMS Program
Pittsburgh, Pennsylvania
Adjunct Professor
George Washington University EMS Program
Washington, District of Columbia

PART I
Foundations

CHAPTER 1

Principles of Pharmacology

OBJECTIVES

1. Explain the difference between a drug's generic name and trade name.
2. Explain the concepts of pharmacology, pharmacokinetics, receptor interactions, and pharmacodynamics.
3. Explain the dose-response relationship.
4. Define *enteral* and *parenteral medications*, and identify the routes of administration for each.
5. Explain first-pass metabolism.
6. Explain the process of drug metabolism and excretion.
7. Define *passive diffusion, carrier-mediated facilitated diffusion, active transport*, and *passive transport*.
8. Explain the difference and relationship between an agonist drug and an antagonist drug.
9. Explain the role of the autonomic nervous system and alpha$_1$, alpha$_2$, beta$_1$, and beta$_2$ receptors.
10. Discuss medications used to stimulate the adrenergic receptors: epinephrine, norepinephrine (Levophed), dopamine, dobutamine, and phenylephrine (Neo-Synephrine).
11. Discuss medications used to block the adrenergic receptors: atropine sulfate and scopolamine (Transderm Scop).

MEDICATIONS THAT APPEAR IN CHAPTER 1

Dopamine (Intropin)
Norepinephrine (Levophed)
Dobutamine (Dobutrex)
Phenylephrine
  (Neo-Synephrine)

Epinephrine
Propranolol (Inderal)
Labetalol (Normodyne,
  Trandate)
Metoprolol (Lopressor, Toprol XL)

Atropine sulfate
Scopolamine (Transderm
  Scop)

CASE STUDY

Your unit is dispatched to a medical call with the report of a 42-year-old woman who has collapsed. The information you receive from the dispatcher is that her brother found her prone on the floor and that she is nonresponsive to his attempts to awaken her. The patient's brother is not aware of any preexisting medical conditions. When you arrive, you find a 42-year-old woman lying on the floor approximately 4 feet from a flight of stairs. Her family has moved her to the supine position. Some vomit has pooled next to her head, and she has some vomit on her face.

An unresponsive person, or "man down," presents several challenges. What are the potential causes of this patient's altered level of consciousness? Cardiac arrhythmia, diabetic emergency, seizure, toxic ingestion or overdose, stroke, and traumatic brain injury are only a few of the potential causes. The treatment of each of these conditions requires unique pharmacologic interventions.

The treatment priorities for the patient in the preceding scenario are the same for all patients: scene safety, airway, breathing, and circulation. You kneel down next to the patient and ensure that her airway is patent and free of vomitus. Her respirations are spontaneous and unlabored. Your partner checks her oxygen saturation reading and reports that it is 93%. While you place a nonrebreathing oxygen mask, you also place her on the cardiac monitor and learn that she is in sinus tachycardia. She begins to have a violent tonic-clonic seizure. Your partner protects her head and closely monitors her airway.

Seizures have several causes, but your immediate priorities include ensuring airway patency and protecting the patient from harm. As the paramedic in charge, you consider your options for stopping the current seizure, preventing additional seizures, preventing potential metabolic complications of seizures, and investigating the potential causes of the seizure that may require emergency treatment. What are the appropriate drugs for the treatment of seizures? What is the most rapid way of delivering those drugs? What if the routes of drug administration cannot be obtained or fail? Are additional routes of drug administration available? Is the patient taking any medications that may interact with the emergency medications? What are some of the adverse effects of the emergency medications to monitor for during and after administration? Does the patient have any allergies or conditions that contraindicate any medications? Does the patient have kidney or liver disease that may require a reduction in drug dosages?

▶ Introduction

Pharmacology can be a challenging topic for any healthcare professional to master. Thousands of drugs are in use, all of which have specific actions, indications, dosages, and **adverse effects**. Several methods of administering drugs exist as well, depending on the drug and the patient. Providing drug therapy to patients in hectic emergency situations in which little time is available to reflect or consult a reference text is particularly challenging.

Try not to approach pharmacology as a topic that requires memorization of a multitude of facts and dosages. Instead, approach it as an opportunity to synthesize and apply all the information you have learned while studying anatomy, physiology, and the management of specific diseases. As you read this text, intermittently stop and reflect on how you will use the information to take action during an emergency. Get comfortable reciting the names and dosages of these medications. Imagine a singer who practices a song to become familiar with the lyrics. The first time you say "epinephrine 1 mg IV push" should not be at the bedside of a critical patient. When you go through this text, practice saying the names of these drugs and their dosages. Take time to study the photographs of the drugs, and imagine yourself requesting a particular medication, getting it out of a box, and administering that medication to a patient.

Athletes and surgeons often visualize each step of a particular event or operation before their performance. As a prehospital provider, patients' lives depend on your optimal performance. Mental rehearsal will make the topic of pharmacology more interesting and familiar.

▶ Drug Names

Many medications have complex-sounding names. You do not need to know every name of every medication you might encounter while providing emergency care. However, you must be able to recognize, document, and communicate important information about various medications that patients may be taking and that you may be administering.

All drugs have at least two names: a generic name and a trade name. The **generic name** is usually an abbreviated version of the drug's chemical name. The generic name is registered with the U.S. Food and Drug Administration (FDA) and listed in a directory of medications known as the **United States Pharmacopeia-National Formulary (USP-NF)**. Generic drug names are written in lowercase and are also known as *nonproprietary names*.

A drug's **trade name** is created by pharmaceutical companies. When a pharmaceutical company discovers a new drug, scientists assign it a chemical name that describes its chemical structure, which is often long and difficult to remember. The manufacturer proposes a generic (nonproprietary) name to the FDA for approval. The company then creates a memorable and descriptive trade name (also known as a *proprietary* or *brand name*). Trade names always begin with a capital letter. In this text, the generic name is listed first, with the trade name in parentheses after it. The *Physician's Desk Reference* is an example of a reference that provides an exhaustive catalog of drug information. **TABLE 1-1** shows examples of the generic and trade names of several common drugs, including their indications for use.

▶ General Principles

Discussions about pharmacology are all too often approached as chemistry lessons. However, the information regarding any drug is relatively constant no matter which drug is being discussed.

When approaching pharmacology in general terms, consider the following questions:

- How does the drug get into the body?
- How does the drug move around in the body?
- Which tissues can the drug reach?
- What makes the drug work?
- How is the drug broken down?
- How is the drug removed from the body?

TABLE 1-1 Examples of Generic and Trade Names

Generic Name	Trade Name	Indication
albuterol	Ventolin	Asthma
nitroglycerin	Nitrostat	Angina
sotalol hydrochloride	Betapace	Ventricular arrhythmia
tamsulosin hydrochloride	Flomax	Benign prostatic hypertrophy

Four major concepts address these topics: pharmacology, pharmacokinetics, receptor interactions, and pharmacodynamics. **Pharmacology** is the study of the biochemical and physiologic properties of medications (the suffix -*ology* means "the study of"; therefore *pharmacology* means "the study of drugs"). Some of the properties of medications include mechanism of action, indications, adverse effects, contraindications, and toxicity.

The pharmacology of a medication is different from its pharmacokinetics. *Kinetic* refers to movement, so **pharmacokinetics** refers to how the body acts on a medication, including how the drug is absorbed into the bloodstream (absorption), how the drug is distributed throughout the body (distribution), how the body metabolizes the drug (biotransformation), and finally, how the body eliminates the drug (excretion).

Receptors are the sites on various tissues to which some drugs bind to exert their desired physiologic effects. When explaining receptors, the analogy to a lock and key is often made—the drug is the key, and the receptor is the lock. Drug–receptor interactions "unlock" the cell receptors to act on the target tissue.

Pharmacodynamics explains how a drug works and interacts with various receptors, other drugs, and **enzyme** systems within the body (what the drug does to the body).

Absorption is the movement of a medication from the point of administration (e.g., gastrointestinal [GI] tract, skin, muscle) into the bloodstream for movement throughout the body. Two factors that affect the absorption of a drug are the dosage and the route of administration. (Absorption is discussed in greater detail later in the chapter.)

Medication Dosage

The **dose** of a medication is the amount of medication administered, often indicated by a unit of measure such as milligram (mg) or gram (g). The **dosage** of a medication is the size, frequency, and number of doses to be administered, such as 50 mg every 4 hours. Dosage is important in determining the concentration of the drug at the site of action. Typically, the higher the dosage, the higher the concentration of the medication at the site of action. The greater the amount of drug at the site of action, the greater the physiologic effect. Typically, as the dosage of a medication increases, so does the physiologic effect manifested by the drug. This effect continues to increase with increasing doses of the medication up to a point at which increasing the medication no longer produces an increase in the desired physiologic effect. This phenomenon is referred to as a **dose-response relationship** or **dose-response curve** (**FIGURE 1-1**).

Medication Forms and Routes

Medications come in different forms, and a single medication commonly comes in a variety of forms. The appropriate form of medication often is determined by the nature and urgency of the medical problem that the drug is being used to treat. To introduce the concept of the various forms of medications, consider the following patient.

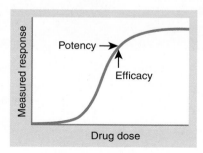

FIGURE 1-1 Dose-response curve: Increasing the dose of a medication increases the physiologic effect. The physiologic effect increases to a point at which an increase in dose does not result in any further increase in the desired physiologic effect.

Someone having an asthma attack needs immediate relief. Oral medications, such as a capsule or tablet, need to be swallowed, digested, absorbed, and then circulated through the body; the patient may not get relief for 30 minutes to 1 hour. Therefore, in the emergent circumstance of an asthma attack, an oral medication is inappropriate. Oral medications are appropriate for the treatment of stable, chronic conditions such as hypertension or acute, non-life-threatening conditions. Aspirin is perhaps the most commonly recognized oral medication. We understand that when taking aspirin for a headache or muscle ache, a certain amount of time will elapse before we feel any relief. This delay is because aspirin must be swallowed and travel to the stomach, where it is broken down, absorbed in the intestine, passed through the bloodstream, and delivered to the desired site of action. This delay of 20 to 60 minutes for administration of an oral medication for symptomatic relief could be problematic, even catastrophic, for patients having an asthma attack. Asthma medications that are given orally (e.g., montelukast [Singulair], zafirlukast [Accolate], theophylline) are typically not used during an acute asthma attack and would be inappropriate for the patient described in the preceding scenario.

Medications that are given enterally (**enteral administration**) are absorbed through the GI tract. Enteral medications, which are given orally or rectally, have several disadvantages. To swallow oral medications, the patient must be conscious and cooperative. Medications absorbed through the GI tract must first pass through the liver before being distributed throughout the body. At this point, the drug is often partially metabolized, which reduces the amount of medication available for distribution to the body. This process is called **first-pass metabolism**. Enteral administration has other disadvantages, including a variable rate of absorption, potential irritation of the stomach's or intestine's mucous lining, and patient noncompliance.

Enteral medication administration also has many advantages. It is by far the most common and safest route of drug administration. The delivery of the medication into the circulation is slow after oral administration. The slow absorption of medications into the bloodstream prevents rapid and high blood levels that often lead to adverse effects. An additional advantage of oral medications is the convenience of delivering medications without a need for sterile technique.

Parenteral medications are drugs that bypass the GI tract. **Injectable medications** are parenteral medications that can be injected directly into a muscle (**intramuscular [IM]**), a vein (**intravenous [IV]**), the bone (**intraosseous [IO]**), or the subcutaneous tissue (**subcutaneous**). Injectable medications are rapidly available and circulate throughout the body, often in minutes. The drawback of injectable medication administration is that it requires special training and, in the case of IV medications, special equipment. The IV route is the preferred route of administration for cardiac medications in advanced life support situations. An example of an IV medication is epinephrine, which is a powerful drug capable of stimulating the heart to function better and faster, as well as causing relaxation of the smooth muscle that surrounds the bronchial tree. Epinephrine is typically used in the treatment of cardiac arrest, asthma attacks, and anaphylaxis. These life-threatening emergencies require rapid and dependable delivery of this medication. Administration of epinephrine by an IV route allows the medication to be delivered much more rapidly than if it could be given enterally.

Noninjectable parenteral routes include topical, intranasal, and inhalational (discussed in Chapter 3).

To achieve a rapid therapeutic concentration of some drugs in a life-threatening emergency, a **loading dose** must be administered. Factors that determine a particular loading dose are the desired serum concentration of the drug and the volume of distribution. In emergency situations, loading doses are administered intravenously to achieve rapid 100% bioavailability of the drug. **Bioavailability** is the percentage of an administered drug that is available in the bloodstream to act at the target tissue. To illustrate this concept, consider the net (or take-home) pay on your paycheck. We are painfully aware that the amount of money on the top line of our paycheck is not the amount we get to take home to pay the rent and buy groceries. For the sake of this example, suppose our paycheck has a gross amount of $1,000. From that initial $1,000, federal and state income taxes are paid, decreasing the amount of money available to take home.

Gross pay	$1,000
−Federal taxes	$350
−State taxes	$150
Net pay (take-home)	$500

When an enteral medication is administered (orally or rectally), not all of that medication is absorbed by the GI tract, and of the percentage that is absorbed, a fraction is broken down and metabolized by the liver. The fraction of the medication that is available in the bloodstream, or *bioavailable fraction*, is similar to net pay.

If 1,000 mg of a particular medication (medication X) is administered as a tablet (enteral administration), perhaps 35% is not absorbed by the intestine; 15% gets metabolized by the liver. That leaves only 50% (i.e., 500 mg of medication X) of the administered medication available to the bloodstream and ultimately the target tissue.

Dose administered	1,000 mg
−Amount not absorbed by the intestine	350 mg
−Amount metabolized in the liver first-pass	150 mg
Bioavailable dose	500 mg

In an emergency, when a medication is given as an IV bolus, the administered dose is delivered directly into the bloodstream. IV administration of medications increases the bioavailability of the dose by removing factors such as variability in absorption from the GI tract and first-pass metabolism.

Maintenance doses ensure an average concentration of a drug at serum-steady states. In the absence of a loading dose, five half-lives must pass to achieve a steady state of the drug concentration.

A **half-life** of a medication is the time required for the concentration of a medication in the bloodstream to decrease to half of its original level. Half-life is different from the duration of action. **Duration of action** is the amount of time a single dose of a medication produces the desired effect. A car filled with gasoline may be able to drive 500 miles before running out of gas. When the gas gauge is on half a tank, the level of gasoline is at half of its original level. The distance the car could drive until the amount of gas in the tank is decreased to half a tank would be the equivalent of half-life. Despite having only a half tank of gas, the car is still able to run at full speed until there is not enough gas to power the engine, or an empty tank. The distance that the car can run using the gasoline in the tank is the duration of action. Therefore, in the car example, the half-life is 250 miles, and the duration of action is 500 miles. Although this example simplifies these concepts, it does illustrate the terms. Clearly, there are differences between gasoline in an automobile and the concentration of a medication in a patient's blood. The engine of a car will run until the tank is empty, but a medication will lose its desired biologic effect long before the serum concentrations are zero.

Let us go back to our hypothetical drug, medication X. The usual dose of medication X is 1,000 mg administered intravenously every 12 hours. Medication X has a half-life of 12 hours. Without a loading dose, it takes approximately five doses for the level of the medication in the blood to approach a steady state of drug concentration. To illustrate the concept of loading doses and half-life, observe what happens to the serum drug levels at the end of each half-life when a medication is administered without a loading dose.

Dose Number	Amount of Drug Administered	After Dose	Serum Concentration at End of Half-Life
Dose 1	1,000 mg	1,000 mg	1,000 mg/2 = 500 mg
Dose 2	1,000 mg	500 mg + 1,000 mg = 1,500 mg	1,500 mg/2 = 750 mg
Dose 3	1,000 mg	750 mg + 1,000 mg = 1,750 mg	1,750 mg/2 = 875 mg
Dose 4	1,000 mg	875 mg + 1,000 mg = 1,875 mg	1,875 mg/2 = 938 mg
Dose 5	1,000 mg	938 mg + 1,000 mg = 1938 mg	1,938 mg/2 = 969 mg
Dose 6	1000 mg	969 mg + 1,000 mg = 1,969 mg	1,969 mg/2 = 985 mg

© Jones & Bartlett Learning.

This example demonstrates that it takes approximately five doses of medication X before the serum levels at the end of a half-life begin to stabilize and approach a steady serum concentration.

Next, administer a loading dose of 2,000 mg of medication X, and then start a maintenance dose of 1,000 mg.

Medication X: 1,000 mg every 12 hours with a loading dose of 2,000 mg:

Dose Number	Amount of Drug Administered	Serum Concentration After Dose	Serum Concentration at End of Half-Life
Dose 1 (Loading)	2,000 mg	2,000 mg	2,000 mg/2 = 1,000 mg
Dose 2	1,000 mg	1,000 mg + 1,000 mg = 2,000 mg	2,000 mg/2 = 1,000 mg
Dose 3	1,000 mg	1,000 mg + 1,000 mg = 2,000 mg	2,000 mg/2 = 1,000 mg
Dose 4	1,000 mg	1,000 mg + 1,000 mg = 2,000 mg	2,000 mg/2 = 1,000 mg
Dose 5	1,000 mg	1,000 mg + 1,000 mg = 2,000 mg	2,000 mg/2 = 1,000 mg
Dose 6	1,000 mg	1,000 mg + 1,000 mg = 2,000 mg	2,000 mg/2 = 1,000 mg

© Jones & Bartlett Learning.

This example clearly demonstrates that by administering a loading dose of 2,000 mg, appropriate serum concentrations of the medication are rapidly obtained and maintained.

For a patient having an asthma attack, IV medications can provide rapid relief. However, a patient with asthma can have several attacks a day, both at home and away from home.

Starting an IV line or giving an IM injection for each asthmatic episode would be impractical. Therefore, **inhaled medications** are often used to deliver medication to patients with asthma. Inhaled medications are rapidly active, easy to administer, and often convenient. Most patients with asthma have prescribed **inhalers**, which contain medication in a fine powder that immediately acts on the lungs when administered. Inhalation is a rapid route of administration in which the medications can act directly on receptors in the lung, as well as be absorbed in the bloodstream. Albuterol (Proventil, Ventolin) is an example of an inhaled medication that is rapidly delivered to a patient having an asthma attack. Other examples include anesthetics administered to patients undergoing surgery.

Inhaled medications can also be given in liquid form. Liquid medication is **nebulized**, or made into small particles, by a delivery device and then delivered to the patient by inhalation. Nebulized medications are inhaled, but they require a device to deliver the medication called a **nebulizer**. Patients with asthma may have a small machine at home that delivers the nebulized medication (**FIGURE 1-2**). Ambulances and hospitals use a small nebulization chamber powered by an oxygen source.

Some medications are delivered by absorption across mucous membranes or the skin. For example, in **buccal administration**, glucose gel is administered between the cheek and gums of a conscious diabetic patient with low blood sugar. The gel is rapidly absorbed and quickly increases the patient's serum glucose level.

Nitroglycerin is a medication available in a variety of forms and can be absorbed in several ways. One form is compressed powder, which is made into tablets. A nitroglycerin tablet can be placed under a patient's tongue, where it is rapidly absorbed through the oral mucous membranes. Alternatively, nitroglycerin is available in a form that can be sprayed under a patient's tongue for **sublingual administration**. A third method of nitroglycerin delivery is **transdermal administration**, which occurs across the skin. Patients may also receive IV nitroglycerin infusions in healthcare facilities or during interfacility patient transport.

Gas is another form that medications can take. The drug most commonly used by prehospital providers is oxygen, which is a gaseous form of a drug. Inhaled nitrous oxide is another drug in the gaseous form that is often used in the prehospital setting. Helium, another gas, is blended with oxygen when certain critically ill patients are placed on ventilators and have difficulty maintaining adequate oxygen despite aggressive ventilator settings.

Chapter 3 provides detailed, step-by-step explanations for delivering drugs by various routes, and Chapter 5 covers the administration of IV drugs.

FIGURE 1-2 An example of a portable nebulizer system for home use.
© spline_x/iStock/Getty Images.

▶ Drug Metabolism and Excretion

Drug **metabolism** is the breakdown and change of a drug by various chemical reactions throughout the body. Within the body, many drugs undergo a process called biotransformation. **Biotransformation** is the action of various biologic systems within the body making changes to the chemical structure of many types of drugs. This transformation may change an active drug to an inactive chemical through a series of chemical reactions. Biotransformation may also convert an inactive (or less active) medication into a new chemical compound with a more significant clinical effect. Awareness of biotransformation is important in many poisoning and overdose situations where other active or toxic substances can remain in the body, even though levels of the original medication or chemical begin to decline.

As previously mentioned, one disadvantage of administering a drug orally is first-pass metabolism. When a drug is absorbed by the GI tract, the drug must first go to the liver. Once in the liver, medications are metabolized (broken down) in a series of complex chemical reactions into either an active or an inactive compound. Enzymes are proteins that act as catalysts to assist and increase the rate of a medication's breakdown; the liver is a source of plentiful enzymes and the site for the majority of drug metabolism. The kidneys and lungs are other sites of drug metabolism. Metabolism changes the chemical nature of a medication, usually making it inactive. Therefore, factors that alter drug metabolism can change the effectiveness of an administered medication. Factors that increase drug metabolism break down a drug at a faster rate and perhaps render the drug less effective or completely ineffective. Therefore, patients whose drug metabolism is increased will often require increased or more frequent dosing for a medication to be effective.

The opposite is also true; a slowed metabolic rate results in a decrease in the breakdown of a given medication. With slower drug metabolism, medications can potentially reach toxic levels and have an adverse effect on a patient. A given dosage of a medication can affect individual patients differently, in part because of differences in the ways patients metabolize drugs. The following are some factors that alter drug metabolism:

- Patient's age
- Drug administration route
- Dosage
- Patient's genetic predisposition
- Diet or starvation
- Preexisting or concurrent disease states

These specific factors are further explained in Chapter 19.

Drugs administered orally require absorption in the intestine and then proceed through the liver for first-pass metabolism. The result of first-pass metabolism is that a medication given orally requires a significantly higher dose than the same medication given by a parenteral route. For example, the IV dose of propranolol is 1 mg; however, the dose of the same medication given orally is 40 mg.

Drug **excretion** is the removal of a drug or metabolite from the body. The kidney typically is the organ responsible for removal of drugs and drug by-products. Many chemicals can be eliminated only by the kidneys after biotransformation or metabolism by the liver. Factors such as underlying kidney function, urine or serum pH, perfusion to the kidney, and overall fluid volume status impact the kidney's ability to excrete various chemicals. The liver can also excrete drugs from the body, although it does so less frequently. When the liver metabolizes medications, by-products are excreted by the liver into the bile. Smaller quantities of medications are eliminated through sweat, saliva, expired air, and breast milk.

▶ Pharmacokinetics

Paramedics administer medications to patients to produce a desired clinical effect. That clinical effect may be to slow a heart that is beating too fast, accelerate a heart that is beating too slowly, or provide relief to a patient in pain. All medications have adverse effects. Adverse effects may range from mild or imperceptible to immediately life threatening, depending on the particular medication or situation. Occurrence or severity of adverse reactions may vary greatly from one patient to the next. In many situations, it is possible to predict adverse reactions based on the medication, dose, route, or patient characteristics. In other situations, adverse reactions occur completely unexpectedly and dramatically alter the patient's predicted clinical course. The goal of drug therapy is to administer a medication to obtain the desired clinical effect while minimizing the likelihood of adverse effects.

Pharmacokinetics is the study of drug absorption, distribution, and excretion. As previously discussed, absorption is the movement of a drug from the site of administration into the bloodstream, where it can be transported throughout the body. Drug absorption determines, to a large degree, how rapidly a medication becomes available for a therapeutic effect. The more rapidly the medication is absorbed, the more quickly it will assist a patient. Absorption occurs from any site at which a medication is administered.

Absorption of most medications by any route other than the IV route (e.g., oral, rectal, IM, subcutaneous, transdermal) follows **first-order kinetics**, which is often called **exponential kinetics of absorption**. In first-order kinetics, a constant fraction of the medication is absorbed into the bloodstream. For example, an oral medication is absorbed from the intestine at a rate of 50% of the administered medication over a period of 20 minutes. Therefore, if the patient takes 10 mg of this particular medication, 5 mg is absorbed at the end of 20 minutes, and 5 mg remains within the intestine. At the end of an additional 20 minutes (40 minutes after administration), an additional 50% (2.5 mg) is absorbed into the bloodstream. Therefore, 40 minutes after administration, 7.5 mg (5 + 2.5 mg) has been absorbed across the intestine and is now circulating in the bloodstream, and 2.5 mg remains within the intestine waiting to be absorbed. After the third 20-minute interval, or 60 minutes after administration, an additional 50% is absorbed. Because only 2.5 mg of the medication remained, 1.25 mg is absorbed during this third 20-minute interval. Compared to the first-order metabolism illustrated here, in which the rate of absorption is 50% over a 20-minute period, some medications may have a much lower absorption rate over a much longer period. These rates of absorption differ from medication to medication.

In contrast to first-order kinetics, after administration of an IV drug, a constant amount of the drug is absorbed and circulates within the bloodstream. Because the medication is administered directly into the bloodstream, absorption is not delayed; 100% of the medication is available in a brief period. This type of absorption is known as **zero-order kinetics**.

Distribution of a drug refers to its transportation through the bloodstream to various tissues in the body and ultimately to the target site. Several factors determine how rapidly and to what magnitude a medication can accumulate in any given tissue. Drugs are rapidly delivered to organs such as the brain, heart, kidney, and liver because they have rich blood supplies. Drugs that are lipid or fat soluble can easily cross the membranes that separate the various body compartments, whereas drugs that are lipid insoluble take longer to cross into the various body compartments. The **volume of distribution** is the space that the drug would occupy; it is expressed as mg/L or such. A drug with a high volume of distribution is fat soluble and can easily pass through membranes and into the various body compartments.

The bioavailability of a drug is the fraction of the drug that reaches circulation. The following factors may alter the bioavailability of a particular drug:

- How rapidly the medication is broken down and absorbed in the intestinal tract
- Patient's dietary habits
- Tablet's size
- Medication's formulation

How a particular medication is absorbed through the intestinal tract largely depends on the drug's physical and chemical properties. Drugs can cross the body's various membranes by several different mechanisms: passive diffusion, carrier-mediated facilitated diffusion, active transport, passive transport, and endocytosis. **Passive diffusion** (also known as *passive* *transport*) occurs when medications penetrate cells by simply crossing through the cell's membrane. Factors that determine whether the medication is capable of diffusing through the cell membrane include the chemical nature of a particular drug, such as the molecular size, the chemical charge, fat or water solubility, and the drug's concentration within the body. This method does not require or consume energy.

In **carrier-mediated facilitated diffusion**, the transportation of a drug into a particular cell depends on a second molecule to carry the drug molecule into the cell. One way of visualizing carrier-mediated facilitated diffusion is to imagine a large group of people who need to be transported from one point to another by a series of buses. When a bus arrives, the people get on the bus, which takes them to their destination. Once at the destination, the people get off the bus and are free to move to their final destination. Applying this example to the transportation of medications into the cell, the administered drug accumulates at the outside of the cell membrane (the bus stop). There, the medication loads (or binds) with a carrier macromolecule (bus). The carrier molecule (bus) then transports the bound medication (passengers) to its destination inside the cell. Once inside the cell, the bound medication disassociates from the carrier molecule (passengers get off the bus). Inside the cell, the drug molecules go to their target site to produce the desired effect.

Carrier-mediated facilitated diffusion is a **saturable process**. As the concentration of the drug outside the cell increases, the rate of transporting the drug into the cell also increases. Eventually a point is reached at which increasing the concentration of a drug outside the cell does not result in an increase in transportation of the drug into the cell. By definition, a saturable process is one in which the external concentrations of the drug can reach a point at which increasing the concentration does not result in an increase in the rate of transportation into the cell. Returning to the bus example, assume that each bus, when full, can carry a maximum of 50 passengers. If a bus comes once an hour and only 20 people are at the bus stop, the bus will transport 20 people an hour. If 40 people are at the bus stop, the bus has the capacity to transport 40 people in an hour. If the number of passengers at the bus stop increases to 60, the bus can load and transport only 50 passengers in an hour. Whether 70, 80, or 100 passengers are at the bus stop, that one bus can still carry only 50 passengers. This is an example of a saturable process. Applying the preceding metaphor, a saturable process is one in which the external concentrations (the number of passengers waiting for a bus) do not increase the rate of influx (the number of passengers transported by the bus in an hour).

Active transport (also a saturable process) is another method by which drug molecules are capable of crossing cell membranes. In many ways, active transport and carrier-mediated facilitated diffusion are similar. Both mechanisms require a macromolecule to assist in transport. Both processes require specific binding of the drug molecule to the macromolecule, and both are capable of reaching a point of saturation. An example that illustrates active transport would be the bilge pump in a boat. A bilge pump pumps water from the bottom of a boat back into the lake or ocean. For the pump to work, it requires energy. The molecules that transport drugs by active transport also require energy.

Passive transport occurs when a drug molecule moves down a concentration gradient. This means that a drug moves from an area of high concentration to an area of low concentration. Factors that determine to what degree and how rapidly a drug may move by passive transport include the size of the drug molecule, the ease with which a particular drug dissolves in either water or fat, and the concentration of the drug in the various body compartments.

Endocytosis is a minor method of drug movement. In endocytosis, a cell essentially forms a sac around the drug molecule with the cell's membrane, and the cell membrane folds inward, bringing the drug into the cell.

With most medications, an amount of time elapses from when the drug is administered until the patient exhibits the desired effect. This interval can range from seconds to hours, even days in some cases. The **onset of action**, or **latent period**, is the time interval from administration to desired effect. A drug may produce its desired effect for varying periods. Duration of action is the period from which the drug initially exhibits its desired action to the point when the effect is no longer perceptible.

As discussed previously, duration of action is different from biologic half-life. The half-life of the particular drug is determined by the rate of transformation and excretion of a drug. A half-life is the period required to eliminate half the administered medication from the body and is not affected by the dose of the drug. In a given patient, the half-life of a medication is the same regardless of the dose of medication administered. Excretion is the process of eliminating a drug or its metabolites from the body. Some drugs are rapidly metabolized and excreted from the body, whereas others can linger for days.

The **therapeutic index (TI)** is the measurement of the relative safety of a drug. Two factors are used to determine the safety or TI of a medication. To calculate TI, the **effective dose 50 (ED50)** and the **lethal dose 50 (LD50)** must be known. The LD50 is the dose that is fatal in 50% of the laboratory animals tested. To obtain this value, researchers intentionally overdose animals to the point at which half the animals die at the administered test dose. In contrast, the ED50 is the dose that produces a therapeutic effect in 50% of laboratory animals tested. Once these two factors are determined, the TI is calculated by the following equation:

$$TI = LD50/ED50$$

This ratio provides a numeric value between 0 and 1. The closer this value is to 1, the more dangerous a drug is when administered. In contrast, the closer this number is to 0, the safer the drug.

▶ Pharmacodynamics

Simply stated, pharmacodynamics explains how drugs work. Having an understanding of how a particular drug works allows you to administer it confidently, with an awareness of its effectiveness, **side effects**, and interactions. The way a drug works at the target tissue is often called the **mechanism of action**. Drugs typically work by one of the following three mechanisms:

1. Drug–receptor interactions
2. Drug–enzyme interactions
3. Nonspecific drug interactions

Drug–Receptor Interactions

Many drugs work much like a key opening a lock. A drug, like a key, has a complex shape, and that shape determines its function. The drug binds to a receptor, as with a key in a lock. The combined drug–receptor interaction then essentially unlocks the drug to act on the target tissue. **Reversible binding** occurs when the drug is able to separate from the cell's receptor, as in removing a key from a lock. When the drug is removed from the receptor, the effect of the drug stops. With some medications, once the drug binds to the receptor, it cannot separate from the receptor; this is known as **irreversible binding**. **FIGURE 1-3** illustrates the concepts of reversible and irreversible binding.

An **agonist** is a drug that produces the desired physiologic effect upon binding with the receptor. Agonists turn things on. In contrast, an **antagonist** is a drug that either diminishes or eradicates the physiologic effect of the agonist. That is, antagonists turn things off. **Pharmacologic antagonism** occurs when an antagonist binds to a receptor and prevents the biologic effect of an agonist. Antagonists can be either competitive or noncompetitive. **Competitive antagonists** can bind to the receptor in a reversible fashion. With increasing concentration of agonists, the competitive antagonist can be displaced by the agonists. Therefore, providing additional agonists is one strategy for overcoming the effect of a competitive antagonist. A **noncompetitive antagonist** irreversibly binds to the receptor. Regardless of how much of the agonist is given, the effect of the noncompetitive antagonists on the receptor cannot be overcome. **Partial agonist** medications bind to a receptor site and initiate a reduced amount of cellular activity compared to other chemicals or medications that may also be present at the cells, reducing the efficacy of other agonist chemicals.

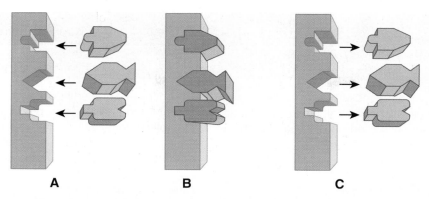

FIGURE 1-3 A. Drugs and their cell receptors have a very specific and complex structure. A drug binding to a specific receptor is like a key fitting into a lock. **B.** Irreversible binding occurs when the drug is not able to separate from the receptor, and the drug will have a prolonged effect. **C.** Reversible binding occurs when the drug separates from the cell receptor; this is similar to removing a key from a lock. Once the drug separates from the receptor, the drug's effect stops.

Drugs and receptors also have some degree of chemical attraction toward one another, similar to the attraction between two magnets. This attraction between drug and receptor is known as **affinity**. Consider two magnets of opposite polarity. The stronger the attraction between two magnets, the greater the likelihood they will bind to each other if placed in proximity to each another. The weaker the attraction between two magnets, the closer they need to be to allow the same magnitude of attraction as two stronger magnets.

Efficacy is the ability of a drug to produce the desired biologic effect by binding to and unlocking a given receptor. For example, aspirin and morphine are two medications known to produce the desired effect of analgesia, or relief of pain. Of the two, morphine has a greater efficacy in relieving pain. Each medication has a "maximal efficacy," which will not be surpassed by increasing the dose or concentration of that medication. A medication such as aspirin will have a maximal efficacy much lower than that of morphine. An excessive dose of aspirin will not provide the same level of analgesia as even a therapeutic dose of morphine.

Potency is a term used to compare the different doses of two medications in producing the same effect. Morphine and fentanyl are both narcotics that produce analgesia. A fentanyl dose of 100 mcg produces the same effect as 10 mg of morphine. Both drugs produce the same effect; however, a much smaller dose of fentanyl is required. In this example, fentanyl would be considered a more potent medication. The potency of a particular medication is independent of that medication's efficacy. For the purposes of selecting medications, efficacy is more important than potency.

When a patient is given two drugs that produce similar effects, the combined effects of these two drugs may be enhanced. **Summation** occurs when two medications with the same effect given together produce an effect in equal magnitude to the effects of the two drugs when given independently. In other words, the observed effect is equal to the effect of drug A plus the effect of drug B (1 + 1 = 2). In some cases, the observed effect of the two medications when given concurrently is greater than the effects of the medications when given individually. This phenomenon is known as **synergism**. With synergism, the combined effect is greater than the effect of drug A plus the effect of drug B (1 + 1 > 2).

The final enhancement of a drug's effect is known as potentiation. **Potentiation** occurs when a drug lacking an effect of its own increases the effect of a second drug (**TABLE 1-2**).

Drug–Enzyme Interactions

Enzymes are chemicals or compounds that control various chemical changes and reactions within the body. Drugs interact with enzymes and either increase or decrease the enzyme's mediated chemical reaction. Drugs are capable of binding or interacting with various enzymes and either accelerating or arresting their actions. An enzyme works by binding to the

TABLE 1-2 Medication Interactions

Type of Interaction	Description	Example
Addition or summation	Two medications with a similar effect combine to produce an effect equal to the sum of the individual effect of each medication (e.g., $1 + 1 = 2$).	The antipyretic properties of acetaminophen (Tylenol) and the antipyretic properties of ibuprofen (Motrin, Advil) combine to reduce a fever in patients with fevers that could not be controlled by either medication alone.
Synergism	Two medications with a similar effect combine to produce an effect greater than the sum of the medications' effects.	Patients experience profound sedation when IV opioid medications such as fentanyl (Sublimaze) are given with IV benzodiazepines such as midazolam (Versed), greater than the expected sum of these two medications.
Potentiation	The effect of one medication is greatly enhanced by the presence of another medication, which does not have the ability to produce the same effect.	Promethazine (Phenergan) is given to increase the effects of codeine or other antitussives (cough suppressants) for more improved relief of cough than is achieved with the antitussive alone.
Altered absorption	The action of one medication increases or decreases the ability of another medication to be absorbed by the body. For example, medications that increase or decrease the gastrointestinal pH or motility may increase or decrease the absorption of other medications that are taken orally.	Ranitidine (Zantac), an H_2 blocker, can reduce absorption of ketoconazole (an antifungal) or certain cephalosporin antibiotics.
Altered metabolism	The action of one medication increases or decreases the metabolism of another medication within the body. For example, many medications (and certain foods) alter the performance of the cytochrome P-450 system in the liver, which is responsible for the metabolism of a variety of other medications.	Fluconazole (Diflucan), an antifungal medication, inhibits the function of cytochrome P-450 enzyme CYP3A4, significantly increasing bleeding risks associated with warfarin (Coumadin), an anticoagulant medication.
Altered distribution	The presence of one medication alters the area available for the distribution of another medication in the body, which becomes important when both medications are bound to the same site, such as plasma proteins. If proteins are already occupied by one medication, toxic levels of the other medication may develop.	The anticonvulsant medication valproic acid (Depakote, Depakene) competes with another anticonvulsant medication, phenytoin (Dilantin), causing potentially increased or decreased serum levels and possibly unpredictable clinical effects.
Altered elimination	Medications may increase or decrease the functioning of the kidneys or other route of elimination, influencing the amount of or duration of another medication's effect in the body.	Ethanol decreases the metabolism of warfarin (Coumadin), which may predispose the patient to bleeding risk.

Type of Interaction	Description	Example
Physiologic (drug) antagonism	Two medications, each producing opposite effects, are present simultaneously, resulting in minimal or no clinical changes.	Sodium nitroprusside (Nipride) and dobutamine (Dobutrex) are often given simultaneously for cardiogenic shock. By itself, dobutamine increases cardiac output, possibly causing an elevated blood pressure. Sodium nitroprusside causes vasodilation and possibly hypotension. When given together, these medications can be titrated to maintain a normal patient blood pressure.
Neutralization	Two medications bind together in the body, creating an inactive substance.	Digoxin-specific antibodies (Digibind, Digifab) are administered to patients with toxicity to the medication digoxin. These medications combine, rendering digoxin molecules inactive.

Abbreviations: H_2, histamine-2 receptor antagonist; IV, intravenous

Data from: Schelleman H, Bilker WB, Brensinger CM, Han X, Kimmel SE, Hennessy S. Warfarin with fluoroquinolones, sulfonamides, or azole antifungals: interactions and the risk of hospitalization for gastrointestinal bleeding. *Clin Pharmacol Ther.* 2008 (Nov);84(5):581–588.

starting compound, known as the **substrate**. Some drugs that act on enzyme systems work by mimicking the substrate molecule, binding with the enzyme system, and essentially clogging the chemical reaction regulated by that particular enzyme. Other drugs can bind enzymes and accelerate a chemical reaction.

Nonspecific Drug Interactions

Nonspecific drug interactions occur when a drug acts on a target organ or tissue in a method that does not require binding of a drug with either a receptor or an enzyme. Nonspecific drug interactions often occur when a drug directly acts on a cell or the cell's membrane. Medications may produce a wide variety of clinical effects without directly interacting with enzymes or receptor sites. Certain medications, known as **chelating agents**, are administered to bind with heavy metals in the body. Other medications contain electrolytes or are administered to manipulate fluid and electrolyte concentrations within the body. Medications may be administered to alter the hydrogen ion concentration (pH) in various body fluids, which can improve cellular function, alter metabolism, and promote excretion of other toxic substances. Certain types of medications, such as antibiotics and antifungals, are carefully designed to target microorganism cells, altering cellular reproduction or causing cell death.

▶ Drug Actions and Effects

Medications are administered to patients to achieve desired physiologic effects or actions. Unfortunately, medications often produce unwelcome physiologic side effects as well. Side effects often are considered nothing more than benign annoyances, such as headaches, nausea, and drowsiness. They are often treated by reducing the dosage or eliminating the offending medication.

However, medications also can cause adverse effects, which are considered serious, undesired effects of a medication. On occasion, adverse effects are serious enough to warrant hospitalization. Examples of adverse effects include renal failure, bleeding, bone marrow suppression, and progression of heart disease. An **idiosyncratic response** is a rare and unpredicted response to a medication. Idiosyncratic responses may be caused by a patient's genetic abnormalities or a subtle alteration in a particular enzyme within the body.

An **allergic response** typically occurs when a patient mounts an antibody response to a medication to which he or she had previously been sensitized. When the patient is reexposed to the medication, he or she responds with signs and symptoms such as rash, itching, and swelling. A patient with one drug allergy can be predisposed to manifest an allergic reaction to another medication of the same class or with similar chemical features. An **anaphylactic reaction** is an allergic reaction with life-threatening manifestations in which the patient can have swelling of the airway, inability to breathe, hypotension, and shock. This topic is further explained in Chapter 8.

Drug interaction occurs when the effects of one drug are modified by or interfere with the effects of a second drug administered concurrently. The result of a drug interaction often is that the effect of one drug is increased by the second drug.

Essentially two types of drug interactions occur: those that alter the plasma levels of the particular medication and those that alter the effects of a medication. Although essentially thousands of drug interactions are clinically relevant, most result in the prolongation of either the effect or half-life of a second medication. A large number of drugs are metabolized by the liver enzyme **cytochrome P-450**. Examples of such drugs include theophylline (Theo-24, Theolair, Uniphyl), warfarin (Coumadin), cimetidine (Tagamet), and antidepressants. Drugs are also able to interact with food and alcohol. Drug interactions with food and alcohol can occur by way of the cytochrome P-450 system, as well as through competition with the drug's binding site. Perhaps the most common drug and food interaction is with a class of drugs known as **monoamine oxidase inhibitors**. This class of drug cannot be taken with aged cheeses or many processed foods. Patients may intentionally attempt to manipulate metabolism or excretion of a particular medication by altering their dietary intake of certain foods known to alter cytochrome P-450 function.

A large element of drug therapy is the manipulation of various physiologic functions. Depending on the disease state, the provider may need to manipulate a given patient's heart rate, blood pressure, respiratory effort, or even bowel functions. Under normal conditions, the autonomic nervous system provides minute-to-minute control of these wide-ranging functions. Therefore, in the attempt to control various disease states and reestablish a state of normal, a clinician needs to be familiar with the autonomic nervous system.

▶ Autonomic Nervous System

The role of the **autonomic nervous system** is to control and integrate many major body functions. This function is in contrast to the **somatic nervous system**, which controls skeletal muscles and movement. The autonomic nervous system provides involuntary control of many internal body functions. It is composed of two divisions: the **sympathetic nervous system** and the **parasympathetic nervous system** (**FIGURE 1-4**). Both the sympathetic and parasympathetic nervous systems innervate the heart, bronchial smooth muscle, iris of the eye, salivary glands, and urinary bladder. The sympathetic nervous system also innervates the vascular smooth muscle, sweat glands, and adrenal medulla.

The sympathetic nervous system readies the body to handle stress through the **fight-or-flight response**. Most people have experienced a situation in which they felt threatened by a real or perceived risk. The physiologic changes that occur to the body when faced with that threat, such as violence or an accident, are responses to the actions of the sympathetic nervous system. Medications that exert effects on the sympathetic nervous system use **adrenergic receptors** and are called **adrenergic agonists**.

The parasympathetic nervous system is responsible for the routine housekeeping chores of the body, such as slowing the heart rate, producing acid for the stomach, and emptying the

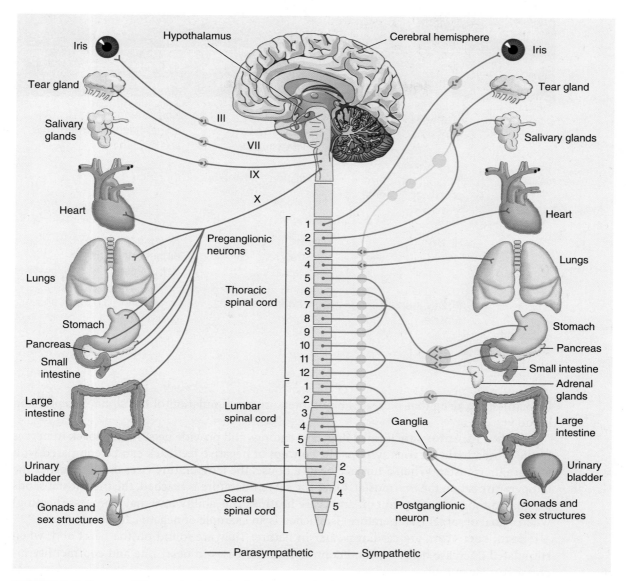

FIGURE 1-4 Pathways of the sympathetic and parasympathetic nervous system.

bladder and bowels. Drugs that act on the parasympathetic nervous system are referred to as **cholinergic agonists**.

Adrenergic Receptors and Activating Drugs

Adrenergic receptors, which get their name from adrenaline, are commonly manipulated by medications. Adrenaline, more commonly known as epinephrine, is responsible for increasing the heart rate, increasing the contractility of the heart, increasing blood pressure, and dilating the bronchioles of the lungs. The net result of these effects is to ready the person for the fight-or-flight response. Epinephrine regulates these effects through a series of adrenergic receptors: alpha$_1$, alpha$_2$, beta$_1$, and beta$_2$. Each receptor has unique properties, locations, and biologic effects when stimulated. A summary of these receptors is found in **TABLE 1-3**. Medications that can mimic and interact with adrenergic receptors have many effects and applications to prehospital care. Remembering the location and effects of each of these receptors can help you understand these drugs and their uses in prehospital care.

Alpha$_1$ receptors are primarily located on the peripheral blood vessels. Stimulation of these receptors results in vasoconstriction and elevation of systemic blood pressures.

TABLE 1-3 Properties of Adrenergic Receptors

Receptor	Locations	Effects	Examples of Receptor Agonists
Alpha$_1$	Peripheral blood vessels	Vasoconstriction, elevation of systemic blood pressure	Norepinephrine, epinephrine, phenylephrine, and dopamine
Alpha$_2$	Presynaptic and postsynaptic nerve terminals	Vasodilation, anesthesia	Clonidine
Beta$_1$	Heart	Increase in heart rate and strength of cardiac contraction	Norepinephrine, epinephrine, and dobutamine
Beta$_2$	Airway, smooth muscle	Bronchodilation	Epinephrine, albuterol, and terbutaline

© Jones & Bartlett Learning.

Dopamine is a drug that increases blood pressure by stimulation of the alpha$_1$ receptors on blood vessels.

Alpha$_2$ receptors are located on nerve endings and provide negative feedback to nerves in the sympathetic nervous system. The concept of negative feedback can be compared with a house thermostat. When a furnace heats a house, the temperature rises until it reaches the temperature set on the thermostat. Once the set temperature is reached, the thermostat sends a signal to the furnace to shut off and cease heating. This ability to signal a process (heating) when a goal or target (temperature) is reached is an example of negative feedback.

Beta$_1$ receptors are cardiovascular in nature. They are found on the heart and, when stimulated, increase heart rate and contractility. Increases in heart rate and contractility increase cardiac output.

Beta$_2$ receptors are located on the bronchial smooth muscle. Stimulation of beta$_2$ receptors relaxes bronchial smooth muscle and increases the diameter of the bronchial tree. Drugs that stimulate the beta$_2$ receptors are often used in respiratory emergencies.

Blood Vessels

The tone of the vascular smooth muscle is principally under the control of adrenergic receptors. Vascular smooth muscles contract and decrease the diameter of blood vessels, resulting in an increase in blood pressure or the shunting of blood from one area of the body to another. Stimulation of alpha$_1$ receptors by drugs such as dopamine results in vasoconstriction and increased blood pressure. Drugs that block the beta receptors are known as **beta blockers**. When a patient is given a beta blocker such as labetalol (Normodyne, Trandate), blood vessels relax, resulting in a decrease in systemic blood pressure.

Heart

Beta agonists are capable of mediating their effect on the heart through the action of the beta$_1$ receptor. Beta$_2$ agonists exert their effects primarily on the bronchial smooth muscles. When a cardiac beta receptor is stimulated by a beta agonist, the heart rate increases. Stimulation of beta receptors in the heart also increases cardiac output.

You can remember the distinction between beta$_1$ agonists and beta$_2$ agonists by remembering that human beings have one heart (beta$_1$) and two lungs (beta$_2$).

Eyes

The eye muscles responsible for pupil dilation are stimulated by alpha agonists. Drugs that act on both alpha and beta receptors can alter the pressure inside the eye, which is clinically significant in patients with glaucoma.

Respiratory Tract

Stimulation of the bronchial smooth muscles' beta$_2$ receptors results in relaxation of these muscles and dilation of the airway. Inhaled bronchodilators commonly used by patients with asthma stimulate beta$_2$ receptors.

Drugs That Stimulate Adrenergic Receptors

Remember that adrenergic receptors work through a receptor mechanism similar to a lock and key. These drugs must mimic the shape and structure of the native agonists of the adrenergic receptors. Drugs that mimic the actions of the sympathetic nervous system are referred to as **sympathomimetic drugs**. Epinephrine and norepinephrine are two examples of sympathomimetic drugs. The following medication profiles include some of the more common sympathomimetic drugs that may be used by the prehospital provider. More detailed discussion of these agents is provided in later chapters in regard to their use in specific diseases.

In the body's natural production of sympathomimetic hormones, dopamine is the **precursor** to norepinephrine, and norepinephrine is the precursor to epinephrine. A precursor is a substance or drug that precedes another substance in the development of a substance or drug. When the body makes epinephrine, a molecule goes through a series of modifications before becoming epinephrine.

Dopamine → Norepinephrine → Epinephrine

Dopamine primarily stimulates the heart's beta$_1$ receptors and causes the release of norepinephrine from the autonomic nervous system. As a beta$_1$ agonist, dopamine can increase heart rate and cardiac output. As the dose of dopamine is increased, it begins to stimulate alpha receptors, resulting in vasoconstriction. Therefore, at higher doses dopamine acts much like an epinephrine infusion.

Norepinephrine is similar to epinephrine in its action on beta$_1$ receptors, but it has less potency on the alpha receptors and essentially no action on beta$_2$ receptors.

Dobutamine is a synthetic sympathomimetic drug that stimulates the beta$_1$ receptors. It is used to improve cardiac performance in patients with congestive heart failure, which it accomplishes with less of an increase in myocardial oxygen consumption than do other sympathomimetic agonists. This effect is caused by the drug's ability to improve cardiac output without significant increases in heart rate or systolic blood pressure.

Phenylephrine is a pure alpha agonist capable of increasing blood pressure. Because of its pure alpha activity, it is used as a vasopressor in conditions such as septic shock.

Epinephrine binds both alpha and beta receptors. The effects on the heart are mediated primarily by beta receptors. Epinephrine administration results in increases in blood pressure, heart rate, cardiac contractility, and cardiac output. Administration of epinephrine can result in cardiac arrhythmias. Alpha stimulation causes vasoconstriction and elevation of blood pressure.

DOPAMINE (INTROPIN)

Classification: Adrenergic agonist, inotropic, vasopressor.

Action: Stimulates alpha and beta adrenergic receptors. At moderate doses (2 to 10 mcg/kg per minute), dopamine stimulates $beta_1$ receptors, resulting in inotropy and increased cardiac output while maintaining dopaminergic-induced vasodilatory effects. At high doses (> 10 mcg/kg per minute), alpha adrenergic agonism predominates, and increased peripheral vascular resistance and vasoconstriction result.

Indications: Hypotension and decreased cardiac output associated with cardiogenic shock and septic shock, hypotension after return of spontaneous circulation following cardiac arrest, symptomatic bradycardia unresponsive to atropine.

Adverse Effects: Tachycardia, arrhythmias, skin and soft tissue necrosis, severe hypertension from excessive vasoconstriction, angina, dyspnea, headache, nausea/vomiting.

Contraindications: **Pheochromocytoma**, ventricular fibrillation (VF), ventricular tachycardia (VT), or other ventricular arrhythmias, known sensitivity (including sulfites). Correct any hypovolemia with volume fluid replacement before administering dopamine.

Dosage:

- **Adult:** 2 to 20 mcg/kg per minute IV line, IO infusion. Starting dose 5 mcg/kg per minute; may gradually increase the infusion by 5 to 10 mcg/kg per minute to desired effect. Cardiac dose is usually 5 to 10 mcg/kg per minute; vasopressor dose is usually 10 to 20 mcg/kg per minute. Little benefit is gained beyond 20 mcg/kg per minute.
- **Pediatric:** Same as adult dosing.

Special Considerations:

Half-life 2 minutes

Pregnancy class C

© Jones & Bartlett Learning.

NOREPINEPHRINE (LEVOPHED)

Classification: Adrenergic agonist, inotropic, vasopressor.

Action: Norepinephrine is an $alpha_1$, $alpha_2$, and $beta_1$ agonist. Alpha-mediated peripheral vasoconstriction is the predominant clinical result of administration, resulting in increasing blood pressure and coronary blood flow. Beta adrenergic action produces inotropic stimulation of the heart and dilates the coronary arteries.

Indications: Cardiogenic shock, septic shock, severe hypotension.

Adverse Effects: Dizziness, anxiety, cardiac arrhythmias, dyspnea, exacerbation of asthma.

Contraindications: Patients taking monoamine oxidase inhibitors (MAOIs), known sensitivity. Use with caution in hypovolemia.

Dosage:

- **Adult:** Add 4 mg to 250 mL of D_5W or D_5NS, but not normal saline alone; 0.1 to 0.5 mcg/kg per minute as IV line, IO, titrated to maintain blood pressure > 80 mm Hg. Many settings still use non-weight-based dosing of 2 to 4 mcg per minute titrated upward for the desired clinical effect. Refractory shock may require doses as high as 30 mcg per minute.
- **Pediatric:** 0.05 to 2 mcg/kg per minute IV line, IO infusion, to a maximum dose of 2 mcg/kg per minute.

Special Considerations:

Do not administer in same IV line as alkaline solutions.

Half-life 1 minute

Pregnancy class C

DOBUTAMINE (DOBUTREX)

Classification: Adrenergic agent, inotropic.
Action: Acts primarily as an agonist at beta$_1$ adrenergic receptors with minor beta$_2$ and alpha$_1$ effects. Consequently, dobutamine increases myocardial contractility and stroke volume with minor chronotropic effects, resulting in increased cardiac output.
Indications: CHF, cardiogenic shock.
Adverse Effects: Tachycardia, premature ventricular contractions, hypertension, hypotension, palpitations, arrhythmias.
Contraindications: Suspected or known poisoning/drug-induced shock, systolic blood pressure < 100 mm Hg with signs of shock, idiopathic hypertrophic subaortic stenosis (IHSS), known sensitivity (including sulfites). Use with caution in hypertension, recent myocardial infarction (MI), arrhythmias, hypovolemia.

Dosage:
- **Adult:** Initial 0.5 to 1 mcg/kg per minute IV line, IO. Maintenance infusions are typically 2 to 20 mcg/kg per minute. At doses > 20 mcg/kg per minute, increases of heart rate of > 10% may induce or exacerbate myocardial ischemia.
- **Pediatric:** Same as adult dosing.

Special Considerations:
Half-life 2 minutes
Pregnancy class C

PHENYLEPHRINE (NEO-SYNEPHRINE)

Classification: Adrenergic agonist.
Action: Stimulates the alpha receptors, causing vasoconstriction, which results in increased blood pressure.
Indications: Neurogenic shock, spinal shock, cases of shock in which the patient's heart rate does not need to be increased, drug-induced hypotension.
Adverse Effects: Hypertension, VT, headache, excitability, tremor, MI, exacerbation of asthma, cardiac arrhythmias, reflex bradycardia, soft tissue necrosis.
Contraindications: Acute MI, angina, cardiac arrhythmias, severe hypertension, coronary artery disease, pheochromocytoma, narrow-angle glaucoma, cardiomyopathy, MAOI therapy, known sensitivity to phenylephrine or sulfites.

Dosage:
- **Adult:** 100 to 180 mcg per minute IV line, IO. Once the blood pressure has been stabilized, the dose can be reduced to 40 to 60 mcg per minute.
- **Pediatric (2 to 12 years):** 5 to 20 mcg/kg IV line, IO followed by 0.1 to 0.5 mcg/kg per minute IV line, IO (max dose: 3 mcg/kg per minute IV line, IO).

Special Considerations:
Pregnancy class C

EPINEPHRINE

Classification: Adrenergic agent, inotropic.
Action: Binds strongly with both alpha and beta receptors, producing increased blood pressure, increased heart rate, bronchodilation.

(continues)

EPINEPHRINE (continued)

Indications:
Bronchospasm, allergic and anaphylactic reactions, restoration of cardiac activity in cardiac arrest.

Adverse Effects: Anxiety, headache, cardiac arrhythmias, hypertension, nervousness, tremors, chest pain, nausea/vomiting.

© Jones & Bartlett Learning.

© Jones & Bartlett Learning.

Contraindications:
Arrhythmias other than VF, asystole, pulseless electrical activity (PEA); cardiovascular disease; hypertension; cerebrovascular disease; shock secondary to causes other than anaphylactic shock; closed-angle glaucoma; diabetes; pregnant women in active labor; known sensitivity to epinephrine or sulfites.

Dosage:
Cardiac Arrest:
- **Adult:** 1 mg (1:10,000 solution) IV line, IO; may repeat every 3 to 5 minutes.
- **Pediatric:** 0.01 mg/kg (1:10,000 solution) IV line, IO; repeat every 3 to 5 minutes as needed (max dose: 1 mg).

Symptomatic Bradycardia:
- **Adult:** 2 to 10 mcg per minute (1:10,000 solution) as a continuous IV infusion; usual dosage range: 2 to 10 mcg per minute IV line; titrate to effect.
- **Pediatric:** 0.01 mg/kg (1:10,000 solution) IV line, IO; may repeat every 3 to 5 minutes (max dose: 1 mg). If giving epinephrine by ET tube, administer 0.1 mg/kg.

Asthma Attacks and Certain Allergic Reactions:
- **Adult:** 0.3 to 0.5 mg (1:1,000 solution) IM or subcutaneous; may repeat every 10 to 15 minutes (max dose: 1 mg).
- **Pediatric:** 0.01 mg/kg (1:1,000 solution) IM or subcutaneous (max dose: 0.5 mg).

Anaphylactic Shock:
- **Adult:** 0.5 mg (1:1,000 solution) IM repeated as needed every 5 to 15 minutes, or transition to IV infusion of 1 to 4 mcg per minute, titrated to effect.
- **Pediatric:** 0.01 mg/kg IM, repeated as needed every 5 to 15 minutes, or transitioned to continuous IV infusion rate of 0.1 to 1 mcg/kg per minute (1:10,000 solution); titrate to response.

Special Considerations:
Half-life 1 minute
Pregnancy class C

Drugs That Block Adrenergic Receptors

Stimulation of adrenergic receptors influences physiologic responses in different organ systems. Medications capable of binding and blocking adrenergic receptors have several therapeutic applications. Beta adrenergic receptor blockers, or beta blockers, prevent naturally occurring beta agonists from stimulating the receptor. When most beta blockers bind to the receptor, they essentially render that receptor nonfunctional. **Nonselective beta blockers** are capable of binding to both beta$_1$ and beta$_2$ receptors, whereas **selective beta blockers** bind and block either beta$_1$ or beta$_2$ receptors but not both.

Beta blockers have both negative chronotropic and inotropic effects. **Chronotropic drugs** affect the heart rate. Positive chronotropic drugs increase heart rate, and negative chronotropic drugs decrease heart rate. **Inotropic drugs** affect the magnitude of the squeeze of the heart muscle. Positive inotropic drugs make the squeeze of the heart stronger, whereas negative inotropic drugs decrease the intensity of the cardiac squeeze.

Reduction of heart rate and inotropy are useful in patients with cardiac disease. Oxygen is the fuel for the heart, and that fuel is delivered by the coronary arteries (a process known as myocardial oxygen consumption). When the heart beats fast, it burns more fuel (oxygen). With heart disease, the coronary arteries narrow, decreasing the amount of oxygen that can be delivered to the heart. To conserve oxygen, beta blockers or negative chronotropic drugs are administered to patients.

Imagine driving a car, and the needle on the gas gauge is resting in that area below the large E for empty. How would you drive to the nearest gas station? Do you punch the pedal to the floor and speed to the next station? No, because that action would consume fuel at a greater rate. When trying to conserve fuel, drive with gradual accelerations and avoid excessive speed. This is similar to a concept applied to the sick heart. The consumption of oxygen by the heart is similar to the use of gas in an automobile. By placing patients on drugs such as beta blockers, the rate of the heart's acceleration is limited and the amount of oxygen delivered to the heart is conserved.

The blockage of beta$_2$ receptors can result in bronchoconstriction in patients with asthma. Although beta-blocking drugs selective for the beta$_1$ receptor are advantageous in the treatment of heart disease, administration of a nonselective beta blocker to patients with asthma or chronic obstructive pulmonary disease can aggravate these pulmonary conditions. Propranolol (Inderal), a nonselective beta blocker, is capable of binding to both beta$_1$ and beta$_2$ receptors and can decrease both heart rate and cardiac output. Labetalol is another example of a nonselective beta blocker. Beta$_1$ selective blockers are advantageous because they provide the desired effect of reducing heart rate and consumption of oxygen by the heart without adversely affecting lung function.

Selective beta$_1$ blockers such as metoprolol (Lopressor, Toprol XL) and atenolol (Tenormin) are used in some prehospital settings for the treatment of hypertension. A more detailed discussion of these agents is found in Chapter 12.

PROPRANOLOL (INDERAL)

Classification: Beta adrenergic antagonist, antianginal, antihypertensive, antiarrhythmic class II.
Action: Nonselective beta antagonist that binds with both the beta$_1$ and beta$_2$ receptors. Propranolol inhibits the strength of the heart's contractions, as well as heart rate. This results in a decrease in cardiac oxygen consumption.
Indications: Angina; narrow-complex tachycardias that originate from either a *reentry mechanism* (reentry supraventricular tachycardia [SVT]) or an *automatic focus* (junctional, ectopic, or multifocal tachycardia) uncontrolled by vagal maneuvers and adenosine in patients with preserved ventricular function; AF and atrial flutter in patients with preserved ventricular function; hypertension; migraine headaches.

Adverse Effects: Bradycardia, atrioventricular (AV) block, bronchospasm, hypotension.
Contraindications: Cardiogenic shock, heart failure, AV block, bradycardia, pulmonary edema, sick sinus syndrome, known sensitivity. Use with caution in chronic lung disease (asthma and chronic obstructive pulmonary disease [COPD]).
Dosage:
- **Adult:** 1 to 3 mg IV line, IO at a rate of 1 mg per minute; may repeat the dose 2 minutes later.
- **Pediatric:** 0.01 to 0.1 mg/kg slow IV line, IO over a 10-minute period.

Special Considerations:
Monitor blood pressure and heart rate closely during administration.
Pregnancy class C

LABETALOL (NORMODYNE, TRANDATE)

Classification: Beta adrenergic antagonist, antianginal, antihypertensive.

Action: Binds with both the beta$_1$ and beta$_2$ receptors and alpha$_1$ receptors in vascular smooth muscle. Inhibits the strength of the heart's contractions, as well as heart rate. This results in a decrease in cardiac oxygen consumption.

Indications: Acute coronary syndrome (ACS), SVT, severe hypertension.

Adverse Effects: Usually mild and transient; hypotensive symptoms, nausea/vomiting, bronchospasm, arrhythmia, bradycardia, AV block.

Contraindications: Hypotension, cardiogenic shock, acute pulmonary edema, heart failure, severe bradycardia, sick sinus syndrome, second- or third-degree heart block, asthma or acute bronchospasm, cocaine-induced ACS, known sensitivity. Use caution in pheochromocytoma, cerebrovascular disease or stroke, poorly controlled diabetes, with hepatic disease. Use with caution at lowest effective dose in chronic lung disease.

Dosage:

Cardiac Indications:

Note: Monitor blood pressure and heart rate closely during administration.

- **Adult:** 10 mg IV line, IO over a 1- to 2-minute period. May repeat every 10 minutes to a maximum dose of 150 mg or give initial bolus and then follow with infusion at 2 to 8 mg per minute.
- **Pediatric:** 0.4 to 1 mg/kg per hour to a maximum dosage of 3 mg/kg per hour.

Severe Hypertension:

- **Adult:** Initial dose is 20 mg IV line, IO slow infusion over a 2-minute period. After the initial dose, blood pressure should be checked every 5 minutes. Repeat doses can be given at 10-minute intervals. The second dose should be 40 mg IV line, IO, and subsequent doses should be 80 mg IV line, IO, to a maximum total dose of 300 mg. The effect on blood pressure typically will occur within 5 minutes from the time of administration. Alternatively, may be administered via IV infusion at 2 mg per minute to a total maximum dose of 300 mg.
- **Pediatric:** 0.4 to 1 mg/kg per hour IV line, IO infusion with a maximum dose of 3 mg/kg per hour.

Special Considerations:

Pregnancy class C

METOPROLOL (LOPRESSOR, TOPROL XL)

Classification: Beta adrenergic antagonist, antianginal, antihypertensive, class II antiarrhythmic.

Action: Inhibits the strength of the heart's contractions, as well as heart rate. This results in a decrease in cardiac oxygen consumption.

Indications: ACS, hypertension, SVT, atrial flutter, AF, thyrotoxicosis.

Adverse Effects: Tiredness, dizziness, diarrhea, heart block, bradycardia, bronchospasm, drop in blood pressure.

Contraindications: Cardiogenic shock, AV block, bradycardia, known sensitivity. Use with caution in hypotension, chronic lung disease (asthma and COPD).

Dosage:

Cardiac Indications:

- **Adult:** 5 mg slow IV line, IO over a 2-minute period; repeat at 5-minute intervals up to a total of three infusions totaling 15 mg IV line, IO.
- **Pediatric:** Oral dosing only.

Special Considerations:

Blood pressure, heart rate, and electrocardiographic activity should be monitored carefully. Use with caution in patients with asthma.

Pregnancy class C.

Cholinergic Receptors and Activating Drugs

Receptors of the parasympathetic nervous system are known as **cholinergic receptors**. The term *cholinergic* comes from the name of the principal neurotransmitter of the parasympathetic nervous system, **acetylcholine**. Acetylcholine is the neurotransmitter used by the parasympathetic nervous system to act on the various organs of the body. It can act on the heart to slow the heart rate in addition to having a negative inotropic effect. Acetylcholine is also used in the sympathetic nervous system to relay messages, not as a neurotransmitter.

Two types of cholinergic receptors are at work within the parasympathetic nervous system: **nicotinic** and **muscarinic receptors**. Nicotinic receptors are found in the central nervous system, autonomic ganglia, and striated muscle. Muscarinic receptors are found on the cardiac and smooth muscle, exocrine glands, and brain.

Several drugs bind and stimulate cholinergic receptors, although few have a role in the prehospital setting. Atropine competes with acetylcholine for the opportunity to bind muscarinic receptors, which results in an increase in heart rate. As a prehospital drug, atropine commonly is used for the treatment of bradycardia. When treating symptomatic bradycardia, the dosage guidelines must be strictly followed. In smaller doses, atropine can cause further slowing of the heart. Higher doses of atropine lead to the desired acceleration of heart rate. In high enough dosages, atropine also exerts effects on the pulmonary system by causing bronchodilation and a reduction of secretions. Consequently, atropine is the drug of choice in nerve agent and organophosphate poisoning.

ATROPINE SULFATE

Classification: Anticholinergic (antimuscarinic).
Action: Competes reversibly with acetylcholine at the site of the muscarinic receptor. Receptors affected, in order from the most sensitive to the least sensitive, include salivary, bronchial, sweat glands, eye, heart, and GI tract.
Indications: Symptomatic bradycardia, asystole or PEA, nerve agent exposure, organophosphate poisoning.
Adverse Effects: Decreased secretions resulting in dry mouth and hot skin temperature,

© Jones & Bartlett Learning.

intense facial flushing, blurred vision or dilation of the pupils with subsequent **photophobia**, tachycardia, and restlessness. Atropine may cause paradoxical bradycardia if the dose administered is too low or if the drug is administered too slowly.
Contraindications: Acute MI; myasthenia gravis; GI obstruction; closed-angle glaucoma; known sensitivity to atropine, belladonna alkaloids, or sulfites. Will not be effective for infranodal (type II) AV block and new third-degree block with wide QRS complex.
Dosage:
Symptomatic Bradycardia:
- **Adult:** 0.5 mg IV line, IO every 3 to 5 minutes to a maximum dose of 3 mg.
- **Adolescent:** 0.02 mg/kg (minimum 0.1 mg/dose; maximum 1 mg/dose) IV line, IO up to a total dose of 2 mg.
- **Pediatric:** 0.02 mg/kg (minimum 0.1 mg/dose; maximum 0.5 mg/dose) IV line, IO, to a total dose of 1 mg.
Nerve Agent or Organophosphate Poisoning:
- **Adult:** 1 to 6 mg IV line, IM; repeat if needed every 5 minutes until symptoms dissipate.
- **Pediatric:** 0.05 mg/kg IV line, IM every 10 to 30 minutes as needed until symptoms dissipate.
- **Infants <15 pounds:** 0.05 mg/kg IV line, IM every 5 to 20 minutes as needed until symptoms dissipate.

(continues)

ATROPINE SULFATE   (continued)

Special Considerations:
Severe organophosphate exposures may require *massive* amounts of atropine, well beyond what
    is carried in most EMS vehicles.
Half-life is 2.5 hours.
Pregnancy class C; possibly unsafe in lactating mothers.

SCOPOLAMINE (TRANSDERM SCOP)

Classification: Neurologic antivertigo, antimuscarinic.
Action: Antagonizes acetylcholine at muscarinic receptors.
Indications: Motion sickness.
Adverse Effects: Dry mouth, drowsiness, dilated pupils and blurred
vision, hallucinations, confusion.
Contraindications: Glaucoma, cardiac arrhythmias, coronary artery
disease, known sensitivity.
Dosage:
  • **Adult and children older than 12 years:** 1 disc applied to
    skin behind the ear.
Special Considerations:
Half-life 8 hours
Pregnancy class C

Scopolamine
Transdermal system
1 mg/3 days
Formulated delivery of approximately
1 mg over three days
**Motion Sickness and
Post-operative
Nausea & Vomiting
Prevention Patches**
NDC 12345-678-90   **Rx only**

Scopolamine is another drug that competitively binds with the muscarinic receptor.
Compared with atropine, scopolamine does not have as potent an effect on the heart and
lungs. Scopolamine commonly is used for the treatment of motion sickness. Although dispensing a scopolamine patch would be highly unlikely for a paramedic, being dispatched to
an interstate or airport for a medical call in which a patient has taken this drug is possible.

▶ Review Questions

1.   Explain the difference between a drug's generic name and trade name.
2.   List the properties of a medication.
3.   Explain the dose-response relationship.
4.   Why would an oral medication be inappropriate for an acute emergency such as an
     asthma attack?
5.   Explain first-pass metabolism.
6.   List the factors that alter drug metabolism.
7.   Explain the similarities between active transport and carrier-mediated facilitated diffusion.
8.   Define *half-life*.
9.   List two factors in determining (calculating) the therapeutic index.
10. What are the roles of the agonist and antagonist in the action of a drug?
11. What is a drug interaction?
12. What are two types of drug interactions?
13. What are the physiologic effects of epinephrine?
14. What is the effect on the heart when stimulating beta$_1$ receptors?
15. What are the effects on the lungs when stimulating beta$_2$ receptors?
16. What is the effect of giving too small a dose of atropine?

CHAPTER 2

Legal Aspects and Risk Management

OBJECTIVES

1. Describe the importance of the publication *To Err Is Human: Building a Safer Health System*.
2. Define the four elements of negligence: duty to act, breach of duty to act, causation, and harm to the patient.
3. Describe the principal goal of Good Samaritan laws.
4. List the steps a provider can take to minimize the risk of a medication mistake.
5. Explain the benefits of protocols in preventing mistakes in medication administration.
6. Describe Schedule I, II, III, IV, V, and VI medications and the abuse potential for each.
7. Discuss the importance of properly storing, securing, and maintaining medications.
8. List the parts of the $A^3E^3P^3$ refusal guidelines.
9. Discuss the effect of living wills and advance directives on prehospital providers.
10. List the *dos* and *don'ts* of documenting medication administration.
11. Discuss the importance of properly documenting and reporting medication errors.

▶ Introduction

The administration of medications by prehospital providers in the field can have a tremendously positive effect on patients. To reduce risk and liability, however, medication administration ideally should be performed in a more controlled environment. The administration of drugs in the field can present obstacles such as low light levels and unstable environmental conditions that test the skills of even the most competent caregiver. Nonetheless, medication administration in the field is a skill that must be mastered, and paramedics can learn to avoid mistakes that can harm patients and open the door to lawsuits.

This chapter describes the legal context of medication administration in the field and the legal basis for negligence lawsuits. It discusses the most common liability areas associated with prehospital medication administration and strategies for minimizing the two key risk areas: **harm to the patient** and likelihood of a lawsuit.

Skill, knowledge, sound judgment, and strict adherence to protocols and procedures can reduce the possibility of a bad patient outcome or a lawsuit.

CASE STUDY

Your paramedic unit is dispatched to a local department store in response to a medical call. While en route, the dispatcher informs you that the patient is a 33-year-old woman with a history of diabetes. When you arrive, you find the patient sitting in a chair and holding her head in her hands. She answers all your questions, and her mental status is clear. She tells you that she is an insulin-dependent diabetic. She was rushed this morning getting her kids ready for school; she took her morning dose of insulin but failed to eat a complete breakfast. She began to run some errands and became dizzy, weak, and diaphoretic. She believes she had a hypoglycemic episode but feels a little better after having some juice. You assess the patient and measure her blood glucose level. The glucometer reads 60 mg/dL. You administer some glucose gel, and the patient reports feeling much better. She is more talkative. She looks at her watch and starts to gather her belongings, saying that she is going to be late to pick up her daughter at preschool. The patient tells you she feels fine and appreciates your concerns. You recommend that she be transported to the hospital for further evaluation. She refuses any further medical care or transport even after you have provided some initial therapy and evaluation.

What type of refusal is this? As a paramedic your job is done, right? Wrong. You tell her that she should not drive. You tell her that you would prefer she call her husband to drive her home. She responds with a prompt no. She does not want her husband to know about this incident. She has provided you with a partial refusal, but what are the legal obligations and potential liabilities in partially treating a patient? Are you obligated to call her husband, or would that be violating her privacy? Is not transporting her to the hospital negligent? What if she has another episode while driving the car, with or without her kids? Is the patient medically and legally competent to refuse additional care? Does the patient understand the potential risks of refusing therapy? Have you explained these concerns in a simple, nonmedical fashion so that the patient can understand? What are the protocols for patients providing consent or refusing emergency medical care?

▶ Scope of Potential Legal Liability

On a national scale, errors in medication administration are a serious problem, even in the more controlled environment of a hospital. A medication error is a preventable occurrence caused by inappropriate use of a medication that has the potential to result in patient harm. The public first became aware of the extent of medication errors after a landmark publication by the National Academy of Medicine (then called the Institute of Medicine) titled *To Err Is Human: Building a Safer Health System.*[1] This report revealed the following findings:

- Approximately 45,000 to 100,000 Americans die each year from general medical errors.[1]
- Medical errors are the third leading cause of death, ranking higher than stroke, diabetes, breast cancer, and human immunodeficiency virus (HIV).[2]
- Approximately 7,000 people die each year from medication errors alone.[3]

Emergency medical services (EMS) is not immune to the problem of medication errors, and in many cases the problem is made worse by the environmental conditions and other situational factors inherent in the field setting that are not present in a hospital. Little research has described the scope of the problem, but in one study, researchers at Western Carolina University assessed the medication calculation skills of a group of practicing paramedics, including the types of computations they found most difficult and the relationships between drug calculation skills and various demographic characteristics. The study involved a 10-item drug calculation examination administered to a group of 109 practicing paramedics who represented a cross-section of EMS system characteristics in North Carolina. The researchers found that the overall performance on the drug calculation examination was poor. The mean score was 51.4%. Intravenous (IV) flow rate and medication bolus calculation problems were answered correctly in 68.8% of the cases, followed by non-weight-based medication infusions (33.9%), weight-based medication infusions (32.5%), and percentage-based medication infusions (4.5%). The examination scores were higher among paramedics with a college-level education but lower among paramedics with more years of experience.[4]

The results of this study were similar to findings in other allied health professions: medication calculation skills were lacking. The paramedics in this study also reported infrequent opportunities to perform drug calculations in the clinical setting, such as during hospital skill rotations, and that medication calculations were not a routine part of EMS continuing education programs.

▶ Principles of Negligence

The same principles of negligence that can lead to liability in other areas of emergency medicine apply to medication administration. **Ordinary negligence**, or basic negligence, is defined as the failure to exercise the degree of care that another reasonable person would exercise in the same or similar situation in which harm to another person results. The average, ordinary person or professional is held to that standard when a negligence lawsuit arises. Applying this concept to medical care, actions that would be considered ordinary negligence are acts that caused harm to the patient and "deviated from good and acceptable medical standards."[5]

Negligence is defined by the following four elements, all of which must be proven in court for the plaintiff to prevail:

1. Duty to act
2. Breach of duty to act
3. Causation
4. Harm to the patient

Duty to Act

Duty to act is a simple concept: Did you have a duty to provide the care to the patient? This is generally an easy element for the plaintiff to prove. Because an ambulance service or EMS organization promotes itself to the public as capable of responding to emergency requests, the service has a duty to respond to the patient and provide the level of care that paramedics are reasonably expected to provide.

However, the duty to act must be a legal duty. The defendant must have a legal obligation to respond, treat, and transport the patient before the duty to act can be breached.

CASE STUDY

A paramedic is on his way to work the night shift at ABC Ambulance and Rescue. He hears on his scanner that a serious motor vehicle accident has occurred just a few blocks away from his location. He chooses not to respond to that call in his private vehicle and continues on his way to work.

In this case, the paramedic has no duty to act because he is not legally obligated to respond until he has officially begun work. Had he been at the station and on duty, he would have had a duty to act.

Breach of Duty to Act

If a paramedic fails in any way to provide the level of care that the EMS agency or local protocols dictate, he or she may be guilty of **breach of duty to act**. This is the point at which the **standard of care** comes into play; that is, if a person failed to act, was the failure to act inconsistent with local protocol or other direction to provide care? In such cases, expert witnesses are used to testify to the standard of care for EMS personnel in the community in which they serve. The key question is what would a reasonably prudent paramedic do in this same situation?

CASE STUDY

A paramedic is at the end of her shift and is very tired—so tired that all she cares about is going home. However, right before the shift ends, a call comes in for a possible heart attack. She responds and is directed by medical command to administer 4 mg of morphine sulfate IV for pain. But the paramedic does not want to deal with all the paperwork that comes with administering a narcotic agent, so she decides not to give the patient the morphine and transports him to the hospital.

In this case, the paramedic clearly breached her duty to act by not administering the medication to the patient as ordered by medical command. She did not provide the standard of care expected by her EMS agency and the community.

Causation

Causation refers to the fact that the plaintiff must prove that the paramedic's conduct was a substantial factor in bringing about harm to the patient. This is a difficult element to prove in most EMS cases because, at the outset, the "wheels of harm" to the patient were set into motion before EMS was even activated. The paramedic responds to a patient who has already incurred harm and is merely intervening in an attempt to reduce the effect of that harm. The question the jury would have to answer is whether the paramedic's conduct was the *cause* of the harm to the patient. This is referred to as **proximate cause**. If the patient's harm can be shown to have come from other sources and not the paramedic's conduct, the causation requirement would not be met.

CASE STUDY

A patient with severe chest pain calls 9-1-1. First responders arrive and find an unconscious patient. The automatic external defibrillator shows a shockable rhythm, and a shock is administered. The patient's pulse and respirations return. EMS then responds, and a paramedic assesses the patient. The paramedic administers a cardiac medication but gives a dose that is too high. After receiving the excessive dose, the patient has a seizure. He is later found to have incurred brain damage.

If the drug administration error in this case can be shown to have caused the seizure and subsequent brain damage, proximate causation would be proven. But in defending the paramedic or EMS agency, the defense attorney would likely argue that the patient had the seizure and incurred brain damage as a result of the heart attack and cardiac arrest itself, not the medication error.

In some cases, medication errors and their effects on the patient can be isolated from the initial insult to the patient. For example, if a patient has a heart attack and is given a medication to which he is allergic, which subsequently leads to an anaphylactic reaction and death, it may be relatively simple to demonstrate that the paramedic's intervention was a substantial factor in the patient's outcome. The question would be whether the patient would have suffered an anaphylactic reaction in the absence of the paramedic's intervention. In this situation, the answer would clearly be no, and this element of negligence would be proven.

Harm to the Patient

A successful lawsuit based on negligence requires that the patient experienced some harm—that is, physical or emotional injury that caused damage to the patient.

Damage can be shown in the form of the patient's own testimony, the testimony of expert witnesses, and other evidence that points to the extent of harm to the patient. The cost of this harm can be translated into medical costs for treatment, recovery, and rehabilitation; pain and suffering; and other compensatory damages. To prove negligence, the plaintiff typically must show that the harm was of the type that could have been caused by the EMS provider.

CASE STUDY

Washington County Fire Department paramedics respond to a motor vehicle crash. On arrival, paramedics find the driver of the vehicle walking around with no apparent injuries. His vehicle incurred minor damage when it struck a parked car. One of the paramedics approaches the patient, who refuses treatment and says he is fine. The paramedic obtains an informed refusal form, which the patient signs. The patient goes home and goes to sleep. The next day he wakes up with a throbbing headache and goes to the emergency department (ED). He is admitted with a cerebral aneurysm that requires surgery; he also has developed some paralysis. The patient sues the municipality, stating that the paramedics were negligent in not transporting him to the hospital.

In this case, although the patient incurred harm from the accident, that harm did not result from the paramedics' acts or omissions. The paramedic was wise to ask the patient to sign an informed refusal.

▶ The Immunity Defense

Many states provide certain **immunities** under the law that make proving negligence against an EMS provider difficult for a plaintiff. These immunities are based on the age-old principle of the Good Samaritan, which encourages others to assist ill and injured people to the best of their ability without fear of a lawsuit if they make any mistakes.

Nearly every state has some form of **Good Samaritan legislation**. Many of these laws merely protect bystanders or people without medical training from getting sued for providing assistance in an emergency. Some of these laws protect physicians and nurses who render care at the scene of an emergency outside their work environment. These laws are designed to encourage off-duty health professionals to assist in an emergency without the fear of liability, which could cloud their judgment or prevent them from lending help.

Other state laws extend the immunity to EMS personnel and other emergency responders. For example, Pennsylvania's immunity statute for EMS personnel states the following:

> *No* first responder, emergency medical technician [EMT] or EMT-paramedic, or health professional who in good faith attempts to render or facilitate emergency medical care authorized by this act *shall be liable* for any civil damages as a result of any acts or omissions, *unless guilty of gross or willful negligence* [italics added for emphasis].[6]

Do Good Samaritan laws provide complete immunity from a negligence lawsuit? Usually they do not. The type of immunity that these laws embody is not full immunity, but rather **qualified immunity**. That is, the immunity has a qualification: the caregiver may not act in a reckless, wanton manner in total disregard to the patient. Acting in this manner would be considered **gross negligence**. Most immunity statutes provide a caregiver immunity from a negligence lawsuit unless his or her actions could be shown to constitute gross negligence.

Gross negligence is difficult to prove in many cases because actions or inactions must be found to be more than a mere mistake to be considered grossly negligent acts. As the Supreme Court of Pennsylvania described it, gross negligence is substantially more than "ordinary carelessness, inadvertence, laxity, or indifference." It is behavior that is "flagrant, grossly deviating from the ordinary standard of care."[7]

Volunteer EMS personnel often have legal protection for their conduct. The underlying philosophy is that if a person volunteers to save a person's life or assist the person in a medical crisis, that volunteer should not have to worry about getting sued. Otherwise, people may not be willing to act as Good Samaritans and help in an emergency. In many cases, these state laws require that volunteers have a minimal level of training, such as cardiopulmonary resuscitation or first aid, and that they render assistance only within the level of that certification or training.

Some states limit immunity protection to volunteer personnel and do not apply it to paid EMS personnel. Lawmakers in those states believe that healthcare providers owe a higher duty to the people they are obligated to serve as part of their profession. Because responding to emergencies is part of a paramedic's responsibility as an emergency professional, paramedics should be better prepared for these situations than Good Samaritans.

> Check state laws carefully to determine whether immunity statutes apply to paid, or career, EMS personnel. If the state has no immunity statute, the standard for evaluating conduct likely will be based on ordinary negligence, which is easier to prove than gross negligence.

How does a paramedic avoid committing gross negligence? First and foremost, paramedics should function within their certification level. They should not perform skills or administer medications outside of their **scope of practice** (the legally approved skills that may be performed and the medications authorized to administer), as defined by state law. For example, if you are not authorized under state law and your medical director to administer paralytic agents to combative patients who need to be intubated, you should not use that medication—even if it is available in the drug box.

Second, always act in good faith. The best way to do this is to always treat patients as though they were your own close relatives. Function in a reasonable and prudent manner with the interest of the patient in your heart and mind. Common sense often helps in this area. Ask yourself the question, "Is this the right thing to do in this situation?" If the answer is no, reevaluate the plan of action. Failure to verify a patent vein when administering IV medication and failure to check the vial of medication to verify its concentration and expiration date are examples of not acting in good faith.

Third, do not take actions or fail to take actions that could be construed as grossly negligent. Function within your scope of practice, and do what the public would expect you to do. Do not commit an action or omit an action that you had a recognized duty to do or not do, knowing or having reason to know that the act or omission could create a substantial risk of harm to the patient. Remember the first rule of medical care: do no harm. If your actions could harm the patient, do not initiate them in the first place.

▶ Medication Errors: Mistake or Negligence?

Mistakes occur every day in the prehospital field. It is a challenging working environment, and providers need to be vigilant and alert at all times. Even the smallest mistake can lead to serious harm to the patient. Still, a mistake does not necessarily mean negligence under the law. The successful plaintiff must prove by a preponderance of the evidence that all four elements of negligence were present; this usually is demonstrated by showing that a provider deviated from the standard of care and that his or her conduct was a substantial factor in causing the harm to the patient.

Negligence is difficult to prove, but in many cases juries are sympathetic to the plaintiff or the plaintiff's surviving family members. Many jurors view paramedics as professionals who are no different from nurses and other healthcare professionals who work in hospitals; they do not always take into account the less-controlled nature of the prehospital setting or the relative roles and training levels of prehospital providers. Jurors who are sympathetic to the plaintiff's emotional appeals or who hold unreasonable expectations for prehospital care providers do not always decide cases on the basis of the law. Compounding this risk to providers, in the U.S. court system, the manner in which a jury decides a negligence case is not subject to review on appeal unless clear errors occurred in trial procedures, such as evidence being admitted when the judge should have disallowed it or the jury acting on instructions that do not reflect the current state of the law. A clear basis for appeal would be tampering with the jury or juror misconduct, but even then, winning an appeal on these issues is rare.

Jurors can be influenced by many factors and make their decisions based on many sources of information. Assessment of witness credibility, opinions of the plaintiff or defense counsel, and the jurors' life experiences all weigh in on the jury's decision of liability. Other more tangible factors include the extent of harm to the patient, life expectancy of the patient, effect of the harm on the patient's activities of daily living, and other emotional issues that are part of the case. Juries are expected to follow the law and abide by the instructions read to them by the judge. However, the biases, prejudices, and persuasiveness of the attorneys greatly affect the final decision.

In all aspects of their work, prehospital care providers must avoid conducting themselves in a manner that others could construe as negligent. These providers can take the following steps to minimize the risk of a medication mistake that can harm a patient and result in a lawsuit:

- *Be well educated.* Know drugs and everything about them, including contraindications to administration, possible side effects, and drug interactions. The U.S. Food and Drug Administration approves new medications at an increasingly rapid pace, and the treatment protocols for specific situations are constantly changing.
- *Be well rested.* Providers are more apt to make a mistake when tired and stressed. In emergency services, failure to be in the best possible physical condition can lead to serious errors. Medication administration requires providers to be sharp and at their best. Many aspects of this skill require intact thought processes and mental skill. Studies have shown that failure to be well rested can lead to mistakes in patient care, and medication errors are more likely to occur when providers are tired and unable to think clearly.[8,9]
- *Know protocols and follow them.* In negligence cases, the standard of care is examined. The standard of care in a lawsuit is determined by that state's scope of practice and other supplemental sources, including training program curricula, textbooks, and medical expert reports and testimony. That standard is also often defined by local medical protocols, which can become direct evidence of legally authorized scope of practice and the standard of medical care for the community. Deviating from these protocols can be considered deviating from the standard of care.
- *Maintain knowledge and skills.* As the North Carolina study mentioned earlier suggests, drug calculation and other medication administration skills should be practiced on a regular basis to keep the provider from getting rusty. Lack of practice leads to a greater likelihood of making mistakes.

Maintaining medication knowledge and administration skills is especially important to avoid mistakes when treating pediatric patients, who are seen less frequently than adults (thus, most paramedics have less practice treating pediatric patients). A recent study, involving over 1,000 paramedics, highlighted significant gaps in both initial training and subsequent performance by paramedics related to pediatric medication administration. Most

FIGURE 2-1 Broselow system.

Courtesy of Armstrong Medical Industries.

paramedics indicated that they did not feel that that they had received enough initial training on pediatric medication administration. One third of these paramedics had not administered medication to a pediatric patient within the past year, and there was great variability regarding how weights were obtained or estimated for pediatric patients.[10] Errors in pediatric drug administration can occur for a variety of reasons, including misplaced decimal points when performing calculations and rushed calculations and medication administration. A number of commercial devices, systems, and electronic reference sources use the child's height (or length when lying supine) to estimate the child's weight. This approach uses the estimated weight to further identify the proper medication dosages, probable size of various resuscitation supplies, expected vital signs, appropriate dose for electrical therapy, and other details. With doses and sizes predetermined, EMS providers do not need to focus on complicated calculations during resuscitation. This approach improves reliability and eliminates guesswork in these very high-stress situations.[11,12] Even the novel use of color-coded prefilled syringes, based on the Broselow system, has been shown to improve accuracy of medication doses during simulated pediatric resuscitation (**FIGURE 2-1**).

Pediatric patients require medication dosages that are not often administered in the prehospital setting. In addition, dealing with a seriously ill or injured child is an added stressor. The liability that can result from a medication error in a pediatric patient can be extensive. The emotional impact on the jury when a child is harmed by a healthcare provider and the young age of the patient generally translate to higher damage awards in pediatric cases. The court can award damages for loss of future income of the child, as well as the loss of affection for the parents. As such, the economic value of the harm to the patient or loss of life can be tremendous.

A paramedic can never be too cautious when administering medication to a pediatric patient. Always double-check procedures and have your partner or another healthcare professional check as well. Stay in close touch with online medical command if possible, and seek guidance and direction when you are unsure of yourself or if protocols require it. Be mindful that administering prehospital medications to a child is an infrequent occurrence for the prehospital provider. Therefore, the likelihood of committing an error is greater.

▶ Protocols as a Risk Management Tool

Established advanced life support (ALS) protocols are an excellent safeguard to prevent mistakes in medication administration. In some ALS systems, online medical direction is extremely important, with most medication orders coming from an emergency physician in the ED. In situations in which medication orders are given over the radio or by telephone, *the paramedic must make certain that the correct medication and dosage were heard and should repeat the order to the physician for confirmation.* Online medical direction can give the paramedic a degree of comfort in knowing that administering a particular medication in the proper amount is not the sole decision of the field provider.

In other ALS systems, medication administration is accomplished by adherence to either standing orders or ALS protocols. Standing orders serve as advance orders from medical direction that are developed ahead of time and are followed by all paramedics in that particular ALS system. They are directives to be followed in the event that certain medical conditions are determined by the paramedic. Standing orders are used routinely, and in these cases online medical direction is not necessary. The paramedic typically provides a report to medical direction either en route or on arrival in the ED to communicate the medication(s) administered, dose, route, and effect on the patient. An example of a standing order is shown in the area shaded in red in **FIGURE 2-2.**

In most cases, **protocols** are orders designed to be followed in the event that online medical direction is not available for certain reasons. These reasons are spelled out as part of protocol development and can include situations such as communication systems failure and limited access to online medical direction because of system design. These protocols define what should be done for the patient in particular situations. An example of a protocol is shown in Figure 2-2.

Medication administration is a critical element of most ALS protocols because remembering the medications and doses to administer to a particular patient in a particular situation can be difficult in the often stressful field environment. Committing protocols to memory is important to help prevent administration of the wrong drug or the wrong dose of the drug.

Both standing orders and protocols are typically developed after much thought and study. In many ways, they represent the standard of care for prehospital ALS in a given community or region. These procedures can be invaluable tools for the paramedic in the field and serve as a safeguard to avoiding errors in medication administration.

Most protocols are based on an either/or analysis and often are written as a flowchart or decision tree. At a particular point in the protocol, a choice must be made. For example, a protocol for cardiac arrest or ventricular fibrillation may state that if a patient is in ventricular fibrillation, epinephrine 1 mg should be administered by IV push every 5 minutes. The first decision is to determine whether the patient is in ventricular fibrillation. If the answer is yes, the protocol to administer the epinephrine should be followed.

An important aspect of standing orders and protocols is that they tend to be rigid and do not allow for unique patient conditions or situations. Most ALS systems require that these orders be followed exactly, except in extremely unusual situations. Because they represent the standard of care for particular patient conditions, failure to follow orders to the letter can put a paramedic at a disadvantage in court. Unfortunately, the clarity of standing orders and protocols can be quickly used against the paramedic in court if he or she did not follow them as any other reasonable and prudent paramedic would have, given the same situation. These documents are commonly entered into evidence in lawsuits through a fact witness (someone involved in the situation, such as a paramedic or emergency physician) or an expert witness hired to provide an opinion on whether the protocols were appropriate, reflected the standard of care in the community, and were properly followed.

Standing orders and protocols are important considerations in lawsuits. They work in the clinician's favor by providing direction in managing patients in difficult and stressful situations in which clarity of thinking and judgment can be skewed.

The following actions can help ensure that protocols involving medication administration work favorably for the paramedic and the patient:

■ *Keep protocols up to date.* Protocols need to change as the standard of medical care changes. This process frequently happens in EMS as treatment modalities are reevaluated by national physician groups, such as the American Heart Association's Emergency Cardiac Care Committee. When medical authorities revise their standards in patient care,

Protocol for Allergic Reactions

History
1. Exposure, ingestion, or contact (stings, drugs, foods, etc.)
2. Prior allergic history
3. Current medications

Symptoms
4. Itching
5. Rash
6. Swelling
7. Respiratory distress
8. Abdominal pain
9. Nausea, vomiting
10. Syncope
11. Weakness
12. Anxiety
13. Choking sensation
14. Cough

Signs
15. Vital signs: Vary (routine or shock*)
16. Skin: Rash, redness, urticaria (hives), generalized or local edema
17. HEENT: Tongue or upper airway (uvula) edema*
18. Respiratory: Wheezing, stridor, hoarseness,* cough, upper airway noise
19. Neurologic: Varies

Basic Life Support
20. Secure airway in accordance with airway protocol
21. **Administer supplemental oxygen, maintain saturation between 90% and 100%**
22. Record and monitor vital signs
23. Assist patient in self-administration of previously prescribed Sub-Q epinephrine (autoinjector)
24. Nothing by mouth

Advanced Life Support
25. Advanced airway/ventilatory management as needed
26. Initiate cardiac monitoring, record and evaluate ECG strip
27. Record and monitor O_2 saturation
28. Microstream capnography (if available), if any acute respiratory symptoms
29. If BP < 90 mm Hg systolic, **administer boluses of 0.9% NaCl at 250–500 mL to maintain systolic BP > 90 mm Hg**
   • *Contraindicated if evidence of congestive heart failure (e.g., rales)*
30. Mild Reaction (Itching/Hives)
   a) **Diphenhydramine** (Benadryl) **1 mg/kg IV** (Maximum 50 mg)
      i) May be administered IM if no IV access available
31. Moderate Reaction (Dyspnea, Wheezing, Chest tightness)
   a) **Albuterol** (Proventil) **2.5 mg/3 mL via aerosolized**
      i) May repeat Albuterol (Proventil) × 2
   b) **Diphenhydramine** (Benadryl) **1 mg/kg IV** (Maximum 50 mg)
      i) May be administered IM if no IV access available
   c) **Methylprednisolone** (Solu-Medrol) **125 mg, slow IV bolus**
32. Severe Systemic Reaction (BP < 90 mm Hg, Stridor, Severe respiratory distress)
   a) **Epinephrine 1:1000 0.3 mg Sub-Q**
   b) **Albuterol** (Proventil) **2.5 mg/3 mL via aerosolized**
      i) May repeat × 2
   c) **Methylprednisolone** (Solu-Medrol) **125 mg, slow IV bolus**
   d) **Diphenhydramine** (Benadryl) **1 mg/kg IV** (Maximum 50 mg)
      i) May be administered IM if no IV access
33. Cardiopulmonary Arrest Imminent
   a) **Epinephrine 1:10,000 0.5 mg IVP** (instead of 1:1000 Sub-Q)
   b) **Albuterol** (Proventil) **2.5 mg/3 mL via aerosolized**
   c) **Diphenhydramine** (Benadryl) **1 mg/kg IV** (Maximum 50 mg)
      i) May be administered IM if no IV access available

FIGURE 2-2 Example of a protocol. A protocol is a series of orders and instructions that outline the treatment required for a specific medical condition. The area in red is an example of a standing order. Standing orders are provided in advance by medical direction for providers to use in specific circumstances. A standing order is usually one element of a series of standing orders or instructions, referred to as a protocol.

a community's ALS system needs to evaluate these changes to determine whether they should be implemented. The ALS system must provide the most current treatment modalities. Failure to keep pace with the changes in prehospital medicine can have a negative effect on patients' clinical outcomes and can work against clinicians in a negligence action. This failure can be used by the plaintiff's attorney to demonstrate what the standard of care should be in that particular case and to show that a system did not follow the appropriate standard of care. In most cases, the individual paramedic is not found liable for performing treatment in accordance with outdated protocols. However, the EMS agency carries a great risk for liability in these situations.

■ *Know the protocols.* Paramedics must know their ALS treatment protocols inside and out. Frequent reviews of these protocols and drills that test knowledge (such as a simulated cardiac arrest situation, or "mega code") are essential. Proper protocol use leads to positive patient outcomes and reduced risk of negligence lawsuits.

▶ Laws Governing Prehospital Pharmacology

Numerous laws govern the use of medications and pharmacologic agents in the field. The basic laws that address the manufacturing, packaging, and labeling of medications have their roots in the early 20th century. At that time, many deaths were caused by improperly manufactured drugs, as well as the lack of education for physicians and patients about contraindications, side effects, and proper administration and use.

The federal Food, Drug, and Cosmetic Act, enacted in 1938, required detailed labeling of all medications. From this law evolved the package insert required in all medication packaging. This insert describes in detail the generic and common names of the drug, indications and contraindications for administration, directions for its use, recommended dosages, and potential side effects. This law alone eliminated scores of medication errors through proper and accurate labeling.

Narcotic agents are afforded extra scrutiny under the law because of their potential for abuse. The federal Comprehensive Drug Abuse Prevention and Control Act of 1970 classified potentially dangerous and habit-forming drugs into five different classes, or schedules, with safeguards for their prescription, use, and control.

The more dangerous drugs have a lower schedule number. **Schedule I** drugs are the most dangerous and have the highest abuse potential. Drugs in this class have no recognized medical use; examples include heroin, lysergic acid diethylamide (LSD), methaqualone, and marijuana (cannabis). Marijuana is a particular anomaly in the U.S. Drug Enforcement Administration (DEA) Drug Scheduling system. While the federal government has taken a restrictive approach to marijuana, many states have elaborate programs allowing medical and even recreational use of marijuana. **Schedule II** drugs are recognized as having a high potential for abuse, but they are safe and have accepted medical uses. Schedule II drugs include narcotics, stimulants, and depressant drugs. They are available only by a written prescription, and their distribution is carefully monitored by the DEA. Some medications administered in the prehospital field, such as morphine sulfate and meperidine, are Schedule II drugs, as are stimulants (e.g., amphetamines) and depressants (e.g., secobarbital). **Schedule III** drugs have less abuse potential than do Schedule I and II drugs. Abuse of Schedule III drugs may lead to moderate or low physical dependence. Examples of Schedule III drugs include narcotics such as codeine, common stimulants such as benzphetamine, and depressants such as talbutal. **Schedule IV** and **Schedule V** agents are less habit forming and pose a lesser risk of harm from overdose. Examples of Schedule IV drugs include diazepam (Valium) and alprazolam (Xanax). Cough medications with codeine are an example of Schedule V drugs.

The Controlled Substances Act is enforced by the DEA. Only physicians, physicians' assistants, and licensed nurse practitioners registered with the DEA and those who have approved DEA numbers may prescribe scheduled medications. The physician's DEA number must appear on the prescription form, and serious criminal penalties can be levied for misusing this number.

In addition to the federal drug control laws, most states have enacted their own laws that address the use and misuse of medications. As with federal laws, many of these laws mandate criminal penalties for violation; so in many cases of abuse, theft, misuse, and illegal sale of scheduled drugs, both the federal and state criminal codes may have been violated.

State EMS laws also govern the use of prehospital medications. Most states have approved drug lists that outline the medications that an EMT-Intermediate or paramedic may administer in the field. Ultimately, the local EMS system's medical director dictates which of those drugs may be used in the system. EMS agencies *must* maintain and use only the medications approved by the state EMS office and local medical director.

In many cases, state EMS laws mandate disciplinary sanctions against emergency personnel who misuse approved medications. Violations of the regulations that control drug administration in the prehospital setting can result in a hearing and disciplinary action, such as suspension or revocation of certification. Care must be taken at all times to follow state laws carefully and report any violations to the EMS agency's management, the medical director, and the appropriate state or local authority.

▶ Operational Considerations

Medications used by paramedics are lifesaving tools that can stabilize the heart or treat anaphylactic shock. As a comparison, consider the traditional tools commonly required for search and rescue. These tools might include hydraulic spreaders/cutters and rams to extricate victims from motor vehicle collisions or ropes and rappelling gear for high-angle rescues. Because the lives of the victim and rescuer depend on this vital equipment, it should be meticulously stored and maintained. Because drugs are the paramedic's tools, they also must be carefully stored, secured, and maintained.

Storage and Security

Because of the mandate to provide proper patient care and adhere to the strict legal controls over drugs used in the prehospital setting, every EMS organization must ensure the safety and security of the medications within its control. Medications must be properly ordered, inventoried, stored, and dispensed when needed. A central storage location at the organization that is kept secure with double locking systems is often the best method for ensuring this protection.

Special care must be taken to ensure the security of narcotic agents because of the potential for theft and misuse. Narcotics should be signed in and signed out at each shift, with clear documentation of the narcotics' transfer of custody from one EMS crew to the next. Appropriate logbooks should be maintained at all times so that, in the event of lost or missing narcotics, determining who had the responsibility for protecting the drug at that time is possible (**FIGURE 2-3**). All transfers of narcotics from one crew to the next should be witnessed so that at no time does only one person have access to the narcotic agents.

Drug Currency

All medications have a varying **shelf life**, the period of time a medication can be stored and remain suitable for use. The length of a medication's shelf life depends on many factors, such as the chemical composition of the drug, its stability or volatility, and its expected period of effectiveness. Shelf life varies significantly across the spectrum of drugs used in the prehospital setting, so expiration dates must be constantly checked and rechecked. Outdated medications have no place in the prehospital setting; they will likely not have the intended beneficial effects for patients. In addition, courts look poorly on organizations and health professionals who use outdated drugs. If the use of an outdated medication can be proven in court, the plaintiff has an easier time proving a case of negligence against the EMS agency or the individual care provider.

NARCOTIC LOG

Date	Patient Name	Drug Given	Amount of Drug Given	Name of Person Administering Drug	Signature of Authorizing Physician
3/16/19	S. Thomas	midazolam	1.0 mg	J. Roberts, EMT-P	MLK

FIGURE 2-3 Example of a logbook. A medication, or narcotic, log is a record of controlled substances administered in the prehospital setting. The log allows the tracking of narcotic inventory and usage.

The potential for using outdated drugs exists when the drugs are infrequently used. For this reason, daily checklists must be used to ensure that no medication carried by the EMS unit is outdated or damaged. All outdated medications should be properly disposed of according to the organization's policies. Medications also should be disposed of when they appear to have been damaged, if the seals on the packaging are broken, or if the medication may have been exposed to environmental conditions that contradict the manufacturer's instructions for storage.

Environmental Issues

Prehospital ALS is provided in all types of weather and in a wide range of environmental conditions. In addition, the nature of emergency response necessitates that medications are portable and ready to go in a given moment. The U.S. Food and Drug Administration has strict requirements on the environmental parameters within which a medication is effective, and storage temperature ranges are established for virtually all medications.

Administering a medication that has been rendered ineffective because of exposure to excessive heat or cold does not benefit the patient and is a risk factor for liability. This is a common area in which liability is assessed against the ALS system in negligence cases. Strict adherence to medication storage and use requirements is absolutely essential.

Where should medications be stored to ensure that they are maintained in the proper environmental conditions according to the manufacturer? Medications often are stored in sealed drug boxes in the ambulance or response vehicle. If the vehicle is parked outside rather than in an environmentally controlled garage, the vehicle itself must be appropriately connected to systems that maintain an appropriate temperature. If drugs are exposed to excessive heat or cold while in use, as in the case of a mountain rescue or other extended-time situation, they should be properly discarded and replaced on return.

▶ Exposure to Bloodborne Pathogens

Safety of self, crew members, and other responders is always a top priority. Medication administration must be conducted in a manner that is as risk free as possible. The Occupational Safety and Health Act provides clear guidelines for EMS personnel in dealing with the potential exposure to bloodborne pathogens, which can occur when administering medications by the IV route or being exposed to bodily fluids. The threat of HIV, hepatitis, and other diseases spread through the blood warrants strict adherence to all safety requirements and procedures.

Recently, the federal Occupational Health and Safety Administration has intensified its interest in the safety of healthcare providers and EMS providers in particular. Recent regulatory changes require all EMS agencies to review their sharps devices and obtain the best possible devices to minimize the risk of exposure. The regulations require that EMS agencies involve their personnel in the selection of safe devices.

The federal Ryan White Law provides safeguards for EMS personnel in the event of a needlestick. The law establishes a mechanism of reporting so that, if a patient tests positive for HIV, EMS personnel are advised through the medical director of the necessary precautions and other steps that should be taken.

▶ Consent Issues and Limitations

The U.S. Supreme Court has upheld the right of every patient to self-determination regarding medical care and the application of lifesaving or life-sustaining measures. Every person has the right to determine whether to accept or reject any type of medical care or treatment (including any form of "laying on of hands" by healthcare providers) as long as he or she is capable of making that decision as a competent adult.

This principle of self-determination applies in the prehospital environment just as it does within a hospital. However, the likelihood of a patient not being competent to make decisions is higher in the prehospital setting because of a variety of factors, such as shock, substance abuse, and decreased level of consciousness. Prehospital professionals need to ensure that their patients give **consent** for every assessment and treatment provided. All competent adults have the right to consent to or refuse care and treatment, even in emergency situations. This includes the right to refuse parts of the care and treatment.

Patients are often leery of medication administration in the field, particularly older patients who are accustomed to traditional health care only and may consider an ambulance as merely a transportation system. Some patients will consent to an assessment and noninvasive treatment but will refuse invasive therapies such as parenteral medications. The patient may simply dislike needles or be opposed to the administration of specific medications. Remember, prehospital professionals have an obligation to inform the patient about what medication is being administered, as well as the reason for administration.

What should paramedics do when a patient refuses to consent to administration of a medication? First, ensure the patient is competent to make that refusal. Any refusal of consent to care must be carefully documented. Failure to properly assess the patient's ability to give consent and improper documentation of a refusal of consent are significant liability risks that open the door to claims of abandonment or negligence.

Refusals can be complete or partial. A **complete refusal** occurs in situations in which the patient refuses all aspects of treatment. This probably is the most common type of refusal situation. A **partial refusal** occurs when a patient agrees to some, but not all, of the treatment offered. If a patient refuses a portion of treatment, such as the administration of a specific medication, the paramedic can still provide other treatment that the patient does consent to receive. In these situations, the paramedic should obtain written documentation of the refusal, even if it is just a partial refusal, when possible.

A³E³P³ Refusal Guidelines

Consent and the refusal of consent must be properly handled to minimize liability. One set of guidelines, termed the **A³E³P³** ("A three, E three, P three") **refusal guidelines**, helps EMS providers remember the key considerations when faced with refusal situations. A³E³P³ stands for *a*ssess, *a*dvise, *a*void; *e*nsure, *e*xplain, *e*xploit; *p*ersist, *p*rotocols, *p*rotect.

Assess

Assess the patient's legal and mental capacity to refuse care. The patient must be a legally recognized adult (older than age 18 years) or deemed by law to be considered an adult (as with an emancipated minor or other special circumstances). However, proof that the patient is emancipated is difficult to obtain because no common form of identification exists that indicates this status. Some states, such as California, place this notation on the person's driver's license if the Division of Motor Vehicles is provided with court documentation that the minor is emancipated. Therefore, always err on the side of treatment whenever doubtful of whether the patient can legally refuse treatment.

Only competent adults can consent to care or refuse care. Minors are permitted by most state laws to consent to medical treatment, but they may not refuse treatment. In other words, allowing a minor to refuse care in a case in which it is clearly needed would pose significant risk of a claim for patient abandonment; minors usually are not considered legally competent to refuse treatment. However, state laws may permit minors to consent or refuse in certain situations. It is possible for minors to be allowed to consent for reproductive/pregnancy services such as birth control or treatment of a sexually transmitted disease, but not for other types of medical treatment. Minors living apart from their parents, and minors with minor children themselves, may have additional rights pertaining to consent and refusal in certain states. When doubt or confusion exists, it is often helpful to consult with online medical control (discussed further in Chapter 3), particularly in unusual situations.

Does the patient have a mental condition that might prevent him or her from making an informed decision? Examples include permanent conditions such as Alzheimer disease and situational conditions such as shock, alcohol or drug intoxication, and decreased level of consciousness from a head injury or other trauma.

Advise

Advise the patient of his or her medical condition and the proposed treatment. Although prehospital care providers do not make diagnoses, they are required to tell a patient what is going on regarding his or her medical condition and how the care provider proposes to help so that the refusal decision is informed. Do not be afraid to tell the patient the truth about what is happening.

Avoid

Avoid the use of confusing terminology when talking to patients; speak to them in terms they can understand. For example, rather than say, "You appear to be having a myocardial infarction with premature ventricular contractions that could cause you to go into ventricular fibrillation at any moment," explain to the patient, "You are probably having a heart attack, and you have very irregular heartbeats that could cause your heart to stop beating at any time. That is why we need to put this medication into your vein—to calm down those irregular beats."

Ensure

Ensure that the patient's decision to refuse care is the result of his or her own informed decision making and not the result of improper influence or coercion by others. Make sure the patient is not merely parroting what a family member is telling him or her to say.

Explain

Explain the alternatives to the patient if he or she refuses care and transport. Make sure the patient knows all the options, such as calling 9-1-1 again, calling his or her physician, and going to the ED if the symptoms continue or worsen.

Exploit

Exploit uncertainty. Many patients are unsure about whether they should go to the hospital, and that uncertainty should be used to the care provider's advantage in advising the patient to obtain the necessary care. For example, when a patient expresses uncertainty, he or she typically expresses it with the idea that the healthcare professional will help make the necessary decision. For example, a patient may say, "I'm not sure I need to go to the hospital." The care provider could reply, "Well, if I were you, I would certainly go to the hospital, where a doctor could check me out and where all the necessary equipment is there if it's needed." The care provider can use a variety of creative positive statements to encourage the patient to allow further care. This situation requires good communications skills.

Persist

Persist in trying to persuade the patient to obtain the necessary care. The prehospital professional may need to make several attempts to convince a patient that he or she should consent to EMS treatment and transport to the hospital. A well-documented refusal helps demonstrate this persistence in the event of a lawsuit.

Protocols

Protocols are meant to be followed. If your service or EMS system has protocols in place regarding patient refusals, be sure to adhere to them. This is especially important regarding medication administration because of the many risks associated with deviating from the traditional treatments.

Protect

Protect yourself with adequate documentation of the refusal (**FIGURE 2-4**). Write a thorough narrative explaining all the steps in the process, obtain the patient's signature to verify his or her understanding of the decision when possible, and try to get the names and addresses of witnesses who observed the refusal process. Describe the specifics of any partial refusal of care.

Living Wills and Advance Directives

All states have living will statutes that allow people to designate in advance the level of medical intervention they want to receive in the event of a terminal illness. These legal documents

Refusal of Services

I hereby refuse the emergency medical services and/or transportation offered and advised by the above-named service provider and its emergency personnel, _____ hospital, and the emergency medical and nursing personnel from said hospital giving directions to the service provider. I understand that my refusal may jeopardize the health of the patient, and hereby release the above-named parties from any and all claims of liability in connection with my refusal.

_____
Signature of patient or legally authorized representative

_____
Signature of EMT/field RN

_____
Witness

FIGURE 2-4 A release from liability form.

provide **advance directives**, or specific orders to the caregiver, regarding what level of treatment the patient wants to receive in such a situation. Many advance directives provide limitations on treatment in the event of a cardiac arrest or coma. These directives typically allow the healthcare provider to treat the patient with palliative or comfort measures and restrict the use of resuscitative measures such as cardiopulmonary resuscitation, endotracheal **intubation**, and medication administration.

Most state laws have strict verification requirements to ensure that the directive being followed is proper. Some states require that patients wear identification tags (similar to medic alert tags that are used to identify patients with allergies or medical conditions), whereas others require a document signed by the patient's attending physician. In some states, these orders are found in a red envelope on the kitchen refrigerator. Some states require that online medical direction be consulted before an advance directive can be recognized. Even if the patient has an advance directive in place, however, he or she can overrule it at any time. A competent patient has the right to void the directive by changing his or her mind during the course of treatment.

Restrictions on medication administration should be clearly delineated in the directive. For example, the directive could state that "no advanced cardiac life support medications" are to be administered. Or the directive could be specific to certain medications, such as stating that epinephrine and atropine should be withheld. In many situations involving terminally ill patients with cancer, morphine sulfate and other pain medications are specifically permitted to be given via the IV route, but all other medications are to be withheld. Check state laws and local protocols for the correct procedures to follow when confronted with an advance directive.

The vast majority of states have some form of **Medical Order for Life-Sustaining Treatment (MOLST)** or Physician Order for Life-Sustaining Treatment (POLST) form. These forms are designed to convert patient wishes into actionable medical orders that are then followed by various medical professionals, including EMS providers, as patients move throughout the healthcare system. Patients collaborate with their medical provider(s) to outline particular interventions that the patient does or does not want to receive during a medical crisis. These forms are particularly useful when patients have a serious medical condition but do not wish to receive interventions that are part of the normal standard of care for this condition.

▶ Documentation

Clear and accurate documentation is required for quality patient care and is a necessity in a litigious society. The patient care record (PCR) is closely scrutinized in malpractice and negligence trials, so ensure that documentation is thorough and specific. If you are called to the witness stand, you will be cross-examined by the plaintiff's counsel about the quality of your documentation. If your documentation of patient care is sloppy or incomplete, this fact will reflect negatively on your credibility as a competent caregiver, even if your documentation contains no gross errors.

The following are some important dos and don'ts to consider when documenting medication administration:[13]

Dos

- Ensure that the documentation of medication administration is an accurate reflection of your prehospital capabilities and your scope of practice.
- Write legibly and in complete sentences with proper abbreviations so that all personnel can adequately read your report.
- Document the time, medication given, dose, method, and route of administration in the treatment section of the PCR.

- Document a medication refusal by the patient and state why the patient refused the medication. Document every attempt you make to persuade the patient, and ask for the patient's signature.
- Document why you gave the patient a particular medication.
- Document known medication allergies and any untoward reactions to medication you administer, as well as the treatment you provided in response.
- Document vital signs before and after administration of all medications.
- Document any changes in vital signs, especially if the patient's condition worsens.
- Document the name of the physician or medical director who gave the medication order and the time of the order.

Don'ts

- Scribble or write illegibly.
- Misspell words or medication names.
- Forget to check the patient's response to the medication.
- Make up abbreviations or use inappropriate acronyms in documentation. Use only approved standard abbreviations.
- Assume that other crew members will take care of your documentation. If you gave the medication, you are responsible for documenting that fact.
- Prepare your report late if you can avoid it. Document any late entries or errors if changes or entries are made after the original report is completed and submitted.

Always prepare your documentation as though it will be presented in a court of law. Ask yourself, "Is my documentation for this patient the best it can be and how I would want my own care documented?" Strive to answer yes to this question in every situation; if you can, your reports will accurately document the care you provide, hold up in court, validate your credibility, and positively reflect your care.

▶ Scope of Practice Issues

Critical patient care situations in the field can be stressful, especially for novice prehospital providers or the sole EMT-Intermediate or paramedic available to provide ALS treatment. Many ALS systems have worked hard to encourage basic life support (BLS) personnel participation in the ALS care of patients through "paramedic assist" courses and other programs. EMTs and first responders are quite willing to assist paramedics with specific ALS procedures.

However, EMT-Intermediates and paramedics should proceed extremely cautiously when involving BLS personnel in ALS procedures. Even when a paramedic does not have enough hands to do everything at once, assigning to BLS personnel a procedure that can be performed legally only by an advanced-level caregiver is risky. At all times, BLS and ALS personnel must function within the limitations of their respective scopes of practice, which is defined by each state's EMS act.

A good example of how scope of practice can become a problem is with establishing an IV line. Should you allow an EMT or first responder to set up the IV bag and tubing, as well as flush the line of any air? No. Allowing this level of assistance (unless BLS personnel are permitted to establish IV lines under state law) is a risk that should not be taken. Unless the EMS provider is certified to provide that level of care, allowing BLS personnel to perform any part of a procedure that requires advanced training is improper. Although properly identifying the IV solution, maintaining a sterile field when removing protective covers, hooking up the IV tubing, and flushing the line may seem like simple tasks, they do involve a level of advanced training that only EMT-Intermediates and paramedics typically receive. A paramedic who permits a basic-level EMS provider to perform an advanced skill could be considered negligent for improperly delegating the skill. In addition, the basic-level EMS provider can be in violation of his or her state's EMS act by performing a skill outside the scope of practice for the person's level of certification.

What can the basic-level provider do to assist in this situation? In a nutshell, everything short of providing a skill considered restricted to a more advanced care provider. With the example of starting an IV line, this could include getting the solutions and IV start supplies, removing them from their packages (but not exposing sterile surfaces), tearing tape, and preparing other material to be used to secure the IV site and tubing.

When administering any medication, EMT-Intermediates and paramedics must *personally* complete all the steps necessary to administer the medication properly. The following steps should be taken each time a medication is administered:

1. Ask the patient about any known allergies to medications, and check for a MedicAlert bracelet or tag.
2. Determine the patient's medical history and current medications to avoid drug interactions.
3. Verify that you have the correct medication in the correct concentration. Although recent packaging procedures have significantly lowered this risk, one of the common medication errors in the field is administering the right medication in the *wrong* concentration (e.g., administering the concentrated form of the medication intended for an IV drip infusion as a direct IV bolus, or vice versa).

> A commonsense rule to avoid mistakes is to check the label on the medication at least four times: when selecting the medication, when preparing to draw it up, after drawing it up, and finally, while administering it.

4. Verify and repeat any order received to administer a medication. The technical quality of radio and telephone communications in the field can be unreliable.
5. Examine the packaging of the medication for discoloration and any other unusual characteristics.
6. Examine the packaging of the medication and the vial or ampule itself for the expiration date.
7. Open the medication and prepare it for administration, following proper procedures for ensuring sterility.
8. Administer the medication according to the proper procedure or protocol for the particular drug.
9. Observe the patient for any untoward reactions and any improvement or other change in condition. Report any changes to medical direction or hospital staff on arrival.

A common question that arises regarding scope of practice is whether an EMT or first responder should document on the BLS PCR interventions or assessments performed by the paramedic. This may be an issue in which EMS is provided in tiered systems; that is, when BLS and ALS are provided by separate organizations (e.g., BLS responds in a transporting ambulance and ALS responds in a nontransporting paramedic intercept or fly car unit). In some systems, the practice may be to document that the ALS provider applied a cardiac monitor and what electrocardiographic rhythm was displayed on the monitor. Some EMTs also document that the paramedic started an IV, how many attempts were necessary to establish the line, what medications and solutions were administered through the IV, and other information about the ALS care provided.

As a general rule, EMS providers should document according to their scope of practice and should not attempt to document skills beyond what they are trained and certified to perform themselves. Too great a risk for inconsistent and inaccurate records is posed when a provider documents beyond his or her scope of practice. In addition, such documentation could impair the credibility of the EMS provider if he or she becomes a witness in a lawsuit. If an EMT documents a particular cardiac rhythm, for example, that provider is vulnerable to a damaging cross-examination about his or her training and qualifications, or lack thereof, to make such determinations and why he or she would document care beyond the scope of practice. An EMT who is not able to answer questions in a deposition or on the witness stand about all the documentation, including the EMT-documented ALS care, could find his or her quality of treatment and credibility called into question.

This is not to suggest that EMTs should not document any facts regarding the ALS treatment. For example, the EMT should certainly document the fact that the paramedic provided patient care in addition to the EMT's role in the care. If the paramedic intubated the patient, and the EMT handled the bag-mask ventilation, the BLS patient care report should reflect that. Other general observations on a BLS patient care report, such as "paramedic performed a patient assessment," "paramedic intubated the patient," "paramedic applied a cardiac monitor," and "IV medications administered by the paramedic," are also appropriate, as long as the EMT refrains from describing details such as the intubation technique used, tube size used, particular cardiac rhythm displayed on the monitor, and the names and dosages of specific medications administered by ALS.

In many areas, the provision of EMS is a team effort between BLS and ALS providers, with both groups performing specific responsibilities and playing valuable roles in patient care. Just as EMS providers must render all patient care within their respective scope of practice, their documentation should likewise be limited to their scope of practice.

▶ Misdirection of Medications

A less common liability issue with respect to medication administration in EMS is "misdirection," or theft, of controlled substances. Federal and state laws place strict requirements on the purchase, storage, and use of medications, particularly controlled substances. Serious criminal penalties exist for the misappropriation of certain types of medications, such as narcotic agents, and healthcare providers who misuse medications entrusted to them are judged harshly.

The medication supply system should be closely monitored, with clearly defined purchase and security procedures in place. Common criminal activity includes stealing a medication from the storage device and replacing it with water or another substance (known as tampering). As a result of this crime, providers appear to be actually administering the medication, when in fact the patient is getting nothing more than a placebo. Ethically, this is a particularly heinous crime because the replacement can go undetected for quite some time, and vast numbers of patients can be harmed by not receiving medication. Medication *diversion* may occur at the time of administration or wasting, where the provider misdirects a portion or all of the medication away from its intended destination.[14] This method of medication theft can also be extremely difficult to prevent or identify.

Unfortunately, because the EMS environment is a less-controlled environment than the traditional hospital setting, weaknesses often exist in the medication supply system that require close attention and monitoring. At a minimum, no person should have sole access to the medication supply system. Appropriate checks and balances should be in place. The medication supply and control system should be periodically audited by people who are not directly associated with it.

▶ Incident Reporting

Every medication error must be properly documented and reported. This is essential for patient care and quality assurance to prevent the error from happening again. The ALS provider who makes a medication error and fails to properly document and report it is in violation of the law, as well as general principles of ethics.

Making these reports is a professional duty even when you know that you could be subjected to disciplinary action or other negative consequences. The failure to report errors demonstrates a lack of professionalism and can jeopardize a patient's life. Being a professional requires a high degree of self-regulation, and the prehospital care provider must adhere to all rules of conduct, particularly when a mistake is made.

National formats for reporting medication errors are available for other healthcare professions, but no national standard has been developed in EMS. Every EMS system should have its own standardized system for documenting medication errors. The system medical director should be involved in the review of any medication errors.

EMS agencies should have a policy on "unusual occurrence reporting," which defines what occurrences should be reported and the procedures for reporting them. Medication errors, such as errors in drug choice, dosage, or route of administration, are high on the list of reportable occurrences.

Incident reports should be completed promptly while the care provider's memory is fresh, providing the essential details of the incident. Once the incident report is completed, it should be submitted to the immediate supervisor. Attaching the incident report to the PCR is not advised, because anything attached to the PCR can become part of the medical record. Of course, the PCR should clearly indicate any known errors that occurred in patient care and the steps that were taken to remedy the error. However, the details of how the error occurred are best left for the separate incident report.

The incident should then be promptly investigated by appropriate management personnel and the system's medical director. Appropriate corrective action should be taken when a medication error has occurred. Corrective action can include additional continuing education for the person and sometimes disciplinary action. Most state EMS laws may also have requirements that certain medication errors be reported to the EMS office, and a standard incident report format may be in place at that agency.

In many cases of medication errors, problems in the system may have contributed to the error. Every medication error should be reviewed from a quality assurance and risk management perspective to ensure that system problems are identified and corrected. Otherwise, the risk of a future error is not reduced, and another care provider in the system may be just as likely to make the same mistake. Systemwide education may ultimately be required after the error is closely reviewed. Although medication and other treatment errors are unfortunate occurrences, these errors provide an opportunity to review the system critically and make positive changes to improve overall prehospital patient care.

Risk reduction is the key to avoiding liability in medication administration. The two primary goals should always be to eliminate or reduce the risk of harm to the patient and eliminate or reduce the risk of a successful lawsuit against the EMS organization. Improving overall patient safety is the general theme that encompasses the actions taken to reduce errors. This theme must be applied to every aspect of medication administration.

In 2001, the EMS Division of the National Highway Traffic Safety Administration sponsored a roundtable to discuss EMS patient safety and error reduction strategies. The participants discussed the types of error reduction activities occurring in other sectors of medicine, considered how errors could be reduced, and identified which patient safety activities should be pursued. The participants recognized that EMS providers need greater insight into the human factors that affect patient safety and a better reporting system when errors occur.

Accepting responsibility for the human factors that can affect your ability to function error free is the key to a professional approach to avoiding medication errors in the field. By taking this responsibility seriously, you can reduce the risk of harm to your patients and minimize the risk of liability for your EMS organization.

▶ Review Questions

1. Define ordinary negligence.
2. What is the principal goal of Good Samaritan laws?
3. If a paramedic makes an honest mistake in a medication administration, is he or she negligent?

4. Define standing orders and protocols.
5. What are the medical uses for medications categorized as Schedule I?
6. Define shelf life and explain the importance of checking a drug's expiration date.
7. What is the Ryan White Law?
8. Who decides what medications will be used by a particular EMS system?
9. What should a prehospital provider do when a patient refuses a medication or treatment?
10. Define a partial and a complete refusal.
11. Generally speaking, can a minor refuse treatment in most states?
12. What treatment levels are acceptable under advance directives?
13. List the don'ts of documenting medication administration.
14. Should an incident report be attached to a PCR?

References

1. Institute of Medicine. *To Err Is Human: Building a Safer Health System.* Washington, DC: National Academies Press; 2000.
2. Makary MA, Daniel M. Medical error—the third leading cause of death in the U.S. *BMJ.* 2016 May 3;353:i2139. doi: https://doi.org/10.1136/bmj.i2139.
3. U.S. Food and Drug Administration. Strategies to Reduce Medication Errors: Working to Improve Medication Safety. https://permanent.access.gpo.gov/lps1609/www.fda.gov/fdac/features/2003/303_meds.html. Updated November 17, 2017. Accessed July 3, 2018.
4. Hubble MW, Paschal KR, Sanders TA. Medication calculation skills of practicing paramedics. *Prehosp Emerg Care.* 2000;4(3):253–260.
5. *Hoffman v. Brandywine Hospital,* 661 A.2d 397 (Pa. Super. 1995).
6. Emergency Medical Services Act, 35 PA Stat § 6931(j) (1989).
7. *Albright v. Abington Memorial Hospital,* 696 A.2d 1159 (Pa. 1997).
8. Scott LD, Arslanian-Engoren C, Engoren MC. Association of sleep and fatigue with decision regret among critical care nurses. *Am J Crit Care.* 2014;23(1):13–23.
9. Basner M, Dinges DF, Shea JA, et al. Sleep and alertness in medical interns and residents: An observational study on the role of extended shifts. *Sleep.* 2017;40(4). https://doi.org/10.1093/sleep/zsx027.
10. Hoyle JD Jr, Crowe RP, Bentley MA, Beltran G, Fales W. Pediatric prehospital medication dosing errors: A national survey of paramedics. *Prehosp Emerg Care.* 2017;21(2):185–191.
11. Moreira ME, Hernandez C, Stevens AD, et al. Color-coded prefilled medication syringes decrease time to delivery and dosing error in simulated emergency department pediatric resuscitations. *Annals Emerg Med.* 2015;66(2):97–106.e3. http://doi.org/10.1016/j.annemergmed.2014.12.035
12. Antevy P. Handtevy method helps providers rapidly calculate pediatric drug dosages. *J Emerg Med Serv.* https://www.jems.com/articles/print/volume-38/issue-8/features/handtevy-method-helps-providers-rapidly.html. Published August 20, 2013. Accessed September 17, 2018.
13. Bruce ML, Sones SS, Peck B. Medication safety. Implications for EMS. *Emerg Med Serv.* 2003;32:97.
14. Gleason W, Richmond N. Best practices for controlled substance monitoring. *J Emerg Med Serv.* https://www.jems.com/articles/print/volume-42/issue-11/features/best-practices-for-controlled-substance-monitoring.html. Published November 2, 2017. Accessed September 17, 2018.

CHAPTER 3

Drug Administration: Safety and Procedures

OBJECTIVES

1. Define *standing orders, one-time orders,* and *as-needed (prn) orders.*
2. Discuss the nine patient rights of drug administration.
3. Explain the routes of enteral medications (oral, rectal, sublingual, and buccal), and demonstrate the proper procedure for each.
4. Explain the routes of parenteral medications (intravenous, intramuscular, subcutaneous, intraosseous, transdermal/topical, intranasal, inhalation, endotracheal tube), and demonstrate the proper procedure for each.

▶ Introduction

Administration of medication in the prehospital field can significantly improve patient outcome. To make the best use of this important patient care tool, prehospital professionals must be cognizant of rules regarding medication orders and guidelines regarding patient and provider safety. This chapter gives step-by-step instructions for safe and accurate medication administration by a variety of routes. Chapter 5 provides instructions for the administration of intravenous (IV) drugs and intraosseous (IO) infusions.

CASE STUDY

You are dispatched to a medical call for an unresponsive person at a local shopping mall. Just before arriving on the scene, the dispatcher informs you that mall security has used an automated external defibrillator on the patient. At the scene, you find an approximately 70-year-old man who is unresponsive. You immediately reach for your defibrillator pads while your partner moves to the patient's head and begins bag-mask ventilation. The screen on the cardiac monitor displays ventricular tachycardia. You immediately defibrillate the patient, and he converts to a sinus rhythm. To prevent him from returning to ventricular tachycardia, you administer a bolus of amiodarone 150 mg IV over 10 minutes.

▶ Medication Orders

A paramedic requires an order from a medical direction physician to administer a medication. **Medical direction** is the process by which physicians direct and monitor the care given in the prehospital environment within an EMS system. Medical direction can be provided either online or offline. **Online medical direction**, sometimes referred to as online medical control, occurs when the prehospital provider is able to consult and obtain direction and orders in real time by radio or telephone communication (**FIGURE 3-1**). **Offline medical direction** occurs when the physician medical director is not available for real-time interactions. The majority of medical direction cases are offline. The medical director approves a series of protocols detailing the care that the prehospital professional is to provide in a given clinical scenario.

Orders can take several forms: standing orders, one-time orders, and as-needed orders. All medication orders follow a standard form and include the following four elements:

1. Name of drug
2. Dose: a quantity followed by a unit of measure (e.g., 5 mg)
3. Route: oral, rectal, sublingual, buccal, endotracheal (ET), intramuscular (IM), subcutaneous, transdermal/topical, inhalation, intranasal, IV, or IO
4. Frequency: a one-time order, as needed, or for a duration of time

Standing Orders

Standing orders are instructions for treatment that are usually specific to a particular patient presentation and may or may not require consultation with medical direction. Standing orders are most appropriate for life-threatening conditions that require immediate intervention. In such circumstances, medication standing orders are part of a larger treatment protocol, or a series of interventions and drugs used to treat an emergency condition. For example, EMS systems typically have standing orders for the treatment of life-threatening cardiac arrhythmias, which often are a component of the advanced cardiac life support (ACLS) treatment guidelines. Standing orders also exist for a variety of other conditions, such as generalized tonic-clonic seizures, asthma, and anaphylaxis. In the preceding scenario, the paramedic was not required to confer with medical direction

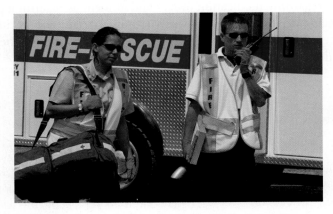

FIGURE 3-1 A paramedic online with medical direction.
© Jones & Bartlett Learning. Courtesy of MIEMSS.

before administering an ACLS drug, because most EMS systems have standing orders for such medications.

One-Time Orders

One-time orders occur when a paramedic has consulted medical direction and has received an order for immediate drug intervention for the treatment. In the preceding scenario, the paramedic was given a one-time order to administer morphine to the injured patient. This is in contrast to a standing order, in which the local protocol prescribes use of a drug without consulting medical direction. With a one-time order, the paramedic cannot repeat the order without again consulting medical direction.

As-Needed Orders

As-needed orders are often referred to as **prn orders** (*prn* is an abbreviation for the Latin phrase *pro re nata,* which means "as the situation demands"). As-needed orders are typically given for a specific patient condition or physiologic parameter. They are commonly given for pain and abnormalities in blood pressure, heart rate, and blood sugar. As-needed orders can be obtained from medical direction to treat a condition if it develops. For example, a paramedic crew is transporting a patient with an open fracture, and the patient is in extreme pain after the initial 50 mcg of IV fentanyl. The paramedic contacts medical direction to obtain an order for morphine. Medical direction orders fentanyl 100 mcg by IV line and gives an additional order of fentanyl 50 mcg by IV line as needed for pain. The second part of that order is an example of an as-needed order.

Communication with Medical Direction

When orders are received from medical direction, communication must be concise and clear. When an order is given, the paramedic should write it down and then read the order back to medical direction. The physician serving as medical direction should then confirm that the order the paramedic read back is either correct or incorrect. If medical direction does not confirm the order, the paramedic should request confirmation before proceeding.

CASE STUDY

You are transporting a 54-year-old man who threw gasoline on a fire while burning brush. The fire flashed on the patient, and he sustained burns on approximately 25% of his total body surface area. You have started an IV line and began to transport the patient. He is screaming in pain and reports the severity of pain as 10 on a scale of 0 to 10. You get on the radio to medical direction. After reporting your assessment and treatment, you request an order for morphine to treat the patient's pain.

Communication Example
Medical direction: "Go ahead and give the patient morphine 4 mg IV."
Paramedic: "Copy. Read back: morphine 4 mg IV push times one. Check?"
Medical direction: (no response)
Paramedic: "Morphine 4 mg IV push times one. Please confirm."
Medical direction: "That's correct."
Paramedic: "Copy."

When taking verbal orders, always read the order back and await acknowledgment that your order read back was correct. This method reduces communication errors regarding medication orders and improves patient safety.

Other Types of Medication Orders

EMS providers will encounter patients in homes, community treatment centers, long-term care facilities, and other healthcare settings during responses to 9-1-1 calls or when performing interfacility patient transports. Patients in these various settings will often be receiving medications or have prescriptions with many different types of administration schedules. These medications may be administered at a set time or frequency each day, associated with a particular activity or event, or may occur at intervals of multiple days, weeks, or months, depending on the medication or clinical situation. EMS providers may also encounter patients in home or community settings who are receiving long-term intermittent or continuous IV medication infusions. Healthcare settings typically document patient medication orders, schedules, and time of administration in a paper or electronic document known as the **medication administration record (MAR)**. Healthcare providers in these settings will often use the abbreviations listed in **TABLE 3-1** when discussing medication administration schedules and sites.

TABLE 3-1 Medication Administration Abbreviations

Abbreviation	Latin Origin	Meaning	Example
ac	*ante cibum*	before meals	Certain fluoroquinolone antibiotics that are taken 1 hour ac to maximize absorption in the stomach
al, as	*aurio laeva, aurio sinister*	left ear	Eardrops for an ear infection only administered into the affected ear
am	*ante meridiem*	morning, or every morning	Diuretic medications taken once a day in the morning to decrease the need to void/urinate during the nighttime
ATC		around the clock	Topical or transdermal patch left in place to maintain a steady medication state

Abbreviation	Latin Origin	Meaning	Example
au	*auris utrae*	both ears	Eardrops placed in both ears for bilateral ear infections
bid	*bis in die*	twice daily	Antibiotics administered twice a day
h, hr	*hora*	hour	IV pain medication given every hour
hs	*hora somni* (hour of sleep)	at bedtime	"Sleeping pill" taken before bed to help a patient sleep
noct	*nocte*	at night	Sequential compression devices or continuous positive airway pressure machine used only at night
od	*oculus dexter*	right eye	Antibiotic eye ointment administered only into the affected eye
os	*oculus sinister*	left eye	Antibiotic eye ointment administered only into the affected eye
ou	*oculus uterque*	both eyes	Eyedrops for glaucoma administered into both eyes
p, per	*per*	by or through	Liquid medication given through a patient's nasogastric tube (PNGT)
pc	*post cibum*	after meals	Antibiotic taken 2 hours after meals to promote absorption
po	*per os*	oral	Blood pressure medication taken by mouth
pr	*per rectum*	administered into rectal cavity	Acetaminophen (Tylenol) suppository
prn	*pro re nata*	as needed	Narcotic pain medicine given as needed for severe pain
q1h, q2h, etc.	*quaque* (number) *hora*	every (specify number) hour(s)	Antibiotic medication taken every 6 hours (q6h)
qad	*quoque alternis die*	every other day	Anticoagulant medication taken every other day
qam	*quaque die ante meridiem*	every morning	Diuretic medication taken every morning
qd	*quaque die*	every day	Antidepressant medication taken every day
qh	*quaque hora*	every hour	Hourly measurement of blood glucose level for patients on an insulin infusion
qhs	*quaque hora somni*	every night at bedtime	Antihypertensive medication taken before bed every night
qid	*quarter in die*	four times a day	Analgesic medication taken every 6 hours
qod	*quaque altera die*	every other day	Oral iron supplements taken every other day
stat or STAT	*statim*	immediately	Aspirin given STAT for patients having myocardial ischemia
tid	*ter in die*	three times a day	Antibiotic medication administered every 8 hours

Sources: Every Patient's Advocate. Master list of prescription abbreviations. https://www.everypatientsadvocate.com/columns/prescriptionabbreviations.pdf. Accessed July 4, 2018; Marotta R. A technician's guide to pharmacy abbreviations. *Pharmacy Times.* http://www.pharmacytimes.com/technician-news/a-technicians-guide-to-pharmacy-abbreviations. Published November 25, 2015. Accessed July 4, 2018.

▶ Issues

Patient Safety

To ensure patient safety regarding medication administration, a checklist known as the **nine patient rights of drug administration** is used that contains the elements shown in **FIGURE 3-2**. Historically, this list contained either five or six rights of medication administration, but the list has grown to eight, nine, or ten different items, depending on the author or source as the evolution of patient safety practices in health care continues.[1-3]

Run through this checklist before administering any drug to reduce the likelihood of a medication error.

Right Patient

Is the person to whom you will administer the medication the person you think he or she is? This question is perhaps more relevant in a setting where one provider may be caring for several patients. You must ensure that the medication you will administer is meant for the correct patient. If administering or assisting with prescription medications, read the medication label and check whether the name on the medication bottle is the name of the patient you are treating.

Right Drug and Right Indication

There are two extremely important considerations when confirming whether you are administering the correct medication. The first regards the *name* of the medication you are preparing to administer. Before administering a drug, confirm that the drug in your hand is the drug you have been ordered to give. This order may come from treatment guidelines, a department/agency protocol, or communication with online medical control.

The second essential consideration is whether the medication order or protocol is appropriate for this particular clinical situation or patient condition. Ask yourself, "Why are we giving this medication?" If you do not know the answer, then you must pause to consider the overall clinical situation. In tense moments and uncontrolled environments, it is easy for protocols and treatment algorithms to overlap or blend together. Inexperienced providers frequently focus on memorizing protocols without having the depth of understanding to recognize the indications and implications of each proposed intervention. This is also the optimal

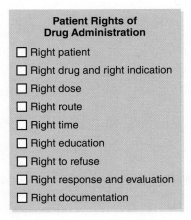

Patient Rights of Drug Administration

- ☐ Right patient
- ☐ Right drug and right indication
- ☐ Right dose
- ☐ Right route
- ☐ Right time
- ☐ Right education
- ☐ Right to refuse
- ☐ Right response and evaluation
- ☐ Right documentation

FIGURE 3-2 Nine patient rights of drug administration. Running through this checklist before drug administration will reduce the likelihood of a medication error and improve patient safety.

time to consider patient allergies or other contraindication(s). As an example, aspirin may be appropriate for a patient with acute coronary syndrome; however, if the patient has a known severe allergy or other contraindication, administering it would be extremely harmful to the patient, despite the normal anticipated benefits. As you consider administering a proposed medication, do a brief review of any significant contraindications that might be present in this particular patient or situation. Even something basic like supplemental oxygen may be contraindicated in certain patients.

Drugs used in ACLS and other emergency situations are commonly supplied in unassembled, preloaded syringes in color-coded boxes. However, several patient care providers often are at an emergency scene, and the person who pulls the medications from the medication drawer and removes them from their color-coded boxes may not be the same person who administers them. One provider can pass a rather generic-looking preloaded syringe to a second provider to administer the medication to the patient. Remember, this may all occur quickly in a tension-filled environment. Therefore, the person who actually administers the medication should never assume that the medication he or she has been handed is indeed the medication ordered. When a medication has been passed to you for administration, read the label on the syringe and confirm the order out loud with the team leader or medical direction.

When receiving a verbal order in person or on the radio, read back the order and wait for confirmation that the order heard is correct. A common source for potential error is mistakenly giving a medication that either looks similar or has a similar name to the medication meant to be administered. The process of stating the order out loud double-checks the name of the medication with those giving the order, as well as other providers in the vicinity. Many other industries, such as fast-food restaurants and drive-through automobile service centers, use this practice to minimize mistakes in noisy, fast-paced environments. In team resuscitation situations, this practice keeps everyone in the room informed about key activities and allows every provider the opportunity to recognize and stop potential errors before they occur.

The pharmaceutical industry has moved toward **tall man lettering** to minimize potential confusion between medications with similar-sounding names. Tall man lettering uses a combination of uppercase and lowercase letters, with the uppercase letters highlighting the key distinctions of a particular drug name. For example, dopamine and dobutamine are similar-sounding names for medications used to treat circulatory system dysfunction. Packaging and print materials often display these two medications with the text *DOBUTamine* and *DOPamine*. The Institute for Safe Medication Practices has compiled a larger list of medication pairs or groups with similar-sounding names that use tall man lettering.[4] Consider doing an extra double-check when administering medications that are known to be easily confused with other similar-sounding medications.

Right Dose

Ensure that the patient is getting the correct dose of the medication. Repeat the dose verbally before administration. If you are not directly administering the medication, listen to the dose being administered. If you question the dose, call for a "stop" or "timeout" to confirm the dosage. Patient safety is everyone's responsibility. Medication dosing often varies significantly based on administration route, with more than a 10-fold difference in medication groups such as beta-adrenergic blockers. A correct IV dose may be significantly incorrect if that same medication is given by the oral, IM, or intranasal route, or via ET tube. Many healthcare facilities perform formal two-person double-checks on high-risk medications. These checks include details such as the dose, concentration, rate, and route as an additional measure of safety, particularly for vulnerable patient groups such as pediatric or neonatal patients.

Right Route

Check the route of administration and whether the route is accessible. If the ordered route is oral, can the patient swallow the medication? Can the medication be crushed? Some oral medications formulated as a sustained-released medication cannot be crushed to assist in oral administration. Administering a sustained-release oral medication in a crushed form may result in overdose.

Right Time

For hospital providers, the *right time* typically refers to administering a medication at the right time of day. This usually is not a significant problem for the prehospital professional. However, the time can also refer to the time it takes to safely administer a bolus of an IV medication. When administering an IV medication as a bolus, questioning over what period the bolus should be given is in the interest of patient safety. In general, any medication ordered as slow IV push (SIVP) should be administered over at least 2 minutes, with the EMS provider actually using a watch or timer to administer it safely. If certain medications are administered too rapidly, serious adverse effects such as hypotension and bradycardia frequently occur. Beta-adrenergic blocking agents, many antiarrhythmic agents, promethazine (Phenergan), prochlorperazine (Compazine), and certain anticonvulsant medications are prone to these issues. Conversely, adenosine (Adenocard) is quickly metabolized in the bloodstream and should be given as rapidly as possible, using a coordinated effort for medication push and immediate flush through a large-bore proximal IV. Slow or uncoordinated administration of adenosine may decrease its efficacy.

Right Education

Inform the patient of the medication name and indication prior to administration whenever possible. This may not be possible in true emergency situations. Include any anticipated side effects or adverse effects of the medication as well as any unusual sensations the patient may experience during or following administration. This is also an excellent opportunity to reconfirm any patient allergies (or significant contraindications) immediately prior to administration. In this discussion, make sure to include the likely implications for the patient if he or she chooses to decline or refuse a particular medication or treatment option.

Right to Refuse

Patients, the parents or legal custodians of most minor patients, or the patient's designated healthcare decision maker may consent to or refuse medication administration. Failure to follow refusal from a patient with decision-making capacity can result in malpractice claims and either civil or criminal penalties for battery. Patient refusal may also be demonstrated in healthcare advance directives and POLST/MOLST forms (discussed in Chapter 2), particularly in the context of life-sustaining interventions or medications.

Right Response and Evaluation

Observe how the patient tolerated the medication. Did a change in the cardiac rhythm or vital signs occur? It is important to document follow-up vital signs after administering any medication that is known to alter heart rate, blood pressure, respirations, or oxygenation. Consider a medication's time of onset and duration of action when monitoring vital signs and overall patient condition. Did the medication improve the patient's condition, did it have no effect, or did it possibly make the situation worse? Did new signs or symptoms such as nausea, vomiting, rash, itching, or changes in mental status occur? Observe the IV site for signs of infiltration or occlusion, which may indicate potential harm to a patient after many prehospital IV medications such as dextrose, vasopressors, and certain antiemetics. Be sure to alert receiving facility personnel that the medication has been administered so appropriate patient monitoring will continue after patient handoff.

Right Documentation

Document the medication given, dose, time of administration, route, and any changes in the patient's condition. Follow the documentation instructions outlined in Chapter 2. Document any orders received from online medical direction, and indicate which EMS provider actually administered the medication.

CASE STUDY

You are back at the first scene of the unresponsive man at the shopping mall. The shift supervisor has arrived. As you are preparing to load the patient onto the cot, the patient develops a bradycardia that rapidly degenerates into asystole. The supervisor instructs you to administer epinephrine 1:10,000, 1 mg IV line, in accordance with your standing order per ACLS guidelines. Another paramedic at the scene pulls epinephrine from the drug box and hands you a preloaded glass syringe. You look at the syringe and read the contents, calling out, "Epinephrine 1:10,000, 1 mg IV push." The team leader responds, "Yes, that's correct," confirming that you have the correct drug in your hands. You administer the drug as intended.

All too often, the person running a code gives an order and is not sure that someone has heard the order or carried it out. Always acknowledge and verify medication orders.

Provider Safety

The first rule of providing emergency care in the field is to ensure your personal safety. A fundamental concept taught to all prehospital providers is scene safety. Paramedics are taught to position emergency vehicles in areas of high visibility and physically protect the scene. When responding to a shooting or stabbing call, standard practice is for an ALS unit to delay arrival on the scene until law enforcement has determined that the scene is safe, weapons are secured, and the assailant is not in the vicinity. The practice of wearing appropriate personal protective equipment (PPE) and following standard precautions is designed to reduce the likelihood that a provider will be infected by a pathogen when exposed to infectious blood, body fluids, or respiratory droplets. These efforts are meant to protect providers from the pathogens with no cure: human immunodeficiency virus (HIV), hepatitis B virus (HBV), and hepatitis C virus (HCV).

Standard precautions are designed with the assumption that all blood, body fluids, and patient materials are contaminated with HIV, HBV, or HCV. When observing standard precautions, a provider dons PPE, specialized clothing or equipment to protect the provider from contamination. Gloves are a standard component of PPE. Gloves will not prevent needlesticks, but they will act as a barrier between a contaminated body fluid and an open wound on the provider's hand. Masks are another element of PPE; they should be worn when a splash of the patient's body fluids may get into the eyes, nose, or mouth of the provider. When a provider wears a mask, the mucous membranes of the eyes must be protected with goggles (**FIGURE 3-3**). A mask is required when intubating a patient, dealing with a patient who is actively bleeding, or drawing blood. Goggles must have side shields to prevent blood from entering the eye from the side. If prescription glasses are used as eye protection, those glasses must have side shields, and a plan must be in place to decontaminate the glasses if they become contaminated.

The most obvious risk of blood contamination to a provider is being accidentally stuck by a needle, scalpel, or other sharp object. A provider should never attempt to recap or bend a needle. Immediately after using a needle or sharp, it should be placed in an approved puncture-resistant and leak-proof needle box (**FIGURE 3-4**). Never should the sharp be set on the ground, stuck into a mattress, or left loose on the ambulance bench.

The EMS community was alarmed by studies published in the 1990s suggesting poor rates of compliance with standard precautions among paramedics. Most paramedics complied with the use of gloves but properly handled sharps in only 37% of cases. The rate of appropriate use of additional protective devices such as goggles, masks, and gowns was unacceptable. Goggles were used in only 6% of the cases in which they were indicated, and gowns were never used when appropriate.[5] More recent studies have

FIGURE 3-3 A paramedic wearing appropriate mask and goggles.

© Jason Joelson/123RF.

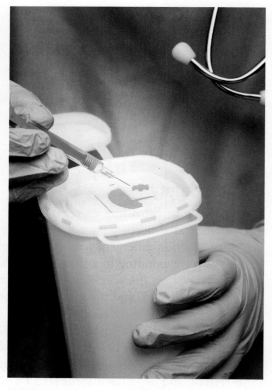

FIGURE 3-4 Sharps should be discarded in an appropriate container.

© Maica/E+/Getty Images.

FIGURE 3-5 PPE—including eyewear, mask, gown, and gloves—provides adequate body substance isolation.

http://medicsbk.com/2014/10/22/ebola-awareness-part-3-ems-response/

demonstrated that EMS providers in busy metropolitan areas still demonstrate significant gaps in compliance with standard precautions, despite having adequate training and knowledge related to exposure risks and PPE use.[6,7] **FIGURE 3-5** shows a provider wearing appropriate PPE.

▶ Enteral Drug Administration Procedures

Chapter 1 explains that medications can be given either enterally or parenterally. Enteral medications enter the bloodstream through the **gastrointestinal (GI)** tract. In the prehospital care environment, enteral medications are given orally, rectally, sublingually, and buccally.

Administration of Oral Medications

The majority of medications prescribed by physicians are taken orally in a solid form, such as a pill, tablet, or capsule, or in a liquid form. The oral route has several limitations when treating medical emergencies in the prehospital environment. Oral medications are not practical or safe to administer to patients with an altered or depressed level of consciousness. In addition, because oral medications require absorption in the GI tract, they often do not produce the rapid effects necessary for treatment of life-threatening emergencies.

Orders for oral medications are often described as "PO," which is an abbreviation for the Latin *per os*, meaning "by mouth."

Assisted medication administration occurs when a prehospital professional helps a patient take his or her own prescribed medication. Assisted medication administration should be performed after consultation with medical direction or based on agency or system protocols. Certain patient home medications, such as epoprostenol (Flolan), require continuous IV infusion. Sudden, unexpected discontinuation is an emergency situation. System or agency protocols may allow paramedics to restart this medication prior to contacting medical control. Albuterol and aspirin are other home medications that EMS providers may be allowed to assist a patient in administering based on protocol, rather than online medical control. Before helping a patient with his or her own medication, read the label. Verify that the medication you are helping the patient administer is indeed his or her own. Read the prescription bottle to ensure that the name on the bottle is the name of the patient, and confirm that the medication and dose are the medication and dose that you intend to administer. Also, be sure the medication has not expired. If a patient has stored multiple medications in the same bottle and you cannot confirm the identification of a medication, do not help the patient take it.

ORAL MEDICATION ADMINISTRATION

Equipment Needed:
Medication, medication cup, gloves, drinking water
Procedure:
1. Observe standard precautions.
2. Verify drug order.
3. Confirm right patient, right medication, right dose, right route, and right time.
4. Confirm with the patient that he or she has no allergies to the medication, and document allergies to any other medication.
5. If a pediatric seizure, make an attempt to educate caregiver of what you are doing.
6. When possible, explain to the patient what medication you are going to administer and why. Obtain informed consent from the patient if the patient is capable of providing consent; otherwise, obtain consent from the patient's healthcare decision maker if one is available.
7. Open the medication container and tap out the prescribed number of pills into a medication cup, the patient's hand, or your gloved hand.
8. *Do not crush solid medication.* Some pills and capsules are formulated as time-released medications. By crushing a tablet, the active ingredient can be absorbed into the bloodstream all at once rather than over a period of hours, which may result in an unintentional overdose. Before crushing any solid medication, consult a drug reference or medical direction.
9. Place the patient in the sitting position.
10. Ask the patient to swallow the medication with 4 to 5 ounces of water.
11. Record the time of drug administration in the patient care record.
12. Evaluate the patient for desired effects of the medication and for any adverse effects. Continued reevaluation should occur throughout transport.

Administration of Rectal Medications

Rectal medications are not frequently used in the prehospital setting, but some indications for their use may arise. **Rectal administration** is used most commonly in situations in which oral administration would be ideal but cannot be tolerated by the patient because of nausea or vomiting. In some emergency settings, the rectal route is optimal for rapidly delivering a medication to a patient who is not able to take an oral medication, such as the rectal administration of diazepam (Valium) or lorazepam (Ativan) for the treatment of pediatric seizures.

Medications formulated to be given as rectal suppositories often have a butter-like consistency. That is, the medication is a solid at room temperature, but once the suppository is placed in the rectum, the body temperature melts the medication into a liquid form, allowing more rapid absorption by the rectal mucosa.

RECTAL MEDICATION ADMINISTRATION

Equipment Needed:
Gloves, suppository or medication to be administered, lubricant (if time permits)
Procedure:
1. Observe standard precautions.
2. Verify drug order.
3. Confirm right patient, right medication, right dose, right route, and right time.
4. Confirm with the patient that he or she has no allergies to the medication, and document allergies to any other medication.
5. When possible, explain to the patient what medication you are going to administer and why. Obtain informed consent from the patient if the patient is capable of providing consent; otherwise, obtain consent from the patient's healthcare decision maker if one is available.
6. Help the patient disrobe. For legal protection, ask a person (not a family member) of the patient's sex to be present.
7. Ask the patient to lie on one side and draw his or her knees up toward the chest.
8. Remove the suppository from its wrapper and hold it at the rectum. Gently hold pressure at the anal sphincter for a few seconds while the patient takes a slow, deep breath and gently bears down. This maneuver will relax the anal sphincter muscles and help introduce the suppository.
9. Advance the suppository into the rectum approximately 1 inch.
10. Once the suppository has been placed, keep the patient on his or her side for approximately 20 minutes if possible.
11. Record the time of drug administration in the patient care record.
12. Evaluate the patient for desired effects of the medication and for any adverse effects. Continued reevaluation should occur throughout transport.

Details on how to administer rectal diazepam are provided in Chapter 15.

Administration of Sublingual Medications

Medications can be applied to mucous membranes, where the drug can be rapidly absorbed and transported by the bloodstream. For certain medications, this method of drug delivery is extremely fast and effective. For example, nitroglycerin is administered to the mucous membranes beneath the tongue, or sublingually, where a rich network of blood vessels facilitates rapid absorption and distribution.

ADMINISTRATION OF NITROGLYCERIN: SPRAY AND SUBLINGUAL

Equipment Needed:
Medication, PPE
Procedure:
1. Observe standard precautions.
2. Obtain baseline vital signs if not already done.
3. Verify drug order.
4. Confirm right patient, right medication, right dose, right route, and right time.
5. Confirm with the patient that he or she has no allergies to the medication, and document allergies to any other medication.
6. When possible, explain to the patient what medication you are going to administer and why. Obtain informed consent from the patient if the patient is capable of providing consent; otherwise, obtain consent from the patient's healthcare decision maker if one is available.
7. Instruct the patient to lift his or her tongue. Place one tablet under the tongue and ask the patient to close his or her mouth. Instruct the patient to not chew the tablet and to leave it under the tongue until it is completely dissolved.

8. If the patient uses nitroglycerin spray, spray once under the tongue or in the buccal membrane per protocol. Instruct the patient to close his or her mouth quickly.
9. Take the patient's blood pressure within 2 minutes of administration.
10. Record the time of drug administration in the patient care record.
11. Reassess and record vital signs.
12. Evaluate the patient for desired effects of the medication and for any adverse effects.

Administration of Buccal Medications

The **buccal area** is the mucous membrane on the inside of the check. Medication such as glucose gel for hypoglycemic patients can be administered here (termed *buccal administration*) by prehospital providers. However, this route of administration is safe only for conscious patients with an intact gag reflex.

ORAL GLUCOSE MEDICATION ADMINISTRATION

Equipment Needed:
Medication, gloves, tongue depressor or other appropriate applicator, PPE
Procedure:
1. Observe standard precautions.
2. Verify drug order.
3. Confirm right patient, right medication, right dose, right route, and right time.
4. Confirm with the patient that he or she has no allergies to the medication, and document allergies to any other medication.
5. When possible, explain to the patient what medication you are going to administer and why. Obtain informed consent from the patient if the patient is capable of providing consent; otherwise, obtain consent from the patient's healthcare decision maker if one is available.
6. Place the medication between the patient's gum and cheek near the location of the molar teeth (**FIGURE 3-6**).
7. Advise the patient not to drink any fluids while the medication is dissolving and being absorbed.
8. Record the time of drug administration in the patient care record.
9. Evaluate the patient for desired effects of the medication and for any adverse effects. Continued reevaluation should occur throughout transport.

FIGURE 3-6 Oral glucose administration. Medications, such as glucose gel, can be administered in the buccal area on the inside of the cheek. This method of administration is only safe in conscious patients with an intact gag reflex.

▶ Parenteral Drug Administration Procedures

The **parenteral route** is the most common route of drug administration used by paramedics. This type of route includes any route of drug administration other than absorption from the GI tract. Parenteral routes include an IV line, **IM injection**, intradermal injection, subcutaneous injection, **IO infusion**, **transdermal/topical administration**, **inhalation administration**, **intranasal**, and **ET tube** administration. Parenteral drug administration is a more effective route in the prehospital environment, because medications given via IV line produce blood levels that are reliable and are available almost immediately. The limitation of parenteral drug administration is the need to have special training and equipment for drug delivery. Chapter 5 explains IV and IO methods of administration.

Equipment

Syringes

A **syringe** is a medical instrument used for injecting fluid into or withdrawing fluid from the body. Syringes can be made of glass or plastic, but plastic syringes are used primarily in the prehospital setting. Syringes are used for a variety of purposes and come in a wide spectrum of sizes from 1 to 60 mL. They have three parts: the tip, barrel, and plunger.

The **tip** of the syringe attaches the needle. With **Luer-lock syringes**, the tip is threaded, allowing a needle to be screwed into the tip. The Luer lock allows the needle to be attached to the barrel with greater security. This type of syringe is required for use in needleless IV systems. With **non-Luer-lock syringes**, the needle fits tightly on the tip.

The **barrel** of the syringe contains the medication. Syringe barrels come in a variety of volumes. Volume markings are etched on the surface of most syringes, typically in milliliters. **Insulin syringes** are calibrated so that the user is able to draw up and measure the units of insulin.

The **plunger** is the inner portion of the syringe that pushes the liquid medication to the tip of the syringe and out the needle.

Needles

Needles (also called *sharps*) are a critical—and potentially dangerous—tool in drug administration. Needles have various parts and come in different sizes. A needle is composed of a hub, shaft, and bevel (**FIGURE 3-7**).

The **hub** typically is made of plastic and, in the case of a non-Luer-lock syringe, tightly fits over the tip of a syringe. When a Luer-lock syringe is used, the needle is attached to the syringe by screwing the hub into the Luer-lock.

The **shaft** of the needle is attached to the hub.

The **bevel** is the angled surface at the end of a needle. The longer the bevel on a needle, the easier the needle will pierce the skin.

Needles also have different gauges, which are determined by their diameter. The larger the needle diameter, the smaller the gauge (e.g., a 16-gauge needle is much larger than a 25-gauge needle).

FIGURE 3-7 Various parts of the needle.

Butterfly needles are small, short needles with plastic tabs that resemble the wings of a butterfly. Attached to the needle of a butterfly needle is a small piece of clear plastic tubing with an IV connector that can be attached to a syringe or IV tubing. Butterfly needles are used to withdraw blood or establish an IV line in children and adults with small or difficult-to-access veins. The needle is inserted into the vein while the wings of the butterfly are held. Access to the vein is confirmed by a small return of blood into the tubing.

Safety Features

IV catheters, needles, and butterfly needles may have other integrated safety devices. Different manufacturers have designed systems that can retract the needle into the housing, deploy a blunt tip, or use some other method to minimize the likelihood of a needlestick. Many needles now contain a plastic needle cover attached to the hub of the needle by a plastic syringe. These systems allow this cover to be swung over the needle. Once in place, this plastic cover cannot be removed. Certain IV catheters have tiny one-way valves that prevent backflow of blood as the needle is removed, minimizing EMS provider exposure to the patient's blood.

Needle safety guidelines include the following:

- Never resheath a needle.
- Never remove a plastic needle sheath with the teeth. Such maneuvers pose a serious risk of injury.
- Do not let needles lie around. No one ever means to get stuck with a contaminated needle. Typically, a needle is put down and someone either forgets about it or is not aware of it.
- Once a needle is used, it should immediately be safely secured, sheathed, and discarded in an appropriate sharps container.
- Ensure that sharps containers are changed before they are full. Injuries can occur when the sharps container is full and someone tries to add one more needle.
- Carefully consider risk versus benefit of starting an IV line or handling an exposed needle in a moving ambulance. With vehicle movement and unexpected stops or turns, it is very easily to injure yourself or others. If an IV start or injection is necessary while the vehicle is moving, alert the driver to avoid any sudden moves, turns, or stops if possible. Make sure that everybody is aware of what you are doing and the presence/location of any active sharps.
- Never stick a needle and syringe in the cushion of a cot or bench of an ambulance. Not only is doing so nonsterile, it is also abusive to the equipment.

Administration of Inhalation Medications: Nebulizers and Metered-Dose Inhalers

Many medications used in the treatment of respiratory emergencies are administered via the inhalation route. The most common inhaled medication is oxygen. Beta$_2$ agonist bronchodilators (e.g., albuterol [Ventolin, Proventil], isoetharine [Bronkosol], metaproterenol [Alupent]) are often administered in the prehospital setting for patients experiencing respiratory distress caused by certain obstructive airway diseases, such as asthma, bronchitis, and emphysema. Other medications, such as ipratropium bromide (Atrovent)—an anticholinergic bronchodilator—are also administered via the inhalation route. Check your drug reference guide or the package insert for the indications, contraindications, and precautions before giving any of these medications.

A patient with a history of respiratory problems will usually have a **metered-dose inhaler (MDI)** to use on a regular basis or as needed (**FIGURE 3-8**). MDIs are usually administered by

FIGURE 3-8 Some medications are inhaled into the lungs with an MDI so that they can be absorbed quickly into the bloodstream.
© Jones & Bartlett Learning.

A   **B**

FIGURE 3-9 A. In children, an MDI and spacer can be used with or without a mask. **B.** Children as young as 6 months can use a mask and spacer device.

© Jones & Bartlett Learning.

the patient using the patient's own prescribed medications, but paramedics must know how to administer via this route because they may assist the patient with administration. Medications administered by the MDI can be delivered through a mouthpiece held by the patient or by a mask—with or without a spacer device—for young children and patients who are unable to hold the mouthpiece (**FIGURE 3-9**).

MDI ADMINISTRATION

Equipment Needed:
Metered-dose inhaler, gloves, PPE
Procedure:
1. Take standard precautions.
2. Obtain an order from medical control or follow local protocol.
3. Assemble the needed equipment.
4. Ensure you have the right medication, right patient, right dose, right route, and that the medication is not expired.
5. Ensure the patient is alert enough to use the inhaler.
6. Check whether the patient has already taken any doses.
7. Obtain baseline breath sounds for comparison after a few minutes of inhaler use.
8. Ensure the inhaler is at room temperature or warmer.
9. Shake the inhaler vigorously several times.

10. Stop administering supplemental oxygen and remove any mask from the patient's face.
11. Ask the patient to exhale deeply and, before inhaling, to put his or her lips around the opening of the inhaler.
12. If the patient has a spacer, then attach it to allow more effective use of the medication.
13. Have the patient depress the handheld inhaler as he or she begins to inhale deeply.
14. Instruct the patient to hold his or her breath for as long as he or she comfortably can to help the lungs absorb the medication.
15. Resume administering supplemental oxygen if needed.
16. Allow the patient to breathe a few times, then give the second dose per direction from medical control or according to local protocol.
17. Monitor the patient's condition, and document the medication given, route, administration time, and response of the patient.[8]

Administration of Intranasal Medications

Intranasal (within the nose) medications include nasal spray for congestion or solutions to moisten the nasal mucosa. In recent years, this route of medication administration has become more popular in the prehospital setting. Intranasally administered medications are rapidly absorbed, providing a more rapid onset of action than IM injections. For example, some studies suggest that intranasal fentanyl has an equal onset and duration to IV morphine. Administration of emergency medications via the intranasal route is performed with a mucosal atomizer device (MAD). The MAD attaches to a syringe and allows you to spray (atomize) select medications into the nasal mucosa.

Owing to the molecular structure of drugs, only a few emergency medications can be given intranasally, including naloxone (Narcan), midazolam (Versed), glucagon (GlucaGen), ketorolac (Toradol), flumazenil (Romazicon), and fentanyl citrate. Typically, intranasal medications require 2 to 2.5 times the dose of IV medications. Follow local protocol, or consult with medical control about the appropriate doses of these medications and any other medications that may be administered intranasally.[8]

MAD ADMINISTRATION

Equipment Needed:
Medications, syringe, needle, atomizer device, gloves, PPE
Procedure:
1. Take standard precautions.
2. Determine the need for the medication based on patient presentation.
3. Obtain a history, including any drug allergies and vital signs.
4. Assemble the needed equipment, including the MAD.
5. Ensure you have the right medication, right patient, right dose, right route, and that the medication is not expired. To ensure it has not expired, check that it is not cloudy or discolored and that the expiration date has not passed.
6. Draw up the appropriate dose of medication in the syringe, dispel air, and reconfirm the medication.
7. Dispose of the needle properly.
8. Attach the MAD to the syringe, maintaining a sterile technique.
9. Explain the procedure to the patient (or to a relative if the patient is unresponsive) and the need for the medication.
10. Stop ventilation of the patient if necessary; remove any masks.[8]
11. Insert the MAD into the larger and less deviated or less obstructed nostril.
12. Quickly spray the medication dose into a nostril.
13. Dispose of the MAD and syringe in the appropriate container.
14. Monitor the patient's condition. Document the medication given, route, time of administration, and response of the patient.

Administration of Intramuscular Injections

IM injection is a method of administering medication directly into muscle tissue, where it is absorbed in the general circulation. Several muscles of varying sizes are appropriate sites for injection. The size of the needle used for an IM injection depends on the location of the injection and the size of the muscle group. IM injections involve placing a needle deep in the muscle tissue. A needle accidentally placed into a nerve can result in permanent pain and disability. To prevent such injuries, care providers must know the proper location for placement of IM injections. Muscles used for IM injections include the deltoid, thigh, and hip.

The **deltoid muscle** is at the top of the shoulder. This muscle is an excellent choice for IM injection of emergency medications because the deltoid has a rich blood supply, allowing injected medications to be rapidly absorbed. In adults, the deltoid can tolerate an injection volume of 2 mL. The appropriate area for an IM injection of the deltoid is a triangular area on the lateral aspect (**FIGURE 3-10**). One structure that can be damaged from an improper IM injection to the deltoid is the radial nerve.

The muscles of the thigh provide another site for IM injections. The appropriate area of injection of the thigh can be located by placing one hand on the upper thigh and one hand on the lower thigh. The area between the two hands on the anterior surface of the thigh is the correct area for an IM injection, the **vastus lateralis** (**FIGURE 3-11**). In adults, up to 5 mL can be injected into this site. This is the preferred site for IM injections in infants until the muscle of the deltoid becomes more developed.

Injections into the hip are termed **dorsogluteal injections**. This area is the upper outer quadrant of the buttocks. This technique of IM injection should not be used in patients younger than 2 years or in patients who are very thin or emaciated. Place the patient on his or her side with the knees flexed toward the chest, and ask the patient to rotate the toes inward. Locate the posterior iliac spine, which is where the hemipelvis meets the sacrum, and then locate the greater trochanter of the femur. Imagine a line between these two points. This is the upper outer quadrant of the buttock. An IM injection in this area is a dorsogluteal IM injection (**FIGURE 3-12**).

Because of variation in the sizes of muscles in children, a **ventrogluteal injection** is the preferred site. Place the patient on his or her side. Put your hand on the side of the hip with the heel of your hand resting on the greater trochanter (hip joint), the thumb toward the umbilicus, the index finger on the anterior iliac spine tubercle, and the middle finger on the posterior iliac crest. With the index finger, point to the anterior iliac spine. The area of injection is in the V formed by your hand (**FIGURE 3-13**).

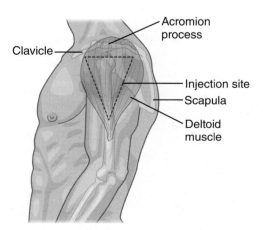

FIGURE 3-10 The injection site for the deltoid muscle is roughly formed by an inverted triangle, with the acromion process as the base. The muscle may be visible in well-developed patients.

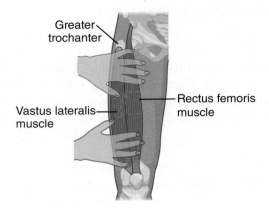

FIGURE 3-11 The injection sites for the vastus lateralis muscle and the rectus femoris muscle can be defined by landmarks. One hand is placed below the greater trochanter. The other hand is placed above the knee. The space between the two hands defines the middle third of the underlying muscle. The rectus femoris is on the anterior thigh. The vastus lateralis is on the lateral side.

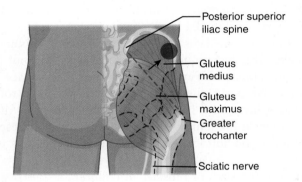

FIGURE 3-12 The posterior superior iliac spine and the greater trochanter are located by palpation. An imaginary line is drawn between the two. The injection site should be above and out from that line.

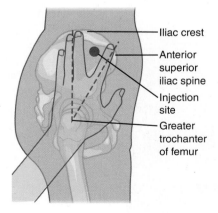

FIGURE 3-13 The injection site for the ventrogluteal muscle is defined by placing the palm of one hand on the trochanter of the femur. A V is then made with the fingers of that hand. One side runs from the greater trochanter to the anterior superior iliac spine. The other side runs from the greater trochanter to the iliac crest. The injection is made into the center of the V.

INTRAMUSCULAR MEDICATION ADMINISTRATION

Equipment Needed:

21-gauge 1½ needle, syringe with desired amount of drug, alcohol wipe, gloves, sharps container, adhesive bandage, PPE

Procedure:

1. Observe standard precautions.
2. Verify the drug order.
3. Confirm right patient, right medication, right dose, right route, and right time.
4. Confirm with the patient that he or she has no allergies to the medication, and document allergies to any other medication.
5. When possible, explain to the patient what medication you are going to administer and why. Obtain informed consent from the patient if the patient is capable of providing consent; otherwise, obtain consent from the patient's healthcare decision maker if one is available.
6. Determine the appropriate muscle site for the IM injection.
7. Identify landmarks for the injection.
8. Prepare the area for injection with alcohol.
9. Insert the needle with a rapid, dartlike motion. Insert the needle at a 90-degree angle to the surface of the skin (**FIGURE 3-14**).
10. Inject the medication.
11. Remove the needle.
12. Immediately dispose of the needle and syringe in an approved sharps container.
13. Apply pressure to the area.

Massaging the area may produce pain, especially if a large volume of fluid was injected.

14. Record the time of drug administration in the patient care record.
15. Evaluate the patient for desired effects of the medication and for any adverse effects. Continued reevaluation should occur throughout transport.

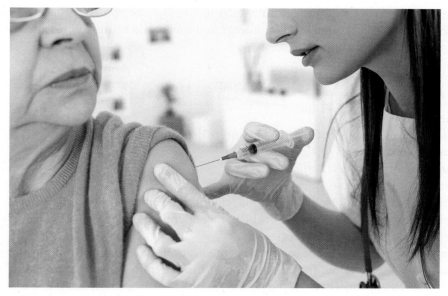

FIGURE 3-14 Appropriate site for an intramuscular injection.
© Phovoir/Shuttterstock.

Some medications used in IM injections are irritating to the soft tissues and can result in permanent staining of the skin. Hydroxyzine (Vistaril) is one drug that can permanently stain the skin. Such medications should be injected by the **Z-track technique** of injection, which can be used at any site and with any medication. This method allows delivery of the medication to the deep muscle tissue, preventing it from leaking back into the soft tissues and skin.

INTRAMUSCULAR MEDICATION ADMINISTRATION: Z-TRACK TECHNIQUE

Equipment Needed:
Medication, gloves, syringe, needle, alcohol prep, dressing, sharps container, PPE

Procedure:
1. Observe standard precautions.
2. Verify the drug order.
3. Confirm right patient, right medication, right dose, right route, and right time.
4. Confirm with the patient that he or she has no allergies to the medication, and document allergies to any other medication.
5. When possible, explain to the patient what medication you are going to administer and why. Obtain informed consent from the patient if the patient is capable of providing consent; otherwise, obtain consent from the patient's healthcare decision maker if one is available.
6. Determine the appropriate muscle site for IM injection.
7. Identify landmarks for injection.
8. Prepare the area for injection with alcohol.
9. Stretch the skin to one side approximately 1 inch (**FIGURE 3-15A**).
10. Insert the needle with a rapid, dartlike motion at a 90-degree angle to the surface of the skin (**FIGURE 3-15B**).
11. Inject the medication slowly, and wait approximately 5 seconds.
12. Remove the needle and let the skin slide back into place (**FIGURE 3-15C**).
13. Immediately dispose of the needle and syringe in an approved sharps container.
14. Apply pressure to the area. Do not massage the area.
15. Record the time of drug administration in the patient care record.
16. Evaluate the patient for desired effects of the medication and for any adverse effects. Continued reevaluation should occur throughout transport.

Intradermal medications are administered just below the epidermal layer of skin. The intradermal route is most often used for allergy and tuberculin testing. Local anesthetics may be administered by this route.

INTRADERMAL MEDICATION ADMINISTRATION

Equipment Needed:
Medication, gloves, syringe, needle, alcohol prep, dressing, sharps container, PPE

Procedure:
1. Observe standard precautions.
2. Verify the drug order.
3. Confirm right patient, right medication, right dose, right route, and right time.
4. Confirm with the patient that he or she has no allergies to the medication, and document allergies to any other medication.
5. When possible, explain to the patient what medication you are going to administer and why. Obtain informed consent from the patient if the patient is capable of providing consent; otherwise, obtain consent from the patient's healthcare decision maker if one is available.
6. Calculate the dose, and withdraw the appropriate amount of medication in a syringe (usually less than 0.5 mL).

FIGURE 3-15 Z-track injection technique. **A** and **B.** Pull the tissue laterally. **C.** Insert the needle straight down into the muscle and inject the medication. **D.** Release the tissue as the needle is withdrawn; this allows the skin to slide over the injection track and seal the medication inside.

7. Determine the appropriate site for intradermal injection. Use the skin on the anterior surface of the forearm.
8. Cleanse the site with an antiseptic wipe. Begin at the desired site and cleanse outward in a circular motion.
9. Tell the patient that he or she will feel a brief discomfort during the injection.
10. Retract the skin below the site and hold it taut. Insert the needle bevel-up into the skin at a 10- to 15-degree angle. Pull back on the plunger to aspirate and ensure that you have not entered a vein. If no blood appears, inject the drug just below the surface of the skin until a small bump appears.

11. Remove the needle and discard into an appropriate sharps container.
12. Apply an adhesive bandage to control any bleeding.
13. Explain to the patient the need to report back for the test to be read within a specific time frame.
14. Record the time of drug administration in the patient care record.
15. Evaluate the patient for desired effects of the medication and for any adverse effects.

Administration of Subcutaneous Injections

The **subcutaneous space** is the tissue between the dermis of the skin and the underlying muscle. This space does not tolerate a volume of injection greater than 2 mL. The dose is usually less than 0.5 mL. The subcutaneous space does not have a rich blood supply; therefore, medications injected into this space have a slow onset of action and a prolonged duration of action. Subcutaneous injections are easy and quick to perform; are performed by patients to self-administer medications, such as diabetic patients who self-administer daily insulin injections and patients with a history of allergies who commonly carry an EpiPen for rapid **subcutaneous administration** if necessary.

Small syringes and needles are used for subcutaneous injections. The sites used for subcutaneous injections in the field are the upper arms, upper back, and scapular regions (**FIGURE 3-16**). Patients who self-administer subcutaneous injections commonly use the abdomen and anterior thigh as sites. Because the volumes of medications administered subcutaneously usually are small, the medications must be potent.

SUBCUTANEOUS MEDICATION ADMINISTRATION

Equipment Needed:
Medication, gloves, syringe, needle, alcohol prep, dressing, sharps container, PPE
Procedure:
1. Observe standard precautions.
2. Verify the drug order.
3. Confirm right patient, right medication, right dose, right route, and right time.
4. Confirm with the patient that he or she has no allergies to the medication, and document allergies to any other medication.

FIGURE 3-16 Technique for subcutaneous injection. **A.** Pinch the skin and inject the needle at a 45-degree angle to the skin. **B.** Cross-section view showing proper placement of the needle in the subcutaneous tissue.

5. When possible, explain to the patient what medication you are going to administer and why. Obtain informed consent from the patient if the patient is capable of providing consent; otherwise, obtain consent from the patient's healthcare decision maker if one is available.
6. Determine the appropriate muscle site for subcutaneous injection.
7. Draw the medication into the syringe.
8. Prepare the area for injection with alcohol.
9. Hold the skin at the site of the proposed subcutaneous injection flat with one hand.
10. Insert the needle at a 45-degree angle (see Figure 3-16). When injecting in the scapular and abdominal areas, grasp a small roll of skin and insert the needle at a 90-degree angle.
11. Aspirate before injection *except* when injecting **heparin**. Aspirating back before injection of heparin leads to bruising after administration.
12. Inject the medication.
13. Remove the needle.
14. Immediately dispose of the needle and syringe in an approved sharps container.
15. Apply pressure to the area.
16. Record the time of drug administration in the patient care record.
17. Evaluate the patient for desired effects of the medication and for any adverse effects. Continued reevaluation should occur throughout transport.

Administration of Topical Medications

Topical medications are administered to the skin for direct treatment of a skin condition or systemic absorption through the skin and transportation through the bloodstream. The most common topical medication used by prehospital providers is nitroglycerin ointment.

Appropriate areas to apply nitroglycerin ointment are the chest, upper arm, and flank. Shaving the skin is not appropriate because it can create small nicks and irritate the skin. Ointments and creams should be applied with a tongue depressor. Nitroglycerin is now supplied with small pieces of applicator paper.

Topical patches are becoming an increasingly popular method of drug delivery for a variety of medical conditions. In identifying patches, keep in mind that patients may use more than one patch at the same time and may hide patches in unusual locations. Practice routinely assessing patients for the presence of one or more medication patches, which can complicate ongoing medical care if not promptly identified and removed. Patients may also attempt to conceal medication patches in an effort to increase the amount of narcotic medications or other controlled substances they are receiving. Medication patches often contain a massive quantity of medication that is intended to release slowly through the skin. Accidental or intentional ingestion of these patches may cause profound or catastrophic clinical effects, especially in younger children. Store and dispose of these patches in a secure manner.

TOPICAL MEDICATION ADMINISTRATION

Equipment Needed:
Medication, gloves, alcohol prep, template, adhesive dressing
Procedure:
1. Observe standard precautions.
2. Verify the drug order.
3. Confirm right patient, right medication, right dose, right route, and right time.

FIGURE 3-17 Patch with nitroglycerin ointment applied to the skin.
© Van D. Bucher/Science Source.

4. Confirm with the patient that he or she has no allergies to the medication, and document allergies to any other medication.
5. When possible, explain to the patient what medication you are going to administer and why. Obtain informed consent from the patient if the patient is capable of providing consent; otherwise, obtain consent from the patient's healthcare decision maker if one is available.
6. Clean the skin with an alcohol prep.
7. Apply the applicator with the nitroglycerin ointment to the skin, with the ointment side facing down (**FIGURE 3-17**).
8. Do not rub the medication into the skin.
9. Record the time of drug administration in the patient care record.
10. Evaluate the patient for desired effects of the medication and for any adverse effects. Continued reevaluation should occur throughout transport.

Administration of Medications Through an ET Tube

In life-threatening emergencies, such as during cardiac arrests or critical resuscitation situations, patients often require medications immediately—even before IV or IO access has been established. If the patient is intubated, paramedics can administer several drugs through the ET tube until reliable IV access is established. These include lidocaine (Xylocaine), epinephrine, atropine, naloxone (Narcan), and vasopressin.

The lungs have a large surface area with a rich blood supply. When a medication is given through an ET tube, the drug is immediately delivered to the basic lung units, the alveoli, where it is rapidly absorbed by the numerous blood vessels that cover each **alveolus**.

Remember which drugs can be given through an ET tube with the mnemonic NAVEL:
N naloxone
A atropine
V vasopressin
E epinephrine
L lidocaine

When a medication is administered through an ET tube, 2 to 2.5 times the dose of medication given via the IV route is required. In addition, to help with rapid absorption, the medication should be diluted in 10 mL of normal saline or sterile water for adult patients and 5 mL of normal saline or sterile water for pediatric patients. Medication administration by this route is appropriate only until reliable IV or IO access has been established, so do not abandon attempts to secure IV or IO access. With increasing use of IO access in adults, the role of ET medication administration is becoming rare in clinical practice. ET tubes remain an acceptable route for aerosolized bronchodilator medication administration in mechanically ventilated patients.

MEDICATION ADMINISTRATION THROUGH AN ET TUBE

Equipment Needed:
Medication, gloves, syringe, normal saline or sterile water
Procedure:
1. Observe standard precautions.
2. Verify the drug order.
3. Confirm right patient, right medication, right dose, right route, and right time. Remember to double the dosage for this route of administration.
4. Confirm that the patient has no allergies to the medication, and document allergies to any other medication.
5. If the patient is awake, explain to the patient what medication you are going to administer and why. If the patient is not awake due to illness or injury, inform his or her family or surrogate healthcare decision maker if present.
6. Dilute the medication in 10 mL of normal saline or sterile water for adult patients and 5 mL of normal saline for pediatric patients.
7. If possible, remove the needle from the syringe.
8. If cardiopulmonary resuscitation is in progress, hold compressions.
9. Ask another EMS provider to grasp the ET tube firmly, and then remove the bag mask. Be careful not to tug or remove the ET tube when disconnecting the bag mask.
10. Administer the medication into the ET tube.
11. "Push" the medication down the tube with two or three strong ventilations with the bag mask.
12. Resume compressions if required.
13. Continue to try to obtain an IV line for additional medication if required.
14. Record the time of drug administration in the patient care record.
15. Evaluate the patient for desired effects of the medication and for any adverse effects. Continued reevaluation should occur throughout transport.

▶ Review Questions

1. For what conditions do standing orders usually exist?
2. Who would the paramedic contact for an as-needed order?
3. List the nine patient rights of drug administration.
4. Why is the parenteral route of drug administration more effective than the enteral route in the prehospital setting?
5. What is the disadvantage of administering oral medications in a medical emergency?
6. List the precautions that should be followed when handling a needle.
7. Explain the rationale of the Z-track technique of IM injections.
8. What medications can be administered through an ET tube?
9. Explain the dosage preparation for a medication for ET delivery.

References

1. Bonsall L. Eight rights of medication administration. NursingCenter Blog. https://www.nursingcenter.com/ncblog/may-2011/8-rights-of-medication-administration. Published May 27, 2011. Accessed July 4, 2018.
2. Elliot M, Liu Y. The nine rights of medication administration: an overview. *Br J Nurs.* 2010;19(5):300–305.
3. Nwagwu V. Ten rights of medication administration and management. Developmental Disabilities Administration. https://ucedd.georgetown.edu/DDA/documents/NursingRTMarch2016.pdf. Accessed July 4, 2018.
4. Look-alike drug names with recommended tall man letters. Institute of Safe Medication Practices. https://www.ismp.org/recommendations/tall-man-letters-list. Published November 20, 2016. Accessed July 4, 2018.
5. Eustis TC, Wright SW, Wrenn KD, Fowlie EJ, Slovis CM. Compliance with recommendations for standard precautions among prehospital providers. *Ann Emerg Med.* 1995;25(4):512–515.
6. Wrentz-Hudson DA. Emergency medical service worker knowledge of and compliance with occupational exposures to infectious diseases. Walden Dissertations and Doctoral Studies. https://scholarworks.waldenu.edu/cgi/viewcontent.cgi?referer=&httpsredir=1&article=3056&context=dissertations. Published 2015. Accessed July 4, 2018.
7. Bledsoe BE, Sweeney RJ, Verkeley RP, et al. EMS provider compliance with infection control recommendations is suboptimal. *Prehosp Emerg Care.* 2014;18(2). doi: 10.3109/10903127.2013.851311.
8. Widmeier K. Medication administration. In A. Pollack, ed. *Nancy Caroline's Emergency Care in the Streets.* 8th ed. Burlington, MA: Jones & Bartlett Learning; 2018.

CHAPTER 4
Medication Math

OBJECTIVES

1. Identify the basic units of measure for weight, length, and volume.
2. Accurately convert milliliters to cubic centimeters, kilograms to pounds, and milligrams to grams (and micrograms).
3. Apply the four basic formulas (single dose, infusion of a measured amount of fluid in a set amount of time, drip infusion not based on weight, and drip infusion based on weight) to solve drug problems and determine dosages.

▶ Introduction

Medication math can be made simple by mastering only a few basic formulas. The purpose of this chapter is to remove the mystery of medication math and instill confidence to easily calculate drug dosages.

Anaphylaxis, as presented in the following case, is a life-threatening condition that is easily treated. However, without a grasp of the concepts of medication math, you cannot properly administer the medication epinephrine. A thorough knowledge of the concepts of pharmacology and dosing of medications is useless without the ability to make conversions of weight and volume and calculate volumes of drug to be administered based on concentration of the drug. As illustrated in the following case, to administer a simple and common medication such as epinephrine, you will need to make several calculations. To perform these calculations in a potentially life-threatening emergency requires a complete grasp of medication math principles.

CASE STUDY

You and your partner are dispatched to a residence on a call for an allergic reaction. You arrive and are directed to the kitchen, where you find a 6-year-old girl who is sitting in a chair in obvious respiratory distress. The child's mother tells you she stepped on a bee while running barefoot in the backyard. The mother states that the child does not have any known allergies, but she has never been stung by a bee before. The child has stridor and a rapid respiratory rate. She is holding and rubbing a markedly swollen left foot and appears quite anxious.

(continues)

CASE STUDY (continued)

Your assessment of this situation is that the child is having an anaphylactic reaction from a bee sting. You determine that epinephrine should be administered as quickly as possible, and you do not think waiting to get intravenous (IV) access before administering the epinephrine is prudent. You decide that the best course of action is to administer intramuscular (IM) epinephrine (1:1,000). You ask the mother how much the child weighs, and the mother replies 50 pounds. The pediatric dose for IM epinephrine is 0.01 mg/kg (1:1000). The concentration of the epinephrine (1:1,000) is 1 mg/mL. How many milliliters of epinephrine (1:1,000) must be administered to this child?

Several questions must be answered before determining how many milliliters to administer.

1. What is the weight of the child in kilograms?
   - The child weighs 50 pounds. To convert to kilograms, you must know that 1 kg equals 2.2 pounds.

$$\frac{50 \text{ lb}}{2.2 \text{ kg/lb}} = \frac{50 \text{ \cancel{lb}}}{2.2 \text{ kg/\cancel{lb}}} = 22.7 \text{ kg}$$

2. What is the weight-based dose of IM epinephrine (1:1,000)?
   - IM dose of epinephrine (1:1,000) is 0.01 mg/kg.

$$\text{Dose} = \frac{0.01 \text{ mg}}{\text{kg}} \times \frac{22.7 \text{ kg}}{1} = \frac{0.01 \text{ mg}}{\cancel{\text{kg}}} \times \frac{22.7 \text{ \cancel{kg}}}{1} = 0.01 \text{ mg} \times 22.7 = 0.23 \text{ mg}$$

3. What is the volume of epinephrine (1:1,000) that needs to be administered IM by the syringe?
   - Concentration of epinephrine 1 mg/mL

$$\text{Milliliters to administer} = \frac{\text{desired dose}}{\text{dose on hand}} \times \frac{\text{volume/quantity}}{1}$$

$$\text{Milliliters to administer} = \frac{0.23 \text{ mg}}{1 \text{ mg}} \times \frac{1 \text{ mL}}{1}$$

$$\text{Milliliters to administer} = \frac{0.23 \text{ \cancel{mg}}}{1 \text{ \cancel{mg}}} \times \frac{1 \text{ mL}}{1}$$

$$\text{Milliliters to administer} = 0.23 \text{ mL}$$

You administer 0.23 mL epinephrine (1:1,000) IM. Shortly after administration, the child's breathing becomes less labored and she is less anxious. You start a peripheral IV line, repeat your assessment, and prepare for transport. (Chapter 8 covers drug therapy for anaphylaxis in detail.)

▶ Systems of Measurement

The first system of measurement for drugs was the **apothecary system**. In that system, the weight of drugs was measured in grains. Linear measures included inches, yards, and miles. **Volume** (i.e., the measurement of fluids and liquids) was measured in minims.

The **metric system** currently is the preferred system for drug measurement and calculation. It is logical and well organized, based on a basic unit and its multiples or submultiples of 10. It is similar to the U.S. monetary system: one dollar is the basic unit of measurement, written as $1.00. It can be divided into 10 dimes (written as $0.10), which can be further divided into 10 pennies (written as $0.01). This analogy is helpful when determining drug dosages.

TABLE 4-1 Common Prefixes Used in Medication Calculation

Prefix	Calculation	Examples of Equivalents	Reverse (Also True) of a Basic Unit	Multiple or Part
kilo	1,000 × basic unit	1 kg = 1,000 g	1,000 g = 1 kg	Multiple
centi	1/100 of a basic unit	1 cm = 1/100 m	1/100 m = 1 cm	Part
milli	1/1,000 of a basic unit	1 mg = 1/1,000 g	1/1,000 g = 1 mg	Part
micro	1/1,000,000 of a basic unit	1 mcg = 1/1,000,000 g	1/1,000,000 g = 1 mcg	Part

© Jones & Bartlett Learning.

Just as the apothecary system has basic units of measure for weight, length, and volume, so does the metric system, as follows:

- Weight (solids or mass): gram (g)
- Length: meter (m)
- Volume (liquid or fluid): liter (L)

In addition, several prefixes are commonly used in medicine to distinguish multiples or smaller parts of these units. The four commonly used in drug calculation are **kilo**, **centi**, **milli**, and **micro**. They are defined in **TABLE 4-1** along with calculations and examples of equivalents.

Most drugs administered in the field are measured in the following units: **gram (g)**, **milligram (mg)**, and **microgram (mcg)**. Drugs present in solutions can be measured in **milliliters (mL)**. At times, volumes of solutions are also reported in cubic centimeters (cc). Milliliters and cubic centimeters refer to the same volume.

▶ Conversions

The ability to convert one unit of measure to another is vital to ensure that the intended dose of medication is administered to the patient. Failure to understand and use unit conversions may lead to overdosing the patient inadvertently or providing the patient with a less than optimal dose. Most IV medications are supplied as solutions expressed as a concentrations (e.g., milligrams per milliliter [mg/mL]). Medications are dosed as a mass (e.g., milligrams), and drug doses are often determined based on a patient's weight (e.g., pounds or kilograms) or body surface area (square meters). As mentioned in Chapter 2, lack of experience in the performance of drug calculations and conversions is a common cause of medical error, patient injury, and legal action against the prehospital professional.

Millimeters and Cubic Centimeters

The milliliter is a measurement of volume (liquids or fluids in this case) and is equal to 1/1,000 of a liter. The cubic centimeter is also a measurement of volume, but it is based on the centimeter, which is equal to 1/100 of a meter. Because 1 cc equals 1 mL, the terms are often used interchangeably.

For example, you may receive an order to administer 2 mL of morphine sulfate. The same order may be given as 2 cc of morphine sulfate. These two doses are considered equivalent. A box with dimensions of 1 cm × 1 cm × 1 cm has a volume of cubic centimeter. If the box

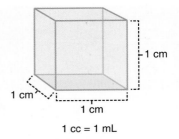

1 cm

1 cm

1 cm

1 cc = 1 mL

FIGURE 4-1 Volume is equal to the space created. The term *cc* represents cubic centimeter. A cubic centimeter is 1 cm wide, 1 cm long, and 1 cm high. One milliliter (mL) is the equivalent volume of a cubic centimeter. To avoid confusion, the term *milliliter* is preferred over cc, or cubic centimeter.

were filled with 1 mL of water at a temperature of 4°C, the water would exactly fill the box. Therefore, the *volume* is equal to the *space* that was created (**FIGURE 4-1**).

> Remember: 1 cc = 1 mL, but 1 mL does *not* equal 1 mg. *Gram* refers to the weight of a powdered drug, not its volume or the space that it occupies.

Never take medication orders in dosages of volume. For example, you are transporting a 43-year-old man with a severe open femur fracture incurred after he fell off a roof. You call medical direction for an order for morphine, and medical direction gives the order for 3 mL (or 3 cc) of morphine sulfate. Many drugs, morphine included, come in several different concentrations. Injectable morphine comes in concentrations of 2, 4, 5, 8, and 10 mg/mL. For instance, if medical direction thought that the advanced life support (ALS) drug box was stocked with morphine sulfate with a concentration of 2 mg/mL, the intended order to give 2 mL would have resulted in 4 mg being administered. If the drug box was supplied with 4 mg/mL, the order of 2 mL would have resulted in the patient getting 8 mg of morphine, or twice the intended dose. Although most drug boxes are supplied with standardized concentrations of medications, administering medications on the basis of volume alone (not concentration) is poor practice and not safe.

Kilograms and Pounds

The next conversion commonly used to calculate drug dosages is kilograms (kg) to pounds (lb). Note that these units refer to the *patient's* weight, not the weight of the drug. Many drug dosages, particularly those administered to pediatric patients, are based on the patient's weight in kilograms to ensure safety from overdose.

The equivalent to remember is 1 kg = 2.2 lb. Therefore, to convert weight in pounds to weight in kilograms, divide the number of pounds by 2.2.

Converting Kilograms to Pounds: Example

If a patient weighs 154 lb, divide 154 lb by 2.2 lb/kg to determine the weight in kilograms.

$$\frac{154 \text{ lb}}{2.2 \text{ lb/kg}} = \text{weight in kilograms}$$

First, cross out "like terms" in the problem; in this case, *lb.*

$$\frac{154 \cancel{\text{ lb}}}{2.2 \cancel{\text{ lb}}/\text{kg}} = \text{weight in kilograms}$$

Now, work the problem.

$$\frac{154}{2.2\,\text{kg}} = 70\,\text{kg}$$

Milligrams, Micrograms, and Grams

The next conversion is from milligrams to grams and, in reverse, from grams to milligrams. This process also includes converting milligrams to micrograms and micrograms to milligrams.

> Remember: *milli* means 1/1,000 of a basic unit; in this case, grams. The equivalent is 1,000 mg = 1 g.

To use an everyday example, when changing a dollar into coins (e.g., dimes or pennies), the *larger unit* (dollar) is changed into an equivalent sum in *smaller units* (dimes or pennies). Therefore, to get the total number of the smaller unit, multiply the number of dollars (e.g., 5 dollars) by the number of dimes or pennies *per dollar*.

Converting to Smaller Units: Example 1

To convert to dimes, you must know there are 10 dimes for every 1 dollar.

$$\frac{5\,\text{dollars} \times 10\,\text{dimes}}{\text{dollar}} = \text{number of dimes}$$

Cross out like terms; in this case, *dollar*.

$$\frac{5\,\cancel{\text{dollars}} \times 10\,\text{dimes}}{\cancel{\text{dollar}}} = \text{number of dimes}$$

Now, work the problem.

$$5 \times 10\,\text{dimes} = 50\,\text{dimes}$$

Converting to Smaller Units: Example 2

To convert to pennies, you must know there are 100 pennies for every 1 dollar.

$$\frac{5\,\text{dollars} \times 100\,\text{pennies}}{\text{dollar}} = \text{number of pennies}$$

Cross out like terms; in this case, *dollars*.

$$\frac{5\,\cancel{\text{dollars}} \times 100\,\text{pennies}}{\cancel{\text{dollar}}} = \text{number of pennies}$$

Now, work the problem.

$$5 \times 100\,\text{pennies} = 500\,\text{pennies}$$

Note that when converting a pocket full of change into dollar bills, *smaller units* (coins) are being changed into *larger units* (dollars). The result will be *fewer* larger units (dollars) than smaller units (coins). So, when converting between units, ask yourself, "Am I changing small units for larger units, or large units for smaller units?" This question also applies in practice; you should have an initial sense of whether the numbers and units should be increasing or decreasing in magnitude.

Converting to Larger Units: Example

To convert grams to milligrams, multiply grams by 1,000. Remember that every 1 g contains 1,000 mg; this can be written as 1,000 mg/g.

$$\frac{5\,g \times 1{,}000\ mg}{g} = \text{number of milligrams}$$

Cross out like terms; in this case, *g*.

$$\frac{5\,\cancel{g} \times 1{,}000\ mg}{\cancel{g}} = \text{number of milligrams}$$

Now, work the problem.

$$5 \times 1{,}000\ mg = 5{,}000\ mg$$

This can be quickly accomplished by moving the decimal point to the right the same number of spaces as there are zeros in the number. For example, because 1,000 mg has 3 zeros, move the decimal point three decimal places to the right.

$$5\ g = 5{,}\underline{000}\ mg$$

The same process can be used to convert milligrams (mg) to micrograms (mcg).

milli means × 1,000, or add 3 zeros

micro means × 1,000,000, or add 6 zeros

To convert milligrams (3 zeros) to micrograms (6 zeros), simply move the decimal point three more places to the right, for a total of 6 zeros.

$$5{,}000\ mg = 5{,}000{,}\underline{000}\ mcg$$

To convert milligrams to grams (smaller to larger), divide the number of grams by 1,000, or simply move the decimal point three places to the left. This is the same as changing 100 pennies back to dollars. The 100 actually means 100 cents. Therefore, move the decimal point to the left the same number of places as there are zeros in the equivalent of $1.00 (100 pennies—therefore 2 zeros, or 2 spaces).

$$100\ \text{pennies (cents)} = 1.00\ \text{dollar}$$

The following are some practice problems. Be sure to master the art of conversion before moving on so that you will understand the rest of the chapter.

Practice Problems

Convert grams to milligrams and milligrams to grams.

1. 1 g = _____ mg
2. 1,000 mg = _____ g
3. 250 mg = _____ g
4. 400 mg = _____ g
5. 500 mg = _____ g
6. 0.75 g = _____ mg
7. 1.25 g = _____ mg
8. 10 g = _____ mg
9. 2 g = _____ mg
10. 2,500 mg = _____ g

Convert milligrams to micrograms and micrograms to milligrams.

1. 1 mg = _____ mcg
2. 500 mcg = _____ mg
3. 250 mcg = _____ mg
4. 400 mg = _____ mcg
5. 0.2 mg = _____ mcg
6. 800,000 mcg = _____ mg
7. 800 mg = _____ mcg
8. 200 mg = _____ mcg
9. 1,000 mcg = _____ mg
10. 200,000 mcg = _____ mg

BOX 4-1 Basic Conversions

1 g = 1,000 mg
1 mg = 1,000 mcg
1 L = 1,000 mL or 1,000 cc
1 kg = 2.2 lb
2.5 cm = 1 in.
Remember: 1 mg does not equal 1 mL or 1 cc.

© Jones & Bartlett Learning.

Answers

Convert grams to milligrams and milligrams to grams.

1. 1 g = 1,000 mg
2. 1,000 mg = 1 g
3. 250 mg = 0.25 g
4. 400 mg = 0.4 g
5. 500 mg = 0.5 g
6. 0.75 g = 750 mg
7. 1.25 g = 1,250 mg
8. 10 g = 10,000 mg
9. 2 g = 2,000 mg
10. 2,500 mg = 2.5 g

Convert milligrams to micrograms and micrograms to milligrams.

1. 1 mg = 1,000 mcg
2. 500 mcg = 0.5 mg
3. 250 mcg = 0.25 mg
4. 400 mg = 400,000 mcg
5. 0.2 mg = 200 mcg
6. 800,000 mcg = 800 mg
7. 800 mg = 800,000 mcg
8. 200 mg = 200,000 mcg
9. 1,000 mcg = 1 mg
10. 200,000 mcg = 200 mg

BOX 4-1 summarizes basic conversions that are useful in drug calculations.

▶ Drug Preparations and Concentrations

Regarding drug dosage calculations, understanding that drugs are supplied in various concentrations with differing preparations is important. The same drug can come in various concentrations, and dosages must be calculated according to the particular preparation. For example, atropine sulfate, a medication commonly used to increase a slow heart rate, comes packaged in two ways in prefilled syringes: 0.5 mg/10 mL and 1 mg/10 mL. The second preparation is twice as concentrated as the first and therefore requires a dose of only half the amount. Another drug, dopamine, which is used by prehospital professionals in certain situations in the field to raise blood pressure, comes in three different concentrations: 0.8, 1.6, and 3.2 mg/mL.

▶ Formulas

Formulas are used to solve drug problems or determine dosages for patients. They should be used in conjunction with the basic conversions explained previously. Four basic formulas can be used to solve all prehospital pharmacology math problems:

Formula 1

Single dose (e.g., bolus of lidocaine or IM injection of Benadryl):

$$\frac{\text{desired dose}}{\text{dose on hand}} \times \frac{\text{volume/quantity}}{1} = X$$

Formula 2

Infusion of a measured amount of fluid in a set amount of time (e.g., fluid challenge):

$$\frac{\text{total volume} \times \text{drops/mL of IV set}}{\text{time in minutes}} = \text{drops/min}$$

Formula 3

Drip (infusion) not based on weight (e.g., lidocaine drip):

$$\frac{\text{dose desired}}{\text{dose on hand}} \times \frac{\text{drops/mL of IV set}}{1} = \text{drops/min}$$

Formula 4

Drip (infusion) based on weight (e.g., dopamine drip):

$$\frac{\text{dose desired}}{\text{kg}} \times \frac{\text{wt (lb)}}{2.2 \text{ lb/kg}} = \text{dose desired}$$

$$\frac{\text{dose desired}}{\cancel{\text{kg}}} \times \frac{\text{wt (}\cancel{\text{lb}}\text{)}}{2.2 \, \cancel{\text{lb}}/\cancel{\text{kg}}}$$

$$\frac{\text{dose desired}}{\text{dose on hand}} \times \frac{\text{drops/mL of IV set}}{1} = \text{drops/min}$$

Application of Formula 1

The first of the four formulas is used to calculate the amount of a drug to give a patient in a single dose on the basis of the desired dose (DD), or the amount ordered by medical direction; the dose on hand (DH), or the amount of the weight of the drug (grams, milligrams, micrograms); and the volume (V) or quantity (Q), or the amount of solution in which the drug is dissolved.

CASE STUDY

A 64-year-old woman is enjoying a round of golf when she suddenly steps in a hornets' nest and is stung multiple times. Because she is allergic to bee stings, she quickly heads back to the clubhouse and asks for help. A paramedic unit is dispatched. On arrival, the patient is in mild distress, with large hives appearing on her face and neck. Because of her age and the relatively mild signs and symptoms at this point, the paramedics avoid epinephrine and choose to administer diphenhydramine (Benadryl) 25 mg IM. Their prefilled syringe reads 50 mg/mL. How many milliliters should they administer?

Step 1: Choose the proper formula.

$$\frac{\text{desired dose}}{\text{dose on hand}} \times \frac{\text{volume (quantity)}}{1} =$$

Step 2: Fill in known values.

$$\frac{25 \text{ mg} \times 1 \text{ mL}}{50 \text{ mg}} =$$

Step 3: Cross out like terms; in this case, *mg*.

$$\frac{25 \, \cancel{\text{mg}} \times 1 \text{ mL}}{50 \, \cancel{\text{mg}}} = \frac{25 \times 1 \text{ mL}}{50} = \frac{25}{50} \text{ mL} = 0.5 \text{ mL}$$

Step 4: Administer 0.5 mL of Benadryl IM to the patient.

Remember, whenever the dosage is less than 1, always place a zero before the decimal point.

Formula 1 Practice Problems

Remember the steps: cross out like terms and multiply across.

1. Administer epinephrine (Adrenalin) 1:1,000 0.3 mg Sub-Q. The prefilled syringe reads 1 mg/mL. How many milliliters should you administer?
2. Administer furosemide (Lasix) 20 mg IV line. Furosemide is supplied in a concentration of 40 mg/5 mL. How many milliliters should you administer?
3. Administer atropine sulfate 0.5 mg rapid IV push. The prefilled syringe reads 1 mg/10 mL. How many milliliters should you administer?
4. Administer verapamil (Isoptin) 5 mg slow IV push. The prefilled syringe reads 5 mg/2 mL (2.5 mg/mL). How many milliliters should you administer?
5. Administer adenosine 12 mg rapid IV push. The prefilled syringe reads 6 mg/2 mL. How many milliliters should you administer?

Formula 1 Answers

$$1.\ \frac{DD:0.3\ \cancel{mg} \times V(Q):1\ mL}{DH:1\ \cancel{mg}} = 0.3 \times 1\ mL = \frac{0.3 \times \cancel{1}\ mL}{\cancel{1}} = \mathbf{0.3\ mL}$$

$$2.\ \frac{DD:20\ \cancel{mg} \times V(Q):5\ mL}{DH:40\ \cancel{mg}} = \frac{20 \times 5\ mL}{40} = \frac{100}{40}\ mL = \mathbf{2.5\ mL}$$

$$3.\ \frac{DD:0.5\ \cancel{mg} \times V(Q):10\ mL}{DH:1\ \cancel{mg}} = \frac{0.5 \times 10\ mL}{1} = \frac{5\ mL}{1} = \mathbf{5\ mL}$$

$$4.\ \frac{DD:5\ \cancel{mg} \times V(Q):2\ mL}{DH:5\ \cancel{mg}} = \frac{5 \times 2\ mL}{5} = \frac{10}{5}\ mL = \mathbf{2\ mL}$$

$$5.\ \frac{DD:12\ \cancel{mg} \times V(Q):2\ mL}{DH:6\ \cancel{mg}} = \frac{12 \times 2\ mL}{6} = \frac{24}{6}\ mL = \mathbf{4\ mL}$$

Application of Formula 2

Formula 2 is used to calculate the amount of a drug to give a patient when infusing a measured amount of fluid in a set amount of time, such as in fluid challenges.

CASE STUDY

Your ALS unit is called out during a snowstorm to attend to an older man who has had the flu since yesterday. His daughter tells you that he has been vomiting, has had diarrhea for more than 24 hours, and has not been able to keep any fluids down. Your patient is weak and warm to the touch. He has elevated respiratory and pulse rates but a blood pressure of 88/60 mm Hg. His lung sounds are present bilaterally and clear. Medical direction tells you to administer a fluid bolus of 200 mL normal saline over a 20-minute period and then reevaluate the patient and call back. You decide to use a macrodrip infusion set that delivers 10 gtt (drops)/mL.

Step 1: Choose the proper formula.

$$\frac{\text{total volume} \times \text{gtt/mL of IV set}}{\text{time (in minutes)}} = \text{gtt/min}$$

Step 2: Fill in known values.

$$\frac{200 \text{ mL} \times 10 \text{ gtt/mL}}{20 \text{ min}} = \text{gtt/min}$$

Step 3: Cross out like terms.

$$\frac{200 \text{ mL} \times 10 \text{ gtt/mL}}{20 \text{ min}} = \text{gtt/min}$$

Step 4: Multiply across.

$$\frac{200 \times 10 \text{ gtt}}{20 \text{ min}} = \frac{2,000 \text{ gtt}}{20 \text{ min}} = \frac{100 \text{ gtt}}{\text{min}}$$

Sometimes a measured amount of fluid is ordered to be given over a period of hours. To make this conversion, change hours to minutes by multiplying by 60 (e.g., 5 hour × 60 min/hr = 300 minutes) and continue as before.

(*continued*) You reassess the patient during and after the fluid challenge. His lungs remain clear, his pulse begins to drop to a normal range, his respirations are less frequent, and his blood pressure rises to 96/70 mm Hg. Medical direction tells you to continue the IV infusion at a keep-open rate and transport the patient to the hospital.

Formula 2 Practice Problems

Remember the steps: cross out like terms and multiply across.

1. Administer 60 mL of fluid containing a medication over a 10-minute period. Use a microdrip IV infusion set that delivers 60 gtt/mL. How many drops per minute should be administered?
2. Administer 120 mL of Ringer's lactate as a fluid challenge over a 20-minute period with an IV infusion set that delivers 20 gtt/mL. How many drops per minute should be administered?
3. Administer 150 mL of normal saline over a 30-minute period with an IV infusion set that delivers 10 gtt/mL. How many drops per minute should be administered?
4. Administer 300 mL of Ringer's lactate over a 30-minute period with an IV infusion set that delivers 10 gtt/mL. How many drops per minute should be administered?
5. Administer 1,000 mL of normal saline over a 5-hour period with a macrodrip IV infusion set that delivers 15 gtt/mL. How many drops per minute should be administered?

Formula 2 Answers

$$1. \ \frac{60 \text{ mL} \times 60 \text{ gtt/mL}}{10 \text{ min}} = \frac{60 \times 60 \text{ gtt}}{10 \text{ min}} = \frac{3,600 \text{ gtt}}{10 \text{ min}} = 360 \text{ gtt/min}$$

$$2. \ \frac{120 \text{ mL} \times 20 \text{ gtt/mL}}{20 \text{ min}} = \frac{120 \times 20 \text{ gtt}}{20 \text{ min}} = \frac{2,400 \text{ gtt}}{20 \text{ min}} = 120 \text{ gtt/min}$$

$$3.\ \frac{150\ \cancel{mL} \times 10\ gtt/\cancel{mL}}{30\ min} = \frac{150 \times 10\ gtt}{30\ min} = \frac{1{,}500\ gtt}{30\ min} = 50\ gtt/min$$

$$4.\ \frac{300\ \cancel{mL} \times 10\ gtt/\cancel{mL}}{30\ min} = \frac{3{,}000\ gtt}{30\ min} = 100\ gtt/min$$

$$5.\ \frac{1{,}000\ \cancel{mL} \times 15\ gtt/\cancel{mL}}{300\ min} = \frac{15{,}000\ gtt}{300\ min} = 50\ gtt/min$$

Application of Formula 3

Formula 3 is used to calculate the amount of a drug to give a patient by drip (infusion) when the dosage is based not on weight but on dose of medication per minute.

CASE STUDY

You are called to respond to the home of the base commander. On arrival, you find a 62-year-old man complaining of heart palpitations. You connect the cardiac monitor to find the patient with a narrow-complex supraventricular tachycardia at a rate of 178 beats/min. You have attempted to correct the arrhythmia with vagal maneuvers and adenosine to no avail. Medical direction orders you to administer an infusion of procainamide at 20 mg/min.

You have a peripheral IV line in place capable of delivering 60 gtt/mL. Your secondary premixed bag of procainamide reads 100 mg/mL. At how many drops per minute should you run the procainamide to administer the proper dose?

Step 1: Choose the proper formula.

$$\frac{DD\,(in\ minutes) \times gtt/mL\ of\ IV\ set}{DH} = gtt/min$$

Step 2: Fill in known values.

$$\frac{20\ mg/min \times 60\ gtt/mL}{100\ mg/mL} = gtt/min$$

Step 3: Cross out like terms. In this case, both *mg* and *mL* can be crossed out.

$$\frac{20\ \cancel{mg}/min \times 60\ gtt/\cancel{mL}}{100\ \cancel{mg}/\cancel{mL}} = gtt/min$$

Step 4: Multiply across for drops per minute.

$$\frac{20/min \times 60\ gtt}{100} = \frac{20/min \times 60\ gtt}{100} = \frac{1{,}200}{100}\ gtt/min = 12\ gtt/min$$

Formula 3 Practice Problems

Remember the steps: cross out like terms and multiply across.

1. Administer an epinephrine infusion at 4 mcg/min. Add 1 mg epinephrine to a bag of 250 mL normal saline. Use a microdrip infusion set that delivers 60 gtt/mL. What is the drip rate in drops per minute?
2. Administer a procainamide infusion at 3 mg/min. Prepare the infusion by adding 1 g procainamide to a bag of 250 mL normal saline. Use a microdrip infusion set that delivers 60 gtt/mL. What is the drip rate in drops per minute?

3. Administer an epinephrine infusion at 2 mcg/min. Prepare the infusion by adding 1 mg epinephrine to a bag of 500 mL normal saline. What is the drug concentration (DH)? What is the drip rate if a microdrip infusion set that delivers 60 gtt/mL is used?

Formula 3 Answers

1. 1 mg = 1,000 mcg, so the DH (drug concentration) is 1,000 mcg/250 mL = 4 mcg/mL.

$$\frac{\text{DD}: 4\,\text{mcg/min} \times 60\,\text{gtt/mL}}{\text{DH}: 4\,\text{mcg/mL}} = \frac{4\,\cancel{\text{mcg}}/\text{min} \times 60\,\text{gtt}/\cancel{\text{mL}}}{4\,\cancel{\text{mcg}}/\cancel{\text{mL}}} = \frac{4/\text{min} \times 60\,\text{gtt}}{4}$$

$$= \frac{240}{4}\,\text{gtt/min} = 60\,\text{gtt/min}$$

2. 1 g = 1,000 mg, so the DH is 1,000 mg/250 mL = 4 mg/mL.

$$\frac{\text{DD}: 3\,\text{mg/min} \times 60\,\text{gtt/mL}}{\text{DH}: 4\,\text{mg/mL}} = \frac{3\,\cancel{\text{mg}}/\text{min} \times \text{gtt}/\cancel{\text{mL}}}{4\,\cancel{\text{mg}}/\cancel{\text{mL}}} = \frac{3/\text{min} \times 60\,\text{gtt}}{4}$$

$$= \frac{180}{4}\,\text{gtt/min} = 45\,\text{gtt/min}$$

3. 1 mg = 1,000 mcg, so the DH is 1,000 mcg/500 mL = 2 mcg/mL.

$$\frac{\text{DD}: 2\,\text{mcg/min} \times 60\,\text{gtt/mL}}{\text{DH}: 2\,\text{mcg/mL}} = \frac{2\,\cancel{\text{mcg}}/\text{min} \times 60\,\text{gtt}/\cancel{\text{mL}}}{2\,\cancel{\text{mcg}}/\cancel{\text{mL}}} = \frac{2/\text{min} \times 60\,\text{gtt}}{2}$$

$$\frac{120}{2}\,\text{gtt/min} = 60\,\text{gtt/min}$$

Application of Formula 4

Formula 4 is used to calculate the amount of a drug to give a patient by drip (infusion) when the dosage is based on weight.

CASE STUDY

You are transporting an older woman with a history of multiple cardiac events to the hospital. En route, her blood pressure begins to drop even though her cardiac rhythm shows only sinus tachycardia at a rate of 120 beats/min. You contact medical direction and are told to begin a dopamine infusion at 2 mcg/kg per minute and to titrate it until her blood pressure is approximately 90 mm Hg systolic. Prepare the infusion by adding 800 mg of dopamine to a 500-mL bag of normal saline. The patient weighs 110 lb.

In this last formula, one more step in the process must be calculated to determine what the desired dose is on the basis of the patient's weight in kilograms. Remember that 1 kg = 2.2 pounds.

Step 1: Choose the proper formula.

$$\frac{\text{DD}}{\text{kg}} \times \frac{\text{lb}}{2.2\,\text{lb/kg}} = \frac{\text{DD}}{\cancel{\text{kg}}} \times \frac{\cancel{\text{lb}}}{2.2\,\cancel{\text{lb}}/\cancel{\text{kg}}} = \text{DD}$$

$$\frac{\text{DD}}{\text{DH}} \times \frac{\text{drops/mL of IV set}}{1} = \text{drops per minute}$$

Step 2: Determine the patient's weight in kilograms by dividing the weight in pounds by 2.2.

$$\frac{110\,\text{lb}}{2.2\,\text{lb/kg}} = \frac{110\,\cancel{\text{lb}}}{2.2\,\cancel{\text{lb}}/\text{kg}} = 50\,\text{kg}$$

Step 3: Multiply the weight in kilograms by DD/kilograms and cross out like terms to determine the DD, *with weight adjustment.* Because this patient weighs 50 kg, and the DD is 2 mcg/kg per minute, the calculation is as follows:

$$\frac{50 \text{ kg} \times 2 \text{ mcg}}{\text{kg/min}} = \frac{50 \cancel{\text{ kg}} \times 2 \text{ mcg}}{\cancel{\text{kg}}/\text{min}} = \frac{50 \times 2 \text{ mcg}}{\text{min}} = 100 \text{ mcg/min}$$

Step 4: Prepare the infusion and calculate the DH (drug concentration). Set the calculation up so that 800 mg = 800,000 mcg, to be added to 500 mL normal saline:

$$\frac{800,000 \text{ mcg}}{500 \text{ mL}} = 1,600 \text{ mcg/mL}$$

Step 5: Determine the drip rate with a microdrip IV infusion set that delivers 60 gtt/mL.

$$\frac{100 \text{ mcg/min} \times 60 \text{ gtt/mL}}{1,600 \text{ mcg/mL}} = \text{gtt/min}$$

Step 6: Cross out like terms and multiply across.

$$\frac{100 \cancel{\text{ mcg}}/\text{min} \times 60 \text{ gtt}/\cancel{\text{mL}}}{1,600 \cancel{\text{ mcg}}/\cancel{\text{mL}}} = \text{gtt/min}$$

Note: The zeros can be crossed out if only one above and one below the line are crossed out at a time, as in this example:

$$\frac{10\cancel{0} \cancel{\text{ mcg}}/\text{min} \times 6\cancel{0} \text{ gtt}/\cancel{\text{mL}}}{1,6\cancel{00} \cancel{\text{ mcg}}/\cancel{\text{mL}}} = \text{gtt/min}$$

If the problem is rewritten by leaving out everything that has been crossed out, it becomes much simpler:

$$\frac{10/\text{min} \times 6 \text{ gtt}}{16} = 3.75 \text{ gtt/min} \left(\text{round up to } 4 \text{ gtt/min}\right)$$

▶ Practical Application Problems

Answers to the problems in this section are found in Appendix E.

CASE STUDY

Ventricular Fibrillation

You are assisting in the resuscitation of a 49-year-old man who is unresponsive and apneic. The cardiac monitor shows ventricular fibrillation, and the paramedic in charge has directed you to prepare and give the medications. Cardiopulmonary resuscitation (CPR) is being performed, defibrillation has been appropriately accomplished, the patient has been successfully intubated and is being bagged with 100% oxygen, and an IV line has been established.

1. The first medication to administer is epinephrine 1:10,000 1 mg IV push. Your prefilled syringe reads epinephrine 1:10,000 1 mg/10 mL. How many milliliters should you administer?

(continued) Five minutes later, you are asked to repeat the previous dose of epinephrine, but you discover that your IV line has infiltrated. The paramedic directs you to administer twice the dose through the endotracheal tube. The patient has good lung sounds bilaterally with bagging.

2. You begin to prepare 2 mg of epinephrine 1:1,000. With prefilled syringes containing 1 mg/mL each, how many milliliters of the epinephrine will you administer?

(*continued*) After additional ventilating and CPR, the ventricular fibrillation continues. Another IV line has been established and is patent. You are now ordered to administer amiodarone 300 mg IV line.

3. Your prefilled syringe reads amiodarone 50 mg/mL. How many milliliters should you administer?

(*continued*) CPR, artificial ventilation, and defibrillation continue, and the epinephrine has been appropriately repeated. You are now ordered to administer 150 mg of amiodarone IV.

4. With another prefilled syringe that reads amiodarone 50 mg/mL, how many milliliters should you administer this time?

(*continued*) Attempts to resuscitate have resulted in the patient establishing a rhythm and pulse.

CASE STUDY

Pulseless Electrical Activity

You have responded to a call for help from the daughter of an 81-year-old man who has fallen. As you pull in the driveway, the dispatcher reports that the daughter called again to say that her father is now unresponsive. On arrival, you assess the patient and find that he is apneic and pulseless. You begin CPR, ventilating with 100% oxygen, and apply the quick-look paddles only to see a sinus tachycardia on the monitor at 120 beats/min. You once again check for a pulse but do not find one.

Your partners continue CPR, intubate the patient, and start an IV line. You administer a dose of epinephrine and question his daughter regarding his medical history. You learn that he is a heavy drinker and was vomiting blood earlier today but refused to go to the hospital. Medical direction tells you to evaluate for hypovolemia by administering a bolus of 500 mL normal saline over the next 20 minutes. You set up your IV line with a macrodrip IV infusion set that delivers 10 gtt/mL.

5. What is your drip rate per minute?

6. What is your drip rate per second?

(*continued*) You notice that the patient's heart rate has dropped to 50 beats/min on the monitor. Medical direction now tells you to also administer a bolus of atropine 0.5 mg rapid IV push. Your prefilled syringe reads 1 mg/10 mL.

7. How many milliliters will you administer? (Show how your work fits into formula 1.)

CASE STUDY

Acute Coronary Syndromes

You are caring for a patient who reports chest pain that suggests cardiac origin. You and your partner have begun supportive care, including oxygen at 100%, vital signs, IV line of normal saline to keep open, and positioning for comfort. Your protocol says to administer aspirin 320 mg. The bottle of aspirin in your drug box is labeled 160 mg/tablet.

8. How many tablets will you administer? (Hint: Use formula 1.)

CASE STUDY

Symptomatic Bradycardia

You respond to a law firm office for a 55-year-old woman with mild chest pain, dizziness, and shortness of breath that began when she returned from lunch. She is pale, cool, and moist to the touch but is oriented to person, place, time, and event. After beginning your supportive care, you find that the cardiac monitor shows a sinus bradycardia and her vital signs are as follows: blood pressure, 84/50 mm Hg; pulse, 50 beats/min; respirations, 20 breaths/min; lung sounds, clear.

You consider immediate transport, but the building's electric power is out because of a snowstorm and the elevators are not functioning. You decide to attempt to stabilize on scene.

After administering the maximum dosage of atropine without change and after seeing no response to the transcutaneous pacemaker (TCP) that you applied when the patient's heart rate did not improve with the atropine, you are advised by medical direction to initiate a dopamine infusion at 4 mcg/kg per minute. The patient weighs 110 pounds.

Your drug box contains dopamine in a prefilled syringe that reads dopamine 800 mg and bags of 500 mL normal saline. You also choose a microdrip infusion set that delivers 60 gtt/mL.

9. Calculate the DD by changing pounds to kilograms and then multiplying kilograms by the desired dose of 4 mcg/kg per minute.

10. Calculate the DH when you add 800 mg (800,000 mcg) to 500 mL.

11. What will the drip rate be per minute?

12. What will the drip rate be per second?

(*continued*) The dopamine infusion is ineffective, your patient is feeling worse, and the snowstorm is getting worse. Medical direction is depending on you to "bring the emergency department to the patient." They direct you to now try administering an epinephrine infusion by adding epinephrine 1 mg to a bag of 250 mL normal saline and starting the drip at 2 mcg/min. (Hint: You can either add epinephrine 1:1,000 or epinephrine 1:10,000 to the bag; both equal 1 mg, or 1,000 mcg.)

13. What will the DH be?

14. What will the drip rate be in drops per minute?

15. What will the drip rate be in drops per second?

(*continued*) Finally, the epinephrine infusion works.

CASE STUDY

Neurologic and Endocrine Emergencies

Your patient has severe diabetes and takes insulin on a daily basis. However, because of financial constraints, he did not take his insulin yesterday or today. He is confused and disoriented. Because you are not sure whether this is hyperglycemia or hypoglycemia and you do not have access to a glucometer, you choose to start an IV line in a large vein and administer dextrose 50% 25 g (50 mL) IV push. The patient has no response, and you begin to suspect a possible drug overdose. Your next choice is naloxone (Narcan).

Your prefilled syringe contains 0.4 mg naloxone in 2 mL normal saline. The order is for 0.4 mg naloxone. You know that if he shows no response you may need to administer as much as 10 mg naloxone depending on what drug was used. You receive an order to give 0.8 mg of naloxone.

16. How much naloxone should you administer if medical direction orders 0.8 mg?

CASE STUDY

You respond to an 11-year-old girl with grand mal seizures. She weighs approximately 88 pounds and has a history of seizures caused by an injury as an infant. Her mother tells you that she had to stop giving her the usual medications because of financial constraints. Medical direction tells you to administer diazepam 5 mg slow IV push or until the seizures stop. Your prefilled syringe contains 10 mg/mL.

17. How many milliliters will you administer IV push?

CASE STUDY

Your patient is a 51-year-old man newly diagnosed with diabetes. He is exhibiting signs and symptoms of an acute diabetic emergency, and medical direction advises the administration of 50% dextrose (0.5 g dextrose/mL) via IV push. Your partner has established an IV line in a large vein, and you estimate the patient's weight to be approximately 165 pounds.

18. If medical direction wants you to give 25 g of 50% dextrose IV push to this patient, how many milliliters will you give?

CASE STUDY

You have been called by the local police unit to care for a prisoner who is exhibiting signs and symptoms of drug withdrawal while at the local jail. When you discover pinpoint pupils, hypotension, respiratory depression, and nausea, you realize that you are dealing with a patient who has overdosed on a drug. You call medical direction, and they direct you to administer 2 mg of naloxone. Your vial reads 0.4 mg/mL.

19. How many milliliters will you administer?

CASE STUDY

On a cold winter night your unit is called to care for and transport a homeless person found in a stairwell covered only with old newspapers. He appears to be hypothermic, and an empty bottle of an alcoholic beverage is found tucked under his body. He is breathing, has a pulse, and has a readable blood pressure. However, even during your examination, he is unresponsive. His pupils are slow to respond but eventually do constrict in response to light. He appears to be malnourished for his height. No identification or other information is available to you.

You bring him immediately into your warmed ambulance and decide to give him 50% dextrose and thiamine because you suspect that he is an undernourished alcoholic. The thiamine in the drug box is packaged as 100 mg/mL.

Once you move him to the ambulance, you are able to initiate an IV line to administer normal saline at a keep-open rate. Medical direction directs you to administer 200 mg of thiamine and transport as soon as possible.

20. How many milliliters will you administer?

CHAPTER 5

Intravenous Fluids and Administration

OBJECTIVES

1. Define *total body water* and its two main compartments (intracellular fluid and extracellular fluid).
2. Define *osmosis* and explain the difference between isotonic, hypotonic, and hypertonic fluids in terms in osmotic pressure.
3. Discuss colloid solutions used in intravenous (IV) therapy.
4. Define *hypertonic saline solutions*.
5. Discuss electrolyte solutions used in IV therapy: calcium gluconate, sodium bicarbonate, insulin, and 5% dextrose.
6. Define *drop factor, microdrip chambers,* and *macrodrip chambers*.
7. List and discuss various appropriate sites for IV line insertion.
8. Demonstrate the proper procedures for the following: IV insertion, IV push, IV piggyback, IV infusion, and intraosseous infusion.
9. List the complications of IV line infiltration, catheter shear, and phlebitis.

MEDICATIONS THAT APPEAR IN CHAPTER 5

Albumin	Sodium bicarbonate	Dextrose (50%, 25%, 10%)
Hypertonic saline (3% saline)	Insulin, regular (Humulin R,	Potassium chloride
Calcium gluconate	Novolin R)	

▶ Introduction

Intravenous (IV) lines are started to administer IV fluids and to provide access for rapid delivery of emergency medications. Various types of IV fluids are used based on the patient's clinical needs. Not all IV fluids are created equal, but what makes each type unique? The most obvious answer is the electrolytes and concentrations that compose the various IV fluids. The human body is essentially a bag of sea water divided into two compartments: **intracellular fluid (ICF)**, which is fluid found inside the cells, and **extracellular fluid (ECF)**, which comprises **intravascular fluid** and **interstitial fluid** (fluid between the cells and outside the vascular bed).

A common misconception is that administered IV fluids are targeted and remain within the confines of the body's blood vessels. **Isotonic** IV solutions have the same salt concentration as (normal) body cells. Salts are chemical compounds consisting of a substance with a positive electrical charge combined with a substance with a negative electrical charge, resulting in an electrically neutral substance. When salts are dissolved in water, they have the potential to conduct electricity and are known as **electrolytes**. Sodium is the most prominent electrolyte in blood and interstitial fluid. Potassium is the most prominent electrolyte in body cells. Electrolyte changes in one location (intracellular, intravascular, or interstitial) cause alterations of electrolyte concentrations in other locations, either from movement of water or the shifting of electrolytes. By altering the various concentrations of the electrolytes in the IV fluids, especially sodium, the prehospital professional can target the fluid to the body's different fluid compartments. Isotonic fluids are discussed in greater detail later in this chapter.

Blood is an instrument to increase oxygen delivery to peripheral tissues. In addition to oxygen delivery, blood products are frequently administered for intravascular volume expansion, or to improve blood-clotting ability in a wide variety of clinical situations. Indications for blood transfusion have become increasingly stringent. Many air-medical and critical care transport (CCT) programs carry blood products for use outside of the hospital. Paramedics performing interfacility transports may continue blood product transfusions initiated in the sending facility.

This chapter focuses on the different indications for IV fluid replacement and the various types of fluids used. The procedure for initiating IV access is also discussed later in this chapter.

CASE STUDY

You are a ranger with the National Park Service. For the past 2 days, you have been involved in a search for two lost hikers. The hikers are eventually found at the base of a canyon. You attend to the first patient, a 20-year-old man who appears weak and severely dehydrated. He tells you that he and his partner were without water for 2.5 days, and the temperature was in excess of 90°F (32.2°C). He reports that he has not urinated in the past 24 hours, and when he did, his urine was dark. On examination, the patient's skin is warm and dry. He has poor skin turgor. The mucous membranes of his mouth are dry and have an almost tacky appearance. His heart rate is 122 beats/min, blood pressure is 96/78 mm Hg, and respiratory rate is 18 breaths/min. His weight is approximately 175 pounds (80 kg).

The patient arrives at the hospital, and a nurse draws blood for evaluation of his serum electrolytes and renal function. The physicians agree with your assessment that the patient is significantly dehydrated. The laboratory tests indicate some acute renal insufficiency manifested by elevated serum creatine and blood urea nitrogen levels. His serum sodium level is markedly elevated because of the dehydration. The physicians calculate that the patient's free water deficit is approximately 6 L. The physician tells you he will replace only half of that fluid in the next 24 hours. He explains that overly rapid fluid replacement causes the serum sodium level to drop too rapidly, which could lead to a form of brain damage.

This patient appears to be dehydrated from a combination of excessive exposure and lack of hydration. **Dehydration** is a loss of water from the fluid space inside the cells. Dehydration can take hours to days to develop. As the cell dehydrates, it begins to malfunction, leading to poor function of tissues, metabolic acidosis, and eventually organ failure.

Dehydration can be illustrated by imagining that a grape is a cell. The grape slowly loses fluid and dehydrates to form a raisin. With dehydration, the cells lose fluid and essentially wither.

As a general rule, conditions that quickly develop should be quickly corrected, and conditions that slowly develop should be slowly corrected. For example, after acute blood loss, such as in trauma, volume replacement occurs over a short period, often measured in minutes to hours, because the blood loss occurred over a rather brief period. Fluid loss in dehydration occurs over a period of days. When such patients are evaluated at the hospital, the physician often calculates the patient's free water (or fluid) deficit. If a patient has a calculated fluid deficit of 6 L, no more than half of the calculated deficit (3 L) should be replaced in the first 24-hour period.

In the preceding hiking scenario, the patient's dehydration developed over several days; therefore, his dehydration should be corrected in a slow and deliberate fashion. An initial **fluid bolus** of 1 to 2 L of isotonic crystalloid 0.9% sodium chloride (NaCl) would be appropriate, with the balance of the fluid loss replaced over a period of 24 to 48 hours. The purpose of prehospital care in this scenario is to start rehydrating the patient, which begins with choosing an IV fluid that provides rehydration to the intracellular space and expands the volume of fluid within the vascular space. It is extremely important to frequently monitor a patient's serum electrolyte levels during fluid replacement, particularly when there are significant alterations in potassium, glucose, or sodium. Excessively rapid correction or overcorrection can be very harmful.

As previously mentioned, a cell that has become dehydrated is like a grape that has become a raisin. Additionally, the stranded hiker's low blood pressure and tachycardia also indicate that he has some depletion of intravascular volume. *Isotonic crystalloid solutions are the preferred initial treatment for dehydration.*[1]

A basic understanding of the body fluid compartments is required to understand the implications of IV fluid administration and, in this case, treat patients with dehydration.

▶ Body Fluid Compartments

Most of the human body is composed of water. In adults, this amounts to approximately 45% to 65% of the body. In an average man weighing 176 pounds (80 kg), this equals approximately 48 L. The total amount of water in the body is known as the **total body water (TBW)** (**FIGURE 5-1**). TBW is divided into two main compartments: ICF space and ECF space. As discussed previously, ICF is found inside the cells (*intra*cellular), and ECF is found outside the cells (*extra*cellular), between the cells and inside the blood vessels.[2] Two thirds of the TBW is found in the ICF, and one third is in the ECF. Of the ECF, three fourths is found in the interstitial fluid, and one fourth resides in the blood vessels, or the **intravascular space**.

> TBW: 45% to 65% of total body weight
> > ICF: two thirds of TBW
> > ECF: one third of TBW
> > > Intravascular fluid: one fourth of ECF
> > > Interstitial fluid: three fourths of ECF

Interstitial fluid is the space outside the vascular space that is between the cells. For the sake of illustration, consider the blood vessels to be pipes running alongside a brick wall. The volume inside the confines of the pipes is the intravascular space. The bricks are the cells of the body, and the volume of those bricks is the intracellular volume. On a brick wall, mortar is in the narrow space between the bricks. The definition of *interstitial* is "the narrow space between things or parts." Therefore, in this example, the mortar of the wall is the interstitial space—the volume of fluid outside the bricks of cells. The mortar (interstitial fluid) and volume of the pipes (intravascular fluid) both compose the ECF (**FIGURE 5-2**).

Water can move freely from one body fluid compartment to another. The compartments are separated by membranes that water can freely move across. The concentration of particles in a particular body compartment drives the movement of fluids. Particles can be dissolved in salt or a body protein, but they cannot freely pass across the membranes separating the body compartments; cell membranes are quite particular regarding which types of particles they

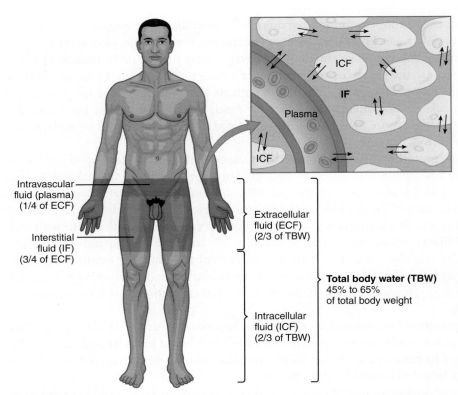

FIGURE 5-1 Body fluid compartments. 45% to 65% of the body is composed of water. Two thirds of this fluid is inside the millions of cells making up the various tissues and organs (intracellular fluid). The remaining one third of the fluid is the extracellular fluid, which is found outside the cells in the blood vessels (intravascular fluid) and between the cells (interstitial fluid).

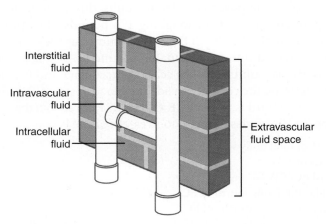

FIGURE 5-2 The extravascular fluid space can be viewed as a brick wall. The bricks represent the cells, and the fluid inside the bricks is the ICF. Interstitial fluid is the fluid that resides between the cells. In this illustration, the mortar of the brick wall represents the interstitial fluid, because the mortar fills the space between the "cellular bricks." The intravascular fluid is the fluid that is within the pipes of the blood vessels.

allow into the internal environment. In the body, the key particle is the electrolyte sodium. Particles that cannot freely pass across a membrane act as magnets for fluid. When particles are trapped on one side of a membrane that is permeable to water, the water will move toward the higher concentration of particles. The movement of water across such a membrane toward a higher concentration of particles is known as **osmosis** (**FIGURE 5-3**).

FIGURE 5-3 Osmosis. The *blue* particles represent water and can move freely across the membrane in the center of the chamber. The *red* particles represent a substance that cannot move across the central membrane. The water moves across the semipermeable membrane toward the higher concentration of the trapped red particles. This process is known as *osmosis*.

FIGURE 5-4 D_5W, which is free of any particles, distributes itself to the various compartments in proportion to each compartment's percentage of total body water (TBW). The extracellular fluid (*red* and *blue*) is one third of the TBW. Therefore, one third of the administered 1000 mL of D_5W (333 mL) is distributed to this space. The intravascular space is only one fourth of the extracellular fluid. Only one fourth of the 333 mL remains in the intravascular space. After administering 1,000 mL of D_5W, only 83 mL will remain in the intravascular space after the fluid has had an opportunity to redistribute between the various fluid spaces.

When "water," or dextrose 5% in water (D_5W), which is free of any particles, is added to one compartment, it is then freely distributed to the various body fluid compartments in proportion to their percentage of TBW. For example, if 1,000 mL of water is administered as an IV bolus to a patient, it will be redistributed to the various compartments in the following way (**FIGURE 5-4**):

    1,000 mL of D_5W IV
       ICF (two thirds of TBW) = 666 mL
       ECF (one third of TBW) = 333 mL
          Extravascular fluid (three fourths of ECF) = 250 mL
          Intravascular fluid (one fourth of ECF) = 83 mL

All this movement of water occurs within 30 minutes of administration of the IV bolus, and less than 9% of it remains in the blood vessels at the end of the 30 minutes. Because the fluid that is administered lacks any particles, the water can freely distribute itself among all the body compartments.

An IV fluid that distributes throughout several body compartments is said to have a large volume of distribution; this type of fluid improves a patient's intravascular and extravascular volume. Chapter 1 discussed the notion that drugs must get to their intended site of action to achieve the desired effect. These same properties apply to IV fluids. If the intention of the provider is to increase the intravascular volume, the provider must choose a fluid that provides maximal expansion of the intravascular space. Attempting to improve a patient's intravascular volume by giving a fluid of which only 9 mL of every 100 mL administered remains in the vascular space is highly inefficient. A better choice of IV fluid would be one in which 25 mL of every 100 mL administered remains in the vascular space. These examples demonstrate the concept of distribution volume. When the treatment goal is fluid resuscitation, a smaller distribution volume is more efficient. By decreasing the distribution volume, a greater proportion of the fluid administered remains in the vascular space.

Infusion of fluids containing particles reduces the distribution volume. That is, limiting the movement of particles limits the distribution volume, and more of the fluid remains in the vascular space. Returning to the previous example, consider a change in the type of fluid from D_5W to a fluid typically used in the prehospital setting, such as normal saline (0.9% NaCl) and Ringer's lactate solution. The salt and electrolytes in these fluids serve as particles. Their sodium concentration approximates that of the extracellular space, and the intracellular space is excluded. As discussed earlier, isotonic solutions have the same sodium concentration as body water.

If the patient is given 1,000 mL of normal saline over a 60-minute period, the resultant increase in the intravascular volume ultimately is only 250 mL, as shown here (**FIGURE 5-5**):

1000 mL of normal saline IV
    ICF (two thirds of TBW): salt particles will not enter = 0 mL
    ECF (one third of TBW) = 1,000 mL
        Interstitial fluid (three fourths of ECF) = 750 mL
        Intravascular fluid (one fourth of ECF) = 250 mL

Predicting the distribution of various types of IV fluids (e.g., 0.45 or 0.23% normal saline) is possible to determine the optimal fluid to administer. **TABLE 5-1** lists the various IV fluids. For example, the patient in the earlier hiking scenario is dehydrated and has depleted intravascular volume. Therefore, the fluid this patient receives should provide some expansion of

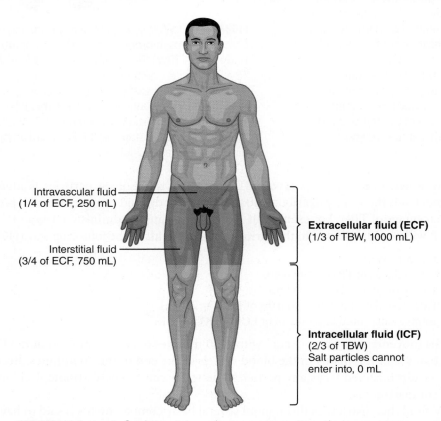

Intravascular fluid
(1/4 of ECF, 250 mL)

Interstitial fluid
(3/4 of ECF, 750 mL)

Extracellular fluid (ECF)
(1/3 of TBW, 1000 mL)

Intracellular fluid (ICF)
(2/3 of TBW)
Salt particles cannot
enter into, 0 mL

FIGURE 5-5 Isotonic fluids contain sodium concentrations that approximate that of the extracellular space. Isotonic fluids have sodium concentrations similar to that of body water, which limits the distribution to the extracellular fluid compartment. The administered 1,000 mL will distribute between the two compartments of the extracellular fluid (intravascular [*red*] and interstitial [*blue*]) in proportion to each compartment's percentage of the extracellular fluid. After distribution, approximately 250 mL of the administered 1,000 mL of isotonic fluid will remain intravascular after redistribution.

TABLE 5-1 Volume of Distribution of Various IV Fluids

1,000-mL Bolus	Intracellular	Extracellular	Interstitial	Intravascular
Normal saline (0.9%) or Ringer's lactate solution (isotonic)	0 mL	1,000 mL	750 mL	250 mL
0.5 Normal saline (0.45%)	333 mL	667 mL	500 mL	167 mL
0.25 Normal saline (0.23%)	500 mL	500 mL	375 mL	125 mL
D_5W	666 mL	333 mL	250 mL	83 mL

© Jones & Bartlett Learning.

TABLE 5-2 Volume of Distribution of 1,000 mL of 0.45% Normal Saline

	500 mL Water	500 mL Saline	Total Fluid
Intracellular fluid	333 mL	0 mL	333 mL
Extracellular fluid	167 mL	500 mL	667 mL
Interstitial fluid	125 mL	375 mL	500 mL
Intravascular fluid	42 mL	125 mL	167 mL

© Jones & Bartlett Learning.

intravascular volume, as well as the fluid in the intracellular space. A good choice of IV fluid in this case is 0.45% normal saline. The following is a description of where this fluid is distributed among the vascular spaces. EMS should avoid attempting to manipulate body sodium concentrations without ongoing electrolyte monitoring and consultation with medical control.

Giving a patient 1,000 mL of 0.45% normal saline is equivalent to giving 500 mL of normal saline and 500 mL of water. Therefore, the fluids would be distributed in the amounts shown in **TABLE 5-2**. Infusion of 0.45% saline is effective in treating a dehydrated patient. This fluid replaces fluid in the vascular space but does not result in much fluid in the intracellular space. As such, this would be ineffective in treating a patient who is acutely hypovolemic from blood loss.

CASE STUDY

You are dispatched to provide assistance to a woman who is reporting severe diarrhea. After your arrival, you learn that the patient ate a buffet dinner approximately 1 hour before feeling ill. She informs you that she had abdominal cramping, followed by two bouts of vomiting, followed by several episodes of severe and watery diarrhea. Your assessment of the patient reveals a 34-year-old woman who is resting on her living room couch. She reports mild abdominal discomfort. She is mildly diaphoretic. Her heart rate is 134 beats/min, blood pressure is 88/66 mm Hg, and respiratory rate is 20 breaths/min. Her mucous membranes are dry. On physical examination, she is tachycardic, lungs are clear, abdomen is soft, and only minimal tenderness is felt on deep palpation.

This patient has acute hypovolemia from vomiting and diarrhea. She is symptomatic, as demonstrated by tachycardia and low blood pressure. The cause of acute hypovolemia must be distinguished from hypovolemia due to acute blood loss. This patient lost fluid that is essentially composed of water and electrolytes. In contrast, acute hemorrhage is from a loss of plasma and red blood cells. A blood sample from the patient with diarrhea would reveal her blood count (hemoglobin concentration and hematocrit) to be elevated. The concentration of red blood cells increases with a decrease in intravascular fluid, whereas the number of red blood cells remains unchanged. In contrast, within several hours of volume loss from acute blood loss, the blood counts (hemoglobin and hematocrit) decrease from the loss of red blood cells and intravascular fluid. Because this patient's condition developed acutely over a period of hours, the treatment needs to take place over a period of hours. The objective of treatment is volume expansion of the intravascular space. This can be accomplished by giving an infusion of an isotonic fluid, such as normal saline or Ringer's lactate, which provides reexpansion of the vascular space.

Volume Expansion

Intravascular volume is often depleted by illness and injury, and restoration of that volume is required to reestablish perfusion to vital organs and tissues. Decreased volume results in a decrease in cardiac output, and decreased cardiac output results in decreased oxygen delivery. In this case, the patient needs a fluid that maximally expands the intravascular volume. Isotonic fluids, normal saline, and Ringer's lactate allow the greatest expansion of the intravascular volume. A general rule is that for any given amount of blood loss, at least three times the amount of crystalloid is required to increase the intravascular volume to compensate for the loss of blood. Because of the large volume of IV fluids distribution, the fluids shift, or leak, out of the vascular space to the interstitial and intracellular spaces. For any significant fluid or blood loss that would produce clinical symptoms of hypovolemia, the amount of required volume replacement is beyond that allowed for by most EMS protocols. From a prehospital perspective, any significant fluid resuscitation is beyond the scope of what can be accomplished in the field. Therefore, hypovolemic patients must be transferred to definitive care in a timely fashion.

After a period of blood loss, the body responds by attempting to autoresuscitate, or shift fluid from both the intracellular space and interstitial space into intravascular space. The result is that cells can become dehydrated and malfunction, causing organ failure. Resuscitation is the administration of IV fluids to patients to replace lost fluids. Shortly after acute blood loss, the body recognizes the need to expand the intravascular volume and responds by shifting fluid from the extravascular space toward the intravascular space. In this manner, the body automatically attempts to resuscitate itself (autoresuscitation).

In the case of acute blood loss, intravascular fluid replacement may need to occur in minutes to resuscitate the patient and prevent multiple organ failure. At the same time, excessive resuscitation can result in edema and pulmonary complications.

Crystalloids are IV fluids in which sodium is the primary particle that controls volume distribution. The most common types of crystalloid fluids used by prehospital providers are Ringer's lactate solution and normal saline. The movement of water through the various fluid compartments is controlled by the biologic principle of osmosis. Osmosis is the diffusion of water across a semipermeable membrane. Particles that are trapped in a particular fluid compartment act like a magnet to attract water to that compartment. In reality, the trapped particles do not attract the movement of water; the difference in concentration gradients between the two compartments does. The greater the concentration of trapped particles, the greater the movement of water. Water moves from the compartment of lower concentration to the compartment of higher concentration. As the water moves into that compartment, the concentration of the trapped particles decreases as they are diluted by the newly added water. Water continues to move down the concentration gradient until a difference in concentration between the two compartments no longer exists.

In the body, the particles in solution that attract water, or exert osmotic pressure, are sodium and serum proteins (e.g., albumin). Fluids that have equal osmotic pressure with the body under normal conditions are called isotonic. Fluids that have less osmotic pressure are hypotonic, and hypertonic fluids have greater than normal osmotic pressure. As previously mentioned, electrolytes (sodium) or large molecules, such as proteins or complex sugars, are added to IV fluids to exert osmotic pressure. Crystalloid solutions are IV fluids that use electrolytes to provide osmotic pressure. **Colloid solutions** use complex molecules such as proteins and complex sugars for osmotic pressure. Isotonic fluids contain sodium and other electrolyte concentrations that closely mimic the concentration of the ECF. In a healthy person, 1 hour after infusion of 1,000 mL of isotonic fluids, only 250 mL of the infused fluid remains in the intravascular space. In critically ill or injured patients, the amount of fluid that remains in the vascular space can be less than 200 mL.[3]

A thorough understanding of hypovolemia and the various forms of volume replacement is required of all advanced prehospital providers. The causes of hypovolemia are numerous and include bleeding, burns, vomiting, diarrhea, diabetic ketoacidosis, sepsis, and bowel obstruction. A healthy person has a remarkable capacity to compensate for intravascular volume loss. Therefore, by the time a patient has symptoms of hypovolemia, the prehospital provider can assume that the magnitude of the volume loss is significant. In the case of acute blood loss, a 154-pound (70-kg) patient will lose greater than 30% of his or her blood volume before exhibiting hypotension.

> (*continued*) Your assessment is that the patient has acute hypovolemia as a result of food poisoning. You believe a fluid bolus is warranted because the patient has clinical signs and symptoms of hypovolemia. You insert a peripheral IV line and determine that an isotonic fluid would be the best choice for this patient because you need to rehydrate both the intravascular and extravascular spaces. You start the fluid bolus of 1,000 mL of Ringer's lactate to run in over a 1-hour period. You arrive at the hospital in approximately 20 minutes, and roughly 350 mL of the fluid bolus has been delivered to the patient. From a clinical standpoint, you observe a slight improvement in vital signs: heart rate of 118 beats/min, blood pressure of 102/78 mm Hg, and respiratory rate of 16 breaths/min.

In the preceding scenario, isotonic fluid is the fluid of choice. Isotonic fluids such as normal saline and Ringer's lactate have large volumes of distribution, and the prehospital provider needs to infuse an amount greater than the estimated fluid loss. The total volume of fluid delivered should be three to five times the amount of blood loss to increase the intravascular fluid. In this scenario, the appropriate fluid choice would be either Ringer's lactate or normal saline.

▶ Delivery of IV Fluids

Rapid fluid losses require rapid replacement. A fluid bolus is a large volume of IV fluid administered as quickly as possible. In extreme situations, an IV fluid bolus is administered through the largest IV catheter possible, simultaneously through multiple IV sites, using commercial pressure bags, squeezing the IV fluid bags, or using a commercial rapid-infuser device (**FIGURE 5-6**). Other strategies include using larger-diameter or shorter IV tubing, using a 10- or 15-drop/mL IV tubing set, elevating the fluids as high as possible above the patient, and eliminating any unnecessary IV tubing connectors, including claves, adapters, and so on

A   B

FIGURE 5-6 A. Rapid-infuser device. **B.** IV pressure bag.

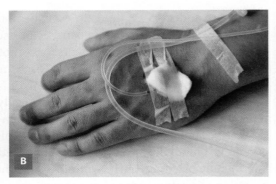

FIGURE 5-7 IV tubing with (**A**) and without (**B**) clave adapters.

(A) © mindfullness/Shutterstock; (B) © iStockphoto/Thinkstock.

(**FIGURE 5-7**). In most situations, EMS providers simply hang the fluids high above the patient with the tubing roller clamp "wide open."

A typical fluid bolus in an adult is 1,000 mL (1 L) administered over a 15- to 60-minute period. Conditions such as septic shock may require boluses of 30 mL/kg in adults. A fluid bolus in a pediatric patient is 10 to 20 mL/kg. Fluid boluses in infants and neonates are typically done with a syringe or commercial infusion pump rather than IV bag, as volume overload can easily occur in these populations.

The key to rapid IV fluid administration for an adult is two large-bore IV catheters, either 14 or 16 gauge. The size of the catheter has a profound effect on the rate at which IV fluids can be given. The rate at which IV fluids can be administered is determined by the length and radius of the catheter. The radius of the catheter, described as "gauge," has a profound effect on determining the rate of fluid administration. Short and fat catheters typically are the most effective for rapid administration of IV fluids or medications. Shorter IV catheters improve the rate of fluid infusion; however, they must be long enough to remain secure within the patient's vein and not allow fluid to escape the intravascular space.

During IV bolus administration, it is extremely important to monitor the IV site for signs of infiltration (discussed later in this chapter). It is also important to not attempt an infusion rate that the patient cannot tolerate; key considerations include the patient's medical condition, such as heart failure or pulmonary edema, and the integrity of the patient's veins near the IV site. Patients may experience hypothermia when large quantities of cool or even room-temperature fluids are infused. Any patient without underlying hyperthermia should have warming measures in place when large volumes of IV fluids or blood products are being administered. Use continuous patient core temperature monitoring if available.

CASE STUDY

You are a paramedic working on the flight crew of an air-medical service, and your aircraft is dispatched to an industrial accident at a sawmill. You arrive to find a 38-year-old man who has had a traumatic amputation of his right leg at the level of the mid-femur. The patient is hemorrhaging from his severed femoral artery. He is awake and alert. His airway is patent, and he is breathing spontaneously. Respiratory rate is shallow and rapid, heart rate is 138 beats/min, respiratory rate is 24 breaths/min, and blood pressure is 78/62 mm Hg. You apply direct pressure to the wound, which slows the rate of hemorrhage. Your partner applies a tourniquet, which stops the bleeding. You place a 14-gauge IV catheter in each arm.

This patient is in hypovolemic shock from rapid blood loss. The objective of fluid therapy in this case is to restore perfusion and oxygen delivery rapidly.

(continued) The victim from the sawmill accident has lost approximately 45% to 50% of his circulating blood volume from the injury to his femoral artery. After your partner applies the tourniquet, you obtain a blood sample and a hemoglobin concentration. Upon arrival at the hospital, the hemoglobin level from the blood that you drew returns as normal despite the patient's profound and life-threatening blood loss.

Colloid Solutions

Colloid solutions contain large molecules that have a preference for the vascular space. The 3:1 rule dictates that paramedics should administer three times the volume of crystalloid for a given loss of blood volume. However, this rule underestimates extravascular fluid shifts.

To carry a significant volume of IV fluids in an ambulance is not problematic. However, military or rural providers are limited by what they can carry. Colloids and hypertonic fluids provide an advantage for these providers by providing greater volume expansion with less fluid administered. Albumin is an IV fluid that can expand the intravascular volume by 80% of the infused volume (compared with 25% for Ringer's lactate and normal saline). The role of albumin and other colloids in the resuscitation of critically ill and injured patients has been the source of great debate for decades, with no current consensus.[1] A variety of other colloid solutions are available; however, their role and use in the prehospital setting remain quite limited. EMS providers who encounter these solutions during interfacility transports should review the dosing, indications, contraindications, risks, and monitoring requirements for the particular solutions commonly used in that setting or area.

The idea that albumin is limited to the intravascular space is a widely held misconception. Under normal conditions, 30% to 40% of albumin is in the intravascular space and 50% to

ALBUMIN

Classification: Volume expander, colloid.
Action: Increases oncotic pressure in intravascular space.
Indications: Expand intravascular volume.
Adverse Effects: Allergic reaction in some patients; an excessive volume of fluid can result in congestive heart failure and pulmonary edema in susceptible patients.
Contraindications: Severe anemia or cardiac failure in the presence of normal or increased intravascular volume, solution appears turbid or after 4 hours since opening the container, known sensitivity.
Dosage: Two preparations: 500 mL of a 5% solution (250 mL of a 5% solution also available) and 100 mL of a 25% solution (50 mL of a 25% solution also available).

- **Adult:**
  - **5% albumin:** 500 to 1,000 mL IV, intraosseous (IO).
  - **25% albumin:** 50 to 200 mL IV, IO.
- **Pediatric:**
  - **5% albumin:** 0.5 to 1 g/kg IV; the initial dose may be repeated in 15 to 30 minutes if the clinical response is inadequate.
  - **25% albumin:** 1 g/kg IV, IO.

Special Considerations:
Patients with a history of congestive heart failure, cardiac disease, hypertension, and pulmonary edema should be given 5% albumin, or the 25% albumin should be diluted. Because 25% of albumin increases intravascular volume greater than the volume administered, slowly administer 25% albumin in normovolemic patients to prevent complications such as pulmonary edema.
Pregnancy class C.

60% is in the interstitial space. The intravascular half-life of albumin is 16 hours, and 2 hours after infusion, 90% of albumin remains in the intravascular space. Albumin, as a colloid, is capable of recruiting extravascular water into the intravascular space; each gram of albumin is capable of "pulling" 18 mL of water.[4]

Hypertonic Saline Solutions

Hypertonic saline solutions have a concentration greater than the isotonic concentration of 0.9%. (Recall that isotonic solutions have the same sodium concentration as body water.) Typical hypertonic solutions are 3, 5, or 7% saline, roughly three to five times higher sodium concentration than standard normal saline. The higher concentration of sodium pulls more volume into the vascular space. Some solutions use particles other than sodium to make the fluid hypertonic. The net effect is that intravascular volume is increased by a greater volume than the total volume infused. Such a notion is attractive to military and rural providers, who are limited in the amount of supplies they can carry.

Critics of hypertonic fluid resuscitation have argued that pulling or mobilizing fluids from the interstitial and intracellular spaces results in the dysfunction of cells and tissues. However, research has shown that during periods of stress and shock, cells actually become fat and swell with additional water. The administration of hypertonic saline results in normalization of cellular water and volume. Although hypertonic fluids were previously believed to reduce cell volume below normal, animal research has demonstrated that administration of 7.5% hypertonic solution rapidly restores both blood pressure and cardiac output in the treatment of hemorrhagic shock. However, these improvements were short-lived; after 30 minutes, both blood pressure and cardiac output were similar to those animals treated with standard normal saline. Research remains active in this area, with the goal of identifying a fluid capable of rapid volume expansion limited to the vascular space and sustained improvement in blood pressure and cardiac output.[5,6]

HYPERTONIC SALINE (3% SALINE)

Classification: Volume expander, electrolyte solution.
Action: The hypertonic nature of this fluid pulls extravascular fluid into the vascular space. Hypertonic saline may therefore be used as a volume expander in cases of hypovolemia or to reduce the edema of the swollen brain. Three percent saline has an electrolyte concentration of 514 mEq/L sodium.
Indications: Reduction of increased intracranial pressure resulting from traumatic brain injury, hypovolemic shock.
Adverse Effects: Increased rate of bleeding, alteration of blood-clotting ability, **osmotic demyelination syndrome**.
Contraindications: Pulmonary congestion, pulmonary edema, known sensitivity. Hypertonic saline should not be administered by the IO route.
Dosage: Note: Hypertonic saline is available in several concentrations from 3% to 5%.

- **Adult:** 100 to 200 mL/hr
- **Pediatric:** 0.1 to 1 mL/kg per hour (off-label for most pediatric indications; consult with online medical control)

Special Considerations:
Hypertonic saline can cause damage to the vein in which it is administered.
Pregnancy class C.

Electrolytes

CASE STUDY

Your paramedic unit is dispatched to a long-term care facility for a medical call. The dispatcher reports that the patient, who has a medical history of renal failure requiring hemodialysis, is reporting nausea, vomiting, and diarrhea. You arrive to find a 78-year-old man lying in his bed. He appears weak and pale and tells you that he has felt ill all afternoon. He has had several episodes of vomiting and one episode of diarrhea. He underwent dialysis 2 days ago. His blood pressure is 146/92 mm Hg, heart rate is 94 beats/min, respiratory rate is 20 breaths/min, and oxygen saturation is 93%. His lungs are clear, and his heartbeat is regular. A dialysis fistula is noted in his left forearm. You place the patient on oxygen, start an IV of normal saline, and place the patient on the cardiac monitor, at which time you note that the patient has peaked T waves.

This case presents one of the few situations in which a prehospital professional may need to treat an electrolyte disorder without the benefit of laboratory tests. Prehospital providers do not have the luxury of laboratory blood tests. In contrast, hospital providers such as nurses and physicians typically treat various electrolyte disorders identified by laboratory blood tests. The paramedic, however, treats electrolyte disorders that have clinical manifestations. With the exception of **hyperkalemia** (elevated levels of potassium), the majority of electrolyte disorders are not immediately life-threatening and often can wait for treatment until confirmation by laboratory tests at a hospital. Hyperkalemia may occur in the presence of renal failure and presents with gastrointestinal symptoms of nausea, abdominal pain, and/or diarrhea. Other causes of hyperkalemia include burns, crush injuries, diabetic keto-acidosis, and severe infections. Patients with hyperkalemia can have cardiovascular signs of initially peaked T waves, widening of the QRS complex, and depression of the ST segment. If left untreated, hyperkalemia can progress to heart block and cardiac arrest. Patients with a rapid rise in potassium levels will experience severe signs and symptoms at lower levels than will patients with chronic or episodic hyperkalemia, such as those with chronic renal failure. Additionally, patients with underlying cardiac dysfunction have a decreased tolerance to increases in potassium.

In the preceding scenario, the paramedic should suspect hyperkalemia because the patient has a history of renal failure and has gone several days without hemodialysis. He has gastrointestinal symptoms of nausea, vomiting, and diarrhea, as well as peaked T waves on electrocardiography. The treatment objectives for this patient are to protect his heart from the effects of hyperkalemia and "hide" the potassium inside the cells. Protection of the potentially life-threatening cardiac complications from hyperkalemia can be achieved temporarily by administering IV calcium. Calcium works by several mechanisms to stabilize cell membranes and suppress cardiac rhythm disturbances caused by excess potassium. The preferred treatment is administering 1 g of 10% calcium gluconate solution. Calcium chloride can also be administered; however, it has three times the concentration of calcium and has the potential to cause calcium toxicity. Administration of calcium does nothing to alter the serum level of potassium.

Potassium can be sequestered in body cells as another temporary measure to prevent patient harm. To "hide the potassium," the potassium must be shifted from the extracellular space into the intracellular space. When available, IV administration of 50% dextrose and insulin is the preferred method of moving excess serum potassium into body cells. Insulin (10 U regular insulin) allows additional potassium to be hidden inside the cells. Dextrose (2.5 g) is given with the insulin to prevent hypoglycemia.

EMS providers can use sodium bicarbonate to also sequester potassium. Sodium bicarbonate rapidly shifts the potassium into the cells within minutes of administration, and the effect lasts up to 12 hours. Sodium bicarbonate works by pushing potassium into the cell in exchange for a hydrogen ion. One to two **ampules** (50 to 100 mEq) are usually required in adults.

Nebulized albuterol has some ability to also sequester potassium. It is not recommended as a primary treatment but can be used as an adjunct to the preceding approaches. The definitive treatment for hyperkalemia is either dialysis or direct removal from the body with diuretic medications or medications that bind and excrete potassium.

CALCIUM GLUCONATE

Classification: Electrolyte solution.
Action: Counteracts the toxicity of hyperkalemia by stabilizing the membranes of the cardiac cells, reducing the likelihood of fibrillation.
Indications: Hyperkalemia, hypocalcemia, hypermagnesemia.
Adverse Effects: Soft tissue necrosis, hypotension, bradycardia (if administered too rapidly).
Contraindications: Ventricular fibrillation, digitalis toxicity, hypercalcemia.
Dosage: Supplied as 10% solution; therefore, each milliliter contains 100 mg of calcium gluconate.
- **Adult:** 500 to 1,000 mg IV, IO administered slowly at a rate of approximately 1 to 1.5 mL/min; maximum dose 3 g IV, IO. It may also be ordered as 60 mg/kg per dose.
- **Pediatric:** 60 to 100 mg/kg IV, IO slowly over a 5- to 10-minute period; maximum dose 3 g IV, IO.

Special Considerations:
Do not administer by intramuscular (IM) or subcutaneous routes, which causes significant tissue necrosis.
Pregnancy class C.

SODIUM BICARBONATE

Classification: Electrolyte replacement.
Action: Counteracts existing acidosis.
Indications: Acidosis, drug intoxications (e.g., barbiturates, salicylates, methyl alcohol).
Adverse Effects: Metabolic alkalosis, hypernatremia, injection site reaction, sodium and fluid retention, peripheral edema.
Contraindications: Metabolic alkalosis, hypocalcemia.
Dosage:
Metabolic Acidosis During Cardiac Arrest:
- **Adult:** 1 mEq/kg slow IV, IO; may repeat at 0.5 mEq/kg in 10 minutes.
- **Pediatric:** Same as adult dosing.

Metabolic Acidosis Not Associated with Cardiac Arrest:
- **Adult:** Dosage should be individualized.
- **Pediatric:** Dosage should be individualized.

Special Considerations:
Do not administer into an IV, IO line in which another medication is being given.
Because of the high concentration of sodium within each ampule of sodium bicarbonate, use with caution in patients with congestive heart failure and renal disease.
Pregnancy class C.

INSULIN, REGULAR (HUMULIN R, NOVOLIN R)

Classification: Hormone.
Action: Binds to a receptor on the membrane of cells and facilitates the transport of glucose into cells.
Indications: Hyperglycemia, insulin-dependent diabetes mellitus, hyperkalemia.
Adverse Effects: Hypoglycemia, tachycardia, palpitations, diaphoresis, anxiety, confusion, blurred vision, weakness, depression, seizures, coma, insulin shock, hypokalemia.
Contraindications: Hypoglycemia, known sensitivity.

Dosage:
Diabetic Ketoacidosis:
- **Adult:** 0.1 U/kg IV, IO, or subcutaneous. Because of poor perfusion of the peripheral tissues, subcutaneous administration is much less effective than the IV, IO route. IV, IO insulin has a very short half-life; therefore, IV, IO insulin without an infusion is not that effective. The rate for an insulin infusion is 0.05 to 0.1 U/kg per hour IV, IO. When dosing insulin, use a U-100 insulin syringe to measure and deliver the insulin. The time from administration to action, as well as the duration of action, varies greatly among different people, as well as at different times in the same person.

Hyperkalemia:
- **Adult:** 10 U IV, IO of regular insulin (Insulin R), coadministered with 50 mL of $D_{50}W$ over 5 minutes.
- **Pediatric:** 0.1 U/kg Insulin R IV, IO.

Special Considerations:
Only regular insulin can be given IV, IO.
Pregnancy class B.

DEXTROSE (50%, 25%, 10%)

Classification: Antihypoglycemic.
Action: Increases blood glucose concentrations.
Indications: Hypoglycemia
Adverse Effects: Hyperglycemia, warmth, burning from IV infusion. Concentrated solutions may cause pain and thrombosis of the peripheral veins.
Contraindications: Intracranial and intraspinal hemorrhage, delirium tremens, solution is not clear, seals are not intact.

Dosage:
Hyperkalemia:
- **Adult:** 25 g of dextrose 50% IV, IO.
- **Pediatric:** 0.5 to 1 g/kg IV, IO.

Hypoglycemia:
- **Adult:** 10 to 25 g of dextrose 50% IV (20 to 50 mL of dextrose solution).
- **Pediatric:**
  - **Older than 2 years:** 2 mL/kg of dextrose 50%.
  - **Younger than 2 years:** 2 to 4 mL/kg of dextrose 10%.

Special Considerations:
Pregnancy class C

Hypokalemia, or low serum concentration of potassium, is a condition that is nearly impossible to diagnose without the benefit of a laboratory blood test. Hypokalemia is typically a result of chronic medical conditions such as reduced dietary intake of potassium, chronic diuretic therapy, diarrhea, short bowel syndrome, vomiting, and burns. Because paramedics lack the benefit of laboratory tests, they must rely on symptoms. Unfortunately, the symptoms of hypokalemia are nonspecific. The clinical manifestations of hypokalemia include muscle weakness (which in its most severe form can lead to paralysis), abdominal distension, and constipation. On an electrocardiogram, the T waves tend to flatten and progress to atrioventricular block and cardiac arrest.

Administration of IV potassium in the prehospital setting is an unlikely occurrence. However, in the hospital setting potassium infusions and supplementation commonly occur. Therefore, the paramedic transporting patients between various facilities may encounter patients who have potassium as a supplement to their IV fluids or who are receiving a potassium infusion.

Potassium replacement in chronic conditions and nonemergent conditions is provided with oral supplements. A medical condition needing oral potassium replacement is often not a medical emergency and does not require intervention by a paramedic. IV administration of potassium can potentially be dangerous because excessively vigorous replacement leads to hyperkalemia. IV potassium should always be diluted and slowly administered to reduce the likelihood of pain from inflammation of the vein (**phlebitis**). Potassium should be administered only to patients with adequate renal function and good urine output. Several forms of potassium can be administered by IV line: potassium chloride, potassium acetate, and potassium phosphate. Potassium chloride is the most commonly used form of potassium administered. Potassium should not be administered to patients who are dehydrated. IV fluids with supplemental potassium should not contain more than 40 mEq/L of potassium, and the rate of administration should not exceed 20 mEq/hr.

POTASSIUM CHLORIDE

Classification: Electrolyte replacement.
Action: Replaces potassium. Slight alterations in extracellular potassium levels can cause serious alterations in both cardiac and nervous function.
Indications: Hypokalemia.
Adverse Effects: Hyperkalemia; atrioventricular block; cardiac arrest; gastrointestinal bleeding, obstruction, or perforation; tissue necrosis if the infusion infiltrates into the soft tissues.
Contraindications: Use with caution in patients with cardiac arrhythmias, renal failure, muscle cramps, severe tissue trauma.
Dosage:
- **Adult:** Dosage must be individualized according to patient serum potassium concentration.
- **Pediatric:** Dosage must be individualized according to patient serum potassium concentration.

Special Considerations:
Pregnancy class C

Other common electrolyte disorders include disorders of calcium, magnesium, and phosphorus (**TABLE 5-3**). Disorders of these electrolytes are usually caused by chronic medical conditions and produce vague and non-life-threatening clinical symptoms. Therefore, prehospital care providers rarely treat any of these conditions in the absence of laboratory blood tests.

TABLE 5-3 Common Electrolyte Problems

Electrolyte Disorder	Causes	Signs and Symptoms
Hypocalcemia	Sepsis, inadequate vitamin D, pancreatitis, parathyroid disease	Irritability, hyperactive deep tendon reflexes, twitching of the face or spasms of the hand, tetany, convulsions, paresthesia, abdominal cramps, muscle cramps, neural excitability
Hypercalcemia	Cancer with metastases and parathyroid disease, overactivity	Weakness, irritability, dehydration, headache, hypertension, renal stone
Hypomagnesemia	Malnutrition, cirrhosis, pancreatitis, diarrhea	Weakness, confusion, irritability, tremors, nausea, hypotension, seizures, and arrhythmias
Hypermagnesemia	Chronic renal failure	Reduced neuromuscular irritability, loss of deep tendon reflexes, sedation, confusion[a]
Hypophosphatemia	Long-term IV nutrition, sustained vomiting or diarrhea, alcoholism parathyroid disease	Weakness, tremors, eventually numbness of the face and fingers, irritability to seizures
Hyperphosphatemia	Chronic renal failure, treatment of acute leukemia and lymphoma	Hypocalcemia

[a] EMS providers should monitor for magnesium toxicity in patients receiving IV magnesium sulfate infusions for conditions such as preeclampsia and preterm labor. When IV magnesium infusions are being administered, providers should have calcium gluconate or calcium chloride immediately available.
© Jones & Bartlett Learning.

▶ IV Therapy: Equipment and Administration

Starting IV lines is a skill that requires a great deal of practice and patience. Starting an IV line in a hospital is much different from starting an IV line in the field or in the back of an ambulance. The paramedic is often starting IV lines in conditions of inclement weather, poor lighting, and unstable movement of the ambulance.

Equipment

Equipment needed to start an IV line includes catheters, tubing sets, and bags of IV solutions. Do not omit the appropriate personal protective equipment (PPE) required to protect yourself from blood and body fluids—eye protection and gloves.

Catheters

Like needles, IV catheters are composed of a hub and catheter shaft. Catheters used for IV infusions have a plastic catheter that fits over a needle. The advantage of over-the-needle catheters is that once the metal needle has been removed from the vein the possibility of puncturing the wall of the vein with prolonged insertion or movement is lessened.

Administration Sets

IV administration sets, or setups, include a bag of IV fluids, **drip chamber, roller clamp**, and administration port (**FIGURE 5-8**). The drip chamber is the compartment immediately

FIGURE 5-8 IV administration setup.

below the IV bag where the IV fluid drips at a predetermined volume. When the IV fluid drips at a uniform rate, the healthcare provider can control the volume and rate of administration with a reasonable degree of accuracy. Drip chambers allow the provider to count the number of drops over a period and calculate the rate of fluid or drug administration. **Drop factor** is the number of drops into the chamber required to administer 1 mL of fluid. Drip chambers come in two forms: microdrip and macrodrip.

Microdrip chambers administer 60 gtt/mL. The number of drops counted per minute equals the rate of infusion in milliliters per hour. Therefore, if 30 drops occur per minute, the infusion rate is 30 mL/hr. These chambers are useful when administering IV medications such as adrenergic agents and cardiac antiarrhythmics. Microdrip chambers are also useful when administering IV fluids to children or other patients who are likely to be sensitive to large amounts of IV fluids. IV infusion rates can still fluctuate significantly with changes in patient position or the height of the IV bag above the patient.

Macrodrip chambers come in a variety of sizes, with drip factors of 10, 12, 15, and 20 gtt/mL. Most EMS agencies carry only one type of macrodrip chamber.

Volume-control chambers are also used to control the amount of fluids delivered (**FIGURE 5-9**). In small children, inadvertent administration of a large volume of fluids can result in significant complications. A volume chamber can be inserted between the drip chamber and the IV bag. A roller clamp between the IV bag and the volume chamber controls the amount of fluid in the chamber. The advantage of the volume chamber is that the provider can set the maximal amount of fluid to be infused by filling the chamber from the IV bag. Once the volume chamber empties, the patient cannot receive any more fluid.

Y-tubing is used in patients who require volume expansion and possibly transfusion of blood products. Y-tubing is also known as a blood solution set. When caring for a trauma patient, start an IV line with Y-tubing and hang a bag of normal saline. With Y-tubing primed with normal saline, a transfusion of blood can be started as soon as blood is available or the patient arrives at the hospital.

IV fluids infused without an **infusion pump** use the force of gravity. In the absence of a pump, many factors can alter the rate of infusion, so the fluid must frequently be verified as

FIGURE 5-9 The volume-control chamber provides an additional level of safety to avoid inadvertent infusion of fluids to a pediatric patient or other volume-sensitive patient.

© Jones & Bartlett Learning.

CASE STUDY

During a violent spring thunderstorm, your unit is dispatched to a structure fire. The house was struck by lightning. When the fire department arrived on the scene, the house was fully engulfed. The owner of the house, a 66-year-old man, ran back into the house to get the keys for his truck, sustaining deep and partial-thickness burns to both arms and the anterior part of his chest. You and your partner remove the burned clothing, stop the burning process, start two IV lines, and obtain orders to administer morphine 6 mg IV push. You estimate the patient has burns on 25% of his body surface area. Once at the hospital, the emergency department physician determines that this patient will need to be transported to the regional burn center by ambulance because of the inclement weather. You and the physician calculate the patient's fluid needs during transport and run the IV fluid rate at 450 mL/hr. When you started the IV line, you used an IV set with a drip factor of 10 gtt/mL. You must determine the drops per minute required to deliver the appropriate amount of IV fluids.

$$\frac{\text{Drop factor of IV set (gtt/mL)}}{60 \text{ min} \times \text{hr}} \times \text{total hourly volume to be infused} = \text{gtt/min}$$

$$\frac{10 \text{ gtt/mL}}{60 \text{ min} \times \text{hr}} \times 450 \text{ mL/hr} = \text{gtt/min}$$

$$75 = \text{gtt/min}$$

You need a drip rate of 75 gtt/min into the chamber to deliver an IV flow rate of 450 mL/hr.

flowing at the intended rate. Factors affecting the drip rate include the height of the IV bag, position of the extremity with the IV, and coiling of the IV tubing. Determination of fluid rates is explained in Chapter 4.

The indication for starting an IV line often determines the rate of fluid administration. When an IV is started on medical calls, it often serves as a vehicle to allow rapid administration of medications as the patient's condition dictates. Under these conditions the fluid rate is often referred to as **TKO** (to keep open) or **KVO** (keep vein open). The KVO rate can typically be achieved with a microdrip set running at 30 to 50 gtt/min, which translates to a rate of

---

BOX 5-1 Pediatric Maintenance Fluids

To determine the appropriate rate of maintenance fluid, the provider must know or estimate the child's weight in kilograms. Remember that 1 kg equals approximately 2.2 pounds.

- For the first 10 kg of weight, the IV fluid rate is 4 mL/hr per kilogram.
  - A 5-kg child has an IV rate of 20 mL/hr (4 mL/hr per kilogram × 5 kg).
  - A 10-kg child has an IV rate of 40 mL/hr (4 mL/hr per kilogram × 10 kg).
- For the second 10 kg of weight (i.e., 10 to 20 kg of body weight), add 2 mL/kg for each additional kilogram.
  - For a 12-kg child, start with a rate of 40 mL/hr for the first 10 kg of body weight and then add 4 mL/hr for the remaining 2 kg. The IV rate then is 44 mL/hr.
    - 10 kg × 4 mL/kg per hour = 40 mL/hr
    - 2 kg × 2 mL/kg per hour = 4 mL/hr
    - Total maintenance rate: 44 mL/hr
- To calculate the IV maintenance rate for children heavier than 20 kg, add an additional 1 mL/hr per kilogram.
  - A 25-kg child will have a maintenance rate as follows:
    - First 10 kg = 40 mL/hr
    - Second 10 kg = 20 mL/hr
    - Remaining 5 kg = 1 mL/kg per hour × 5 kg = 5 mL/hr
    - Therefore, the total maintenance rate is 65 mL/hr.

© Jones & Bartlett Learning.

---

30 to 50 mL/hr. Failure to infuse some fluids slowly can result in the IV line clotting, which means the vein will not be available in the event of an emergency. When caring for small children, be mindful that fluid amounts that would seem small and insignificant in an adult are much more significant in a child. For example, in a 22-pound (10-kg) child, an infusion rate of 50 mL/hr would exceed the child's hourly maintenance rate (**BOX 5-1**).

When caring for patients who have undergone trauma, IV lines are started for rapid administration of fluids or blood to expand the intravascular volume. Considerable debate exists about what constitutes the appropriate rate and magnitude of IV fluid administration in the prehospital setting. Some conditions require the paramedic to administer fluids rapidly. Running fluids wide open means opening the roller clamp all the way to allow for maximal fluid delivery with the aid of gravity. To increase the rate of fluid delivery, the paramedic can place the IV bag in a pressure bag or have someone manually squeeze the bag of fluids. Both methods increase the rate of fluid delivery.

The size of the IV catheter is the principal determinant of the maximal rate of fluid administration that can be achieved. An increase in the radius of the catheter results in a profound increase in IV flow rate. For example, water will flow through a pipe with a 5-inch diameter 2.5 times faster than through a 4-inch diameter pipe of equal length.

The rate that fluid can flow through a tube is defined by the laws of physics with the following formula:

$$\frac{(\text{Change in pressure}) \times \text{Radius}^4}{\text{Length of the catheter}}$$

Based on this formula, increasing the change in pressure by increasing the height of the bag, adding a pressure bag, or manually squeezing the bag increases the rate of fluid delivery. Increasing the length of tubing by adding tubing extension sets actually *decreases* the IV fluid rate.

In helicopters and mobile intensive care units, prehospital providers may encounter a variety of electric infusion pumps. While microdrip chambers can be used for titrating medication infusions, providers who routinely transport medication infusions should use programmable medication infusion pumps. These pumps should ideally have an electronic library that matches medications and concentrations used in that setting. Vasoactive medications should always be administered with an infusion pump; otherwise, dramatic and harmful patient hemodynamic changes are likely to occur. Numerous pumps are available with a variety of features. A well-calibrated pump offers several advantages over microdrip and macrodrip sets. The pump can easily regulate the rate of fluid administration by letting the paramedic directly enter the fluid rate into a keypad rather than count drips per minute and convert that rate to a volume per hour. Many pumps allow the provider to enter the patient's weight and desired dose of a medication, and the pump automatically calculates and sets the rate of delivery. Pumps also allow the user to set a volume to be delivered, and the pump will stop the infusion after delivering the set volume.

Site Selection and Preparation

IV lines are most commonly inserted in the veins of the hands and arms. In cases of trauma or shock, the provider should place the IV line in a larger vein of the antecubital fossa. In less critical cases, starting an IV line in the most distal aspect of the extremity preserves the more proximal veins for later IV access. When possible, avoid starting an IV line in the dominant hand or in an injured extremity. Avoid IV lines in the lower extremities of adults because of potential complications with infections. In children, insertion of an IV line into the dorsal aspect of the foot or the scalp is common.

Depending on local protocols, chlorhexidine gluconate or povidone iodine (Betadine) is most commonly used to prepare a site for the placement of an IV catheter. Start preparing the area by cleansing the proposed site of the IV line. Start and continue in a circular motion with an increasing radius. Allow the site to dry. EMS providers may still use isopropyl pads for intramuscular or subcutaneous injections; however, they are rarely used for IV starts.

Procedures

The following are step-by-step procedures for IV assembly, IV assembly with Volutrol, peripheral IV access, withdrawing medication from a vial, assembly of a preloaded syringe, withdrawing medication from an ampule, IV drug administration, IV infusion (piggyback), and IO infusion (tibial and sternal).

IV ASSEMBLY

Equipment Needed:
IV solution, IV tubing
Procedure:
1. Observe standard precautions.
2. When possible, explain to the patient what procedure you are going to perform and why. Obtain consent as appropriate.
3. Select the appropriate IV fluid.
4. Remove the cover from both the IV part of the IV bag of fluids and the spike on the IV tubing drip chamber.
5. Insert the spike of the tubing drip chamber into the IV tubing part of the bag of IV fluids.
6. Open the roller clamp on the IV tubing to flush the IV fluid through the tubing.
7. Once the tubing has been flushed, close the roller clamp or set the fluid infusion rate as prescribed.

IV ASSEMBLY WITH VOLUTROL

Equipment Needed:
IV solution, IV tubing with Volutrol
Procedure:
1. Observe standard precautions.
2. Confirm with the patient that he or she has no allergies to the medication, and document allergies to any other medication.

3. When possible, explain to the patient what procedure you are going to perform and why. Obtain consent as appropriate.
4. Select the appropriate IV fluid, and spike the bag in the same way you would for a regular IV line.
5. Connect and hang the drip set. Close the flow clamp at the bottom of the volume-control changer.
6. Open the flow clamp above the chamber. Fill the chamber with the appropriate amount of IV solution. Close the clamp. Open the bottom flow clamp and fill the drip chamber and tubing.
7. Cannulate the vein, connect the IV tubing, and set the drip rate by using the flow regulation clamp below the volume chamber.
8. Monitor the fluid in the chamber at all times.
9. When the volume regulation chamber is almost empty, reassess the patient's condition and lung fields to determine whether the procedure should be continued as a premeasured infusion or in a TKO format.
10. Document the medication, dose, route, needle size, and time in the patient care record.
11. Evaluate the patient for desired effects of the medication, as well as any adverse effects. Continued reevaluation should occur throughout transport.

PERIPHERAL IV ACCESS

Equipment Needed:
Alcohol or Betadine prep, tourniquet, IV catheter, IV tubing, IV solution, adhesive tape or dressing to secure IV line, sharps, PPE
Procedure:
1. Observe standard precautions.
2. Confirm with the patient that he or she has no allergies to the medication, and document allergies to any other medication.
3. When possible, explain to the patient what procedure you are going to perform and why. Obtain consent as appropriate.
4. Position the patient to stabilize the extremity where the IV catheter is to be inserted with pillows or a cot that is easily accessible.
5. Ensure that all IV tubing and equipment are assembled and flushed and that all materials required for securing and dressing the catheter are immediately available.
6. Determine the location for IV catheter placement.
7. Apply the tourniquet several inches proximal to the proposed IV site.
8. Prepare the area.
9. Hold the needle in your dominant hand at a 30-degree angle, with the needle bevel up. Insert the needle through the skin approximately 0.5 to 1 inch (1 to 3 cm) distal to the site where it will enter the vein. As you slowly advance the needle through the skin, reduce the angle to approximately 15 degrees while advancing through the soft tissues and into the vein.
10. Once the needle has entered into the vein, blood will flow back into the hub of the needle. Holding the needle still, slowly advance the catheter over the needle and into the vein.
11. Discard the needle immediately into an appropriate sharps container. Some IV catheters restrict the backward flow of blood; in other situations you will need to apply gentle pressure proximal to the insertion site to prevent blood flow out of the back of the catheter.
12. While securing the catheter with one hand, release the tourniquet and connect the hub of the catheter to the preassembled IV tubing set.
13. Open the clamp on the IV tubing and observe the flow in the drip chamber.

14. Secure the IV catheter in place with tape or adhesive dressings. Anchoring an IV line in the older adult or burn and trauma patients can be difficult because adhesive tapes and dressings do not always adhere. In these cases, consider securing the catheter in place with a roller gauze.

In conditions in which adhesive dressings or tapes will not adequately secure an IV line, secure the line with roller gauze.

15. Document the medication, dose, route, needle size, and time in the patient care record.
16. Evaluate the patient for desired effects of the medication, as well as any adverse effects. Continued reevaluation should occur throughout transport.

Once an IV line has been established, prehospital care providers can deliver medications directly into the circulatory system. IV medications can be delivered by three methods:

1. IV push
2. IV piggyback
3. IV continuous infusion

IV Push

IV push involves using a syringe connected to the **injection port** of an IV line so that the provider can rapidly administer medications or slowly empty the syringe over a period of several minutes, depending on the particular medication. Injection ports are areas placed along the IV tubing where the provider can inject the contents of a syringe into the IV line.

Many of the medications used in the prehospital environment are supplied in preloaded syringes. To use a **preloaded syringe**, the paramedic must assemble the syringe by removing the yellow caps on the ends of the two pieces and then screwing the two pieces together. Prefilled tubes of medication are also available to emergency providers to deliver medications rapidly. **Prefilled tubes** are glass syringes or tubes that are rapidly screwed in a plastic or metal tubes. This type of medication delivery is becoming rare as disposable preloaded syringes become more prevalent. Medications not supplied in preloaded syringes are provided in **vials** or ampules. To administer the medication contained within the ampule or vial, the provider must transfer the medication into a syringe. Vials are often glass bottles with a sealed opening, rubber diaphragm, and aluminum rim and cover. Ampules are small glass containers that typically contain a single dose of a medication.

WITHDRAWING MEDICATION FROM A VIAL

Equipment Needed:
Alcohol prep, vial of medication, syringe, needle for syringe, sharps
Procedure:
1. Observe standard precautions.
2. Verify the drug order.
3. Confirm right patient, right medication, right dose, right route, and right time.
4. Confirm with the patient that he or she has no allergies to the medication, and document allergies to any other medication.
5. When possible, explain to the patient what medication you are going to administer and why. Obtain consent as appropriate.
6. Peel back the aluminum lid of the vial to expose the rubber diaphragm.
7. Wipe the rubber diaphragm with an alcohol wipe.
8. Fill the syringe with the volume of air equal to the amount of medication desired to be removed from the vial.

9. With the bevel of the needle facing you, insert the needle into the vial and inject the air from the syringe.
10. Load the medication from the vial into the syringe.
11. When withdrawing a medication from a vial for use by the intramuscular or subcutaneous routes, place a new needle on the syringe before administering the medication.

ASSEMBLY OF A PRELOADED SYRINGE

Equipment Needed:
Medication in preloaded syringe, sharps
Procedure:
1. Observe standard precautions.
2. Verify the drug order.
3. Confirm right patient, right medication, right dose, right route, and right time.
4. Confirm with the patient that he or she has no allergies to the medication, and document allergies to any other medication.
5. Calculate the volume of medication to be administered.
6. Remove the protective cap from the barrel and cartridge.
7. Screw the cartridge into the barrel.
8. Push in the plunger to expel the air.

WITHDRAWING MEDICATION FROM AN AMPULE

Equipment Needed:
Ampule of medication, two pieces of 4 × 4 gauze, syringe, filtered needle for drawing the medication into the syringe, needle for injection, sharps
Procedure:
1. Observe standard precautions.
2. Verify the drug order.
3. Confirm right patient, right medication, right dose, right route, and right time.
4. Confirm with the patient that he or she has no allergies to the medication, and document allergies to any other medication.
5. When possible, explain to the patient what medication you are going to administer and why. Obtain consent as appropriate.
6. Shift all the medication into the lower portion of the ampule by tapping the top half of the ampule.
7. Hold the ampule between your hands by wrapping it with two pieces of gauze. In one hand, hold the top of the ampule in a piece of gauze; with the other hand, hold the lower portion of the glass ampule. Break the top off the ampule by bending it away from you.
8. With a filtered needle to prevent any glass shards from being drawn up, draw the medication up into the syringe. Discard this needle and switch to a different needle if using a needle to administer medication.

Whether you are using preloaded syringes or medication from a vial or ampule, you are now ready to administer the medication as an IV push.

IV DRUG ADMINISTRATION

Equipment Needed:
Alcohol prep, medication loaded in a syringe, needle for the syringe, sharps, PPE
Procedure:
1. Observe standard precautions.
2. Verify the drug order.

3. Confirm right patient, right medication, right dose, right route, and right time.
4. Confirm with the patient that he or she has no allergies to the medication, and document allergies to any other medication.
5. When possible, explain to the patient what procedure you are going to perform and why. Obtain consent as appropriate.
6. Locate the medication port of the IV line and wipe it clean with alcohol.
7. Clamp or pinch the IV tubing above the site of the medication port.
8. Insert the needle of the syringe through the diaphragm of the medication port. If using a needleless system, first unscrew the needle.

> Be careful not to insert the needle through the back wall of the tubing. A short needle can help avoid this problem. Needleless systems in which the syringe is screwed to the port also work well.

9. Gently pull back on the plunger of the syringe until you see a small flow of blood in the IV tubing. This maneuver ensures that the catheter is in the vein and prevents infiltration of the medication into the soft tissues.
10. Inject the medication into the IV line at the rate appropriate for the particular medication.
11. Once all the medication has been injected, remove the needle from the medication port, unclamp the IV tubing, and dispose of the needle and syringe using the appropriate container.
12. Document the medication, dose, route, needle size, and time in the patient care record.
13. Evaluate the patient for desired effects of the medication, as well as any adverse effects. Continued reevaluation should occur throughout transport.

IV Piggyback

IV piggyback infusions are secondary infusions attached to the primary infusion line. Rather than directly injecting the medication into the line as an IV push, the medication is added to a smaller bag of IV fluid and slowly infused through the medication port of the main IV line. Many IV medications are administered over a projected period of 30 minutes to hours. To administer medications via the IV route over such a long period by a syringe would be highly inconvenient and impractical. Using the IV piggyback technique, such medications are given more slowly, by injecting the medication into a smaller bag of IV fluids (100 or 250 mL). The smaller IV bag containing the medication is then connected by an injector port into the main IV line.

IV INFUSION (PIGGYBACK)

I. Preparing Medication for Infusion

Equipment Needed:
Alcohol prep, medication, syringe, needle, small bag of compatible IV fluids (100 or 250 mL), IV tubing, medication label, sharps
Procedure:
1. Observe standard precautions.
2. Verify the drug order.
3. Confirm right patient, right medication, right dose, right route, and right time.

4. Confirm with the patient that he or she has no allergies to the medication, and document allergies to any other medication.
5. When possible, explain to the patient what procedure you are going to perform and why. Obtain consent as appropriate.
6. To prepare the medication for piggyback infusion, draw it into a syringe by the techniques previously explained.
7. Wipe the injection port of the smaller bag of IV fluids being used for the piggyback infusion with alcohol.
8. Inject the medication into the IV bag.
9. Mix the solution by shaking the IV bag.
10. Label the bag with a medication label. Document the name and amount of the medication added.
11. Document the medication, dose, route, needle size, and time in the patient care record.
12. Evaluate the patient for desired effects of the medication, as well as any adverse effects. Continued reevaluation should occur throughout transport.

II. Attaching Infusion Solution to Primary IV Line

Equipment Needed:
Alcohol prep, medication, syringe, commercial Y-site adapter, small bag of compatible IV fluids, IV tubing, medication label, sharps
Procedure:
1. Observe standard precautions.
2. Verify the drug order.
3. Confirm right patient, right medication, right dose, right route, and right time.
4. Confirm with the patient that he or she has no allergies to the medication, and document allergies to any other medication.
5. When possible, explain to the patient what procedure you are going to perform and why. Obtain consent as appropriate.
6. Wipe clean the medication port of the IV line with alcohol.
7. Clamp the IV tubing of the primary line above the site of the medication port.
8. Connect the piggyback medication line to a commercial Y-site adapter or use a needleless Luer-lock connection. *It is unsafe to use a needle on the line containing the piggyback medication placed through the diaphragm of the medication port. The needle may become disconnected during patient transport or movement and risk a needlestick injury or infectious exposure to the EMS provider.*
9. Infuse the medication into the primary IV line at the rate appropriate for the particular medication.
10. Hang the smaller IV bag containing the medication given by piggyback infusion at a level higher than the bag used for the primary IV infusion.
11. Once the infusion of the medication is complete, remove the piggyback infusion and unclamp the tubing of the primary IV line.
12. Document the medication, dose, route, needle size, and time in the patient care record.
13. Evaluate the patient for desired effects of the medication, as well as any adverse effects. Continued reevaluation should occur throughout transport.

Intraosseous Infusions

When providing care in the emergent prehospital environment, starting and maintaining vascular access is essential. IO infusion involves placement of a needle set into the highly vascular **intramedullary space** of the bone and infusion of fluids or medications into this space (**FIGURE 5-10**). In cases of hypovolemic shock, veins often collapse, making access with IV catheters difficult or impossible. However, even in such cases, the intramedullary cavity of the bone remains open. Fluids, blood, and medications administered through

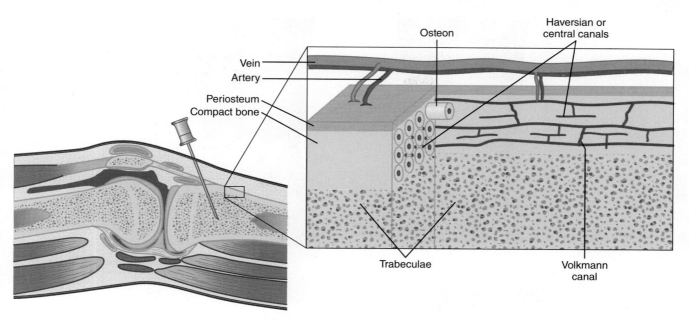

FIGURE 5-10 Bone composition and placement of an IO infusion needle set.

an IO line can be delivered to the central circulation by this route as rapidly as though administered through peripheral or central venous catheters. Once reserved for pediatric patients, IO lines are used across the full age spectrum and have become a powerful tool for EMS, emergency department, and intensive care providers.[7] Use of IO infusions is of great interest to military and civilian EMS because of the ease and reliability of starting such access in suboptimal and hostile conditions. EMS systems may bypass IV attempts completely in critical or cardiac arrest patients and use IOs as the primary method for vascular access in these patients.

The most common site for placement of an IO line is the proximal tibia. This site is ideal because of its flat nature and lack of extensive overlying muscle and soft tissue. Other sites, such as the distal tibia and proximal humerus, are also well studied. To locate the proximal tibia site, palpate the proximal tibia immediately below the knee and feel for a marked bump in the bone. This prominent portion of the tibia is called the **tibial tuberosity**. The optimal location for IO needle placement is medial to the tibial tuberosity on the antero-medial portion of the bone. If possible, avoid placing an IO needle in an extremity with a suspected injury.

Several different types of devices are used to gain access to the intramedullary cavity, including the Jamshidi IO needle and other commercial devices for use in adults and children. These devices vary in their application and techniques. Some devices use manual application, whereas others use spring-loaded devices and even electrical drills. The EZ-IO device is shown in **FIGURE 5-11**. The Jamshidi needle set, which was originally used as a bone marrow aspiration, is the most widely used IO device. The depth of the needle set can be controlled by the end user. The needle set has a stylet that is locked in place with a plastic cap. The IO needle can be further secured by placing two Kerlix rolls on either side of the needle.

In adults, the **sternum** is occasionally used as an IO infusion site because it is thin and flat, contains a high proportion of red marrow, is easy to penetrate and less likely to be fractured in certain situations, and is close to the central circulation.[8] The recommended insertion site is in the manubrium, 1.6 cm below the sternal notch. Use of a specifically designed device is critical for sternal applications.

FIGURE 5-11 The EZ-IO device. **A.** Identify the tibial tuberosity. **B.** Prepare the site in sterile fashion. **C.** Insert the IO needle with the EZ-IO device. **D.** Remove the inner stylus from the needle. **E** and **F.** Attach tubing and flush with sterile normal saline. Attach to IV tubing setup.

IO INFUSION—TIBIAL APPROACH

Equipment Needed:
Betadine or chlorhexidine prep, IO needle set, 10-mL syringe, IV tubing, bag of IV-compatible fluids, several rolls of gauze, tape, sharps, PPE

Procedure:
1. Observe standard precautions.
2. Verify the drug order.
3. Confirm right patient, right medication, right dose, right route, and right time.
4. Confirm with the patient that he or she has no allergies to the medication, and document allergies to any other medication.
5. When possible, explain to the patient what procedure you are going to perform and why. Obtain consent as appropriate.
6. Identify the insertion site.
7. Prepare the insertion site with either Betadine or chlorhexidine.
8. Make sure the angle of needle set insertion is 90 degrees to the bone.
9. Advance the needle set with a back-and-forth screwing motion. Entrance into the intra-medullary cavity will be apparent by a gentle give and a marked decrease in resistance to needle advancement. Avoid excessive insertion pressure.
10. Unlock and remove the stylet. Dispose of the stylet as you would a sharp.
11. Confirm proper placement of the catheter by aspirating marrow back into a syringe that is attached to the catheter or verifying that fluids infuse freely and without any noted swelling (which would indicate infiltration) and that the catheter stands in place without any support.
12. Attach the preassembled administration set to the IO catheter.
13. Secure the IO line in place with bulky dressings. This can easily be done by placing two roller gauze dressings on either side of the IO needle and then wrapping the entire area.
14. Document the medication, dose, route, needle size, and time in the patient care record.
15. Evaluate the patient for desired effects of the medication, as well as any adverse effects. Continued reevaluation should occur throughout transport.

IO INFUSION—STERNAL APPROACH FOR FAST IO

Equipment Needed:
Chlorhexidine or Betadine prep, IO needle, 10-mL syringe, IV tubing, bag of IV-compatible fluids, several rolls of gauze, tape, sharps, PPE

Procedure:
1. Observe standard precautions.
2. Verify the drug order.
3. Confirm right patient, right medication, right dose, right route, and right time.
4. Confirm with the patient that he or she has no allergies to the medication, and document allergies to any other medication.
5. When possible, explain to the patient what procedure you are going to perform and why. Obtain consent as appropriate.
6. Locate the patient's manubrium and prepare the site with aseptic solution.
7. Use the index finger to align the target patch with the patient's sternal notch. Place the target patch.
8. Place the introducer into the target zone on the patch, perpendicular to the skin. Firmly push on the introducer to insert the infusion tube into the correct site and to the right penetration depth. Pull the introducer straight back, exposing the infusion tube and a two-part support sleeve, which falls away.
9. Verify correct placement by observing marrow entering the infusion tube.
10. Connect the IV solution and tubing to the infusion tube on the patch, and adjust the flow rate.

11. Place the protective dome over the site by pressing firmly over the target patch to engage the Velcro fastening.
12. Document the medication, dose, route, needle size, and time in the patient care record.
13. Evaluate the patient for desired effects of the medication, as well as any adverse effects. Continued reevaluation should occur throughout transport.

Complications of IV Therapy

Every medication and therapy has potential complications, and the same is true for IV therapy. Complications of IV therapy include infiltration, catheter shear, phlebitis, infection, and infected phlebitis.

The most troublesome IV complication for the patient is infiltration. **Infiltration** occurs when the tip of the catheter dislodges from the lumen of the vein; the fluid or medication is then delivered to soft tissues around the vein. Infiltration of medications into the soft tissues can result in tissue destruction and necrosis at the site of infiltration.

Infiltration of an IV line can be suspected when the fluid no longer freely drips. Other signs of an IV line infiltration include pain and swelling at the IV site. Often the only treatment required for infiltration is discontinuation of the IV line and starting a new IV line either proximal to the infiltration or in a different, uninjured extremity. Infiltration of a large amount of fluids in areas such as the hand and foot can cause pressure damage to the underlying and adjacent structures. Infiltration in these areas should be treated by elevation of the affected area and serial examinations to evaluate vascular, motor, and sensory function.

If medication infiltration is suspected, clearly communicate that information to the receiving hospital and document the communication. Also document findings about the site, the time of the incident, and any treatment rendered. Many medications and electrolytes that can cause vasoconstriction require injection of medications into the infiltrated site, intensive monitoring, and even surgical debridement and reconstruction.

Catheter shear is a complication that occurs when a segment of the catheter breaks off and is either retained in the vein or, even worse, embolizes through the venous system. This complication can occur when a provider attempts to pull a catheter back over a needle. This typically occurs when blood return appears while starting an IV line. While attempting to advance the catheter into the vein over the needle, the provider either encounters resistance or loses the blood return and tries to salvage the IV line by pulling the catheter back over the needle. After advancing the catheter, the catheter follows the course of the vein, which is at an angle from the needle. When the provider pulls the catheter back over the straight needle, the tip of the needle can cut the catheter into two pieces, and the severed piece of the IV catheter can remain at the site of the attempted IV start. The severed IV catheter can also float away in the vein to a site more proximal in the limb or even the heart and lungs. Sheared catheters can require retrieval by surgery or angiography. If shearing of an IV catheter is suspected, notify medical direction and document the communication.

Less-immediate complications of IV lines include phlebitis, infection, and infected phlebitis. None of these infectious complications will become apparent to the paramedic who starts the IV line in the prehospital setting. However, exercising a strict sterile technique can reduce the incidence of these complications. IV lines started in the field are often started in less than optimal conditions. For this reason, many hospitals have policies about prompt removal of field lines.

Phlebitis is an inflammation of the vein that can manifest as pain, redness, and edema. Many different conditions can irritate the vein and cause the inflammation of phlebitis, including concentrated fluids, certain electrolyte solutions, various medications, and simply the presence of the catheter in the lumen of the vein. When phlebitis causes the blood inside of the lumen to clot, the condition is known as **thrombophlebitis**. When a patient has thrombophlebitis, he or she can often feel the thrombosed vessel along the length of the thrombosis, and palpation of the vein elicits tenderness. On occasion, the thrombophlebitis can become infected. **Suppurative thrombophlebitis** occurs when the clot of thrombophlebitis becomes infected. Suppurative thrombophlebitis is a potentially fatal condition. The treatment for this type of thrombophlebitis is excision of the infected vein.

▶ Review Questions

1. Define *ICF space*. What portion of the TBW is ICF?
2. What types of fluid compose the ECF space?
3. Define *osmosis*.
4. If you give a patient a 1,000-mL bolus of D_5W, how much of that volume will remain within the vascular space?
5. After giving a patient a 1,000-mL bolus of 0.9% normal saline, how much of the volume will remain in the vascular space?
6. What are the differences among crystalloid solutions, colloid solutions, and isotonic fluids?
7. What are some of the causes of hyperkalemia?
8. What is a typical fluid bolus in a pediatric patient?
9. What is the drop factor?
10. When using a microdrip chamber, how many drops compose 1 mL?
11. With a microdrip chamber attached to an IV line, what is the rate of IV fluids in milliliters per hour if you count 60 gtt/min?
12. When administering IV fluids without an infusion pump, what factors can alter the rate of IV fluid delivery?
13. What determines the maximal rate of IV fluid administration?
14. What occurs when an IV line infiltrates?
15. What are the signs that indicate an IV line is infiltrating?
16. How can you prevent IV catheter shear?

References

1. Mandel J, Palevsky PM. Treatment of severe hypovolemia or hypovolemic shock in adults. UpToDate. https://www.uptodate.com/contents/treatment-of-severe-hypovolemia-or-hypovolemic-shock-in-adults. Updated March 12, 2018. Accessed July 13, 2018.
2. Mange K, Matsuura D, Cizman B, et al. Language guiding therapy: the case of dehydration versus volume depletion. *Ann Intern Med.* 1997;127:848.
3. Hauser CJ, Shoemaker WC, Turpin I. Oxygen transport responses to colloids and crystalloids in critically ill surgical patients. *Surg Gynecol Obstet.* 1980;150:811.
4. Granger DN, Gabel JC, Drake RE, Taylor AE. Physiological basis for the clinical use of albumin solutions. *Surg Gynecol Obstet.* 1978;146:97.
5. Velasco IT, Pontieri V, Rocha e Silva M Jr, Lopes OU. Hypertonic NaCl and severe hemorrhagic shock. *Am J Physiol.* 1980;239:H664.
6. Nakayama S, Sibley L, Gunther RA, Holcroft JW, Kramer GC. Small volume resuscitation with hypertonic saline resuscitation (2400 mOsm/liter) during hemorrhagic shock. *Circ Shock.* 1984;13:149.
7. Petitpas F, Guenezan J, Vendeuvre T, Scepi M, Oriot D, Mimoz O. Use of intra-osseous access in adults: a systematic review. *Crit Care.* 2016;20:102.
8. Aehlert B. *ACLS Study Guide*. 3rd ed. St. Louis, MO: Mosby; 2007.

© Andrew Brookes/Getty Images

PART II

Problem-Oriented Pharmacology

CHAPTER 6

Acute Coronary Syndromes

▶ Introduction

Heart disease is the leading cause of death in adults in the United States, accounting for approximately 600,000 deaths annually.[1] **Acute coronary syndrome (ACS)** is a type of heart disease that encompasses the spectrum of conditions that occur when the heart muscle is deprived of oxygen. This deprivation of oxygen is called **ischemia**. Ischemia of the heart can occur as a brief and temporary condition referred to as **stable angina pectoris** or can progress to cause death to a portion of the cardiac muscle, which is referred to as an acute **myocardial infarction (MI)**.

Morbidity and mortality for ACS in the prehospital environment is due to arrhythmias, most of which occur within the first 4 hours after symptom onset. In-hospital deaths are often caused by low cardiac output such as that seen in acute congestive heart failure and cardiogenic shock. Additional causes of in-hospital deaths include recurrent AMI and cardiac wall rupture. The severity of the damage is directly related to the size of the infarction. Therefore, the goal of prehospital therapy is directed at limiting the size of the infarct and preserving left ventricular function.

Great strides have been made in diagnosing and treating **ischemic heart disease**, and developments in EMS over the past decade have allowed prehospital professionals across the country to intervene quickly and efficiently to manage these critical patients. This chapter highlights the current pharmacologic treatments for ACS. Chapters 9, 10, and 12 address the treatment of patients with cardiac arrhythmias, congestive heart failure, and hypertensive emergencies.

▶ Overview of Acute Coronary Syndromes

ACS defines a progression of cardiac disease that results from ischemia. Coronary artery disease begins with early plaque formation within an artery. Plaque formation is an inflammatory response caused by deposition of lipoproteins that carry cholesterol. Rupture of these plaques can cause obstruction of the artery by thrombus formation and can interfere with blood delivery to the heart muscle (**FIGURE 6-1**).

There is a spectrum of pathophysiologic and clinical progression of ACS. Ischemia occurs when the heart is deprived of oxygen. This is a reversible process, and permanent damage does

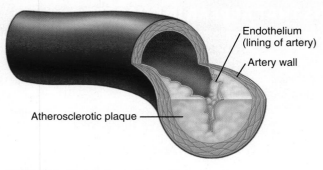

FIGURE 6-1 Plaque formation within an artery.

not occur unless there is prolonged oxygen deprivation. Stable angina pectoris occurs when the oxygen demand of the heart exceeds the oxygen supplied to the heart. The pain associated with stable angina pectoris may be relieved with rest or oxygen supplementation. Unstable angina **pectoris** (UA; occasionally also abbreviated USA) typically occurs when a partially occluding thrombus produces symptoms of ischemia, including chest pain. This chest pain may occur at rest or with little provocation. The UA pain is also longer in duration and may not be relieved by rest or medication. This very serious condition requires immediate attention and may actually cause a non-ST-segment elevation myocardial infarction (NSTEMI). The definition of an NSTEMI is the acute process in which ischemia affects the myocardium with no elevation of the ST segment on the **electrocardiogram (ECG)**. The difference between NSTEMI and UA is that with the NSTEMI, cardiac enzymes will be elevated, indicating necrosis of the cardiac tissue. ST-segment elevation myocardial infarction (STEMI) is the actual infarction of the cardiac tissue secondary to oxygen deprivation. Cell death occurs and there is permanent, irreversible damage to cardiac muscle cells. A STEMI will have elevation of the ST segments on an ECG.

Overview of Stable Angina Pectoris

CASE STUDY

You are dispatched to the home of a man with a chief complaint of chest pain. You arrive to find a 55-year-old man with obesity sitting in a chair. He states the he was shoveling snow and felt pressure in his chest. He continued shoveling, but the pain would not go away, so he went inside the house and sat down. After approximately 10 minutes, just before your arrival, the pain subsided. The patient denies previous episodes of chest pain and states that he has no medical history of coronary artery disease. He denies diabetes, a smoking history, and hypercholesterolemia. He does state that his father died of a heart attack at the age of 62 years, and his mother has coronary artery disease.

Angina means "tightening," not pain. A patient may describe classic **angina pectoris** as squeezing, pressure, burning, heaviness, or bandlike pain. It typically is felt in the center of the chest or on the left side of the rib cage. The sensation may radiate to the jaw or to the right or left arm. Stable angina pectoris is described as periodic chest discomfort that occurs when oxygen demand exceeds the oxygen supply of cardiac muscle. This discomfort is typically predictable and reproducible. The attacks may become more frequent over time. Physical activity, psychologic stress, anemia, arrhythmias, and certain environmental conditions can precipitate an attack of angina. Rest, supplemental oxygen, or the administration of nitroglycerin will typically resolve stable anginal pain. The pain is usually short in duration—usually 2 to 5 minutes. It almost always lasts less than 20 minutes.

The pathophysiology of this condition is a reduction in the diameter of the coronary arteries that supply blood to the heart. This narrowing occurs because of the long-term deposition of atherosclerotic plaque. When the heart muscle is stressed by exertion, an increased need for oxygen occurs. However, because of the decreased diameter of these vessels, delivery of oxygenated blood cannot be increased to accommodate the heart's demands, resulting in ischemia and chest pain, pressure, or discomfort. When the patient rests, the heart's oxygen demand is once again met, and the ischemia and pain subside. The patient in the previous scenario represents the classic presentation of stable angina pectoris.

(*continued*) You recommend to the patient that he should allow you to transport him to the emergency department for further evaluation, but he refuses. He tells you that he often gets this type of pain in his chest when he overexerts himself.

Management

Chest pain that is relieved with rest is an indication that the patient should be evaluated for cardiac damage and coronary artery disease in the emergency department. The patient in the previous scenario should be transported to the emergency department even though he is feeling better at the time of evaluation. The clinical presentation of cardiac ischemia can mislead even the most seasoned prehospital professionals. The consequences of failed or delayed treatment could be catastrophic. For these reasons, the evaluation and treatment of the symptom of chest pain should follow standardized protocols.

After completing the primary assessment of a patient reporting chest pain, oxygen should be administered[2,3] if a patient's oxygen saturation is less than 90% to 94%,[4] the patient has respiratory distress, or the patient has signs suggestive of heart failure. Routine administration of oxygen to nonhypoxemic patients with ACS is no longer recommended. If indicated, oxygen supplementation may be in the form of a nasal cannula or nonrebreather mask and titrated to an oxygen saturation of 94% or greater. The patient should be placed on a cardiac monitor, and intravenous (IV) access should be obtained. A 12-lead ECG should also be completed.

(*continued*) Your attempts to convince the patient to go to the emergency department appear to have failed. The patient argues that he only has heartburn and is too busy to spend the rest of his day in the emergency department. He removes the blood pressure cuff and stands up. As he stands up, he appears weak and puts his right hand on his chest. His color is poor, and he is diaphoretic. You rapidly help him sit back down in the chair. You place an oxygen mask on him while your partner sets up to start an IV line. You administer a 325-mg non-enteric-coated aspirin and instruct him to chew it, then swallow.

Oxygen is a naturally occurring gas that exists in the atmosphere at an approximately 21% concentration. It is odorless, tasteless, and colorless. Oxygen is an important drug used in the management of a large number of medical emergencies. A detailed description of oxygen is covered in Chapter 14. When a patient has angina pectoris, oxygen demand exceeds the body's ability to deliver adequate oxygen to the heart muscle. By providing these patients with supplemental oxygen, the red blood cells become loaded with oxygen for delivery to the heart muscle. The goal is to increase the supply of oxygen to the heart muscle to meet the demand. Oxygen causes coronary artery vasoconstriction and may undermine cardiac perfusion. Additionally, studies have observed that 100% oxygen can decrease cardiac output while increasing systemic vascular resistance.[5] In a larger analysis, there was no demonstrated benefit of the routine use of oxygen in nonhypoxemic patients with ACS.[5,6] EMS providers should follow local or regional treatment protocols regarding the use of oxygen in patients with ACS.

Oxygen has an immediate onset of action, and its duration is less than 2 minutes. People who are new to medicine may not consider oxygen a drug, but oxygen has a clear, beneficial physiologic effect when given at the appropriate dose; when given in excess it can have negative effects.

Aspirin is an **antiplatelet** medication that prohibits platelets from adhering to each other. It can also be used for analgesic, anti-inflammatory, and antipyretic effects. In AMI, reducing clot formation in the coronary arteries is of paramount concern. Aspirin prevents the clot from growing larger by inhibiting the platelets from adhering to one another and preventing clots from forming. In cases of stable angina, such as in the previous scenario, aspirin helps prevent clots from forming and the condition from progressing to an AMI. Prehospital providers do not administer aspirin for its pain-relieving attribute but rather for its antiplatelet properties. Reduction of pain in chest pain is accomplished more commonly with morphine sulfate. This is discussed in greater detail in the next section.

OXYGEN

Classification: Elemental gas.
Action: Facilitates cellular energy metabolism.
Indications: Hypoxia, ischemic chest pain, respiratory distress, suspected carbon monoxide poisoning, traumatic injuries, shock.
Adverse Effects: High concentrations can cause a decreased level of consciousness and respiratory depression in patients with chronic carbon dioxide retention or chronic lung disease. Oxygen causes systemic and coronary vasoconstriction, possibly coronary artery perfusion.
Contraindications: Known paraquat poisoning.
Dosage:
Low-Concentration Oxygen:
- A dose of 1 to 4 L/min by a nasal cannula is appropriate.

High-Concentration Oxygen:
- A dose of 10 to 15 L/min via nonrebreather mask is appropriate.

Special Considerations:
Pregnancy class A.

© Jones & Bartlett Learning. Courtesy of MIEMSS.

ASPIRIN, ASA

Classification: Antiplatelet, nonnarcotic analgesic, antipyretic.
Action: Prevents the formation of a chemical known as thromboxane A2, which causes platelets to clump together, or aggregate, and form plugs that cause obstruction or constriction of small coronary arteries.
Indications: Fever, inflammation, angina, AMI, and patients complaining of pain, pressure, squeezing, or crushing in the chest that may be cardiac in origin.
Adverse Effects: Anaphylaxis, angioedema, bronchospasm, bleeding, stomach irritation, nausea/vomiting.

© ClassicStock/S. FELD/Medical Images.

Contraindications: Gastrointestinal (GI) bleeding, active ulcer disease, hemorrhagic stroke, bleeding disorders, children with chickenpox or flu-like symptoms, known sensitivity.
Dosage: Note: "Baby aspirin" 81 mg, standard adult aspirin dose 325 mg.
Myocardial Infarction:
- **Adult:** 160 to 325 mg orally (PO; alternatively, four 81-mg baby aspirin are often given), 300-mg rectal suppository.
- **Pediatric:** 3 to 5 mg/kg per day to 5 to 10 mg/kg per day given as a single dose.

Pain or Fever:
- **Adult:** 325 to 650 mg PO (one to two adult tablets) every 4 to 6 hours.
- **Pediatric:** 60 to 90 mg/kg per day in divided doses every 4 to 6 hours.

Special Considerations:
Pregnancy class C except the last 3 months of pregnancy, when aspirin is considered pregnancy class D.

(*continued*) After starting the patient on oxygen and administering 325 mg of a non-enteric-coated aspirin, the patient agrees to be transported to the local emergency department. Your partner is able to start the IV line without difficulty, and you place the patient on the ECG and pulse oximeter monitors. You transport him in a position of comfort. During transport, the patient's pain subsides. A week later, you see the patient's wife and ask her about her husband's condition. She tells you that he had a cardiac catheterization and has undergone angioplasty of several vessels. She expresses her gratitude for insisting that her husband go to the hospital and saving his life.

Overview of Unstable Angina Pectoris and Non-ST-Segment Elevation Myocardial Infarction

---

CASE STUDY

You are called to assist a 68-year-old woman with chest pain. You arrive to find the patient sitting at her kitchen table with her hand on her chest. She states the pain has been there on and off for 2 weeks. It usually starts while she is resting and lasts approximately 25 minutes. She describes the pain as "an elephant sitting on my chest." She feels like she cannot catch her breath. Her history is significant for hypertension: smoking, high cholesterol, and a positive family history for MI. Her heart rate is 96 beats/min, blood pressure is 146/98 mm Hg, and respirations are 22 breaths/min.

This patient is displaying symptoms of UA. UA is defined as chest pain or discomfort that occurs with minimal exertion or at rest. It may not follow a pattern. It can also be defined as new-onset angina or a significant change in previously stable angina. Patients may experience chest discomfort with minimal exertion or even while at rest. The episode may also be longer in duration. The patient's description of chest pain at rest that lasts more than 20 minutes is typical for UA/NSTEMI. NSTEMI is an AMI without the characteristic ST-segment elevation seen in AMI.

The characteristics are classic with UA/NSTEMI:

- Symptoms of angina at rest
- New-onset exertional angina
- Recent acceleration of angina
- Variant angina
- Post-MI angina (more than 24 hours)

The patient in this scenario is displaying symptoms of UA or NSTEMI. Additional terms for this condition include rest angina, crescendo angina, and preinfarction angina. UA/NSTEMI differs from stable angina by both the pathophysiology and the duration of the pain. UA/NSTEMI may not follow a pattern. In particular, women may present atypically. Their chief complaint may be weakness, shortness of breath, or fatigue. Variant, or **Prinzmetal's**, angina is a form of UA caused by coronary artery spasm at rest. Little atherosclerotic disease is typically noted in these patients. The pain of **variant angina** is often severe and occurs between midnight and the early hours of the morning. This form of angina can also display characteristics of a STEMI.

The pathophysiology of UA and NSTEMI is the same as that of STEMI. The atherosclerotic changes of coronary artery disease form plaques. These plaques may rupture and a platelet-rich thrombus can form. This thrombus can occlude or partially occlude an artery. Arterial occlusion causes decreased blood flow to a portion of the cardiac muscle. Ischemia occurs, which can lead to infarction.

Management

Every complaint of chest pain or pressure should be treated emergently. All forms of ischemia present similarly and, therefore, must be treated aggressively. Patients with this condition can display all the characteristics of an AMI and should be treated and transported immediately.

Initial management is similar to that of a patient with stable angina pectoris. A thorough history and physical assessment should be performed. The patient should receive IV access, a 12-lead ECG, and aspirin. Supplemental oxygen is based on patient presentation and is administered when patients are hypoxemic (>94% oxygen saturation) or have signs of respiratory distress or heart failure.[4] The patient should be monitored with an ECG and pulse oximeter monitor. In addition, the American Heart Association (AHA) has developed an algorithm for UA/NSTEMI (**FIGURE 6-2**).

Medications that are indicated for UA/NSTEMI include nitroglycerin, beta blockers, antiplatelet medications (clopidogrel), anticoagulant medications (heparin, enoxaparin), **glycoprotein** IIb/IIIa inhibitors, angiotensin-converting enzyme (ACE) inhibitors, and statins.

FIGURE 6-2 Ischemic chest discomfort algorithm.

Many of these medications are not initiated in the prehospital environment but are part of the emergency department and definitive treatment.

Nitroglycerin is a commonly used medication in the treatment of UA/NSTEMI. It is typically administered by the sublingual route, which allows for rapid absorption. Once in the body, the nitroglycerin is converted to nitric oxide, which is a potent vasodilator. The dilation of the venous system reduces the amount of blood returning to the heart with each heartbeat, in turn reducing the workload on the heart and decreasing tension on the walls of the heart. These changes result in a significant reduction in the amount of oxygen consumed by the heart, which helps balance oxygen supply and demand, a classic problem in cardiac ischemia and infarction.

(*continued*) You place the patient on oxygen 4 L/min by nasal cannula. While your partner is starting an IV line, you place her on the cardiac monitor, as well as the pulse oximeter. Her heart rate is 104 beats/min and her blood pressure is 188/98 mm Hg. Her pulse oximeter reads 98% on 4 L/min via nasal cannula. You administer one 325-mg tablet of non-enteric-coated aspirin and instruct her to chew the aspirin before swallowing it. Because she has been having pain for 20 minutes, you are appropriately worried that the patient has myocardial ischemia, and you prepare to administer nitroglycerin.

Although nitroglycerin causes both venous and arterial dilation, the veins dilate more than the arteries. This produces an increase in the diameter of the coronary vessels, and the heart muscle subsequently receives more oxygen-enriched blood flow. These properties make nitroglycerin a desirable choice for a UA/NSTEMI/STEMI. Sublingual nitroglycerin has long been considered the gold standard of drugs used in the treatment of angina. Nitroglycerin has many benefits. It is easy to administer, effective, and safe. Nitroglycerin also reduces blood pressure. Therefore, vital signs must be monitored and blood pressure evaluated after each administration of a sublingual nitroglycerin tablet or a dose of nitroglycerin spray. Chapter 12 includes an additional discussion of nitroglycerin and its various forms.

Before administering nitroglycerine, EMS providers should determine whether patients are taking phosphodiesterase inhibitor medications such as sildenafil (Viagra) and tadalafil (Cialis), commonly prescribed for erectile dysfunction. These medications may cause intractable hypotension when nitroglycerin is administered. Additionally, EMS providers should assess for ECG evidence of a right ventricular infarction prior to administering nitroglycerine. These patients are dependent on adequate blood return to the heart (preload) and may potentially decompensate when given a vasodilator medication such as nitroglycerin.[7]

Morphine sulfate is a medication that is often used for pain control. It is an opioid agonist and is beneficial in treating refractory pain in ACS. In addition to treating pain, it has some vasodilating properties that reduce preload, thus decreasing stroke volume and blood flow to the coronary arteries. Morphine sulfate has not been studied extensively and is still indicated as a Class I recommendation for STEMI. It is a Class IIa recommendation for UA and NSTEMI. Morphine should also be used with caution in patients with signs of a right ventricular infarction, as it may reduce cardiac preload and lead to severe hypotension.[7] Fentanyl and hydromorphone (Dilaudid) are narcotics that are also being used for pain management in ACS.

NITROGLYCERIN (NITROLINGUAL, NITROQUICK, NITRO-DUR)

Classification: Antianginal agent.

Action: Relaxes vascular smooth muscle, thereby dilating peripheral arteries and veins. This causes pooling of venous blood and decreased venous return to the heart, which decreases preload. Nitroglycerin also reduces left ventricular systolic wall tension, which decreases afterload.

Indications: Angina, ongoing ischemic chest discomfort, hypertension, myocardial ischemia associated with cocaine intoxication.

© Sue Heaton/Alamy Stock Photo.

© Allik Camazine/Alamy Stock Photo.

Adverse Effects: Headache, hypotension, bradycardia, lightheadedness, flushing, cardiovascular collapse, methemoglobinemia.

Contraindications: Hypotension, severe bradycardia or tachycardia, right-sided MI, increased intracranial pressure, intracranial bleeding, patients taking any medications for erectile dysfunction (such as sildenafil [Viagra], tadalafil [Cialis], or vardenafil [Levitra]), known sensitivity to nitrates. Use with caution in anemia, closed-angle glaucoma, hypotension, postural hypotension, uncorrected hypovolemia.

Dosage:
- **Adult:**
    - **Sublingual tablets:** One tablet (0.3 to 0.4 mg) at 5-minute intervals to a maximum of three doses.
    - **Translingual spray:** One (0.4 mg) spray at 5-minute intervals to a maximum of three sprays.
    - **Ointment:** 2% topical (Nitro-Bid ointment): Apply 1 to 2 inches of paste over the chest wall, cover with transparent wrap, and secure with tape.
    - **IV infusion:** 5 mcg/min; may increase rate by 5 to 10 mcg/min every 5 to 10 minutes as needed. End points of dose titration for nitroglycerin include a drop in the blood pressure of 10%, relief of chest pain, and return of ST segment to normal on a 12-lead ECG.

- **Pediatric IV infusion:** The initial pediatric infusion is 0.25 to 0.5 mcg/kg per minute IV, intraosseous (IO) titrated by 0.5 to 1 mcg/kg per minute. Usual required dose is 1 to 3 mcg/kg per minute to a maximum dose of 5 mcg/kg per minute.

Special Considerations:
Administration of nitroglycerin to a patient with right ventricular MI can result in hypotension. Pregnancy class C.

MORPHINE SULFATE

Classification: Opiate agonist, Schedule C-II.
Action: Binds with opioid receptors. Morphine is capable of inducing hypotension by depression of the vasomotor centers of the brain, as well as release of the chemical histamine. In the management of angina, morphine reduces stimulation of the sympathetic nervous system caused by pain and anxiety. Reduction of sympathetic stimulation reduces heart rate, cardiac work, and myocardial oxygen consumption.
Indications: Moderate to severe pain, including chest pain associated with ACS, congestive heart failure, pulmonary edema.
Adverse Effects: Respiratory depression, hypotension, nausea/vomiting, dizziness, lightheadedness, sedation, diaphoresis, euphoria, dysphoria, worsening of bradycardia and heart block in some patients with acute inferior wall MI, seizures, cardiac arrest, anaphylactoid reactions.
Contraindications: Respiratory depression, shock, known sensitivity. Use with caution in hypotension, acute bronchial asthma, respiratory insufficiency, head trauma.
Dosage:
- **Adult:** 2 to 10 mg IV, IO, intramuscular (IM), or subcutaneous administered slowly over a period of several minutes. The dose is the same whether administered IV, IO, IM, or subcutaneous.
- **Pediatric <110 pounds (50 kg):** 0.025 to 0.2 mg/kg IV, IO, IM, or subcutaneous.

Special Considerations:
Monitor vital signs and pulse oximetry closely. Be prepared to support patient's airway and ventilations. Patients may report a "flushed" or hot feeling immediately following administration. Assess for signs of allergic reaction; however, this is typically a histamine release.
Overdose should be treated with naloxone.
Pregnancy class C.

Beta Blockers. Beta blockers help the ischemic heart by reducing chronotropic and inotropic activity. These two actions reduce the consumption of oxygen by the heart. Beta blockers should be administered to all patients (lacking a contraindication) with UA/NSTEMI. Beta blockers administered within the first few hours following ischemia have demonstrated decreased myocardial damage and decreased long-term complications.[8] Beta blockers should be administered as soon as possible. The choice of beta blocker is not as important as ensuring that at-risk patients receive beta blockade. When administering IV beta blockers to patients, frequently reevaluate the patient's heart rate, blood pressure, and ECG monitor. In addition, frequently auscultate the patient's lungs to evaluate for the development of rales, bronchospasms, or signs of bronchospasm. Beta blockers should be avoided in patients with current cocaine abuse. Cocaine is a sympathetic stimulant. With beta blockade, unopposed alpha-receptor stimulation can lead to life-threatening hypertension.

Beta blockers should be administered for STEMI patients unless the following contraindications occur:

- Signs of heart failure
- Evidence of low output state

- Cardiogenic shock or increased risk for cardiogenic shock
- Preload-dependent conditions such as right ventricular infarction
- PR interval greater than 0.24 second
- Second- or third-degree heart block
- Active asthma or reactive airway disease

Patients who have atrial fibrillation (AF) or sinus tachycardia should have left ventricular function rapidly evaluated before the administration of IV beta blockers.

Information about specific beta blockers metoprolol (Lopressor), atenolol (Tenormin), esmolol (Brevibloc), and labetalol (Trandate) follows.

METOPROLOL (LOPRESSOR, TOPROL XL)

Classification: Beta adrenergic antagonist, antianginal, antihypertensive, Class II antiarrhythmic.
Action: Inhibits the strength of the heart's contractions, as well as heart rate. This results in a decrease in cardiac oxygen consumption.
Indications: ACS, hypertension, supraventricular tachycardia (SVT), atrial flutter, AF, thyrotoxicosis.
Adverse Effects: Tiredness, dizziness, diarrhea, heart block, bradycardia, bronchospasm, drop in blood pressure.
Contraindications: Cardiogenic shock, atrioventricular (AV) block, bradycardia, known sensitivity. Use with caution in hypotension, chronic lung disease (asthma and chronic obstructive pulmonary disease [COPD]).
Dosage:
Cardiac Indications:

- **Adult:** 5 mg slow IV, IO over a 2-minute period; repeat at 5-minute intervals up to a total of three infusions totaling 15 mg IV, IO.
- **Pediatric:** Oral dosing only.

Special Considerations:
Blood pressure, heart rate, and ECG should be monitored carefully.
Use with caution in patients with asthma.
Pregnancy class C.

ATENOLOL (TENORMIN)

Classification: Beta adrenergic antagonist, antianginal, antihypertensive, Class II antiarrhythmic.
Action: Inhibits the strength of the heart's contractions and heart rate, resulting in a decrease in cardiac oxygen consumption. Also saturates the beta receptors and inhibits dilation of bronchial smooth muscle (beta$_2$ receptor).
Indications: ACS, hypertension, SVT, atrial flutter, AF.
Adverse Effects: Bradycardia, bronchospasm, hypotension.
Contraindications: Cardiogenic shock, AV block, bradycardia, known sensitivity. Use with caution in hypotension, chronic lung disease (asthma and COPD).
Dosage:
ACS:

- **Adult:** Oral dosing only, not administered acutely for ACS.
- **Pediatric:** Not recommended for pediatric patients.

Special Considerations:
Pregnancy class D.

ESMOLOL (BREVIBLOC)

Classification: Beta adrenergic antagonist, Class II antiarrhythmic.
Action: Inhibits the strength of the heart's contractions, as well as heart rate, resulting in a decrease in cardiac oxygen consumption.
Indications: ACS, MI, acute hypertension, supraventricular tachyarrhythmias, thyrotoxicosis.
Adverse Effects: Hypotension, sinus bradycardia, AV block, cardiac arrest, nausea/vomiting, hypoglycemia, injection site reaction.
Contraindications: Acute bronchospasm, COPD, second- or third-degree heart block, bradycardia, cardiogenic shock, pulmonary edema, sick sinus syndrome, known sensitivity. Use with caution in patients with pheochromocytoma, Prinzmetal's angina, cerebrovascular disease, stroke, poorly controlled diabetes mellitus, hyperthyroidism, thyrotoxicosis, renal disease.
Dosage:
- **Adult:** 500 mcg/kg (0.5 mg/kg) IV, IO over a 1-minute period, followed by a 50-mcg/kg per minute (0.05 mg/kg) infusion over a 4-minute period (maximum total: 200 mcg/kg). If patient response is inadequate, administer a second bolus 500 mcg/kg (0.5 mg/kg) over a 1-minute period, and then increase infusion to 100 mcg/kg per minute. Maximum infusion rate: 300 mcg/kg per minute.
- **Pediatric:** 500 mcg/kg (0.5 mg/kg) IV, IO over a 1-minute period, followed by an infusion at 25 to 200 mcg/kg per minute.

Special Considerations:
Half-life 5 to 9 minutes.
Any adverse effects caused by administration of esmolol are brief because of the drug's short half-life.
Resolution of effects usually within 10 to 20 minutes.
Pregnancy class C.

LABETALOL (NORMODYNE, TRANDATE)

Classification: Beta adrenergic antagonist, antianginal, antihypertensive.
Action: Binds with both the beta$_1$ and beta$_2$ receptors and alpha$_1$ receptors in vascular smooth muscle. Inhibits the strength of the heart's contractions, as well as heart rate. This results in a decrease in cardiac oxygen consumption.
Indications: ACS, SVT, severe hypertension.
Adverse Effects: Usually mild and transient; hypotensive symptoms, nausea/vomiting, bronchospasm, arrhythmia, bradycardia, AV block.
Contraindications: Hypotension, cardiogenic shock, acute pulmonary edema, heart failure, severe bradycardia, sick sinus syndrome, second- or third-degree heart block, asthma or acute bronchospasm, cocaine-induced ACS, known sensitivity. Use caution in pheochromocytoma, cerebrovascular disease or stroke, poorly controlled diabetes, with hepatic disease. Use with caution at lowest effective dose in chronic lung disease.

Dosage:
Cardiac Indications:
Note: Monitor blood pressure and heart rate closely during administration.
- **Adult:** 10 mg IV, IO over a 1- to 2-minute period. May repeat every 10 minutes to a maximum dose of 150 mg or give initial bolus and then follow with infusion at 2 to 8 mg/min.
- **Pediatric:** 0.2 to 1 mg/kg to a maximum dosage of 3 mg/kg per hour; may also administer 0.25 to 3 mg/kg per hour as an infusion.

(continues)

LABETALOL (NORMODYNE, TRANDATE) *(continued)*

Severe Hypertension:
- **Adult:** Initial dose is 20 mg IV, IO slow infusion over a 2-minute period. After the initial dose, blood pressure should be checked every 5 minutes. Repeat doses can be given at 10-minute intervals. The second dose should be 40 mg IV, IO, and subsequent doses should be 80 mg IV, IO, to a maximum total dose of 300 mg. The effect on blood pressure typically will occur within 5 minutes from the time of administration. Alternatively, may be administered via IV infusion at 2 mg/min to a total maximum dose of 300 mg.
- **Pediatric:** 0.25 to 3 mg/kg per hour IV, IO infusion with a maximum dose of 3 mg/kg per hour.

Special Considerations:
Pregnancy class C.

(continued) You have administered sublingual nitroglycerin tablets of 0.4 mg three times. The patient states there is a reduction in her pain from an 8 of 10 to a 4 of 10. You arrive at the hospital. Immediately the emergency team prepares the patient for a 12-lead ECG. Oxygen is connected and vital signs are assessed. The patient is asked questions for medical allergies and conditions. The physician orders metoprolol 5-mg IV push and a nitroglycerin drip at 10 mg/min. The patient's heart rate is reduced to 62 beats/min and blood pressure is now 124/84 mm Hg.

Antiplatelets. The development of platelet plugs within the coronary arteries resulting in decreased blood flow to the oxygen-hungry cardiac muscle is the underlying mechanism for ACS. As discussed earlier, aspirin is rapid and effective in reducing aggregation. Clopidogrel (Plavix) is a medication that is categorized as an antiplatelet and anticoagulant medication. Clopidogrel inhibits a specific site on the platelet, rendering it incapable of binding to other platelets. This medication alters the platelet for the remainder of its life span. This makes clopidogrel a powerful anticoagulant. It is often used in conjunction with aspirin, as well as other anticoagulants, in the treatment of UA/NSTEMI. Clopidogrel 75 mg should be added to aspirin in patients with STEMI regardless of whether they undergo reperfusion with fibrinolytic therapy or do not receive **reperfusion therapy**. If coronary artery bypass graft (CABG) surgery is planned, the drug should be withheld for at least 5 days, or preferably 7 days. In patients younger than 75 years who receive fibrinolytic therapy or who do not receive reperfusion therapy, it is reasonable to administer an oral loading dose of clopidogrel 300 mg.

CLOPIDOGREL (PLAVIX)

Classification: Antiplatelet.
Action: Blocks platelet aggregation by antagonizing the GP IIb/IIIa receptors.
Indications: ACS, chronic coronary and vascular disease, ischemic stroke.
Adverse Effects: Nausea, abdominal pain, and hemorrhage.
Contraindications: History of intracranial hemorrhage, GI bleed or trauma, known sensitivity.

NDC 12345-678-90
Clopidogrel Bisulfate
75 mg   Rx only
500 Tablets
Usual adult dosage: See package insert
DISPENSE IN TIGHT, LIGHT-RESISTANT CONTAINER.
Each tablet contains 97.875 mg of clopidogrel bisulfate equivalent to 75 mg of clopidogrel base. Store at 25° C (77° F); excursions permitted to 15°–30° C (59°–86° F) [see USP Controlled Room Temperature]

LOT
EXP

Dosage:
Unstable Angina Pectoris or Non-Q-Wave Acute Myocardial Infarction:

- **Adult:** Single loading dose of 300 to 600 mg PO followed by a daily dose of 75 mg PO.
- **Pediatric:** Not recommended for pediatric patients.

Special Considerations:
Pregnancy class B.

© Dr P. Marazzi/Science Source.

(*continued*) The 12-lead ECG demonstrates T-wave inversion in the lateral leads. There is no ST-segment elevation. The patient is still having pain and rates it a 4 out of 10. Because of this continued pain, the emergency physician provides the patient with clopidogrel 300 mg PO. He is contacting a nearby cardiac center for transfer of this patient for further evaluation.

Anticoagulants. Unfractionated heparin and **low-molecular-weight heparin (LMWH)** are anticoagulants that inhibit thrombin. Heparin acts at multiple sites in the normal coagulation system. Heparin prevents fibrin formation and inhibits the activation of platelets. Enoxaparin (Lovenox) is an LMWH that works by inhibiting two proteins in the clotting cascade. It also inhibits the formation of clots. Compared with unfractionated heparin, which requires a loading dose, IV access, and laboratory monitoring, LMWH has greater bioavailability and is administered daily or twice daily by subcutaneous injection. The only detriment to LMWH is that there is no way to completely reverse its anticoagulant effects. Both medications are considered "blood thinners," but they do not dissolve existing clots. They are both used in ACS. They are typically initiated in the emergency department; however, prehospital providers may transport patients who are receiving these medications. Paramedics performing interfacility transports may also encounter bivalirudin (Angiomax), administered as an IV infusion for patients with STEMI or being transported for a cardiac catheterization.

HEPARIN (UNFRACTIONATED HEPARIN)

Classification: Anticoagulant.
Action: Acts on antithrombin III to reduce the ability of the blood to form clots, thus preventing clot deposition in the coronary arteries.
Indications: ACS, acute pulmonary embolism, deep venous thrombosis.
Adverse Effects: Bleeding, thrombocytopenia, allergic reactions.
Contraindications: Predisposition to bleeding, aortic aneurysm, peptic ulceration; known sensitivity or history of heparin-induced thrombocytopenia, severe thrombocytopenia, sulfite sensitivity.
Dosage:
Cardiac Indications:

- **Adult:** 60 units/kg IV (max 4,000 units), followed by 12 units/kg per hour (max 1,000 units). Once in the hospital, additional dosing is determined based on laboratory blood tests.
- **Pediatric:** 75 units/kg followed by 20 units/kg per hour.

(*continues*)

HEPARIN (UNFRACTIONATED HEPARIN) (continued)

Pulmonary Embolism and Deep Vein Thrombosis:
- **Adult:** 80 units/kg IV, followed by 18 units/kg per hour.
- **Pediatric:** 75 units/kg IV followed by 20 units/kg per hour.

Special Considerations:
Half-life approximately 90 minutes.
Pregnancy class C.

ENOXAPARIN (LOVENOX)

Classification: Anticoagulant.
Action: Acts on antithrombin III to reduce the ability of the blood to form clots, thus preventing clot deposition in the coronary arteries; inhibits factor Xa.
Indications: ACS, acute pulmonary embolism, deep venous thrombosis.
Adverse Effects: Bleeding, thrombocytopenia, allergic reactions.
Contraindications: Predisposition to bleeding, aortic aneurysm, peptic ulceration; known sensitivity or history of heparin-induced thrombocytopenia, severe thrombocytopenia, sulfite sensitivity.
Dosage:
Cardiac Indications:
- **Adult:** 30 mg IV × 1, then 1 mg/kg every 12 hours subcutaneously.
- **Pediatric:** 0.5 to 1.5 mg subcutaneously every 12 hours.

Deep Vein Thrombosis:
- **Adult:** 1 mg/kg every 12 hours.
- **Pediatric:** 0.5 to 1.5 mg subcutaneously every 12 hours.

Special Considerations:
Onset is approximately 3 to 5 hours; duration is approximately 12 hours.
Pregnancy class B.

BIVALIRUDIN (ANGIOMAX)

Classification: Anticoagulant; direct thrombin inhibitor.
Action: Binds with thrombin to inhibit various clotting pathways.
Indications: ACS, cardiac surgery.
Adverse Effects: Bleeding, hypotension, hypertension, allergic reactions.
Contraindications: Predisposition to bleeding, aortic aneurysm, peptic ulceration; intracranial hemorrhage.
Dosage:
Cardiac Indications:
- **Adult:** 0.75 mg/kg bolus followed by intravenous infusion 1.75 mg/kg per hour.

Special Considerations:
Rapid onset. Anticoagulant effects subside approximately 1 hour after discontinuing.
Pregnancy class B.

Glycoprotein IIb/IIIa Inhibitors. Glycoprotein IIb/IIIa inhibitors are medications that are used in patients with UA/NSTEMI/STEMI. They are often used in conjunction with heparin or aspirin to prevent clotting before and during invasive heart procedures. The mechanism of action of these medications is that they inhibit platelet aggregation by inhibiting the integrin glycoprotein IIb/IIIa receptor, as well as the final common pathway of platelet aggregation. These medications are very potent platelet inhibitors.

There are three medications in this class:

■ Abciximab (ReoPro)
■ Eptifibatide (Integrilin)
■ Tirofiban (Aggrastat)

The use of this class has shown definite reduction in death, MI, and the need for revascularization. These medications are used in the emergency department and extensively by cardiology. Currently they are not used in the prehospital environment. However, they remain an important treatment modality for UA/NSTEMI/STEMI, so prehospital professionals may transport patients receiving glycoprotein IIb/IIIa inhibitors.

ABCIXIMAB (REOPRO)

Classification: GP IIb/IIIa inhibitor.
Action: Prevents the aggregation of platelets by inhibiting the integrin GP IIb/IIIa receptor.
Indications: UA/NSTEMI patients undergoing planned or emergent percutaneous coronary intervention.
Adverse Effects: Bleeding from the GI tract, internal bleeding, intracranial hemorrhage, hypotension, stroke, anaphylactic shock.
Contraindications: Bleeding from any source, severe uncontrolled hypertension, surgery or trauma within the previous 6 weeks, stroke within the previous 30 days, renal failure, thrombocytopenia, intracranial mass.

© Bob London/Alamy Stock Photo.

Dosage:
UA/NSTEMI with Planned PCI Within 24 Hours:
- 0.25 mg/kg IV, IO (10 to 60 minutes before procedure), then 0.125 mcg/kg per minute IV, IO infusion for 12 to 24 hours.

Percutaneous Coronary Intervention Only:
- 0.25 mg/kg IV, IO, then 10 mcg/min IV, IO infusion.

Special Considerations:
Pregnancy class C.

EPTIFIBATIDE (INTEGRILIN)

Classification: GP IIb/IIIa inhibitor.
Action: Prevents the aggregation of platelets by binding to the GP IIb/IIIa receptor.
Indications: UA/NSTEMI—to manage medically and for those undergoing percutaneous coronary intervention.
Adverse Effects: Bleeding from the GI tract, internal bleeding, intracranial hemorrhage, hypotension, stroke, anaphylactic shock.
Contraindications: Bleeding from any source, severe uncontrolled hypertension, surgery or trauma within the previous 6 weeks, stroke within the previous 30 days, renal failure, thrombocytopenia.
Dosage:

- **Adult:** Loading dose: 180 mcg/kg IV, IO (max dose: 22.6 mg) over 1 to 2 minutes, then 2 mcg/kg per minute IV, IO infusion (max dose: 15 mg/hr).
- **Pediatric:** No current dosing recommendations exist for pediatric patients.

Special Considerations:
Half-life approximately 90 to 150 minutes.
Pregnancy class B.

Eptifibatide
Injection
NDC 12345-678-90
0.75 mg/mL Single-Dose Container
SINGLE USE VIAL FOR INTRAVENOUS USE ONLY
75 mg/100 mL vial
Rx only

TIROFIBAN (AGGRASTAT)

Classification: GP IIb/IIIa inhibitor.
Action: Prevents the aggregation of platelets by binding to the GP IIb/IIIa receptor.
Indications: UA/NSTEMI—to manage medically and for those undergoing percutaneous coronary intervention.
Adverse Effects: Bleeding from the GI tract, internal bleeding, intracranial hemorrhage, hypotension, stroke, anaphylactic shock.
Contraindications: Bleeding from any source, severe uncontrolled hypertension, surgery or trauma within the previous 6 weeks, stroke within the previous 30 days, renal failure, thrombocytopenia.
Dosage: 25 mcg/kg IV given over 5 minutes; 0.15 mcg/kg per minute IV, IO infusion for 48 hours.
Special Considerations:
Half-life approximately 2 hours.
Pregnancy class B.

Tirofiban
(hydrochloride)
Injection
NDC 12345-678-90
250 mL Single-Dose Container
Sterile Nonpyrogenic
Iso-osmotic
12.5 mg per 250 mL
(50 mcg per mL)
Rx only

Angiotensin-Converting Enzyme Inhibitors. ACE inhibitors are often used to treat patients with congestive heart failure and postinfarction and are usually administered orally. Although these medications are not initiated in all prehospital systems, they are an integral treatment modality for UA/NSTEMI/STEMI treatment. In addition, patients may already be taking a medication from this class. It is currently believed that this class of medications reduces morbidity and mortality in severe ACS. The reduction of future exacerbations of NSTEMI/STEMI has been linked to reduction in plaque rupture and shear force within the artery.

The body produces a hormone called angiotensin I, which is inactive. It is converted to the active form, angiotensin II, by the action of the ACE. Angiotensin II causes significant vasoconstriction and aldosterone secretion. Aldosterone causes retention of salt and water at the kidney with increased excretion of potassium. Both of these actions increase blood volume and blood pressure. Using an ACE inhibitor prevents the conversion of angiotensin I to angiotensin II. This causes a drop in blood pressure and reduces the stress on myocardial tissue.

The medications in this class include the following:

- Captopril
- Enalapril
- Lisinopril
- Ramipril

There has been no documented study to suggest one ACE inhibitor delivers better outcomes.

ANGIOTENSIN-CONVERTING ENZYME (ACE) INHIBITORS: CAPTOPRIL (CAPOTEN), ENALAPRIL (VASOTEC), LISINOPRIL (PRINIVIL, ZESTRIL), RAMIPRIL (ALTACE)

Classification: ACE inhibitors.
Action: Blocks the enzyme responsible for the production of angiotensin II, resulting in a decrease in blood pressure.
Indications: Congestive heart failure, hypertension, post-MI.
Adverse Effects: Headache, dizziness, fatigue, depression, chest pain, hypotension, palpitations, cough, dyspnea, upper respiratory infection, nausea/vomiting, rash, pruritus, angioedema, renal failure.
Contraindications: Angioedema related to previous treatment with an ACE inhibitor, known sensitivity. Use with caution in aortic stenosis, bilateral renal artery stenosis, hypertrophic obstructive cardiomyopathy, pericardial tamponade, elevated serum potassium levels, acute kidney failure.
Dosage:
- **Adult:** Medication is administered orally. Dosage is individualized.
- **Pediatric:** Medication is administered orally. Dosage is individualized.

Special Considerations:
Pregnancy class D.

HMG Coenzyme A Reductase Inhibitors (Statins). HMG coenzyme A reductase inhibitors have been shown to reduce the incidence of morbidity when administered within 24 hours after the onset of ACS. They have also been shown to reduce the incidence of reinfarction, recurrent angina, rehospitalization, and stroke when initiated within a few days after onset of ACS.[9] Although these medications are not typically initiated in the prehospital environment, they are part of the AHA algorithm for UA/NSTEMI. These medications are often referred to as the statins.

HMG COENZYME A STATINS: ATORVASTATIN (LIPITOR), FLUVASTATIN (LESCOL), LOVASTATIN (MEVACOR), PRAVASTATIN (PRAVACHOL), ROSUVASTATIN (CRESTOR), SIMVASTATIN (ZOCOR)

Classification: HMG-CoA reductase inhibitors (statins).
Action: Reduces the level of circulating total cholesterol, low-density lipoprotein cholesterol, and serum triglycerides; reduces the incidence of reinfarction, recurrent angina, rehospitalization, and stroke when initiated within a few days after onset of ACS.
Indications: Acute coronary syndromes/AMI prophylaxis, hypercholesterolemia, hyperlipoproteinemia, hypertriglyceridemia, stroke prophylaxis.

(continues)

HMG COENZYME A STATINS: ATORVASTATIN (LIPITOR), FLUVASTATIN (LESCOL), LOVASTATIN (MEVACOR), PRAVASTATIN (PRAVACHOL), ROSUVASTATIN (CRESTOR), SIMVASTATIN (ZOCOR)   *(continued)*

Adverse Effects: Constipation, flatulence, dyspepsia, abdominal pain, infection, headache, flu-like symptoms, back pain, allergic reaction, asthenia, diarrhea, sinusitis, pharyngitis, rash, arthralgia, nausea/vomiting, myopathy, myasthenia, renal failure, rhabdomyolysis, chest pain, bronchitis, rhinitis, insomnia.
Contraindications: Active hepatic disease, pregnancy, breastfeeding, rhabdomyolysis.
Dosage:
- **Adult:** Medication is administered orally. Dosage is individualized.
- **Pediatric:** Safe use has not been established.

Special Considerations:
Pregnancy class X.

(continued) The patient is started on heparin with a 4,200-U bolus dose followed by an 840-U/kg bolus. A nitroglycerin drip is started at 5 mcg/min. The patient is prepared for transport. During transport the patient develops increased pain. Per medical control, you adjust the nitroglycerin drip to 15 mcg/min. A repeat blood pressure is 130/88 mm Hg. You arrive at the receiving facility and the staff immediately obtains a 12-lead ECG that demonstrates no acute change. The cardiologist arrives and schedules the patient for **percutaneous coronary intervention (PCI)** immediately. He requests abciximab 0.25 mg IV and an infusion of 0.125 mg/kg per hour to be administered. In addition, he requests an initial IV dose of enalapril 1.25 mg IV and atorvastatin 80 mg PO. The patient is prepared for PCI and transferred to the cardiac catheterization laboratory.

Overview of ST-Segment Myocardial Infarction

CASE STUDY

You receive a call for a 61-year-old man with a chief complaint of chest pain. On arrival, you find a man with obesity sitting in a chair. He is dyspneic and diaphoretic. He states that his chest pain has been present for 45 minutes and is "like a ton of bricks on my chest." The patient describes the pain as radiating to his jaw and left arm. He has a history of hypertension, diabetes, smoking, and a positive family history of heart disease. He denies a history of congestive heart failure, COPD, asthma, or emphysema. His last cardiac workup was 3 years ago. His pulse is 96 beats/min, blood pressure is 138/98 mm Hg, and respiratory rate is 24 breaths/min. Your 12-lead ECG demonstrates elevations in leads I, aV_L, V_5, and V_6.

The patient in this scenario has a significant number of risk factors for ACS and infarction. He has chest pain that is pressure-like and lasts longer than 30 minutes. Radiation to the jaw and left arm are also common symptoms relating to anginal pain. He has shortness of breath and diaphoresis. Chest pain itself is a poor predictor of the prehospital diagnosis of AMI; however, diaphoresis in a patient with chest pain is definitely suggestive of ACS and infarction. ST-segment elevation in leads I, aV_L, V_5, and V_6 are specific for a lateral wall STEMI. This patient should be aggressively treated and prepared for transport.

The pathophysiology of STEMI is usually the complete blockage of an artery by a ruptured plaque and thrombus formation. Occasionally, the decreased blood flow can occur secondary to vasospasm. This can be caused by cocaine abuse. Thrombus or vasospasm actually causes blood flow to the heart to stop or diminish considerably. Decreased oxygen delivery causes ischemia. If not reversed, infarction will occur and result in cell death. After heart cells are damaged, they are unable to respond to electrical stimulus, which alters the conduction and contraction of cardiac muscle.

> (*continued*) You place the patient on oxygen 4 L/min by nasal cannula. Your partner places the patient on a cardiac monitor and gets ready to start an IV line while you prepare to administer several medications. You give the patient four 81-mg baby aspirins. You tell him to chew and then swallow the aspirins. You ask the patient whether he is taking any medications for erectile dysfunction or impotence, and the patient denies use of these medications. You administer one sublingual nitroglycerin tablet of 0.4 mg, then reassess the patient, including a complete set of vital signs. The patient reports that he has no reduction in his chest pain. Repeat vitals show heart rate of 92 beats/min, blood pressure 142/96 mm Hg, and respiratory rate of 18 breaths/min. Pulse oximeter reading is 95% on 4 L/min oxygen. Because the patient is still having chest pain after 5 minutes, you administer a second dose of nitroglycerin 0.4 mg sublingually. You take his blood pressure again, and it is 140/96 mm Hg. You then administer morphine sulfate 2 mg slow IV push. On reassessment of the patient, he reports significant improvement in his chest pain.

Management

Initial care for this patient is the same as for patients with UA. Appropriate prehospital care would include starting the patient on oxygen when indicated; initiating an IV; placing the patient on a cardiac monitor; and administering aspirin, nitroglycerin, and morphine sulfate. Additional medications that are used in STEMI treatment include those medications discussed in "Overview of unstable angina pectoris and non-ST-segment elevation myocardial infarction" section. This includes the antiplatelet medications, anticoagulant medications, ACE inhibitors, beta blockers, glycoprotein IIb/IIIa inhibitors, and HMG coenzyme A reductase inhibitors (statins). Reperfusion therapy is also indicated.

Reperfusion Therapy. Reperfusion therapy is the gold standard for the treatment of STEMI. The two methods for reperfusion are pharmacologic reperfusion (fibrinolytics) and PCI. Fibrinolytic treatment is indicated in those patients who have onset of symptoms of less than 12 hours, ST-segment elevation greater than 1 mm in two or more contiguous leads (or bundle branch block obscuring ST-segment analysis), and a history suggesting STEMI (**BOX 6-1**).

BOX 6-1 Reperfusion Therapy: Fibrinolytics or Percutaneous Coronary Intervention?

Fibrinolysis is generally preferred in the following circumstances:

- Invasive strategy is not an option (catheterization laboratory occupied/not available, vascular access difficulties, lack of access to skilled PCI facility).
- Invasive strategy would be delayed (prolonged transport, medical contact-to-balloon or door-to-balloon time >120 minutes, [door-to-balloon time] minus [door-to-needle time] is >1 hour).
- There are no contraindications to fibrinolysis.

An invasive strategy is generally preferred in the following circumstances:

- The diagnosis of STEMI is in doubt.
- A skilled PCI facility is available with surgical backup (medical contact-to-balloon or door-to-balloon time <120 minutes, [door-to-balloon time] minus [door-to-needle time] is <1 hour).
- Contraindications to fibrinolysis exist, including increased risk of bleeding and intracranial hemorrhage.
- There is a high risk from STEMI (such as congestive heart failure).[10]

PCI is preferred if the patient comes to a facility where PCI is available and if it can be accomplished within 90 minutes of the onset of symptoms. It is also preferred if there is increased bleeding risk. Patients with STEMI who come to a hospital with PCI capability should be treated with primary PCI within 90 minutes of first medical contact as a systems goal. Patients with STEMI who come to a hospital without PCI capability and who cannot be transferred to a PCI center and undergo PCI within 120 minutes should be treated with fibrinolytic therapy within 30 minutes.[11,12] Bottom line, faster reperfusion is endorsed.[13]

FIBRINOLYTIC: TISSUE PLASMINOGEN ACTIVATOR (TPA)

Classification: Thrombolytic agent.
Action: Dissolves thrombi plugs in the coronary arteries and reestablishes blood flow.
Indications: ST-segment elevation (≥1 mm in two or more contiguous leads), new or presumed-new left bundle branch block.
Adverse Effects: Bleeding, intracranial hemorrhage, stroke, cardiac arrhythmias, hypotension, bruising.
Contraindications: ST-segment depression, cardiogenic shock, recent (within 10 days) major surgery, cerebrovascular disease, recent (within 10 days) GI bleeding, recent trauma, severe hypertension (systolic blood pressure ≥180 mm Hg or diastolic blood pressure ≥110 mm Hg), high likelihood of left heart thrombus, acute pericarditis, subacute bacterial endocarditis, severe renal or liver failure with bleeding complications, significant liver dysfunction, diabetic hemorrhagic retinopathy, septic thrombophlebitis, advanced age (older than 75 years), patients taking warfarin (Coumadin).
Dosage: Dosing per medical direction.
Special Considerations:
Pregnancy class C.

(*continued*) You arrive at the emergency department. The physician orders a 12-lead ECG. The ST-segment elevation has worsened. The patient is started on a nitroglycerin drip at 10 mcg/min. Heparin is initiated with a bolus of 400 U and a drip of 1,000 U/hr. The patient is given clopidogrel 300 mg PO. Atorvastatin 10 mg PO is given, as well as enalapril 1.25 mg IV. Abciximab is ordered from the pharmacy. The PCI team is in place and the patient is taken to the catheterization laboratory for intervention. On your next call, you stop back to check on your patient. He received a drug-eluting stent in the circumflex artery. He has been placed on atorvastatin and captopril. He will be discharged home in the morning.

ACS represents a spectrum of diseases. The most benign form of ACS is stable angina. This is chest pain that generally occurs with exertion, is relieved by rest, and lasts less than 5 minutes. This may progress to UA, which is pain that follows no pattern. Chest pressure may occur at rest, during sleep, or during activity. This pain typically lasts less than 20 minutes. NSTEMI is very similar to UA in its presentation. The difference is that with NSTEMI there is alteration in cardiac enzymes that reflect myocardial damage. To the prehospital professional, these two conditions will be indistinguishable. STEMI occurs when there is a significant decrease in coronary blood flow. This is often caused by a rupture of the atherosclerotic plaque. A thrombus rich in platelets obstructs blood flow and oxygen delivery to the myocardial cell. This can lead to cell death and loss of cardiac muscle function.

The primary goal of treatment is to minimize the damage to the myocardial cells. This can be accomplished by a variety of medications.

- Oxygen is used to help increase the supply of oxygen to the ischemic cells.
- Nitroglycerin is a vasodilating medication that increases blood flow to the coronary arteries.
- Morphine sulfate, fentanyl, and hydromorphone are narcotic pain medications that reduce the sympathetic response to pain.

- Aspirin is an antiplatelet medication that reduces platelet clumping and formation of a thrombus.
- Clopidogrel is an antiplatelet medication that also inhibits the clumping of platelets and affects the platelet for its entire life.
- Heparin and LMWH affect the clotting cascade and inhibit further clotting at the site of the thrombus.
- Glycoprotein IIb/IIIa inhibitors also prevent the terminal step in platelet aggregation.
- Beta blockers reduce the heart rate and blood pressure, lowering the sheer stress on the myocardial muscle cells.
- ACE inhibitors reduce volume and blood pressure.
- Fibrinolytics are the only medications that actually will break an existing thrombus.
- PCI is the mechanical opening of the blocked artery by either balloon or stent placement.

ACS is a major cause of morbidity and mortality in this country and around the world. Research and development continue to advance the science of the treatment for ACS. With the common goal of reperfusion to minimize cardiac damage as the gold standard, prehospital professionals will continue to be at the forefront of this fascinating change in treating this disease process.

▶ Review Questions

1. List risk factors for acute myocardial ischemia.
2. Why is oxygen administration critical to a patient with stable angina pectoris?
3. Before administering nitroglycerin to a male patient, you should ask whether the patient is taking medications for what condition?
4. Name two benefits of administering morphine to a patient with chest pain.
5. What is the effect of beta blockers on the ischemic heart?
6. Name three contraindications for the use of beta blockers.
7. Explain the role of antiplatelets know as glycoprotein IIb/IIIa receptor antagonists.
8. What are the contraindications for fibrinolytic drug administrations?

References

1. National Center for Chronic Disease Prevention and Health Promotion, Division for Heart Disease and Stroke Prevention. Heart disease links. Centers for Disease Control and Prevention. https://www.cdc.gov/heartdisease/facts.htm. Updated November 28, 2017. Accessed July 16, 2018.
2. Shuvy M, Atar D, Steg PG, et al. Oxygen therapy in acute coronary syndrome: are the benefits worth the risk? *Euro Heart J*. 2013;34(22):1630–1635.
3. Khoshnood A, Carlsson M, Akbarzadeh M, et al. The effects of oxygen therapy on myocardial salvage in ST elevation myocardial infarction treated with acute percutaneous coronary intervention: The Supplemental Oxygen in Catheterized Coronary Emergency Reperfusion (SOCCER) study. *Cardiology*. 2015;132:16–21.
4. American Heart Association. Web-based integrated 2010 and 2015 American Heart Association guidelines for cardiopulmonary resuscitation and emergency cardiovascular care. Part 9: Acute coronary syndromes. https://eccguidelines.heart.org/index.php/circulation/cpr-ecc-guidelines-2/part-9-acute-coronary-syndromes/. Accessed July 16, 2018.
5. Cornet AD, Kooter AJ, Peters MJ, Smulders YM. The potential harm of oxygen therapy in medical emergencies. *Critical Care*. 2013;17(2):313. doi:10.1186/cc12554.
6. Cabello JB, Burls A, Emparanza JI, Bayliss S, Quinn T. Oxygen therapy for acute myocardial infarction. *Cochrane Database Syst Rev*. 2013. doi:10.1002/14651858.CD007160.pub3.
7. Levin T, Goldstein JA. Right ventricular myocardial infarction. UpToDate. https://www.uptodate.com/contents/right-ventricular-myocardial-infarction/print?source=see_link#H12. Updated October 23, 2017. Accessed July 16, 2018.
8. Dészsi CA, Szentes V. The real role of β-blockers in daily cardiovascular therapy. *Am J Cardiovasc Drugs*. 2017;17(5):361–373.
9. American Heart Association. 2005 American Heart Association guidelines for cardiopulmonary resuscitation and emergency cardiovascular care. Part 8: Stabilization of the patient with acute coronary syndromes. *Circulation*. 2005;112:IV89–IV110.

10. Gibson CM, Pinto DS, Cutlip D. Acute ST elevation myocardial infarction: selecting a reperfusion strategy. UpToDate. https://www.uptodate.com/contents/acute-st-elevation-myocardial-infarction-selecting-a-reper-fusion-strategy/print?source=see_link. Updated March 29, 2018. Accessed July 16, 2018.
11. Bouthillet T. AHA changes acceptable time to primary PCI from 90 to 120 minutes for acute STEMI. EMS 12-Lead. http://www.ems12lead.com/2011/12/30/aha-changes-acceptable-time-to-primary-pci-from-90-to-120-minutes-for-acute-stemi. Published December 30, 2011. Accessed September 17, 2018.
12. Muñoz D, Roettig ML, Monk L, Al-Khalidi H, Jollis JG, Granger CB. Transport time and care processes for patients transferred with ST-segment-elevation myocardial infarction: the reperfusion in acute myocardial infarction in Carolina emergency rooms experience. *Circulation*. 2012;5(4):555–562.
13. Antman EM, Hand M, Armstrong PW, et al. 2007 focused update of the ACC/AHA 2004 guidelines for the management of patients with ST-elevation myocardial infarction: a report of the American College of Cardiology/American Heart Association task force on practice guidelines developed in collaboration with the Canadian Cardiovascular Society endorsed by the American Academy of Family Physicians. *J Am Coll Cardiol*. 2008;117(2):296–329.

CHAPTER 7

Analgesia and Sedation

OBJECTIVES

1. Discuss why, despite the frequency of patient reports of pain, pain often is not treated in the field.
2. Discuss the narcotics (opiates) that the prehospital provider may encounter: morphine sulfate and fentanyl citrate (Sublimaze).
3. Discuss the effects of nonsteroidal anti-inflammatory drugs, including ibuprofen and ketorolac (Toradol).
4. List the benefits of nitrous oxide, and demonstrate the proper procedure for administering the drug.
5. Discuss various roles of ketamine (Ketalar) and etomidate (Amidate) in prehospital care.
6. Explain the benefit of the ability of benzodiazepines to induce anterograde amnesia.
7. Discuss the role of sedatives (benzodiazepines) in pain management, including the following drugs: diazepam (Valium), midazolam (Versed), lorazepam (Ativan), flumazenil (Romazicon), and naloxone (Narcan).
8. Explain why antiemetics may be necessary in the treatment of pain.
9. Discuss the effects of the following antiemetics: promethazine (Phenergan), ondansetron (Zofran), and dolasetron (Anzemet).

MEDICATIONS THAT APPEAR IN CHAPTER 7

Morphine sulfate	Ketamine (Ketalar)	Flumazenil (Romazicon)
Fentanyl citrate (Sublimaze)	Etomidate (Amidate)	Naloxone (Narcan)
Ibuprofen	Diazepam (Valium)	Promethazine (Phenergan)
Ketorolac (Toradol)	Midazolam (Versed)	Dolasetron (Anzemet)
Nitrous oxide	Lorazepam (Ativan)	Ondansetron (Zofran)

▶ Introduction

Pain is a common complaint in the prehospital field. Paramedics often encounter reports of headaches, chest pain, pain from trauma such as fractures, and abdominal discomfort. Innumerable medical conditions can present as pain. A variety of agents and treatments are available to reduce a patient's discomfort and even allow a more thorough patient assessment. The term **narcotic** describes the very broad group of chemicals that are known to induce sleep. This term is commonly used to describe illicit drugs or legally controlled medications. In a legal context, cocaine and other stimulant medications are frequently referred to as narcotics despite not having predominant sedative properties. Most true narcotics administered by EMS providers are **opioids**, medications that act upon opioid receptors in the body. The group of opioids includes synthetic medications such as hydromorphone (Dilaudid), fentanyl (Sublimaze), and oxycodone. It also includes morphine, a true **opiate** chemical, meaning it can be derived directly from the opium poppy (*Papaver somniferum*) plant. In addition to opioid medications, EMS providers may administer other sedating and pain-relieving substances such as **nonsteroidal anti-inflammatory drugs (NSAIDs)**, sedatives (benzodiazepines), antiemetics, and other miscellaneous pain medications.

CASE STUDY

Your unit is dispatched to a local park. On arrival, you find a 34-year-old man lying on a paved running path. The patient's distraught wife explains that her husband fell while Rollerblading. The patient is experiencing extreme pain in his left leg. You perform an assessment. The patient has a heart rate of 130 beats/min, blood pressure of 160/102 mm Hg, respiratory rate of 18 breaths/min, and an oxygen saturation level of 97%. The patient has gross deformity of the left thigh, indicating a closed femur fracture. He has good motor and sensory function, as well as pulses distal to the fracture.

▶ Overview of Analgesia and Sedation

Despite the frequency of patient reports of pain, it is often not adequately treated in the prehospital setting.[1,2] Several reasons explain this fact, with the principal one being the concern that administration of **analgesics** (compounds that relieve pain), especially opioids, can cause respiratory depression and hypotension. Providers are also concerned that analgesics may mask the progression of symptoms.

Pediatric patients have been historically undermedicated for pain, due to a combination of communication barriers, lack of validated pain assessment tools, and other related factors.[3,4] Older adult patients have similar challenges related to pain control. Pain assessment in older adults can be complicated by other medical conditions, cognitive decline, depression, acceptance of pain as a normal process, and other factors. EMS providers should be particularly mindful when assessing these groups for the presence or severity of pain.

Another argument against the liberal use of analgesics in the field is that administration of these agents can complicate assessment of the patient after arrival at the hospital. For example, in a patient with a head injury or another neurologic condition, the administration of analgesics or sedatives (calming, quieting drugs) can mask the progression of the condition. In the case of abdominal pain, narcotics have historically been withheld until a diagnosis or a decision for surgery has been made. However, this philosophy originated in an era when the principal method for determining that a patient needed surgery was physical examination of the abdomen. The near-universal use of computer tomographic scanning for the evaluation of abdominal pain makes analgesia less of a concern. Narcotics in excessive doses can reduce the patient's ability to protect the airway and decrease respirations. Fear of these complications results in a lower rate of authorization for narcotics administration. Unfortunately, the result is that patients endure pain that can be easily treated. Apnea and loss of an airway are potentially catastrophic complications. Therefore, the provider must closely monitor the patient's oxygen saturation, ventilations, and airway. If any of these becomes compromised, the paramedic needs to be prepared and equipped to intervene to support oxygenation and ventilation.

A patient's discomfort can be composed of several elements. The most obvious is pain, which can be treated with analgesics. A second element of a patient's distress is often anxiety, which is best treated with sedative drugs. **Sedatives** result in a generalized and nonspecific depression of the **central nervous system (CNS)**. Narcotic drugs such as opioids produce both analgesia and some degree of sedation as a secondary effect.

▶ Management

Opioids

Prehospital providers may encounter opioid chemicals in a variety of situations. Patients may be prescribed opioids for the management of short- or long-term (chronic) pain associated with a diagnosed medical condition. Opioids are also frequently misused or abused for recreational enjoyment, unrelated to any legitimate medical condition. It becomes extremely challenging for EMS and other healthcare providers when patients with a diagnosed medical condition appear to excessively use, misuse, or abuse prescribed or illegally obtained opioids.

Prehospital providers may administer opioid medications, such as morphine sulfate and fentanyl citrate in either the prehospital or interfacility transport setting. Morphine is specifically indicated in the advanced cardiac life support (ACLS) acute coronary syndrome (ACS) algorithm due to its analgesic and generally favorable hemodynamic effects in these patients. EMS providers employed in healthcare facilities may administer additional opioid medications that are not included in this text.

Opioid chemicals bind with **opioid receptors** in the CNS, resulting in a reduction of the pain sensation. At least three types of opioid receptors are present in the body, each activated by certain endogenous or exogenous chemicals. Morphine acts on the mu (μ) opioid receptor. However, opiates do not address the underlying mechanism producing the pain. If the muffler fell off your car, you would be disturbed by the loud noise your car now makes. One solution would be to increase the volume of the car's radio. The result is that you can no longer hear the rumble of your car, so it no longer disturbs you. However, as with the use of opiates, the underlying problem still exists.

The patient in the preceding scenario is reporting severe pain from a fracture of his femur. The administration of a narcotic to this patient will decrease his pain sensation but will do nothing to treat the fracture. Despite subjective improvement after administration of an opiate, the patient still requires specific therapy for the underlying problem, in this case the fractured femur. The fact that opioids can mask the principal problem by altering the patient's perception of pain is one argument for conservative use of prehospital analgesics.

Another example is a patient with abdominal pain from possible appendicitis. The provider may not know that the patient's appendix perforated if the pain is masked by excessive narcotics. Although this is certainly a valid concern, the judicious use of narcotics—versus withholding all analgesia—provides patients with some degree of relief and allows the examiner to obtain a reliable physical examination. *Judicious* is a subjective term and impossible to quantify. A safe practice is to administer small doses with frequent reevaluation between each dose. The administration of several small doses is better practice than administering one large dose.

The patient in the preceding scenario exhibits many of the typical signs of a patient with severe pain: agitation and restlessness, tachycardia, and hypertension. Although the tachycardia could be caused by blood loss associated with the femur fracture, the concomitant presentation of pain and hypertension supports the fact that the patient's elevated heart rate is most likely caused by severe discomfort. Tachycardia from hypovolemia is usually associated with a normal or depressed blood pressure.

Excessive administration of opioid medications can result in respiratory depression, so prehospital providers should give supplemental oxygen and be equipped and skilled to intervene and support a patient's airway in the event of respiratory depression or arrest.

Administration of some narcotics, such as morphine sulfate, can result in hypotension, particularly in hypovolemic patients. For example, some trauma patients can lose 25% of their blood volume without any depression of their blood pressure. Patients can often tolerate such blood loss because they are able to compensate for this decrease of their circulatory volume. However, administration of an opioid to such a patient can result in vasodilation and subsequent hypotension. Therefore, paramedics need to ensure that patients have adequate intravascular blood volume before administering narcotics. This may require administration of several hundred milliliters of an intravascular fluid bolus before administration of opioid medications.

Morphine induces the release of histamine, which causes vasodilation, which in turn produces hypotension. Patients frequently report a hot or flushed feeling with morphine that may be misinterpreted as an allergy. It is worth asking for additional information, and providing additional patient teaching, when contemplating administering morphine. Fentanyl citrate, although rarely used in the prehospital setting, does not result in the release of histamine and therefore is less associated with hypotension after intravenous (IV) administration. For this reason, if a patient who is hypovolemic requires narcotic administration, consider the use of fentanyl instead of morphine.

Meperidine (Demerol) is a synthetic narcotic commonly used to treat moderate to severe pain. Meperidine can decrease cardiac output in higher dosage ranges. It is broken down or metabolized by the liver, and its metabolites can cause confusion, hallucinations, and seizures. However, in a **single dose** it is unlikely that these toxic metabolites will become clinically significant. Paramedics are unlikely to administer meperidine, as it is no longer recommended for acute pain due to its neurologic side effects.[5]

(*continued*) The patient has a femur fracture and is reporting severe pain. His heart rate is elevated at 130 beats/min. You consider that the heart rate could be elevated as a result of blood loss from the fracture. However, given the elevated blood pressure and the patient's agitation from pain, you consult with medical direction. You present the patient's case, mentioning the patient's reported pain, hypertension, and tachycardia. Given the thigh deformity from the fracture, you are concerned that the patient may have had substantial blood loss. Medical direction approves the administration of fentanyl 50 mcg IV push. After administering the fentanyl, you repeat a set of vitals and patient assessment. After 5 minutes, the patient reports that his pain has not changed, and his blood pressure is 182/108 mm Hg, heart rate is 136 beats/min, and oxygen saturation is 98%. Medical control approves a second 50-mcg IV dose. After the second dose, the patient reports that his pain improves from 8 out of 10 to 4 out of 10. His repeat blood pressure is 138/88 mm Hg and heart rate is 110 beats/min. The pulse oximeter displays a saturation level of 95%.

MORPHINE SULFATE

Classification: Opiate agonist, Schedule C-II.
Action: Binds with opioid receptors. Morphine is capable of inducing hypotension by depression of the vasomotor

centers of the brain, as well as release of the chemical histamine. In the management of angina, morphine reduces stimulation of the sympathetic nervous system caused by pain and anxiety. Reduction of sympathetic stimulation reduces heart rate, cardiac work, and myocardial oxygen consumption.
Indications: Moderate to severe pain, including chest pain associated with ACS, congestive heart failure (CHF), pulmonary edema.
Adverse Effects: Respiratory depression, hypotension, nausea/vomiting, dizziness, lightheadedness, sedation, diaphoresis, euphoria, dysphoria, worsening of bradycardia and heart block in some patients with acute inferior wall myocardial infarction (MI), seizures, cardiac arrest, anaphylactoid reactions.

Contraindications: Respiratory depression, shock, known sensitivity. Use with caution in hypotension, acute bronchial asthma, respiratory insufficiency, head trauma.

Dosage:
- **Adult:** 2 to 10 mg IV, intraosseous (IO), intramuscular (IM), or subcutaneous administered slowly over a period of several minutes. The dose is the same whether administered IV, IO, IM, or subcutaneous.
- **Pediatric <110 pounds (50 kg):** 0.025 to 0.2 mg/kg IV, IO, IM, or subcutaneous.

Special Considerations:

Monitor vital signs and pulse oximetry closely. Be prepared to support patient's airway and ventilations.

Patients may report a "flushed" or hot feeling immediately following administration. Assess for signs of allergic reaction; however, this symptom is typically caused by histamine release.

Overdose should be treated with naloxone.

Pregnancy class C.

FENTANYL CITRATE (SUBLIMAZE)

Classification: Narcotic analgesic, Schedule C-II.

Action: Binds to opiate receptors, producing analgesia and euphoria.

Indications: Pain.

Adverse Effects: Respiratory depression, apnea, hypotension, nausea/vomiting, dizziness, sedation, euphoria, sinus bradycardia, sinus tachycardia, palpitations, hypertension, diaphoresis, syncope, pain at injection site.

Contraindications: Known sensitivity. Use with caution in traumatic brain injury, respiratory depression.

© Joe Amon/Contributor/Denver Post/Getty Images.

Dosage: Note: Dosage should be individualized.
- **Adult:** 50 to 100 mcg/dose (0.05 to 0.1 mg) IM or slow IV, IO (administered over 1 to 2 minutes).
- **Pediatric:** 1 to 2 mcg/kg IM or slow IV, IO (administered over 1 to 2 minutes).

Special Considerations:

Pregnancy class B.

Nonsteroidal Anti-inflammatory Drugs

CASE STUDY

On a hot Saturday afternoon, a 42-year-old man mows the lawn and then proceeds to enjoy the remainder of his day watching a baseball game on television and drinking iced tea. You are called to his home because he has a rapid onset of severe left flank pain. He describes the pain as rapid in onset, 10 on a 0 to 10 scale, located on his left side, and radiating down to his left testicle. He passed some bloody urine before your arrival. He denies any chest pain or shortness of breath. He has no significant medical history. His vital signs are heart rate, 122 beats/min; blood pressure, 132/88 mm Hg; respiratory rate, 16 breaths/min; and pulse oximetry reading, 97%.

The patient in this scenario presents with the classic signs and symptoms of **nephrolithiasis**, or kidney stones. Patients with nephrolithiasis typically have flank pain with radiation to the groin and, occasionally, hematuria. An NSAID would be an appropriate drug choice for this patient. NSAIDs work by inhibiting the body's pathways for producing an inflammatory response. They provide pain relief and decrease the inflammation partly responsible for generation of the pain.

The most commonly used NSAIDs are aspirin and ibuprofen. Ketorolac (Toradol) is another powerful analgesic that belongs to this drug class. It is an NSAID that can be delivered IV, IO, or IM. A dose of 60 mg ketorolac IM is equivalent to 800 mg ibuprofen.[6] Ketorolac can provide pain relief at the level traditionally provided by narcotics.[6,7] Additionally, ketorolac holds advantages over narcotics in the treatment of renal colic from kidney stones. NSAIDs block the production of prostaglandins, which subsequently blocks the spasms and peristalsis of the ureter. Conversely, narcotics increase the ureteral spasm and may actually increase the patient's discomfort.

NSAIDs lack the most common and dreaded adverse effect of the narcotic agents: respiratory depression. However, NSAIDs can pose some serious complications, including gastric ulcers, prolongation of bleeding time, and decreased kidney function. Aspirin, another common NSAID medication, is not used as a routine analgesic medication in the prehospital setting, but it remains a valuable tool in the treatment of ACS for its potent antiplatelet properties.

IBUPROFEN

Classification: NSAID.

Action: Inhibits prostaglandin synthesis by inhibiting cyclooxygenase (COX) isoenzymes, resulting in analgesic, antipyretic, and anti-inflammatory effects.

Indications: Mild to moderate pain, fever, osteoarthritis, rheumatoid arthritis.

Adverse Effects: Anorexia, nausea/vomiting, epigastric/abdominal pain, dyspepsia, constipation, diarrhea, gastritis, melena, flatulence, headache, dizziness.

Contraindications: Sensitivity to NSAID or salicylate. Use with caution in asthma, hepatic disease, renal disease, CHF, hypertension, cardiac disease, cardiomyopathy, cardiac arrhythmias, significant coronary artery disease, peripheral vascular disease, cerebrovascular disease, fluid retention, or edema.

© digitalreflections/Shutterstock.

Dosage:

Mild to Moderate Pain:

- **Adult:** 400 mg PO every 4 hours as needed, not to exceed 1,200 mg/day.
- **Pediatric: 6 months to 12 years:** 5 to 10 mg/kg PO every 6 to 8 hours as needed, not to exceed 40 mg/kg per day.

Fever:

- **Adult:** 200 to 400 mg PO every 4 to 6 hours as needed, not to exceed 1,200 mg/day.
- **Pediatric: 6 months to 12 years:** 5 mg/kg PO if baseline temperature is less than 102.5°F (39°C), or 10 mg/kg PO if baseline temperature is greater than 102.5°F (39°C) (max dose: 40 mg/kg per day).

Osteoarthritis or Rheumatoid Arthritis:

- **Adult:** 400 to 800 mg PO 3 to 4 times per day, not to exceed 3,200 mg/day.
- **Pediatric: 1 to 12 years:** 30 to 40 mg/kg per day PO in 3 to 4 divided doses, not to exceed 50 mg/kg per day.

Special Considerations:

Pregnancy class B.

KETOROLAC (TORADOL)

© Allik Camazine/Alamy Stock Photo.

Classification: NSAID.

Action: Inhibits the production of prostaglandins in inflamed tissue, which decreases the responsiveness of pain receptors.

Indications: Moderately severe acute pain.

Adverse Effects: Headache, drowsiness, dizziness, abdominal pain, dyspepsia, nausea/vomiting, diarrhea.

Contraindications: Patients with a history of peptic ulcer disease or gastrointestinal bleed, patients with renal insufficiency, hypovolemic patients, pregnancy (third trimester), nursing mothers, allergy to aspirin or other NSAIDs, stroke or suspected stroke or head trauma, need for major surgery in the immediate or near future (i.e., within 7 days).

Dosage: For patients weighing <110 pounds (50 kg) and/or aged ≥65 years refer to older adult dosing.

- **Adult:**
  - **IV:** 30 mg a single dose or 30 mg every 6 hours not to exceed a maximal total daily dose of 120 mg.
  - **IM:** 60 mg as a single dose or 30 mg every 6 hours not to exceed a maximal total daily dose of 120 mg.
- **Older adult (age ≥65 years or weight <110 pounds [50 kg]):**
  - **IV:** 15 mg as a single dose or 15 mg every 6 hours not to exceed a maximal total daily dose of 60 mg.
  - **IM:** 30 mg as a single dose or 15 mg every 6 hours not to exceed a maximal dose of 60 mg.

For patients with moderate renal impairment, administer half the recommended doses, not to exceed a total daily dose of 60 mg/day IV or IM.

Special Considerations:

Pregnancy class C; class D in third trimester.

Other Pain Medications

The need to induce or maintain an altered level of consciousness may require a variety of medications that are neither narcotic analgesics nor benzodiazepine sedatives. Nitrous oxide is an inhaled agent capable of providing some relief associated with fractures. Ketamine is a drug that provides anesthesia, allowing for the performance of invasive procedures. Ketamine is used by air medical services, combat medics, and prehospital providers in Europe. Etomidate is used in rapid sequence and pharmacologically assisted intubations. Propofol is a sedative agent administered to intubated patients being transported from one hospital to another; because it is rarely used by EMS providers, it is not further discussed in this chapter.

Inhaled nitrous oxide is a long-standing and safe method of providing rapid analgesia for procedure-related pain. Nitrous oxide, commonly known as laughing gas, is routinely used to provide analgesia for dental and surgical procedures. Patient-administered, inhaled nitrous oxide is safe and easy to administer. The agent is delivered by a demand-valve face mask as a 50:50 mixture with oxygen.[8] When the patient begins to near oversedation, the mask falls away from the patient's face and the patient begins to breathe room air.

Once the patient has received an adequate amount of nitrous oxide, the mask simply falls away from the face, preventing the patient from inhaling any additional anesthetic.

Nitrous oxide can provide mild analgesia and sedation. Inhaled nitrous oxide has a rapid onset of action, typically within 30 to 60 seconds. The patient's ability to protect and maintain an airway is preserved.[9] Nitrous oxide has been effectively used in the prehospital setting for analgesia.[8]

NITROUS OXIDE ADMINISTRATION

Equipment Needed:
Nitrous oxide and oxygen cylinders, blender, mask with demand valve, gas scavenger circuit
Procedure:
1. Tell the patient (not the provider) to hold the mask tightly against the face.
2. Instruct the patient not to talk or remove the mask between breaths.
3. Instruct the patient to breathe normally.
4. Monitor the patient's vital signs and pulse oximetry.
5. Continuously assess the patient for lightheadedness, restlessness, and nausea.[10,11]

Providers assisting with nitrous oxide administration must choose their words carefully and control the environment because patients who receive this medication can be open to suggestion after nitrous oxide administration. Keep the environment quiet and avoid any unnecessary conversation.

NITROUS OXIDE

Classification: Inorganic gas, inhaled anesthetic.
Action: Exact mechanism is not known.
Indications: Mild to severe pain.
Adverse Effects: Delirium, hypoxia, respiratory depression, nausea/vomiting.
Contraindications: Use with caution in head trauma, increased intracranial pressure (ICP), pneumothorax, bowel obstruction, patients with COPD who require a hypoxic respiratory drive.
Dosage: Inhaled: 20 to 50% concentration mixed with oxygen.
Special Considerations:
Ensure the safety of healthcare professionals. Use only with a scavenger gas system to ensure that unused gas is collected, or scavenged, and that providers are not exposed to significant levels of the agent.
Pregnancy class not noted.

CASE STUDY

You are a member of a flight crew that is responding to the scene of a burned child. You are told by dispatch that the patient is a 3-year-old child whose clothes caught on fire when she came too close to a fire used to burn trash. When you arrive, you find a child who is essentially being controlled with physical restraint by several adults. She is in extreme pain and is violently thrashing about. You perform your primary assessment. The child's airway is patent, and she is screaming in pain. You cannot obtain a blood pressure. She has good distal pulses. You determine that she has approximately 40% total body surface area burns that are deep, full-thickness burns. You consider placing an IV line, but this seems impractical given the child's violent movements and the severity of pain. Nevertheless, you need to obtain access for fluid resuscitation and pain control, as well as to maintain the child's airway.

Ketamine is a drug that is not often used by the average prehospital provider in the United States. However, it is extremely effective when used by advanced providers in air medical services and providers in the military. Ketamine has an expanding list of possible indications, including airway management, pain refractory to opioid medications, agitation refractory to sedative medications, and as a supplemental bronchodilator in severe asthma patients requiring intubation. Ketamine is a derivative of phencyclidine and is often referred to as a dissociative anesthetic. Dissociative anesthetics cause a state in which the patient feels "dissociated" from their environment. A notable number of patients describe a very unpleasant emergence reaction that may involve delirium, feelings of terror, unpleasant thoughts, and other related symptoms. Consider concomitant administration of a benzodiazepine medication in patients, particularly children, to minimize or prevent these reactions.[12] Ketamine is unique among the anesthetic drugs in that the patient can maintain spontaneous ventilation and airway patency.[13]

Many analgesics and sedatives are relatively contraindicated in hypovolemic patients because many agents cause vasodilation and subsequent hypotension. In contrast, ketamine stimulates the cardiovascular system by increasing heart rate and mean arterial blood pressure.

Etomidate (Amidate) is a hypnotic drug that induces a rapid and brief state of deep sleep or unconsciousness. It is most commonly used as an induction agent for rapid-sequence orotracheal intubation. After a bolus of etomidate, the patient is typically ready for intubation within 1 minute, and the duration of the hypnotic state lasts only 3 to 5 minutes. Despite causing unconsciousness, etomidate provides little analgesia.[14] After a dose of etomidate, the patient becomes unconscious and stops most movement. Administration of etomidate typically does not cause depression of the cardiovascular system.

> Just because a patient is not moving when experiencing a painful procedure does not mean the patient is not feeling pain. This is a common misconception.

KETAMINE (KETALAR)

Classification: General anesthetic, analgesic, sedative.
Action: Produces a state of anesthesia while maintaining airway reflexes, heart rate, and blood pressure.
Indications: Pain and as anesthesia for procedures of short duration.
Adverse Effects: Emergence phenomena, hypertension and sinus tachycardia, hypotension and sinus bradycardia, other cardiac arrhythmias (rare), respiratory depression, apnea, laryngospasms and other forms of airway obstruction (rare), tonic and clonic movements, vomiting.
Contraindications: Patients in whom a significant elevation in blood pressure would be hazardous (hypertension, stroke, head trauma, increased intracranial mass or bleeding, MI). Use with caution in patients with increased ICP or increased intraocular

© Julia Hiebaum/Alamy Stock Photo.

(continues)

KETAMINE (KETALAR) *(continued)*

pressure (glaucoma) and patients with hypovolemia, dehydration, or cardiac disease (especially angina and CHF).

Dosage: Administer slowly over a period of 60 seconds.

IV, IO:
- **Adult:** 1 to 4.5 mg/kg IV, IO; 1 to 2 mg/kg produces anesthesia usually within 30 seconds that typically lasts 5 to 10 minutes.
- **Pediatric:** 0.5 to 2 mg IV, IO over a 1-minute period.

IM:
- **Adult:** 6.5 to 13 mg/kg IM; 10 mg/kg IM is capable of producing anesthesia within 3 to 4 minutes with an effect typically lasting 12 to 25 minutes. In adults, concomitant administration of 5 to 15 mg of diazepam reduces the incidence of emergence phenomena.
- **Pediatric:** 4 to 5 mg/kg IM.

Special Considerations:
Pregnancy class C

ETOMIDATE (AMIDATE)

Classification: Hypnotic, anesthesia induction agent.

Action: Although the exact mechanism is unknown, etomidate appears to have GABA-like effects.

Indications: Induction for rapid sequence intubation and pharmacologic-assisted intubation, induction of anesthesia.

Adverse Effects: Hypotension, respiratory depression, pain at the site of injection, temporary involuntary muscle movements, frequent nausea/vomiting on emergence, adrenal insufficiency, hyperventilation, hypoventilation, apnea of short duration, hiccups, laryngospasm, snoring, tachypnea, hypertension, cardiac arrhythmias.

Contraindications: Known sensitivity. Use in pregnancy only if the potential benefits justify the potential risk to the fetus. Do not use during labor and avoid in nursing mothers.

Dosage:
- **Adult:** 0.2 to 0.6 mg/kg slow IV, IO (over 30 to 60 seconds); 0.3 mg/kg is used in many protocols/references. A typical adult intubating dose of etomidate is 20 mg slow IV. Consider less (e.g., 10 mg) in older adults or patients with cardiac conditions.
- **Pediatric:**
    - **Older than 10 years:** Same as adult dosing.
    - **Younger than 10 years:** Safety has not been established.

Special Considerations:
Etomidate is used to prepare a patient for orotracheal intubation. Both personnel and equipment must be present to manage the patient's airway before administration.

Pregnancy class C.

(*continued*) The child is badly burned and needs IV fluid resuscitation. Additionally, the child cannot be safely placed in the helicopter in such an agitated state. You estimate that the patient weighs approximately 15 kg (33 pounds). The plan is to administer IM ketamine. Once the child is sedated with the ketamine, then you will start an IV line and continue with analgesia and sedation with IV morphine and midazolam (Versed). Because the patient weighs 15 kg, you administer 60 mg IM (4 mg/kg). Within a few minutes, the child begins to calm down and has an almost faraway stare. You place her on the helicopter cot without any objection. You insert a peripheral IV line in her left arm and start some IV fluids. To prevent emergence phenomena and provide some additional sedation, you administer midazolam 0.75 mg IV (0.05 mg/kg). Approximately 15 minutes after administration of the ketamine, the child begins to report severe pain, which you treat with morphine sulfate 2 mg IV push. The remainder of the transport to the hospital goes well. You have to administer 1 mg of morphine immediately before arrival at the hospital.

Sedatives (Benzodiazepines)

CASE STUDY

You are dispatched to assist a despondent woman. Police are on the scene and have informed dispatch that the patient is hysterical after being informed of the death of a relative. You arrive to find an approximately 35-year-old woman who is crying and cannot be consoled. She has no medical or psychiatric history. Her vital signs are all within normal limits. You obtain additional history and learn that she was recently informed of her brother's death in an airplane crash. You try to control the scene by asking law enforcement to clear the scene of any bystanders. You try talking to her calmly, but your efforts fail. She then starts pounding the wall with her fists to the point at which her hands begin to bleed. People on the scene are concerned that the woman is going to hurt herself and perhaps someone else. Law enforcement begins to talk about physically restraining her, but you are concerned that physical restraints will only frustrate her and make matters worse. You contact online medical control and receive an order for an IV sedative/anxiolytic medication.

This case represents a patient who is likely to benefit from the administration of a sedative. The most commonly used class of medications that provide sedation are benzodiazepines. Benzodiazepines are also used to reduce anxiety (anxiolytics), relax muscles, and treat seizures. They cause a generalized depression of the CNS. Benzodiazepines have the added benefit of inducing a state of **anterograde amnesia**, or amnesia regarding events occurring after the trauma or disease that caused the condition. Patients who receive a benzodiazepine before an unpleasant procedure or situation are often unable to recall the objectionable event at a later time.

Commonly used benzodiazepine drugs include diazepam (Valium), lorazepam (Ativan), and midazolam (Versed).

In the preceding case, diazepam could be administered as a sedative. After IV administration, diazepam has a rapid onset of CNS effects. It is considered to have a long duration of action, with clinical effects lasting several hours and a half-life ranging from 20 to 70 hours. Diazepam can be quite irritating at the site of injection and can cause inflammation of the vein, or phlebitis. For this reason, diazepam should be injected into larger veins and administered slowly.

Midazolam is a short-acting benzodiazepine with peak sedation occurring in 30 to 60 minutes and a half-life of approximately 2.5 hours. Onset of action is seen in 3 to 5 minutes after IV administration. In the preceding case, midazolam could also be used to provide sedation. When compared with diazepam, patients will have a briefer period of sedation (30 to 60 minutes) after administration of midazolam. Its rapid onset of action and brief duration of action make midazolam an effective medication for use in the prehospital setting. When administered for ongoing sedation, frequent repeat administration or a continuous infusion is required.

Lorazepam is used by prehospital providers as a sedative, and to reduce anxiety. In healthcare facilities, lorazepam is additionally used for ongoing sedation, for control of seizures, and in the management of acute alcohol withdrawal. Like diazepam, lorazepam has a duration of action measured in hours and a half-life of 10 to 20 hours. It is not unusual for sedation to persist long after lorazepam has been discontinued. Patients may be prescribed oral lorazepam tablets for ongoing treatment of anxiety and other related conditions.

DIAZEPAM (VALIUM)

Classification: Benzodiazepine, Schedule C-IV.
Action: Binds to the benzodiazepine receptor and
enhances the effects of GABA. Benzodiazepines act at the level of the limbic, thalamic, and hypothalamic regions of the CNS and can produce any level of CNS depression required (including sedation, skeletal muscle relaxation, and anticonvulsant activity).
Indications: Anxiety, skeletal muscle relaxation, alcohol withdrawal, seizures.
Adverse Effects: Respiratory depression, drowsiness, fatigue, headache, pain at the injection site, confusion, nausea, hypotension, oversedation.
Contraindications: Children younger than 6 months, acute-angle glaucoma, CNS depression, alcohol intoxication, known sensitivity.
Dosage:
Anxiety:
- **Adult:**
  - **Moderate:** 2 to 5 mg slow IV, IM.
  - **Severe:** 5 to 10 mg slow IV, IM (administer no faster than 5 mg/min).
  - **Low:** Low dosages are often required for older adults or debilitated patients.
- **Pediatric:** 0.2 to 0.3 mg/kg per dose IV, IM every 4 hours to a maximum dose of 0.6 mg/kg.

Delirium Tremens from Acute Alcohol Withdrawal:
- **Adult:** 10 mg IV.

Seizure:
- **Adult:** 5 to 10 mg slow IV, IO every 10 to 15 minutes; maximum total dose 30 mg.
- **Pediatric:**
  - **IV, IO:**
    - **5 years and older:** 1 mg over a 3-minute period every 2 to 5 minutes to a maximum total dose of 10 mg.
    - **Older than 30 days to younger than 5 years:** 0.2 to 0.5 mg over a 3-minute period; may repeat every 2 to 5 minutes to a maximum total dose of 5 mg.
    - **Neonate:** 0.1 to 0.3 mg/kg per dose given over a 3- to 5-minute period; may repeat every 15 to 30 minutes to a maximum total dose of 2 mg. (Not a first-line agent due to sodium benzoic acid in the injection.)
  - **Rectal administration:** If vascular access is not obtained, diazepam may be administered rectally to children.
    - **12 years and older:** 0.2 mg/kg.
    - **6 to 11 years:** 0.3 mg/kg.
    - **2 to 5 years:** 0.5 mg/kg.
    - **Younger than 2 years:** Not recommended.

Special Considerations:

Make sure that IV, IO lines are well secured. Extravasation of diazepam causes tissue necrosis.

Diazepam is insoluble in water and must be dissolved in propylene glycol. This produces a viscous solution; give slowly to prevent pain on injection.

Pregnancy class D.

MIDAZOLAM (VERSED)

Classification: Benzodiazepine, Schedule C-IV.

Action: Binds to the benzodiazepine receptor and enhances the effects of the brain chemical (neurotransmitter) GABA. Benzodiazepines act at the level of the limbic, thalamic, and hypothalamic regions of the CNS to produce short-acting CNS depression (including sedation, skeletal muscle relaxation, and anticonvulsant activity).

Indications: Sedation, anxiety, skeletal muscle relaxation.

Adverse Effects: Respiratory depression, respiratory arrest, hypotension, nausea/vomiting, headache, hiccups, cardiac arrest.

© Dr P. Marazzi/Science Source.

Contraindications: Acute-angle glaucoma, pregnant women, known sensitivity.

Dosage:

Sedation: Note: The dose of midazolam needs to be individualized. Every dose should be administered slowly over a period of 2 minutes. Allow 2 minutes to evaluate the clinical effect of the dose given.

- **Adult:**
  - **Healthy and younger than 60 years:** *Some patients require as little as 1 mg IV, IO. No more than 2.5 mg should be given over a 2-minute interval.* If additional sedation is required, continue to administer small increments over 2-minute periods (max dose: 5 mg). If the patient also has received a narcotic, he or she will typically require 30% less midazolam than the same patient not given the narcotic.
  - **60 years and older and debilitated or chronically ill patients:** This group of patients has a higher risk of hypoventilation, airway obstruction, and apnea. The peak clinical effect can take longer in these patients; therefore, dose increments should be smaller, and the rate of injection should be slower. *Some patients require a dose as small as 1 mg IV, IO, and no more than 1.5 mg should be given over a 2-minute period.* If additional sedation is required, additional midazolam should be given at a rate of no more than 1 mg over a 2-minute period (max dose: 3.5 mg). If the patient also has received a narcotic, he or she will typically require 50% less midazolam than the same patient not given the narcotic.
  - **Continuous infusion:** Continuous infusions can be required for prolonged transport of intubated, critically ill, and injured patients. After an initial bolus dose, the adult patient will require a maintenance infusion dose of 0.02 to 0.1 mg/kg per hour (1 to 7 mg/hr).
- **Pediatric (weight-based):** Pediatric patients typically require higher doses of midazolam than do adults on the basis of weight (in mg/kg). Younger pediatric patients (younger than 6 years) require higher doses (in mg/kg) than older pediatric patients. Midazolam takes approximately 3 minutes to reach peak effect; therefore, wait at least 2 minutes to determine the effectiveness of the drug and the need for additional dosing.

(continues)

MIDAZOLAM (VERSED) *(continued)*

- **12 to 16 years:** Same as adult dosing. Some patients in this age group require a higher dose than that used in adults, but rarely does a patient require more than 10 mg.
  - **6 to 12 years:** 0.025 to 0.05 mg/kg IV, IO up to a total dose of 0.4 mg/kg. Exceeding 10 mg as total dose usually is not necessary.
  - **6 months to 5 years:** 0.05 to 0.1 mg/kg IV, IO up to a total dose of 0.6 mg/kg. Exceeding 6 mg as total dose usually is not necessary.
  - **Younger than 6 months:** Dosing recommendations for this age group is unclear. Because this age group is especially vulnerable to airway obstruction and hypoventilation, use small increments with frequent clinical evaluation. Dose: 0.05 to 0.1 mg/kg IV, IO.

Special Considerations:
Patients receiving midazolam require frequent monitoring of vital signs and pulse oximetry. Be prepared to support the patient's airway and ventilation.
Pregnancy class D.

LORAZEPAM (ATIVAN)

Classification: Benzodiazepine, Schedule C-IV.
Action: Binds to the benzodiazepine receptor and enhances the effects of the brain chemical GABA, an inhibitory transmitter, and may result in a state of sedation, hypnosis, skeletal muscle relaxation, anticonvulsant activity, coma.
Indications: Preprocedure sedation induction, anxiety, status epilepticus.
Adverse Effects: Headache, drowsiness, ataxia, dizziness, amnesia, depression, dysarthria, euphoria, syncope, fatigue, tremor, vertigo, respiratory depression, paradoxical CNS stimulation.
Contraindications: Known sensitivity to lorazepam, benzodiazepines, polyethylene glycol, propylene glycol, or benzyl alcohol; COPD; sleep apnea (except while being mechanically ventilated); shock; coma; acute closed-angle glaucoma.

© Scott Camazine/Science Source.

Dosage: Note: IV, IO lorazepam needs to be administered slowly.
Analgesia and Sedation:
- **Adult:** 2 mg or 0.44 mg/kg IV, IO, whichever is smaller. This dosage will provide adequate sedation in most patients and should not be exceeded in patients older than 50 years.
- **Pediatric:** 0.05 mg/kg IV, IO. Each dose should not exceed 2 mg IV, IO.
Seizures:
- **Adult:** 2 to 4 mg IV, IO given over 2 to 5 minutes; may repeat in 10 to 15 minutes (max total dose: 8 mg in a 12-hour period).
- **Pediatric:** 0.1 mg/kg slow IV, IO given over 2 to 5 minutes (max single dose: 4 mg). May repeat at half the original dose in 10 to 15 minutes if seizure activity resumes.

Special Considerations:
Be prepared to support the patient's airway and ventilation.
Pregnancy class D.

(continued) You administer 2 mg of midazolam slowly by IV to the patient over a 2-minute period. Two to 3 minutes after your initial dose you determine that the patient is still agitated. You decide to give her a second dose of 2 mg of midazolam. She calms down and slowly appears to be falling asleep. You monitor her vital signs; her pulse oximetry reading is 94%. Three minutes later, her pulse oximetry reading decreases to 87%. You apply a jaw thrust, insert a nasopharyngeal airway, and use a bag mask to get her oxygen saturation up to 97%. You retake her vital signs. Her blood pressure has declined from 114/74 to 68/48 mm Hg.

The preceding scenario is that of an inadvertent iatrogenic (caused by the medical treatment itself) benzodiazepine overdose. Airway maintenance, assisted ventilations, and IV fluid bolus are necessary in this case. In addition, the benzodiazepine antagonist, flumazenil (Romazicon), is needed for the treatment of benzodiazepine overdose. Flumazenil works by competing with the same receptor used by the benzodiazepines. Flumazenil is primarily indicated in situations where there are complications following (excessive) benzodiazepine administration by healthcare providers and none of the contraindications outlined in the following drug profile are present or suspected.

Flumazenil does not reverse the excessive sedation or other ill effects of opioids and other nonbenzodiazepine drugs. There are a number of important reasons *not* to administer flumazenil. Flumazenil should not be used for any person with a history of long-term benzodiazepine use, as it may precipitate withdrawal symptoms. Flumazenil should not be administered to any person with an intentional overdose, an overdose of unknown substance(s), or an overdose of any substance or medication known to cause seizures. In the event that seizures occur, flumazenil will interfere with benzodiazepine administration, preventing control of seizures with the medications typically carried by EMS. For obvious reasons, flumazenil should not be given to any patient with a known history of seizures, particularly in the prehospital setting when other types of anticonvulsant medications are not generally available. The duration of action of flumazenil is shorter than many benzodiazepine medications, especially if taken in excessive quantities. Remain vigilant for the return of sedation following flumazenil use.

(*continued*) You administer 0.2 mg flumazenil over a period of 15 seconds and start a bolus of Ringer's lactate. After 1 minute, the patient is still minimally responsive and requires airway and ventilatory assistance. You repeat the dose of 0.2 mg of flumazenil, again over a 15-second period. The patient begins to become more responsive, and her blood pressure begins to improve. You recheck her vital signs. Her blood pressure has improved to 104/76 mm Hg. She is breathing spontaneously, but her respirations remain shallow. You are aware that flumazenil does not reverse the hypoventilation associated with benzodiazepines; therefore, you continue to monitor both her airway and vital signs closely for the duration of the transport.

FLUMAZENIL (ROMAZICON)

Classification: Benzodiazepine receptor antagonist, antidote.
Action: Competes with benzodiazepines for binding at the benzodiazepine receptor, reverses the sedative effects of benzodiazepines.
Indication: Benzodiazepine oversedation.
Adverse Effects: Resedation, seizures, dizziness, pain at injection site, nausea/vomiting, diaphoresis, headache, visual impairment.
Contraindications: Cyclic antidepressant overdose; life-threatening conditions that require treatment with benzodiazepines, such as status epilepticus and intracranial hypertension; known sensitivity to flumazenil or benzodiazepines. Use with caution where there is the possibility of unrecognized benzodiazepine dependence and in patients who have a history of substance abuse, who are known substance abusers, or have a history of seizures.
Dosage:

- **Adult:** Initial dose is 0.2 mg IV, IO over a 15-second period. If the desired effect is not observed after 45 seconds, administer a second 0.2-mg dose, again over a 15-second period. Doses can be repeated a total of four times until a total dose of 1 mg has been administered.
- **Pediatric:** Children older than 1 year, 0.01 mg/kg IV, IO given over a 15-second period. May repeat in 45 seconds and then every minute to a maximum cumulative dose of 0.05 mg/kg or 1 mg, whichever is the lower dose.

NDC 12345-678-90
10 x 5 mL Multiple-Dose Vials
Flumazenil
Injection, USP
0.5 mg/5 mL
(0.1 mg/5 mL)
FOR IV USE ONLY
Sterile   Rx only

(*continues*)

FLUMAZENIL (ROMAZICON) *(continued)*

Special Considerations:
Monitor for signs of hypoventilation and hypoxia for approximately 2 hours.
If the half-life of the benzodiazepine is longer than flumazenil, an additional dose may be needed.
May precipitate withdrawal symptoms in patients dependent on benzodiazepines.
Flumazenil has not been shown to benefit patients who have overdosed on multiple drugs.
Pregnancy class C.

Naloxone (Narcan) is a **narcotic antagonist** that reverses the effects of opiate narcotics in the event of adverse effects such as CNS and respiratory depression. Naloxone is effective in reversing opiate-induced respiratory depression. However, the effects of this narcotic reversal are relatively short lived, lasting approximately 20 minutes.[15] A second dose of naloxone may be required 20 minutes after the initial dose to prevent the patient from again experiencing opiate-induced respiratory depression.

NALOXONE (NARCAN)

Classification: Opioid antagonist.
Action: Binds the opioid receptor and blocks the effect of narcotics.
Indications: Narcotic overdoses, reversal of narcotics used for procedure-related anesthesia.
Adverse Effects: Nausea/vomiting, restlessness, diaphoresis, tachycardia, hypertension, tremulousness, seizures, cardiac arrest, narcotic withdrawal. Patients who have gone from a state of somnolence from a narcotic overdose to wide awake may become combative.
Contraindications: Known sensitivity to naloxone, nalmefene, or naltrexone. Use with caution in patients with supraventricular arrhythmias or other cardiac disease, head trauma, brain tumor.

© Tomas Nevesely/Shutterstock.

Dosage:
- **Adult:** 0.4 to 2 mg IV, IO, endotracheal (ET), IM, or subcutaneous. Alternatively, administer 2 mg intranasally. Higher doses (10 to 20 mg) may be required for overdoses of synthetic narcotics. A repeat dose of one third to two thirds the original dose is often necessary.
- **Pediatric:**
  - **5 years or older or weight >20 kg:** 2 mg IV, IO, ET, IM, or subcutaneous.
  - **Younger than 5 years or weight <20 kg:** 0.1 mg/kg IV, IO, ET, IM, or subcutaneous; may repeat every 2 to 3 minutes.

Special Considerations:
Pregnancy class C.

Antiemetics

CASE STUDY

You are called to the home of a 36-year-old man who reports several hours of excruciating abdominal pain. The patient tells you that he has had the pain for several hours. It is localized to the lower midline portion of the abdomen, and he is unable to stand or walk because of the severity of the pain. Your assessment reveals an otherwise healthy man who is lying in the fetal position in pain. His abdomen is rigid and extremely tender to any type of touch or manipulation. The patient is having dry heaves, which are aggravating his severe discomfort. You consult medical direction and obtain authorization to administer morphine 4 mg IV, as well as an antiemetic. Once inside the ambulance, you administer 12.5 mg of promethazine slow IV push. The patient has significant improvement in his nausea, his dry heaves stop, and his pain is significantly decreased.

Antiemetics are a functional class of medications used to treat nausea and vomiting, which are common adverse effects of the administration of narcotics analgesics. In emergency departments and hospitals, narcotics and antiemetics are often administered simultaneously to prevent the patient from experiencing the discomfort of nausea and vomiting. These agents can also be used to treat nausea and vomiting caused by conditions unrelated to the administration of narcotics. Common antiemetics are promethazine, dolasetron, and ondansetron.

Promethazine (Phenergan) is often used to prevent or control nausea and vomiting. It is also used as an adjunct for the control of pain. Promethazine is notorious for causing mental status alteration in older adults. When administering, dilute the dose in at least 10 mL of normal saline. Administer slowly over at least 2 minutes through a running IV line while observing for any signs of IV infiltration. Promethazine remains in use despite numerous risks and warnings. In many settings, it is being replaced by other medications for first-line treatment of nausea or vomiting.

Dolasetron (Anzemet) and Ondansetron (Zofran) are two **5-HT3 receptor antagonists** used to prevent nausea and vomiting. This class of drugs is typically used for prevention of chemotherapy-associated nausea. Use of these medications is expanding to include nausea and vomiting not associated with chemotherapy. These medications work better at treating nausea and preventing vomiting, rather than resolving active vomiting. They have overall efficacy similar to promethazine without many of the risks and warnings.[16]

PROMETHAZINE (PHENERGAN)

Classification: Antiemetic, antihistamine.
Action: Decreases nausea and vomiting by antagonizing H_1 receptors.
Indications: Nausea/vomiting.
Adverse Effects: Paradoxic excitation in children and older adults.
Contraindications: Altered level of consciousness, jaundice, bone marrow suppression, known sensitivity. Use with caution in seizure disorder.
Dosage:
- **Adult:** 12.5 to 25 mg IV, IO or IM.
- **Pediatric: 2 years and older:** 0.25 to 1 mg/kg IV, IO, IM (maximum rate of IV, IO administration is 25 mg/min).

Special Considerations:
Must dilute to at least 10 mL before IV administration.
Monitor IV site for signs of infiltration.
Use caution in older adults.
Pregnancy class C.

© Allik Camazine/Alamy Stock Photo.

DOLASETRON (ANZEMET)

Classification: Antiemetic.
Action: Prevents/reduces nausea/vomiting by binding and blocking a receptor for the brain chemical serotonin.
Indications: Prevent and treat nausea/vomiting.
Adverse Effects: Headache, fatigue, diarrhea, dizziness, abdominal pain, hypotension, hypertension, electrocardiographic (ECG) changes (prolonged PR and QT intervals, widened QRS), bradycardia, tachycardia, syncope.
Contraindications: Known sensitivity. Use with caution in hypokalemia, hypomagnesemia, cardiac arrhythmias.
Dosage:
- **Adult:** 12.5 mg IV, IO.
- **Pediatric: 2 to 16 years:** 0.35 mg/kg IV, IO (max dose: 12.5 mg).

Special Considerations:
Pregnancy class B.

ONDANSETRON (ZOFRAN)

Classification: Antiemetic.
Action: Prevents/reduces nausea/vomiting by binding and blocking a receptor for the brain chemical serotonin.
Indications: Prevent and treat nausea/vomiting.
Adverse Effects: Headache, fatigue, diarrhea, dizziness, abdominal pain, hypotension, hypertension, ECG changes (prolonged PR and QT intervals, widened QRS), bradycardia, tachycardia, syncope.
Contraindications: Known sensitivity. Use with caution in hypokalemia, hypomagnesemia, cardiac arrhythmias.
Dosage:
- **Adult:** 4 to 8 mg IV, IO, PO.
- **Pediatric: 2 to 16 years:** 0.15 mg/kg IV, IO (max dose: 16 mg).

Special Considerations:
Pregnancy class B.

© Margaret M Stewart/Shutterstock.

▶ Review Questions

1. Analgesics are used to treat what condition?
2. Discuss why, despite the frequency of patient reports of pain, pain is often not treated in the field.
3. How does morphine produce hypotension?
4. Which narcotic is less likely to produce hypotension in a hypovolemic patient?
5. Explain the risks of administering narcotics to a patient with abdominal pain.
6. What NSAID analgesic can be administered parenterally?
7. List the advantages of nitrous oxide administration in pain management.
8. What class of medications is used to produce sedation?
9. Define *antegrade amnesia* and identify the class of medications that can produce this effect.
10. Explain why antiemetics may be necessary in the treatment of pain.

References

1. Phrampus PE, Paris P. A guide to prehospital pain management. *J Emerg Med Serv*. http://www.jems.com/articles/print/volume-41/issue-11/features/a-guide-to-prehospital-pain-management.html. Published November 1, 2016. Accessed July 17, 2018.
2. Rutkowska A, Skotnicka-Klonowicz G. Prehospital pain management in children with traumatic injuries. *Pediatr Emerg Care*. 2015;31(5):317–320.
3. Verghese ST, Hannallah RS. Acute pain management in children. *J Pain Res*. 2010;3:105–123.
4. Kaye AD, Baluch A, Scott JT. Pain management in the elderly population: a review. *The Ochsner J*. 2010;10(3):179–187.
5. Buck ML. Is meperidine the drug that just won't die? *J Pediatr Pharmacol Thera*. 2011;16(3):167–169. doi:10.5863/1551-6776-16.3.167.
6. Turturro MA, Paris PM, Seaberg DC. Intramuscular ketorolac versus oral ibuprofen in acute musculoskeletal pain. *Ann Emerg Med*. 1995;26:117.
7. Cordell WH, Wright SW, Wolfson AB, et al. Comparison of intravenous ketorolac, meperidine, and both (balanced analgesia) for renal colic. *Ann Emerg Med*. 1996;28:151.

8. Oglesbee S, Selde W. Using nitrous oxide to manage pain. *J Emerg Med S*. https://www.jems.com/articles/print/volume-39/issue-4/features/using-nitrous-oxide-manage-pain.html. Published April 1, 2014. Accessed July 17, 2018.

9. Huang C, Johnson N. Nitrous oxide, from the operating room to the emergency department. *Curr Emerg Hosp Med Rep*. 2016;4:11–18.

10. Paris PM, Yealy DM. Pain management. In: Marx J, Hockberger R, Walls R, eds. *Rosen's Emergency Medicine: Concepts and Clinical Practice*. 6th ed. Philadelphia, PA: Mosby; 2005.

11. Munson ES. Transfer of nitrous oxide into body air cavities. *Br J Anaesth*. 1974;46:202.

12. Perumal DK, Adhimoolam M, Selvaraj N, Lazarus SP, Mohammed MAR. Midazolam premedication for ketamine-induced emergence phenomenon: a prospective observational study. *J Res Pharm Pract*. 2015;4(2):89–93. doi:10.4103/2279-042X.155758.

13. Roberts FW. A new intramuscular anesthetic for small children: a report of clinical trials of CI-581. *Anesthesia*. 1967;22:23.

14. Van Hamme MJ, Ghoneim NM, Amber JJ. Pharmacokinetics of etomidate, a new intravenous anesthetic *Anesthesiology*. 1978;49:274.

15. Anderson R, Dobloug I, Refstad S. Postanesthetic use of naloxone hydrochloride after moderate doses of fentanyl. *Acta Anaesth Scand*. 1976;20:255.

16. Patka J, Wu DT, Abraham P, Sobel RM. Randomized controlled trial of ondansetron vs. prochlorperazine in adults in the emergency department. *West J Emerg Med*. 2011;12(1):1–5.

CHAPTER 8

Anaphylaxis

OBJECTIVES

1. List the symptoms of anaphylactic shock.
2. Discuss the role of the immune system in fighting antigens.
3. Define an allergic response.
4. Describe the body's response to a foreign substance.
5. Identify the most common cause of death from anaphylaxis.
6. Discuss medications used to treat anaphylaxis: epinephrine, epinephrine autoinjectors (EpiPen and EpiPen Jr), albuterol (Proventil, Ventolin), diphenhydramine hydrochloride (Benadryl), hydrocortisone (Solu-Cortef), and methylprednisolone (Solu-Medrol).
7. Demonstrate the proper procedure for using an EpiPen.

MEDICATIONS THAT APPEAR IN CHAPTER 8

Epinephrine
Epinephrine autoinjectors
    (EpiPen, EpiPen Jr)
Albuterol (Proventil, Ventolin)

Diphenhydramine
    hydrochloride (Benadryl)
Hydrocortisone sodium
    succinate (Cortef, Solu-Cortef)

Methylprednisolone sodium
    succinate (Solu-Medrol)
Glucagon

▶ Introduction

Anaphylaxis and allergic reactions are included in a wider group of conditions called **hypersensitivity reactions**. Anaphylaxis, an exaggerated hypersensitivity reaction to a previously encountered antigen, is a potentially life-threatening series of events that affects multiple body systems. **Anaphylactic shock** is a serious and rapid allergic reaction that can be severe enough to result in death. The symptoms of anaphylactic shock include shortness of breath, syncope, itching, swelling of the throat, and a sudden drop in blood pressure. Anaphylactic shock causes hundreds of deaths each year in the United States. The allergic responses most often are stimulated by drugs such as penicillin or insect bites and stings. For prehospital providers to give optimal care to the patient experiencing anaphylaxis, they must understand the mechanism and the pharmacologic treatment necessary to prevent and resolve this life-threatening condition.

You respond to a call for a man in respiratory distress. The address is a local football field. It is a warm, sunny day. As you walk on the field, you notice bees swarming around garbage cans and discarded beverage cans. You find the patient, a 32-year-old man, sitting against a concession stand in the shade. He is wheezing audibly and is in obvious distress. His skin is warm and flushed. His wife tells you a bee stung him, and he is allergic to stings. She states that he is supposed to carry a medication pack for this type of situation, but he never got the prescription filled.

▶ Overview of Anaphylaxis

Immune Response

The human body has an elaborate system for protection against external threats. This system, known as the **immune system**, is designed to mitigate the effects of harmful substances that might enter the body and compromise essential body functions. The immune system complements and overlaps many other body systems as it helps to keep humans alive and healthy. It identifies and targets **antigens**, foreign molecules that are capable of generating a specific response. The subsequent response from the immune system is the formation of proteins, called **antibodies** or **immunoglobulins**, that are intended to bind with that specific antigen. Once bound to the antigen, antibodies have a variety of mechanisms to either destroy the antigen or facilitate its removal from the body. In patients with an autoimmune disorder, the immune system uses this same process to attack certain normal body cells and tissues, causing a vast array of harmful effects. The antigen/antibody response is needed to keep humans alive; however, an exaggerated immune response can be equally dangerous.

Allergic Response

An allergic response is brought about by a hypersensitivity to a particular antigen out of proportion to its hazard to the body. The allergic response, not the antigen, is the real threat. Humans can be hypersensitive or allergic to a variety of things: animals, vegetables, and minerals (**BOX 8-1**). In fact, people can be sensitive to almost anything, including medications, foods, and even dust. Materials that can induce a hypersensitivity or allergic reaction are known as **allergens**.

Foreign materials that initiate a normal immune response are antigens; antigens that produce an exaggerated allergic reaction are allergens.

People with allergies to an agent should avoid contact with the allergen and be medically prepared to treat inadvertent exposure. In many people, an accidental exposure to an allergen may cause a rapidly developing, life-threatening condition; these people need to carry medication to be administered in case of exposure.

Mechanisms of an Anaphylactic Reaction

When a person with a hypersensitivity is exposed to the allergen, cells within the body release the chemicals **histamine**, **serotonin**, **bradykinin**, and **slow-reacting substance of anaphylaxis**. The chief chemical among these is histamine. The release of histamine causes vasodilation, increased capillary permeability, and smooth muscle spasm. These effects cause

BOX 8-1 Common Allergens

Foods	Drugs
Milk	Antibiotics (e.g., cephalosporins, tetracyclines, penicillin, streptomycin, neomycin, bacitracin)
Egg whites	Aspirin
Shellfish	**Insect Bites and Stings**
Beans	Honeybees
Nuts	Yellow jackets
Citrus fruits	Wasps
Bananas	Hornets
Fish	Fire ants
Chocolate	
Chamomile tea	
Grains	
Sulfites	

the signs and symptoms of an allergic reaction, and the magnitude of this response determines whether the patient has an allergic reaction or anaphylaxis. Allergic responses can be minor, affecting only one body system, or severe, affecting multiple organ systems and even causing shock from respiratory and circulatory complications. When treatment is missed or delayed, these severe reactions are often fatal. Cardiac arrest can occur within minutes of the initial exposure.[1] The typical allergic response involves skin rashes, hives (urticaria), itching, redness, and edema. The patient can feel warm and flushed, exhibit edema of the lips and eyelids, and have watery eyes.

When confronted with a patient having a mild allergic response, determining whether the patient will progress to anaphylactic shock is not possible. However, always assume the potential for the development of shock and closely monitor the patient so that quick action can arrest or reverse anaphylaxis. Patients in anaphylaxis are having a serious medical event and require immediate intervention.

Although rash and hives are the most common manifestations of an allergic reaction, more severe complications can arise quickly and without warning. The signs and symptoms of a more serious anaphylactic reaction are best understood by reviewing the body's responses to invading foreign substances, including the following (**FIGURE 8-1**):

- After a foreign invader or material has been targeted, various cells attack the invader, releasing various chemicals—principally histamine.
- What distinguishes a normal immune response from an anaphylactic reaction is the magnitude of the chemical release.

FIGURE 8-1 Pathophysiology of anaphylactic shock.

- Histamine causes vasodilation, increased capillary permeability, and smooth muscle spasm.
- Vasodilation results in a drop in the systemic blood pressure and a decrease in peripheral tissue perfusion and oxygen delivery.
- Spasm of smooth muscle produces diarrhea, vomiting, and laryngospasm.
- Increased capillary permeability results in edema of the airway. The most common cause of death from an allergic reaction is obstruction of the airway.

The faster the onset of symptoms of an allergic reaction, the more serious the threat to life.

Most patients begin to show symptoms within minutes to an hour after exposure. The faster the onset of symptoms, the more serious the threat to life. As the condition progresses, laryngoedema, swelling of the vocal cords, can cause varying degrees of airway obstruction along with tightness in the chest, shortness of breath, and lightheadedness. Continuing development of anaphylaxis can be accompanied by a decrease in the level of consciousness, respiratory distress, and circulatory collapse. When a patient having an allergic reaction reports hoarseness or describes a "full feeling," the provider should assume the patient is progressing toward life-threatening anaphylaxis.

The patient's history often confirms the diagnosis of allergic response and anaphylaxis. While monitoring the airway and respiratory status, a history of allergies and any recent exposure should be obtained. In the event that the material the patient has been exposed to is still present, decontamination or removal of the substance from the patient should be accomplished immediately.

Management

With the knowledge that most deaths caused by allergy are the result of airway obstruction, rapid and thorough assessment of the airway and breathing is of utmost importance. Patients with airway or ventilatory deficits should be assisted as their history is obtained. If the patient's airway is rapidly collapsing, intubation must be considered. Rapidly developing edema can make intubation impossible after the airway obstructs.

The first-line medication for anaphylaxis is epinephrine given intramuscularly (IM) as soon as anaphylaxis is suspected or recognized. Epinephrine is a catecholamine that stimulates alpha-adrenergic and beta-adrenergic receptors. This stimulation increases the rate and force of heart contractions, increasing cardiac output, and relaxes bronchial smooth muscle. By relaxing smooth muscle, lung capacity is enhanced. Edema in the bronchioles is reduced by constriction of the arterioles of the bronchioles. Epinephrine also causes peripheral vasoconstriction, which raises the arterial blood pressure.

Epinephrine should be administered as quickly as possible; waiting to start an intravenous (IV) line to administer epinephrine often is not prudent. Therefore, in the treatment of an allergic reaction and anaphylaxis, consider epinephrine administration by an alternative route. Epinephrine 1:1,000 can be given by IM injection. Subcutaneous administration is discouraged because the medication absorption is slower and it results in lower concentrations of epinephrine at the desired sites. Larger patients require longer injection needles to avoid inadvertent subcutaneous administration.[1] The IM route is preferred over IV administration because there is less likelihood of adverse hypertension and cardiac arrhythmias.

> **What is the difference between epinephrine 1:1,000 and 1:10,000?**
> The two forms of epinephrine refer to the concentration, or potency, of the solution. Epinephrine 1:10,000 is 10 times more diluted than the epinephrine 1:1,000 solution. Ratio expressions of "1:1,000" and "1:10,000" are being phased out in the United States, in favor of "mg/mL" labeling to prevent medication errors.[1]
>
> **Why is one preparation used for IV use and another for subcutaneous and IM use?**
> For IV administration, the more diluted preparation of epinephrine is used: 1:10,000. When the medication is injected using subcutaneous or IM methods, it is not being delivered directly to the circulatory system. For subcutaneous and IM injection, use the more concentrated, or more potent, 1:1,000 preparation.

Once patients have a significant allergic reaction, they often are prescribed an epinephrine autoinjector (EpiPen or EpiPen Jr), which is an epinephrine self-injection system. This system allows patients to inject themselves, even through clothing, with an amount of epinephrine that should decrease their symptoms in time to seek medical attention. In many EMS systems, basic and intermediate providers are trained and permitted to help patients self-administer epinephrine with these devices.

USE OF THE EPIPEN

Equipment needed:
EpiPen, sharps, PPE
Procedure:
1. Unscrew the cap from the carrying case and remove the EpiPen.
2. The black tip of the EpiPen is where the needle comes out. Hold the EpiPen with the black tip pointing downward.
3. With the other hand, remove the gray safety release on the other end of the EpiPen.
4. Hold the black tip near the outer portion of the thigh. The autoinjector is designed to work through clothing. Do not inject into any area other than the outer thigh.
5. With a swinging motion of your arm, jab the EpiPen into the outer portion of the thigh so that the EpiPen clicks and the unit is perpendicular to the thigh.
6. Hold the autoinjector in place for 10 seconds. The color in the window of the autoinjector will change from clear to red, indicating completion of the injection.
7. Remove the autoinjector and massage the area for 10 seconds.

The next concern in treating anaphylaxis is maintaining circulatory integrity. Infusions of crystalloids, normal saline, or Ringer's lactate solution should be given to maintain sufficient volume in the vascular space to promote adequate perfusion. This usually means an initial bolus of 1 to 2 L of fluids in patients with hypotension.

EPINEPHRINE

Classification: Adrenergic agent, inotropic.

Action: Binds strongly with both alpha and beta receptors, producing increased blood pressure, increased heart rate, bronchodilation.

Indications: Bronchospasm, allergic and anaphylactic reactions, restoration of cardiac activity in cardiac arrest, persistent bradycardia where pacing is ineffective or unavailable.

Adverse Effects: Anxiety, headache, cardiac arrhythmias, hypertension, nervousness, tremors, chest pain, nausea/vomiting.

Contraindications: Arrhythmias other than ventricular fibrillation, asystole, pulseless electrical activity; cardiovascular disease; hypertension; cerebrovascular disease; shock secondary to causes other than anaphylactic shock; closed-angle glaucoma; diabetes; pregnant women in active labor; known sensitivity to epinephrine or sulfites.

© Jones & Bartlett Learning.

© Jones & Bartlett Learning.

Dosage:

Cardiac Arrest:
- **Adult:** 1 mg (1:10,000 solution) IV, intraosseous (IO); may repeat every 3 to 5 minutes.
- **Pediatric:** 0.01 mg/kg (1:10,000 solution) IV, IO; repeat every 3 to 5 minutes as needed (max dose: 1 mg).

Symptomatic Bradycardia:
- **Adult:** 2 to 10 mcg/min (1:10,000 solution) as a continuous IV infusion; usual dosage range: 2 to 10 mcg/min IV; titrate to effect.
- **Pediatric:** 0.01 mg/kg (1:10,000 solution) IV, IO; may repeat every 3 to 5 minutes (max dose: 1 mg). If giving epinephrine by endotracheal tube, administer 0.1 mg/kg.

Asthma Attacks and Certain Allergic Reactions:
- **Adult:** 0.3 to 0.5 mg (1:1,000 solution) IM or subcutaneous; may repeat every 10 to 15 minutes (max dose: 1 mg).
- **Pediatric:** 0.01 mg/kg (1:1,000 solution) IM or subcutaneous (max dose: 0.5 mg).

Anaphylactic Shock:
- **Adult:** 0.5 mg (1:1,000 solution) IM repeated as needed every 5 to 15 minutes, or transition to IV infusion of 1 to 4 mcg/min, titrated to effect.
- **Pediatric:** 0.01 mg/kg IM, repeated as needed every 5 to 15 minutes, or transitioned to continuous IV infusion rate of 0.1 to 1 mcg/kg per minute (1:10,000 solution); titrate to response.

Special Considerations:

Half-life 1 minute.

Pregnancy class C.

EPINEPHRINE AUTOINJECTORS (EPIPEN, EPIPEN JR)

Classification: Adrenergic agonist, inotropic.

Action: Binds strongly with both alpha and beta receptors, producing increased blood pressure, increased heart rate, bronchodilation.

Indications: Anaphylactic shock, certain allergic reactions, asthma attacks.

Adverse Effects: Headaches, nervousness, tremors, arrhythmias, hypertension, chest pain, nausea/vomiting.

Contraindications: Arrhythmias other than ventricular fibrillation, asystole, pulseless electrical activity; cardiovascular disease; hypertension; cerebrovascular disease; shock secondary to causes other than anaphylactic shock; closed-angle glaucoma; diabetes; pregnant women in active labor; known sensitivity to epinephrine or sulfites.

Dosage:

- **Adult:** An EpiPen contains 0.3 to 0.5 mg epinephrine to be administered IM into the anterolateral thigh area.
- **Pediatric:** For children weighing <66 pounds (30 kg), an EpiPen Jr delivers 0.15 mg IM.

Special Considerations:

Half-life 1 minute.

Pregnancy class C.

© smartstock/iStock Editorial/Getty Images Plus/Getty Images.

(*continued*) After placing the patient on 100% oxygen by a nonrebreather mask, you obtain IV access. Vital signs are respiratory rate of 30 breaths/min and shallow, pulse of 120 beats/min, and blood pressure of 90/60 mm Hg. The patient's continued distress causes you to suspect he is progressing to anaphylaxis, so you prepare to administer 0.3 to 0.5 mg of 1:10,000 epinephrine IV push. You also rapidly infuse 500-mL crystalloids for his hypotension. You follow the epinephrine with 50 mg of diphenhydramine IV push over a 2- to 3-minute period. With his continuing respiratory distress, you choose to administer 2.5 mg albuterol by nebulizer. The patient begins to improve, and you load him into the ambulance. While transporting, you contact medical direction and communicate the patient report. As you continue to monitor the patient, you prepare to repeat dosages of the medications already delivered because your protocol allows at least one repeat dose of the epinephrine and albuterol after 5 minutes if needed.

Second-line medications can include antihistamines, corticosteroids, and bronchodilators. *These medications are helpful, but they do not replace epinephrine. Epinephrine should not be delayed while these other medications are prepared or administered.* Antihistamines should be administered to all patients who have had an anaphylactic reaction. Diphenhydramine (Benadryl) is the most commonly used antihistamine. It controls the histamine release and, in turn, the allergic response to the antigen. Methylprednisolone (Solu-Medrol) and hydrocortisone (Cortef, Solu-Cortef) frequently are used to reduce edema and limit the recurrence of symptoms. Steroids are not helpful in the acute treatment of anaphylaxis, but they do prevent some of the later reactions of an allergic response.

For continuing respiratory distress, nebulizer treatments of bronchodilators such as albuterol frequently are used. Many prehospital protocols do not include the use of steroids, but most use epinephrine, crystalloid infusions, diphenhydramine, and albuterol or other bronchodilating medications. The use of steroids is more prevalent in protocols for extended transport times, such as prolonged interhospital ground transport and air medical services.

Albuterol (Proventil, Ventolin) is a direct-acting beta-adrenergic bronchodilator. By stimulating beta$_2$ receptors, albuterol causes bronchodilation. In the case of the bee sting, victim having an anaphylactic reaction, albuterol relaxes the bronchial smooth muscle that has been thrown into spasm by the release of histamine.

Diphenhydramine hydrochloride is also used to treat anaphylactic reactions because it competes with histamine for H$_1$ receptor sites and has significant anticholinergic properties. Diphenhydramine blocks the effects of histamine, including vasodilation, increased gastrointestinal tract secretions, increased heart rate, and hypotension.

Hydrocortisone is a corticosteroid that has anti-inflammatory properties. It is used in the treatment of allergic reactions, anaphylaxis, asthma, and chronic obstructive pulmonary disease (COPD). Although hydrocortisone generally is not helpful in the acute treatment of anaphylaxis, it does help prevent some of the later complications of laryngoedema and urticaria. As a prehospital drug, hydrocortisone generally is used only during extended transports as a single dose.

Methylprednisolone is a corticosteroid that decreases the body's inflammatory response and suppresses the immune system. It is used to treat severe anaphylaxis, asthma, and COPD.

ALBUTEROL (PROVENTIL, VENTOLIN)

Classification: Bronchodilator, beta agonist.
Action: Binds and stimulates beta$_2$ receptors, resulting in relaxation of bronchial smooth muscle.
Indications: Asthma, bronchitis with bronchospasm, and COPD.
Adverse Effects: Hyperglycemia, hypokalemia, palpitations, sinus tachycardia, anxiety, tremor, nausea/vomiting, throat irritation, dry mouth, hypertension, dyspepsia, insomnia, headache, epistaxis, paradoxical bronchospasm.

© Joseph Gaul/Alamy Stock Photo.

Contraindications: Angioedema, sensitivity to albuterol or levalbuterol. Use with caution in lactating patients, cardiovascular disorders, cardiac arrhythmias.
Dosage:
Acute Bronchospasm:
- **Adult:**
  - **Metered-dose inhaler (MDI):** 4 to 8 puffs every 1 to 4 hours may be required.
  - **Nebulizer:** 2.5 to 5 mg every 20 minutes for a maximum of three doses. After the initial three doses, escalate the dose or start a continuous nebulization at 10 to 15 mg/hr.
- **Pediatric:**
  - **MDI:**

- **4 years and older:** Two inhalations every 4 to 6 hours; however, in some patients, one inhalation every 4 hours is sufficient. More frequent administration or more inhalations are not recommended.
    - **Younger than 4 years:** Administer by nebulization.
  - **Nebulizer:**
    - **Older than 12 years:** The dose for a continuous nebulization is 0.5 mg/kg per hour.
    - **Younger than 12 years:** 0.63 to 2.5 mg every 20 minutes for a maximum of three doses. Alternatively, continuous nebulization at 0.5 mg/kg per hour can be delivered to children younger than 12 years.

Asthma in Pregnancy:

- **MDI:** Two inhalations every 4 hours. In acute exacerbation, start with 2 to 4 puffs every 20 minutes.
- **Nebulizer:** 2.5 mg (0.5 mL) by 0.5% nebulization solution. Place 0.5 mL of the albuterol solution in 2.5 mL of sterile normal saline. Flow is regulated to deliver the therapy over a 5- to 20-minute period. In refractory cases, some physicians order 10 mg nebulized over a 60-minute period.

Special Considerations:
Pregnancy class C.

DIPHENHYDRAMINE HYDROCHLORIDE (BENADRYL)

Classification: Antihistamine.
Action: Binds and blocks H_1 histamine receptors.
Indications: Anaphylactic reactions.
Adverse Effects: Drowsiness, dizziness, headache, excitable state (children), wheezing, thickening of bronchial secretions, chest tightness, palpitations, hypotension, blurred vision, dry mouth, nausea/vomiting, diarrhea.
Contraindications: Acute asthma, which thickens secretions; patients with cardiac histories; known sensitivity.
Dosage:

- **Adult:** 25 to 50 mg IV, IO, IM.
- **Pediatric: 2 to 12 years:** 1 to 1.25 mg/kg IV, IO, IM.

Special Considerations:
Pregnancy class B.

HYDROCORTISONE SODIUM SUCCINATE (CORTEF, SOLU-CORTEF)

Classification: Corticosteroid.
Action: Reduces inflammation by multiple mechanisms. As a steroid, it replaces the steroids that are lacking in adrenal insufficiency.
Indications: Adrenal insufficiency, allergic reactions, anaphylaxis, asthma, COPD.
Adverse Effects: Leukocytosis, hyperglycemia, increased infection, decreased wound healing, increased rate of death from sepsis.
Contraindications: Cushing syndrome, known sensitivity to benzyl alcohol. Use with caution in diabetes, hypertension, congestive heart failure, known systemic fungal infection, renal disease, idiopathic thrombocytopenia, psychosis, seizure disorder, gastrointestinal disease, glaucoma, known sensitivity.

(continues)

HYDROCORTISONE SODIUM SUCCINATE (CORTEF, SOLU-CORTEF) *(continued)*

Dosage:
Anaphylactic Shock:
- **Adult:** 100 to 500 mg IV, IO, or IM.
- **Pediatric:** 2 to 10 mg/kg per day IV, IO, or IM (max: 500 mg).

Special Considerations:
Pregnancy class C.

METHYLPREDNISOLONE SODIUM SUCCINATE (SOLU-MEDROL)

Classification: Corticosteroid.
Action: Reduces inflammation by multiple mechanisms.
Indications: Anaphylaxis, asthma, COPD.
Adverse Effects: Depression, euphoria, headache, restlessness, hypertension, bradycardia, nausea/vomiting, swelling, diarrhea, weakness, fluid retention, paresthesias.
Contraindications: Cushing syndrome, fungal infection, measles, varicella, known sensitivity (including sulfites). Use with caution in active infections, renal disease, penetrating spinal cord injury, hypertension, seizures, congestive heart failure.
Dosage:
Asthma and COPD:
- **Adult:** 40 to 80 mg/day IV in divided doses.
- **Pediatric:** 1 mg/kg (up to 60 mg) IV, IO per day in two divided doses.

Anaphylactic Shock:
- **Adult:** 0.5 to 1 mg/kg IV every 12 hours.
- **Pediatric:** Same as adult dosing.

Special Considerations:
May mask signs and symptoms of infection.
Pregnancy class C.

Glucagon may be helpful in instances where patients are taking beta-blocker medications. It may improve hypotension that persists despite treatment with epinephrine, producing both positive inotropic and chronotropic effects as well as bronchodilation. Glucagon is typically given 1 mg IV or IM in these situations.

GLUCAGON

Classification: Hormone.
Action: Converts glycogen to glucose.
Indications: Hypoglycemia, beta-blocker overdose.
Adverse Effects: Nausea/vomiting, rebound hyperglycemia, hypotension, sinus tachycardia.
Contraindications: Pheochromocytoma, insulinoma, known sensitivity.
Dosage:
Hypoglycemia:
- **Adult:** 1 mg IM, IV, IO, or subcutaneous.
- **Pediatric (<44 pounds [20 kg]):** 0.5 mg IM, IV, IO, or subcutaneous.

Beta Blocker Overdose:
- **Adult:** 3 to 10 mg IV, IO over a 1-minute period, followed by a second dose of 10 mg IV (or IV infusion 3 to 5 mg/hr) if the symptoms of bradycardia and hypotension recur. (Note that this dose is much higher than the dose required to treat hypoglycemia; avoid using the supplied glycerin-based reconstitution solution when larger doses of glucagon are being administered.)
- **Pediatric:** For patients weighing <44 pounds (20 kg), the dose is 0.5 mg.

Special Considerations:
Pregnancy class B.

▶ Review Questions

1. List the symptoms of anaphylactic shock.
2. Explain why the allergic response and not the antigen is the greater threat in a hypersensitivity reaction.
3. What is the principal chemical released by the body that produces many of the symptoms of anaphylaxis?
4. What is the most common cause of death from anaphylaxis?
5. What is the suspected diagnosis of a patient reporting difficulty breathing and swelling of the lips who remembers a reaction to seafood several years ago?
6. What is the first line of drug therapy for the patient in anaphylaxis?
7. What are the effects of epinephrine on smooth muscle and blood vessels?
8. What is the handheld form of epinephrine prescribed to patients for home use?

Reference

1. Campbell RL, Kelso JM. Anaphylaxis: emergency treatment. UpToDate. https://www.uptodate.com/contents/anaphylaxis-emergency-treatment. Updated December 5, 2017. Accessed July 18, 2018.

CHAPTER 9

Cardiac Arrhythmias

▶ Introduction

Cardiac **arrhythmias**, the loss or abnormality of cardiac rhythms, are commonly encountered in the prehospital setting. A particular arrhythmia can be long-standing, such as chronic **atrial fibrillation**, or it can be the reason that 9-1-1 was called, such as a cardiac arrest caused by **ventricular fibrillation (VF)**. Prehospital professionals must be familiar with the most commonly used antiarrhythmic agents and be proficient in administration of medications used to provide advanced cardiac life support (ACLS). In this chapter, we will discuss therapies to manage various cardiac arrhythmias.

CASE STUDY

You receive a 9-1-1 call for a patient who had a syncopal episode. You arrive to find a 72-year-old man who is awake and talking. He reports to you that he feels dizzy, and he denies any chest pain or shortness of breath. You take a pulse while your partner places the patient on the cardiac monitor/defibrillator. The pulse feels slow, and when the patient is on the monitor you note that his rhythm is a sinus bradycardia at a rate of 48 beats/min.

▶ Basic Electrophysiology

The heart is a complex muscular organ composed of four smaller chambers that contract and relax in an organized pattern to pump blood around the body. Each chamber is made up of millions of cardiac muscle cells, and each cell is capable of contracting independently. For the heart to pump blood most efficiently, the muscle cells and the four chambers of the heart must work in a coordinated fashion. The muscle cells composing the four chambers must contract at precise moments. This complex process is coordinated by the heart's electrical system. Under normal conditions, an electrical impulse originates in the sinoatrial (SA) node and travels through the heart's electrical system along a particular pathway through the heart. As each impulse moves through the heart, it signals each portion of the heart to contract in the required organized fashion. These electrical impulses coordinating cardiac contraction give the heart its rhythm. When electrical impulses controlling cardiac contraction are too slow, too fast, or irregular, the heart chambers do not contract in the proper organized fashion, the amount of blood pumped by the heart (cardiac output) drops, and, without other compensatory mechanisms, the patient's blood pressure falls.

▶ Overview of Arrhythmias

In the preceding case, the patient's heart is in sinus bradycardia (**FIGURE 9-1**). Cardiac output (CO) is determined by the patient's heart rate (HR) multiplied by the amount of blood pumped with each heartbeat (stroke volume [SV]).

$$CO = HR \times SV$$

The decrease in the heart rate causes a drop in cardiac output, producing reduced blood flow in the brain, which then causes the patient to experience dizziness and syncope.

A cardiac rhythm that is a common cause for out-of-hospital cardiac arrest is VF (**FIGURE 9-2**). VF has been described as a "bag of worms," referring to a situation in which all the cardiac cells are trying to contract independently and are not cooperating or communicating

FIGURE 9-1 Sinus bradycardia.

FIGURE 9-2 Ventricular fibrillation.

with one another. The aim of **electrical therapy** is to reset the heart and cause all the cardiac cells to pause and restart in an organized fashion. This action often allows a stable rhythm to be reestablished.

Cardiac arrest is usually caused by the sudden onset of a cardiac arrhythmia. The typical prehospital patient in nontraumatic cardiac arrest is found to have VF when initially placed on a cardiac monitor. In the prehospital setting, VF is thought to occur from chronic myocardial ischemia resulting in electrical instability of the heart. In the hospital, a cardiac arrest typically follows an acute myocardial infarction (AMI).[1] The initial management of the victim of a cardiac arrest varies depending on the equipment that is immediately available. Electrical defibrillation, not drug therapy, is without debate the single best method of treatment for the patient with VF. The likelihood that a patient will survive an arrest from VF will significantly diminish the longer this rhythm is not converted using electrical therapy. When defibrillation is applied within 1 minute of the development of VF, the survival rate can be greater than 90%.[2] This rate of successful defibrillation drops by 7% to 10% for each minute defibrillation is delayed.[3]

▶ Management

Bradycardia

A heart rate of less than 60 beats/min is the definition of bradycardia. Many people will have a heart rate of less than 60 beats/min and be physiologically normal. For instance, a well-conditioned athlete such as a marathon runner will have a heart rate of less than 60 beats/min and be symptom free. Other patients may require a high resting heart rate to maintain an adequate cardiac output. Such patients may be accustomed to having a resting heart rate of 90 beats/min, and a decrease of their heart rate to 70 beats/min may be inappropriately slow for them and may produce symptoms. The initial treatment of these symptomatic patients is the same as in any emergency: ensure a patent airway, provide supplemental oxygen if indicated, monitor the cardiac rhythm, evaluate oxygen saturation and blood pressure, and place an intravenous (IV) line. The decreased heart rate will decrease cardiac output and may produce symptoms of decreased mental status, syncope, hypotension, chest pain, congestive heart failure, dyspnea, seizures, or shock.

The treatment of symptomatic bradycardia is both drug and electrical therapy. Current literature and American Heart Association (AHA) ACLS algorithms recommend atropine, an anticholinergic medication known to decrease vagal (parasympathetic) tone, as the first-line therapy for symptomatic bradycardia.[4,5] The initial dose of atropine in adults is 0.5 mg IV. Atropine is used to treat sinus bradycardia because it inhibits the effects of the vagus nerve. The vagus nerve, when stimulated, causes slowing of the heart rate, much like applying the brakes when driving a vehicle. Therefore, a drug that inhibits the vagus nerve will increase the heart rate, as if you took your foot off the brake pedal in the vehicle. Atropine may be repeated to a total dose of 3 mg.

If treatment with atropine is unsuccessful, the electrical therapy for bradycardia is transcutaneous pacing. When confronted with a symptomatic patient with bradycardia, prepare for transcutaneous pacing. Immediately start external pacing for patients with type II second-degree heart blocks and patients with third-degree heart blocks. It usually takes time to apply a transcutaneous pacemaker, so drug therapy may be required while preparing the patient and equipment. Infusions of epinephrine (2 to 10 mcg/min) or dopamine (2 to 10 mcg/kg per minute) may be used while waiting to establish transcutaneous pacing or if pacing is ineffective. Both epinephrine and dopamine are beta-adrenergic drugs, meaning they bind and stimulate the beta$_1$ receptors of the heart. These properties make these drugs chronotropic, which results in an increase in heart rate.

ATROPINE SULFATE

© Jones & Bartlett Learning.

Classification: Anticholinergic (antimuscarinic).
Action: Competes reversibly with acetylcholine at the site of the muscarinic receptor. Receptors affected, in order from the most sensitive to the least sensitive, include salivary, bronchial, sweat glands, eye, heart, and gastrointestinal (GI) tract.
Indications: Symptomatic bradycardia, nerve agent exposure, organophosphate poisoning.
Adverse Effects: Decreased secretions resulting in dry mouth and hot skin temperature, intense facial flushing, blurred vision or dilation of the pupils with subsequent photophobia, tachycardia, restlessness. Atropine may cause paradoxical bradycardia if the dose administered is too low or if the drug is administered too slowly.
Contraindications: AMI; myasthenia gravis; GI obstruction; closed-angle glaucoma; known sensitivity to atropine, belladonna alkaloids, or sulfites. Will not be effective for infranodal (type II) atrioventricular (AV) block and new third-degree block with wide QRS complex.
Dosage:
Symptomatic Bradycardia:
- **Adult:** 0.5 mg IV, intraosseous (IO) every 3 to 5 minutes to a maximum dose of 3 mg.
- **Adolescent:** 0.02 mg/kg (minimum 0.1 mg/dose; maximum 1 mg/dose) IV, IO up to a total dose of 2 mg.
- **Pediatric:** 0.02 mg/kg (minimum 0.1 mg/dose; maximum 0.5 mg/dose) IV, IO, to a total dose of 1 mg.
Nerve Agent or Organophosphate Poisoning:
- **Adult:** 1 to 6 mg IV, intramuscular (IM); repeat if needed every 5 minutes until symptoms dissipate.
- **Pediatric:** 0.05 mg/kg IV, IM every 10 to 30 minutes as needed until symptoms dissipate.
- **Infants <15 lb:** 0.05 mg/kg IV, IM every 5 to 20 minutes as needed until symptoms dissipate.
Special Considerations:
Severe organophosphate exposures may require *massive* amounts of atropine, well beyond what is carried in most EMS vehicles.
Half-life 2.5 hours.
Pregnancy class C; possibly unsafe in lactating mothers.

EPINEPHRINE

Classification: Adrenergic agonist, inotropic.

Action: Binds strongly with both alpha and beta receptors, producing increased blood pressure, increased heart rate, bronchodilation.

Indications: Bronchospasm, allergic and anaphylactic reactions, restoration of cardiac activity in cardiac arrest, persistent bradycardia where pacing is ineffective or unavailable.

Adverse Effects: Anxiety, headache, cardiac arrhythmias, hypertension, nervousness, tremors, chest pain, nausea/vomiting.

© Jones & Bartlett Learning.

Contraindications: Arrhythmias other than VF, asystole, PEA; cardiovascular disease; hypertension; cerebrovascular disease; shock secondary to causes other than anaphylactic shock; closed-angle glaucoma; diabetes; pregnant women in active labor; known sensitivity to epinephrine or sulfites.

© Jones & Bartlett Learning.

Dosage:

Cardiac Arrest:

- **Adult:** 1 mg (1:10,000 solution) IV, IO; may repeat every 3 to 5 minutes.
- **Pediatric:** 0.01 mg/kg (1:10,000 solution) IV, IO; repeat every 3 to 5 minutes as needed (max dose: 1 mg).

Symptomatic Bradycardia:

- **Adult:** 2 to 10 mcg/min (1:10,000 solution) as a continuous IV infusion; usual dosage range: 2 to 10 mcg/min IV; titrate to effect.
- **Pediatric:** 0.01 mg/kg (1:10,000 solution) IV, IO; may repeat every 3 to 5 minutes (max dose: 1 mg). If giving epinephrine by endotracheal tube, administer 0.1 mg/kg.

Asthma Attacks and Certain Allergic Reactions:

- **Adult:** 0.3 to 0.5 mg (1:1,000 solution) IM or subcutaneous; may repeat every 10 to 15 minutes (max dose: 1 mg).
- **Pediatric:** 0.01 mg/kg (1:1,000 solution) IM or subcutaneous (max dose: 0.5 mg).

Anaphylactic Shock:

- **Adult:** 0.5 mg (1:1,000 solution) IM repeated as needed every 5 to 15 minutes, or transition to IV infusion of 1 to 4 mcg/min, titrated to effect.
- **Pediatric:** 0.01 mg/kg IM, repeated as needed every 5 to 15 minutes, or transitioned to continuous IV infusion rate of 0.1 to 1 mcg/kg per minute (1:10,000 solution); titrate to response.

Special Considerations:

Half-life 1 minute.

Pregnancy class C.

DOPAMINE (INTROPIN)

Classification: Adrenergic agonist, inotropic, vasopressor.

Action: Stimulates alpha- and beta-adrenergic receptors. At moderate doses (2 to 10 mcg/kg per minute), dopamine stimulates beta$_1$ receptors, resulting in inotropy and increased cardiac output while maintaining dopaminergic-induced vasodilatory effects. At high doses (>10 mcg/kg per minute), alpha- adrenergic agonism predominates, and increased peripheral vascular resistance and vasoconstriction result.

Indications: Hypotension and decreased cardiac output associated with cardiogenic shock and septic shock, hypotension after return of spontaneous circulation following cardiac arrest, symptomatic bradycardia unresponsive to atropine.

Adverse Effects: Tachycardia, arrhythmias, skin and soft-tissue necrosis, severe hypertension from excessive vasoconstriction, angina, dyspnea, headache, nausea/vomiting.

© Jones & Bartlett Learning.

Contraindications: Pheochromocytoma, VF, **ventricular tachycardia (VT)**, or other ventricular arrhythmias, known sensitivity (including sulfites). Correct any hypovolemia with volume fluid replacement before administering dopamine.

Dosage:

- **Adult:** 2 to 20 mcg/kg per minute IV, IO infusion. Starting dose 5 mcg/kg per minute; may gradually increase the infusion by 5 to 10 mcg/kg per minute to desired effect. Cardiac dose is usually 5 to 10 mcg/kg per minute; vasopressor dose is usually 10 to 20 mcg/kg per minute. Little benefit is gained beyond 20 mcg/kg per minute.
- **Pediatric:** Same as adult dosing.

Special Considerations:

Half-life 2 minutes.

Pregnancy class C.

(*continued*) Because the patient is feeling dizzy with a slow heart rate, you determine that the patient is experiencing symptomatic bradycardia. You place the patient on the cardiac monitor and oxygen while you start an IV line. You feel a weak radial pulse while your partner measures a blood pressure of 92/74 mm Hg. You administer atropine 0.5 mg IV and watch the heart rate on the monitor increase to 88 beats/min. Your partner repeats the blood pressure reading; it has increased to 122/81 mm Hg. The patient reports feeling better.

Tachycardia

CASE STUDY

You receive a 9-1-1 call for a patient with palpitations. Your patient is a 25-year-old woman with no medical problems except that she feels as though her heart is racing. Her ABCs (airway, breathing, and circulation) are intact. You take her pulse, which is 180 beats/min. You attach the cardiac monitor, which shows **supraventricular tachycardia (SVT)** as the rhythm (**FIGURE 9-3**). As you establish the IV line, you try to break the SVT by performing some vagal maneuvers. You perform the Valsalva maneuver on the patient. She remains in SVT, so you try carotid massage, which returns her to a normal sinus rhythm.

FIGURE 9-3 Supraventricular tachycardia.

In young patients with symptomatic SVT, vagal maneuvers and carotid massage can be used to return the patient to normal sinus rhythm. Carotid massage should never be attempted in older people who have a high likelihood of carotid stenosis because of plaque formation. The only vagal maneuver that should be performed in older patients is a Valsalva maneuver. Remember, synchronized cardioversion is indicated if your patient is unstable, such as having altered mental status, hypotension, or chest pain. The following scenario takes a different approach to treating SVT and includes pharmacologic management.

CASE STUDY

You respond to a call for a man with palpitations. Your patient is 65 years old and has many medical problems, including heart disease. His mental status is normal, and he has no abnormal vital signs, except for a pulse rate of 180 beats/min. He is in SVT according to your interpretation of the cardiac monitor. While you establish an IV line, you instruct him through the Valsalva maneuver. His rhythm continues to be SVT. You decide not to use carotid massage because of his age and medical problems. The IV line is established and you decide to administer adenosine 6 mg IV push.

When drug therapy is required, adenosine is the drug of choice for stable patients in SVT. Adenosine (Adenocard) works by altering the movement of potassium in the action potential of the heart, which slows the conduction of the action potential through the SA node. This creates a short period of asystole or ventricular escape beats and is usually seen for a few seconds after adenosine has been given. Short, self-limited episodes of VT are not uncommon. Adenosine's only use is as an antiarrhythmic for SVT. Adenosine has no effect on ventricular arrhythmias. Adenosine also will not resolve atrial fibrillation or atrial flutter; however, it may slow AV conduction enough to identify a particular arrhythmia.

Adenosine has an ultrashort half-life of 5 to 20 seconds and works only when the majority of the administered dose reaches the heart quickly. Consequently, it is given by rapid IV push and immediately followed by a flush solution. The 2015 American Heart Association Emergency Cardiovascular Care Guidelines recommendation is 6 mg IV, followed immediately by a normal saline bolus of 20 mL, and then the extremity should be elevated. If the SVT does not resolve within 1 to 2 minutes, the dose should be increased to 12 mg rapid IV push. A second 12-mg dose is no longer recommended.[6]

ADENOSINE (ADENOCARD)

Classification: Antiarrhythmic.

Action: Slows the conduction of electrical impulses at the AV node.

Indications: Stable reentry SVT. Does not convert AF, atrial flutter, or VT.

Adverse Effects: Common adverse reactions are generally mild and short-lived: sense of impending doom, complaints of flushing, chest pressure, throat tightness, numbness. Patients will have a brief episode of asystole after administration.

Contraindications: Sick sinus syndrome, second- or third-degree heart block, poison-/drug-induced tachycardia, asthma, or bronchospasm.

Dosage: Note: Adenosine should be delivered only by rapid IV bolus with a peripheral IV or directly into a vein, in a location as close to the heart as possible, preferably in the antecubital fossa. Administration of adenosine must be immediately followed by a saline flush, and then the extremity should be elevated.

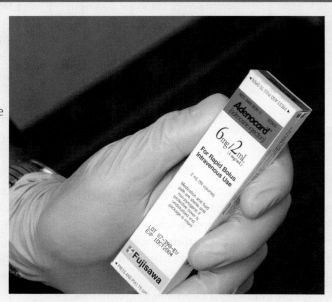
© Jones & Bartlett Learning.

- **Adult:** Initial dose 6 mg rapid IV, IO (over a 1- to 3-second period) immediately followed by a 20-mL rapid saline flush. If the first dose does not eliminate the rhythm in 1 to 2 minutes, administer a second dose of 12 mg rapid IV, IO.
- **Pediatric:**
  - **Children >110 pounds (50 kg):** Same as adult dosing.
  - **Children <110 pounds (50 kg):** Initial dose 0.1 mg/kg IV, IO (max dose: 6 mg) immediately followed by a ≥5-mL rapid saline flush; may repeat at 0.2 mg/kg (max dose: 12 mg).

Special Considerations:

Use with caution in patients with preexisting bronchospasm and those with a history of AF.

Older adults with no history of **paroxysmal SVT (PSVT)** should be carefully evaluated for dehydration and rapid sinus tachycardia requiring volume fluid replacement rather than simply treated with adenosine.

Pregnancy class C.

Antiarrhythmic Drugs

Calcium Channel Blockers

CASE STUDY

A 70-year-old man calls 9-1-1 because of palpitations. He has a long history of atrial fibrillation with a rapid ventricular rate and usually takes the beta blocker atenolol (Tenormin) for rate control, as well as warfarin (Coumadin) for anticoagulation. He has been noncompliant with his atenolol and started feeling as though his heart was racing this morning.

Calcium channel blockers are Class IV antiarrhythmics that bind to calcium channels. They block the influx of calcium into cardiac cells and arterial smooth muscle cells. This slows conduction velocity of the cardiac action potential and prolongs the period of repolarization. The overall effect is that the rapid electrical impulses traveling down from the atria to the ventricles through the AV node are slowed, and the ventricular rate is slowed. In the preceding case, the administration of a calcium channel blocker will decrease the ventricular rate, but the rhythm will remain an atrial fibrillation. Calcium channel blockers also cause peripheral arterioles to dilate. Some calcium channel blockers have more of an ability to result in arteriole dilation than do others. Why is this important to the prehospital provider? If you are administering a calcium channel blocker to treat a rapid heart rate like that in atrial fibrillation with a rapid ventricular rate, be mindful that the medication used to treat the heart rate may have the undesirable effect of dropping the blood pressure. Therefore, following administration for treatment of the heart rate, be sure to observe the patient closely and monitor the blood pressure frequently.

The actions of calcium channel blockers provide many clinical applications in both the acute setting and for long-term therapy. Calcium channel blockers are useful for controlling and/or converting certain supraventricular arrhythmias—stable, narrow-complex reentry SVT, and automatic focus (junctional, **ectopic**, and multifocal) tachycardias not converted or controlled by adenosine or vagal maneuvers. Calcium channel blockers do not convert atrial fibrillation or atrial flutter into a sinus rhythm; they only slow the ventricular rate by slowing conduction through the AV node. Because of their arterial dilatory effects, calcium channel blockers are used to treat hypertension. Because they also block vasospasm, calcium channel blockers can be used to decrease anginal episodes and even decrease the incidence of migraine headaches. Various calcium channel blockers have different proportions of vasodilator, antihypertensive, and antiarrhythmic effects.

Diltiazem (Cardizem) can be used for acute ventricular rate control and the management of hypertension. Advanced life support drug boxes that carry calcium channel blockers invariably use diltiazem. Verapamil (Isoptin) tends to produce more hypotension than diltiazem due to more prominent negative inotropic effects. Both of these medications can be given intravenously for urgent rate control in atrial fibrillation with rapid ventricular response; however, diltiazem is typically the preferred agent.[7]

DILTIAZEM (CARDIZEM)

© Allik Camazine/Alamy Stock Photo.

Classification: Calcium channel blocker, Class IV antiarrhythmic.
Action: Blocks calcium from moving into the heart muscle cell, which prolongs the conduction of electrical impulses through the AV node.
Indications: Ventricular rate control in rapid AF.
Adverse Effects: Flushing; headache; bradycardia; hypotension; heart block; myocardial depression; severe AV block; and, at high doses, cardiac arrest.
Contraindications: Hypotension, heart block, heart failure.
Dosage:
- **Adult:** Optimum dose is 0.25 mg/kg IV, IO over a 2-minute period to control rapid AF; 20 mg is a reasonable dose for the average adult patient. A second, higher dose of 0.35 mg/kg IV, IO (25 mg is a typical second dose) may be administered over a 2-minute period if rate control is not obtained with the lower dose. For continued reduction in heart rate, a continuous infusion can be started at a dose range of 5 to 15 mg/hr.
- **Pediatric:** Not recommended for pediatric patients.

Special Considerations:
Use with extreme caution in patients who are taking beta blockers because these two drug classes potentiate each other's effects and toxicities.
Patients with a history of heart failure and heart block are at a higher risk for toxicity.
Pregnancy class C.

VERAPAMIL (ISOPTIN)

Classification: Calcium channel blocker; Class IV antiarrhythmic.
Action: Blocks calcium from moving into the heart muscle cell, which prolongs the conduction of electrical impulses through the AV node. Also dilates arteries.
Indications: Atrial fibrillation, hypertension, PSVT, PSVT prophylaxis.
Adverse Effects: Sinus bradycardia; first-, second-, or third-degree AV block; congestive heart failure; reflex sinus tachycardia; transient asystole; AV block; hypotension.
Contraindications: Second- or third-degree AV block (except in patients with a functioning artificial pacemaker); hypotension (systolic pressure <90 mm Hg) or cardiogenic shock; sick sinus syndrome (except in patients with a functioning artificial pacemaker); Wolff-Parkinson-White (WPW) syndrome; Lown-Ganong-Levine syndrome; severe left ventricular dysfunction; known sensitivity to verapamil or any component of the formulation; atrial flutter or fibrillation and an accessory bypass tract (WPW, Lown-Ganong-Levine syndrome); in infants <1 year.
Dosage:
- **Adult:** 2.5 to 10 mg IV, IO over 2 minutes (3 minutes in older adults). May repeat at 5 to 10 mg every 15 to 30 minutes to a maximum dose of 30 mg.
- **Pediatric:**
  - **Children 1 to 16 years:** 0.1 mg/kg IV, IO (maximum 5 mg/dose) over 2 minutes. May repeat in 30 minutes to a maximum dose of 10 mg.
  - **Infants <1 year:** Not recommended.
Special Considerations:
Do not administer to patients with heart failure or impaired ventricular function. Pregnancy class C.

Beta Blockers

CASE STUDY

A patient you previously saw with atrial fibrillation calls 9-1-1 on another occasion. He is again in atrial fibrillation with a rapid ventricular rate. This time, however, he also has anginal chest pain. Medical direction asks you to administer a beta blocker rather than a calcium channel blocker.

As discussed in Chapters 1 and 6, beta blockers exert their pharmacologic effects on both beta$_1$ and beta$_2$ receptors. Beta$_1$ receptors are located in the heart and act as the main mediator of rate and contractility. Beta blockers are negative inotropic drugs that decrease the force and velocity of myocardial contractility, thus lowering blood pressure and oxygen consumption. The negative chronotropic effects of beta blockers result in a lower heart rate, automaticity, and conduction. Thus, beta blockers can dramatically decrease cardiac output. Beta$_2$ blockers prevent vasoconstriction and contribute to lowering of blood pressure.[7]

For these reasons, beta blockers are highly effective drugs for people with angina and hypertension. Research has shown that beta blockers decrease mortality rate during and after AMIs.[8]

Beta blockers also decrease infarct size, reduce the risk of recurrent ischemia, and decrease the incidence of sudden death from arrhythmias. Because of their ability to decrease both heart rate and myocardial contractility, beta blockers are useful in the treatment of dissecting aortic aneurysms.[7,9–11]

Beta blockers can also be used as antiarrhythmics, especially in high catecholamine or epinephrine states such as alcohol withdrawal, panic attacks, and hyperthyroidism. Beta blockers are useful for controlling heart rate in SVTs, decrease AV nodal conduction, and depress ventricular automaticity. They may be effective in the rate control of atrial fibrillation, SVT, and sinus tachycardia. They can be used to suppress **premature ventricular contractions** (PVCs), especially in anginal patients, because of their antiarrhythmic effects combined with oxygen-sparing properties.

Numerous beta blockers are available. The most common are propranolol, metoprolol, and the short-acting esmolol. These agents are discussed in detail in Chapter 6.

PROPRANOLOL (INDERAL)

Classification: Beta-adrenergic antagonist, antianginal, antihypertensive, antiarrhythmic Class II.

Action: Nonselective beta antagonist that binds with both the $beta_1$ and $beta_2$ receptors. Propranolol inhibits the strength of the heart's contractions, as well as heart rate. This results in a decrease in cardiac oxygen consumption.

Indications: Angina; narrow-complex tachycardias that originate from either a reentry mechanism (reentry SVT) or an automatic focus (junctional, ectopic, or multifocal tachycardia) uncontrolled by vagal maneuvers and adenosine in patients with preserved ventricular function; AF and atrial flutter in patients with preserved ventricular function; hypertension; migraine headaches.

Adverse Effects: Bradycardia, AV block, bronchospasm, hypotension.

Contraindications: Cardiogenic shock, heart failure, AV block, bradycardia, pulmonary edema, sick sinus syndrome, known sensitivity. Use with caution in chronic lung disease (asthma and COPD).

Dosage:
- **Adult:** 1 to 3 mg IV, IO at a rate of 1 mg/min; may repeat the dose 2 minutes later.

Special Considerations:
Monitor blood pressure and heart rate closely during administration.
Pregnancy class C.

METOPROLOL (LOPRESSOR, TOPROL XL)

Classification: Beta-adrenergic antagonist, antianginal, antihypertensive, Class II antiarrhythmic.

Action: Inhibits the strength of the heart's contractions, as well as heart rate. This results in a decrease in cardiac oxygen consumption. Metoprolol is a selective $beta_1$ type blocker.

Indications: ACS, hypertension, SVT, atrial flutter, AF, thyrotoxicosis.

Adverse Effects: Tiredness, dizziness, diarrhea, heart block, bradycardia, bronchospasm, drop in blood pressure.

Contraindications: Cardiogenic shock, AV block, bradycardia, known sensitivity. Use with caution in hypotension, chronic lung disease (asthma and COPD).

Dosage:
Cardiac Indications:
- **Adult:** 5 mg slow IV, IO over a 2-minute period; repeat at 5-minute intervals up to a total of three infusions totaling 15 mg IV, IO.
- **Pediatric:** Oral dosing only.

Special Considerations:
Blood pressure, heart rate, and ECG should be monitored carefully.
Use with caution in patients with asthma.

ESMOLOL (BREVIBLOC)

Classification: Beta-adrenergic antagonist, Class II antiarrhythmic.

Action: Inhibits the strength of the heart's contractions, as well as heart rate, resulting in a decrease in cardiac oxygen consumption. Esmolol is a beta$_1$ specific or cardioselective blocker.

Indications: ACS, myocardial infarction, acute hypertension, supraventricular tachyarrhythmias, thyrotoxicosis.

Adverse Effects: Hypotension, sinus bradycardia, AV block, cardiac arrest, nausea/vomiting, hypoglycemia, injection site reaction.

Contraindications: Acute bronchospasm, COPD, second- or third-degree heart block, bradycardia, cardiogenic shock, pulmonary edema, sick sinus syndrome, known sensitivity. Use with caution in patients with pheochromocytoma, variant (Prinzmetal's) angina, cerebrovascular disease, stroke, poorly controlled diabetes mellitus, hyperthyroidism, thyrotoxicosis, renal disease.

Dosage:

- **Adult:** 0.5 to 1 mg/kg IV, IO over a 1-minute period, followed by a 50-mcg/kg per minute (0.05 mg/kg) infusion over a 4-minute period (maximum total: 200 mcg/kg). If patient response is inadequate, administer a second bolus 500 mcg/kg (0.5 mg/kg) over a 1-minute period, and then increase infusion to 100 mcg/kg per minute. Maximum infusion rate: 300 mcg/kg per minute.

Special Considerations:

Half-life 5 to 9 minutes.

Any adverse effects caused by administration of esmolol are brief because of the drug's short half-life.

Resolution of effects usually within 10 to 20 minutes.

Pregnancy class C.

Ventricular Antiarrhythmic Drugs

CASE STUDY

You receive a 9-1-1 call for a patient who is unresponsive. When you arrive, you determine the patient is apneic and pulseless. You begin CPR, establish an airway, and ventilate the patient. Once the patient is connected to your cardiac monitor/defibrillator, you see VF on the monitor. He is successfully shocked into a sinus rhythm with a pulse but has multiple PVCs, some of which occur in couplets and triplets.

What antiarrhythmic is best in this situation? Are there other therapeutic options?

A number of drugs can be used to treat patients with ventricular arrhythmias. The Vaughan-Williams classification of antiarrhythmic medications defines four classes based on primary mechanism of action:

1. Class I: Sodium channel blockers. These agents are further divided into subclasses according to their effect on the sodium channel.

   IA: Agents that block the fast sodium channels and depress depolarization.

   IB: Sodium channel blockers that shorten the action potential duration.

   IC: Sodium channel blockers that depress depolarization and conductivity. This subclass of agents is the most potent sodium channel blocker.

2. Class II: Beta blockers.
3. Class III: Potassium channel blocking agents.
4. Class IV: Calcium channel blocking agents.

In the previous scenario, amiodarone would be the drug of choice. Although it is classified as a Class III agent, amiodarone is the only commonly used antiarrhythmic drug that has actions from every class of antiarrhythmics. That is, it has some sodium-blocking effects, some beta-blocking effects, and some calcium-blocking effects in addition to predominant effects on the potassium channels.[7] Amiodarone is used to treat arrhythmias that originate both above and below the AV node. It is widely accepted as the drug of choice in cardiac arrest from VF and **pulseless ventricular tachycardia**.[12]

Amiodarone can also be used to convert acute atrial fibrillation (**FIGURE 9-4**) or **atrial flutter** (**FIGURE 9-5**) pharmacologically.[7,9] Amiodarone increases the duration of the action potential, as well as the refractory period of the atria, AV node, and ventricular tissues. Because amiodarone exerts its effect in both atrial and ventricular tissue, the drug is capable of treating both atrial and ventricular arrhythmias.

When a drug increases the duration of the action potential or the refractory period, what does that mean? To explain this you need to imagine that you are standing on a bridge that passes over an interstate highway. Below you is a constant stream of automobiles speeding down the highway. In the heart, the specialized tissue that conducts electrical impulses or action potential from the SA node through the ventricles, past the SA node, and down into the ventricles is similar to the interstate highway in this example. What determines how many cars rush underneath your bridge in a matter of 1 minute? The velocity of the cars and the distance between those cars are the principal elements that determine the number of cars that can pass underneath the bridge. The speed, or velocity, of the cars rushing down the highway can be likened to the action potential duration. The faster the action potential duration, the faster the action

FIGURE 9-4 Atrial fibrillation.

FIGURE 9-5 Atrial flutter.

potential will move down the conduction system. Various medications and shifts of electrolytes can affect the duration of the action potential and, therefore, how rapidly that particular impulse moves down the system. Let us go back to watching the traffic on the interstate. Between each car on the highway is a certain amount of space. If the cars are all traveling at 55 miles per hour (89 km/hr), the greater the space between the cars, at a given speed, the fewer cars can pass under the bridge. In the heart, each electrical action potential has a period known as the *refractory period*. This refractory period is similar to the space between the cars. The greater the refractory period, the fewer action potentials will travel down through the heart in 1 minute.

Amiodarone is a Class III antiarrhythmic drug that increases the action potential duration and refractory period. It has been shown to decrease short-term mortality rates in patients with congestive heart failure.[13] In cases of chronic heart failure, amiodarone reduces the risk of developing atrial fibrillation and can convert patients who are in atrial fibrillation to a **sinus rhythm**.[10]

> Because of amiodarone's irritating effects to veins and soft tissues, be careful not to allow amiodarone infusions to infiltrate into the soft tissue. It should always be administered by a secure, large-bore IV line.

> Amiodarone is recommended as the first-line antiarrhythmic medication for patients in cardiac arrest from ventricular arrhythmias; lidocaine is recommended as an alternative to amiodarone. However, research remains somewhat inconclusive.[14]

Lidocaine is a Class IB antiarrhythmic because it blocks the sodium channel and it decreases the amount of time required for repolarization. These effects also make lidocaine an excellent short-acting anesthetic.

Procainamide (Pronestyl) is a Class IA antiarrhythmic that works by binding to fast sodium channels and slows almost all phases of the action potential. It slows depolarization, repolarization, and impulse conduction. Procainamide can prolong the PR and QT intervals and at higher dosing can cause the QRS complex to widen. Because it decreases nodal conductivity, it can be used for both atrial and ventricular arrhythmias. It has often been used as the second-line agent of choice for atrial fibrillation, atrial flutter, and SVT in addition to its role as an effective ventricular antiarrhythmic.[7] Procainamide is usually the drug of choice when amiodarone is not effective. However, because it cannot be given rapidly and can take 20 to 40 minutes to work, most out-of-hospital providers do not use procainamide.

AMIODARONE (CORDARONE)

Classification: Antiarrhythmic, Class III.
Action: Acts directly on the myocardium to delay repolarization and increase the duration of the action potential.
Indications: Ventricular arrhythmias; second-line agent for atrial arrhythmias.
Adverse Effects: Burning at the IV site, hypotension, bradycardia.
Contraindications: Sick sinus syndrome, second- and third-degree

© Jones & Bartlett Learning.

heart block, cardiogenic shock, when episodes of bradycardia have caused syncope, sensitivity to benzyl alcohol and iodine.

Dosage:

Ventricular Fibrillation and Pulseless Ventricular Tachycardia:

- **Adult:** 300 mg IV, IO. May be followed by one dose of 150 mg in 3 to 5 minutes.
- **Pediatric:** 5 mg/kg (max dose: 300 mg); may repeat 5 mg/kg IV, IO up to 15 mg/kg.

Relatively Stable Patients with Arrhythmias Such as Premature Ventricular Contractions or Wide-Complex Tachycardias with a Strong Pulse:

- **Adult:** 150 mg in 100 mL D_5W IV, IO over a 10-minute period; once return of spontaneous circulation is accomplished, begin an infusion of 1 mg/min for 6 hours, then decrease to 0.5 mg/min; may repeat in 10 minutes up to a maximum dose of 2.2 g over 24 hours.
- **Pediatric:** 5 mg/kg very slow IV, IO (over 20 to 60 minutes); may repeat in 5-mg/kg doses up to 15 mg/kg (max dose: 300 mg).

Special Considerations:

Pregnancy class D.

LIDOCAINE (XYLOCAINE)

Classification: Antiarrhythmic, Class IB.

Action: Blocks sodium channels, increasing the recovery period after repolarization; suppresses automaticity in the His-Purkinje system and depolarization in the ventricles.

Indications: Ventricular arrhythmias, when amiodarone is not available: cardiac arrest from VF/VT, stable monomorphic VT with preserved ventricular function, stable polymorphic VT with normal baseline QT interval and preserved left ventricular function (when ischemia and electrolyte imbalance are treated), stable polymorphic VT with baseline QT prolongation suggestive of torsades de pointes.

2% Lidocaine
HCl Injection, USP
1,000 mg per 50 mL
For Infiltration and Nerve Block.
Methylparaben as preservative
Not for Caudal or Epidural Use.
25 × 50 mL Multiple-Dose Vials
(20 mg/mL) **Rx only**

Adverse Effects: Toxicity (signs may include anxiety, apprehension, euphoria, nervousness, disorientation, dizziness, blurred vision, facial paresthesias, tremors, hearing disturbances, slurred speech, seizures, sinus bradycardia), seizures without warning, cardiac arrhythmias, hypotension, cardiac arrest, pain at injection site.

Contraindications: AV block; bleeding; thrombocytopenia; known sensitivity to lidocaine, sulfite, or paraben. Use with caution in bradycardia, hypovolemia, cardiogenic shock, Adams-Stokes syndrome, WPW syndrome.

Dosage:

Pulseless Ventricular Tachycardia and Ventricular Fibrillation:

- **Adult IV, IO:** 1 to 1.5 mg/kg IV, IO; may repeat at half the original dose (0.5 to 0.75 mg/kg) every 5 to 10 minutes to a maximum dose of 3 mg/kg. If a maintenance infusion is warranted, the rate is 1 to 4 mg/min.
- **Pediatric IV, IO:** 1 mg/kg IV, IO (maximum: 100 mg). If a maintenance infusion is warranted, the rate is 20 to 50 mcg/kg per minute.

Perfusing Ventricular Rhythms:

- **Adult:** 0.5 to 0.75 mg/kg IV, IO (up to 1 to 1.5 mg/kg may be used). Repeat 0.5 to 0.75 mg/kg every 5 to 10 minutes to a maximum total dose of 3 mg/kg. A maintenance infusion of 1 to 4 mg/min (30 to 50 mcg/kg per minute) is acceptable.
- **Pediatric:** 1 mg/kg IV, IO. May repeat every 5 to 10 minutes to a maximum dose of 3 mg/kg. Maintenance infusion rate is 20 to 50 mcg/kg per minute.

Special Considerations:

Half-life approximately 90 minutes.
Pregnancy class B.

PROCAINAMIDE (PRONESTYL)

Classification: Antiarrhythmic, Class IA.

Action: Blocks influx of sodium through membrane pores, consequently suppresses atrial and ventricular arrhythmias by slowing conduction in myocardial tissue.

Indications: Alternative to amiodarone for stable monomorphic VT with normal QT interval and preserved ventricular function, reentry SVT if uncontrolled by adenosine and vagal maneuvers if blood pressure stable, AF with rapid rate in WPW syndrome.

Adverse Effects: Asystole, VF, flushing, hypotension, PR prolongation, QRS widening, QT prolongation.

Contraindications: AV block, QT prolongation, torsades de pointes. Use with caution in hypotension, heart failure.

Dosage:
- **Adult:** 500 to 600 mg over 25 to 3 minutes IV, or 20 to 50 mg/min slow IV, IO (max total dose: 17 mg/kg until one of the following occurs: arrhythmia resolves, hypotension, QRS widens by >50% of original width).
- **Maintenance:** Infusion (after resuscitation from cardiac arrest): mix 1 g in 250 mL solution (4 mg/mL), infuse at 1 to 4 mg/min.
- **Pediatric:** 10 to 15 mg/kg slow IV, IO over 30 to 60 minutes.

Special Considerations:
Pregnancy class C.

CASE STUDY

You are dispatched to a local apartment building for a 72-year-old man who suddenly collapsed. When you arrive, you find an unresponsive older man in a chair. You rapidly get him to the floor while your partner prepares the defibrillator. The man's daughter is telling you that her father has never had any problems with his heart but does have a history of alcoholism, as well as some problems with his liver. The ECG monitor shows an unusual type of VT. That is, the tachycardia is not monomorphic, with every QRS complex looking the same. Instead, it is polymorphic, with many different-shaped complexes that appear to rotate by 180 degrees over time, almost like it is twisting. You recognize this as **torsades de pointes** (**FIGURE 9-6**).

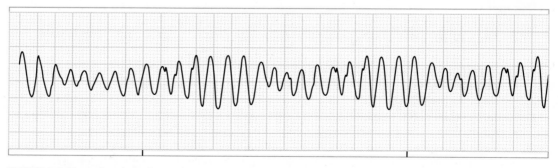

FIGURE 9-6 Torsades de pointes.

Magnesium sulfate is an electrolyte and an extremely effective antiarrhythmic. Magnesium can be used to treat patients with torsades de pointes (such as in the previous scenario) successfully and decrease PVCs caused by a prolonged QT interval.[15] The exact mechanism of how magnesium prevents torsades de pointes is not defined, but it may block the sodium channels. Alcoholics typically have poor diets that cause several nutritional and electrolyte abnormalities that can result in arrhythmias. Therefore, magnesium should always be considered in alcoholics and malnourished patients.

Torsades de pointes is French for the phrase "twisting of points." This rhythm is often confused with VT. It is easier to detect the twisting of points on a printed strip.

MAGNESIUM SULFATE

Classification: Electrolyte, tocolytic, mineral.

Action: Required for normal physiologic functioning. Magnesium is a cofactor in neurochemical transmission and muscular excitability. Magnesium sulfate controls seizures by blocking peripheral neuromuscular transmission. Magnesium is also a peripheral vasodilator and an inhibitor of platelet function.

Indications: Torsades de pointes, cardiac arrhythmias associated with hypomagnesemia, eclampsia and seizure prophylaxis in preeclampsia, status asthmaticus.

Adverse Effects: Magnesium toxicity (signs include flushing, diaphoresis, hypotension, muscle paralysis, weakness, hypothermia, and cardiac, CNS, or respiratory depression).

Contraindications: AV block, GI obstruction. Use with caution in renal impairment.

Dosage:

Pulseless Ventricular Fibrillation/Ventricular Tachycardia with Torsades de Pointes or Hypomagnesemia:
- **Adult:** 1 to 2 g in 10 mL D$_5$W IV, IO administered over 15 minutes or faster with cardiac arrest.
- **Pediatric:** 25 to 50 mg/kg IV, IO over 10 to 20 minutes; may administer faster for torsades de pointes (max single dose: 2 g).

Torsades de Pointes with a Pulse or Cardiac Arrhythmias with Hypomagnesemia:
- **Adult:** 1 to 2 g in 50 to 100 mL D$_5$W IV, IO administered over 5 to 60 minutes. Follow with 0.5 to 1 g/hr IV, IO titrated to control torsades de pointes.
- **Pediatric:** 25 to 50 mg/kg IV, IO over 10 to 20 minutes (max single dose: 2 g).

Eclampsia and Seizure Prophylaxis in Preeclampsia:
- **Adult:** 4 to 6 g IV, IO over 20 to 30 minutes, followed by an infusion of 1 to 2 g/hr.

Status Asthmaticus:
- **Adult:** 1.2 to 2 g slow IV, IO (over 20 minutes).
- **Pediatric:** 25 to 50 mg/kg (diluted in D$_5$W) slow IV, IO (over 10 to 20 minutes).

Special Considerations:
Pregnancy class A.

(continued) Because the patient has been converted back into a sinus rhythm with a pulse and he is having PVCs, it would be prudent to administer an antiarrhythmic drug. You administer amiodarone 150 mg IV over a 10-minute period.

Cardiopulmonary Arrest

There are four arrhythmias associated with cardiac arrest: PEA, asystole, VT, and VF. Although some of the medications used to treat all four rhythms are the same, there are variations.

Pulseless Electrical Activity and Asystole. PEA and asystole are the most dreaded cardiac arrhythmias. PEA is characterized by detectable electrical activity on the monitor but no mechanical cardiac activity as detected by the presence of a pulse or audible heart tones. In asystole, the patient has neither electrical nor mechanical cardiac activity. Only epinephrine is indicated in the treatment of either of these arrhythmias. Epinephrine has very strong inotropic and chronotropic effects on the heart. In an arrest situation, 1 mg IV, IO of epinephrine can be administered every 3 to 5 minutes. In cases in which you are treating an overdose of a beta blocker or calcium channel blocker, high doses up to 0.2 mg/kg may be used. In emergency situations in which the prehospital professional cannot rapidly obtain either IV or IO access, epinephrine can be administered down the endotracheal tube at a dose of 2 to 2.5 mg. In the case of asystole, epinephrine is stimulating the adrenergic receptors, trying to reestablish a rhythm. Vasopressin, another vasoconstrictor medication, has recently been removed from the AHA ACLS Cardiac Arrest algorithm.[16]

Pulseless Ventricular Tachycardia and Ventricular Fibrillation. Epinephrine is also indicated in pulseless VT and VF; however, electrical therapy has proven to be the most effective treatment for patients in cardiac arrest with these rhythms. If a patient in pulseless VT or VF does not respond to defibrillation, epinephrine should be administered as previously indicated. If the patient's rhythm does not change after two or three shocks and administration of a vasopressor, consider administration of amiodarone. If amiodarone is unavailable, lidocaine may be used as a substitute.

▶ Review Questions

1. Why is electrical therapy preferred over drug administration for the initial therapy of cardiac arrest and some arrhythmias?
2. Explain the effect of atropine on the vagus nerve in a patient with bradycardia.
3. What is the half-life of adenosine?
4. List three classes of antiarrhythmic agents.
5. To what drug class do calcium channel blockers belong, and what are their effects on the heart?
6. Explain how beta blockers decrease cardiac output.
7. What is the drug of choice for most ventricular arrhythmias?
8. What drug is indicated for the treatment of torsades de pointes?
9. What is the status of the heart's electrical and mechanical activity in pulseless electrical activity? What is the status of the heart's electrical and mechanical activity in asystole?

References

1. Bergum D, Nordseth T, Mjolstad OC, Skogvoll E, Haugen BO. Causes of in-hospital cardiac arrest—incidences and rate of recognition. *Resuscitation*. 2015;87:63–68. https://doi.org/10.1016/j.resuscitation.2014.11.007.
2. Ibrahim WH. Recent advances and controversies in adult cardiopulmonary resuscitation. *Postgrad Med J*. 2007;83(984):649–654. doi:10.1136/pgmj.2007.057133.

3. American Heart Association. Facts: every second counts; rural and community access to emergency devices. http://www.heart.org/idc/groups/heart-public/@wcm/@adv/documents/downloadable/ucm_301646.pdf. Published March 2013. Accessed July 19, 2018.

4. Homoud MK. Sinus bradycardia. UpToDate. https://www.uptodate.com/contents/sinus-bradycardia?-search=bradycardia&source=search_result&selectedTitle=1~150&usage_type=default&display_rank=1. Updated June 7, 2017. Accessed July 19, 2018.

5. American Heart Association. The ACLS cases: bradycardia. In: *Advanced Cardiovascular Life Support Provider Manual*. Dallas, TX: American Heart Association; 2016.

6. Pozner CN. Advanced cardiac life support (ACLS) in adults. UpToDate. https://www.uptodate.com/contents/advanced-cardiac-life-support-acls-in-adults. Updated March 19, 2018. Accessed July 19, 2018.

7. Ganz LI. Control of ventricular rate in atrial fibrillation: pharmacologic therapy. UpToDate. https://www.uptodate.com/contents/control-of-ventricular-rate-in-atrial-fibrillation-pharmacologic-therapy. Updated May 15, 2018. Accessed September 17, 2018.

8. Rosenson RS, Reeder GS, Kennedy HL. Acute myocardial infarction: role of beta blocker therapy. UpToDate. https://www.uptodate.com/contents/acute-myocardial-infarction-role-of-beta-blocker-therapy/print. Updated July 10, 2017. Accessed July 19, 2018.

9. American Heart Association. *Handbook of emergency cardiovascular care for healthcare providers*. Dallas, TX: American Heart Association; 2006.

10. Deedwania PC, Singh BN, Ellenbogen K, Fisher S, Fletcher R, Singh SN. Spontaneous conversion and maintenance of sinus rhythm by amiodarone in patients with heart failure and atrial fibrillation: observations from the Veterans Affairs Congestive Heart Failure Trial of Antiarrhythmic Therapy (CHF-STAT). *Circulation*. 1998;98:2574.

11. Atkins DL, Dorian P, Gonzalez ER, et al. Treatment of tachyarrhythmias. *Ann Emerg Med*. 2001;37:S91–S109.

12. Pozner CN. Supportive data for advanced cardiac life support in adults with sudden cardiac arrest. UpToDate. https://www.uptodate.com/contents/supportive-data-for-advanced-cardiac-life-support-in-adults-with-sudden-cardiac-arrest/print?sectionName=VF%20or%20VT%20arrest%20and%20vasopressors&anchor=H6&source=see_link. Updated May 16, 2018. Accessed July 19, 2018.

13. Sturmer ML, Talajic M, Thibault B, et al. Management of atrial fibrillation in patients with congestive heart failure. *Am J Geriatric Cardiol*. 2005;14(2):91–94.

14. Sugiyama K, Kashiura M, Hamabe Y. Amiodarone and lidocaine for shock refractory ventricular fibrillation or ventricular tachycardia in out-of-hospital cardiac arrest: are they really effective? *J Thorac Dis*. 2016;8(8);E791–E793.

15. Iseri LT. Magnesium: nature's physiologic calcium blocker. *Am Heart J*. 1984;108:188.

16. American Heart Association. The ACLS cases: cardiac arrest; VF/pulseless VT. In: *Advanced Cardiovascular Life Support Provider Manual*. Dallas, TX: American Heart Association; 2016.

© Andrew Brookes/Getty Images

CHAPTER 10

Congestive Heart Failure

OBJECTIVES

1. Explain the concept of polypharmacy in the treatment of congestive heart failure (CHF).
2. Explain the function of a diuretic.
3. Discuss drugs used for the initial management of CHF: furosemide (Lasix), morphine sulfate, and nitroglycerin (Nitrolingual, NitroQuick, Nitro-Dur).
4. Discuss digoxin (Lanoxin) and its use in the long-term management of CHF.
5. Discuss the role of angiotensin-converting enzyme inhibitors, beta blockers, and calcium channel blockers in treating patients with CHF.

MEDICATIONS THAT APPEAR IN CHAPTER 10

Furosemide (Lasix)
Morphine sulfate
Nitroglycerin (Nitrolingual, NitroQuick, Nitro-Dur)
Digoxin (Lanoxin)

Angiotensin-converting enzyme (ACE) inhibitors: captopril (Capoten), enalapril (Vasotec), lisinopril

(Prinivil, Zestril), ramipril (Altace)
Metoprolol (Lopressor, Toprol XL)

CASE STUDY

You are dispatched to assist a woman who is reporting shortness of breath. You arrive at the apartment of a 78-year-old woman who is in moderate respiratory distress. Her legs are swollen, and she reports shortness of breath that has become more severe over the past few days. She coughs when lying down and has been having difficulty sleeping for the past three nights. She tells you that her breathing has been more comfortable when she has tried to sleep in the chair in the living room. Her blood pressure is 188/92 mm Hg, heart rate is 100 beats/min, and respirations are 20 breaths/min. The patient tells you she is diabetic and hypertensive and has high cholesterol, kidney failure, and congestive heart failure. You administer high-flow oxygen with a nonrebreather face mask, establish an intravenous (IV) line, and administer 40 mg furosemide IV. Before leaving for the hospital, she hands you a plastic bag full of the medications she is taking. They include simvastatin (Zocor), lisinopril (Zestril), metoprolol (Lopressor, Toprol XL), furosemide (Lasix), potassium, and digoxin (Lanoxin).

▶ Introduction

Congestive heart failure (CHF) is one of the few cardiovascular disorders that continues to increase in prevalence, especially among the older adult population. Currently 5 million people in the United States have heart failure, and 550,000 new cases are diagnosed each year.[1] CHF is predominantly a condition of older adults, with 6 to 10% of all people older than 65 years having symptoms consistent with the disease. Paramedics are often called to assist patients with a long-standing disease who are often taking multiple medications. Prehospital care providers must be familiar with the medications used for long-term therapy of CHF, as well as short-term drug therapy for exacerbations of CHF and resultant pulmonary edema.

▶ Overview of Congestive Heart Failure

Heart failure may be the result of ischemic heart disease, diabetes mellitus, hypertension, or disease of the heart valves. The onset of heart failure may be rather acute after a myocardial infarction (MI) or may take years to develop in conditions such as valvular heart disease, hypertension, or diabetes mellitus. Patients with heart failure may have symptoms from accumulation of excess fluid or poor peripheral perfusion and inadequate oxygen delivery to the tissues (**FIGURE 10-1**). Signs of fluid overload include shortness of breath from pulmonary

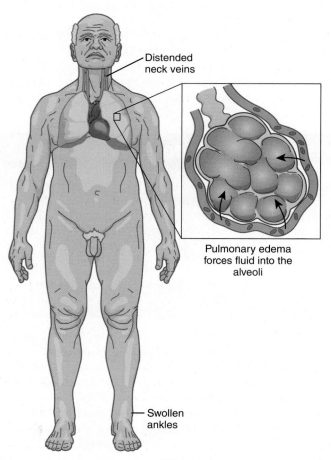

Distended neck veins

Pulmonary edema forces fluid into the alveoli

Swollen ankles

FIGURE 10-1 In congestive heart failure, decreased forward cardiac output by a diseased left ventricle results in the accumulation of blood in the pulmonary vasculature, leading to pulmonary edema. Pulmonary edema occurs when fluid accumulates in the alveoli. This fluid widens the gap between the alveoli and capillary membrane, which makes diffusion of oxygen and carbon dioxide less efficient.

edema, as well as edema of the extremities, especially the lower legs. Poor output of the heart caused by heart failure results in an accumulation or "backing up" of fluid in the lungs, which is known as **pulmonary edema**. Other patients with heart failure may report only fatigue and weakness from poor delivery of oxygen to the tissues as a result of low cardiac output.

The diagnosis of CHF is often suspected in patients with shortness of breath and peripheral edema. Shortness of breath, or dyspnea, can be caused by CHF but can also be the result of chronic obstructive pulmonary disease (COPD). In one study of patients with CHF, dyspnea was present in 93%, and peripheral edema was present in 70%.[2] CHF, as well as a variety of other conditions, can produce peripheral edema. CHF is not easily diagnosed by physical examination. Up to 50% of patients diagnosed with left ventricular dysfunction have no symptoms at all.[3] Children with heart disease can also have heart failure and resultant pulmonary edema.

▶ Management

The American Heart Association provides guidelines for the management of CHF and pulmonary edema. Long-term control of systolic and diastolic hypertension is imperative to control the symptoms seen in CHF. Patients with CHF are often taking medications for the treatment of lipid disorders. **Angiotensin-converting enzyme (ACE) inhibitors** are a class of medication recommended for patients with a history of atherosclerotic vascular disease, diabetes, and hypertension. ACE inhibitors are discussed later in this chapter. Additionally, physicians often place these patients on medications to control heart rate and treat thyroid disorders. The importance of these recommendations in prehospital management is not in the administration of these medications, but in the effects of **polypharmacy** (the administration of many drugs at the same time) on the patient with CHF who is unstable. Additionally, although these medications are often used for the treatment of CHF, drugs such as digoxin, nitrates, or ACE inhibitors may be potentially harmful in patients with CHF from valvular heart disease or with diastolic dysfunction.

The most common treatment protocols for patients with CHF in the prehospital setting include administration of oxygen, furosemide (Lasix), morphine, and nitroglycerin. Oxygen is indicated when patients present in significant respiratory distress or evidence of hypoxemia (oxygen saturation level <90%).[4] Consider a trial of noninvasive positive pressure ventilation prior to endotracheal intubation for patients with profound respiratory distress or failure. Titrate the fraction of inspired oxygen to maintain an oxygen saturation level greater than 90%. Patients with symptoms consistent with CHF or pulmonary edema are treated with sublingual or mucosal nitroglycerin, IV furosemide, and IV morphine or some combination of these drugs.

Drugs Used for Immediate Management

After the administration of oxygen, one of the principal objectives of drug therapy is the reduction of pulmonary edema.

Drugs commonly used for the immediate management of CHF include furosemide, morphine sulfate, and nitroglycerin. Patients with chronic heart failure will typically be taking a diuretic such as furosemide, as well as an ACE inhibitor and a beta blocker.

Furosemide, which is a loop diuretic, is commonly used to reduce pulmonary edema. Diuretics increase urine output, and loop diuretics work by decreasing the absorption of water in the kidneys. This decrease in water absorption increases urine production and decreases intravascular volume. Loop diuretics are more effective than other diuretics in the management of acute and chronic heart failure, as well as life-threatening pulmonary edema. In the management of an adult with CHF, an initial dose of furosemide 20 to 40 mg IV push should be administered.[4] Once administered, the diuretic effects of furosemide do not become apparent until approximately 20 minutes later. Because furosemide is not capable of providing immediate relief to the patient with CHF or dyspnea, the provider must rely on other medications for the 20 minutes of treatment.

Nitroglycerin produces vasodilation and dilates veins to a greater magnitude than it does arteries. Venodilation results in less blood returning to the heart, which produces a reduction in cardiac preload. This effect of nitroglycerin provides some early relief before the onset of the diuretic effects of furosemide. Nitroglycerin also reduces cardiac workload in patients with acute symptoms of congestive heart disease, improves blood flow to ischemic myocardium, and decreases myocardial oxygen demand.

In addition to its common uses for the treatment of pain, morphine sulfate is used in patients with CHF and pulmonary edema to relieve pulmonary congestion by venodilation. Morphine also lowers myocardial oxygen demand and reduces anxiety.

> Because morphine is a respiratory depressant, paramedics need to be skilled and equipped to support the patient's airway and respirations in the event of respiratory failure.

FUROSEMIDE (LASIX)

Classification: Loop diuretic.
Action: Inhibits the absorption of the sodium and chloride ions and water in the **loop of Henle**, as well as the convoluted tubule of the nephron. This results in decreased absorption of water and increased production of urine.
Indications: Pulmonary edema, CHF, hypertensive emergency.
Adverse Effects: Vertigo, dizziness, weakness, orthostatic hypotension, hypokalemia, thrombophlebitis. Patients with anuria, severe renal failure, untreated hepatic coma, increasing azotemia, and electrolyte depletion can develop life-threatening consequences.
Contraindications: Known sensitivity to sulfonamides or furosemide.
Dosage:
Congestive Heart Failure and Pulmonary Edema:
- **Adult:** 20 to 40 mg IV, intraosseous (IO) administered slowly over a 1- to 2-minute period. Begin with 40 mg in emergent situations. If a satisfactory response is not achieved within 1 hour, an additional dose of 80 mg can be given. A maximum single IV dose is 160 to 200 mg.
- **Pediatric:** 1 mg/kg IV, IO, or intramuscular (IM). If the response is not satisfactory, an additional dose of 2 mg/kg may be administered no sooner than 2 hours after the first dose.
Hypertensive Emergency:
- **Adult:** 40 mg IV, IO.
- **Pediatric:** 1 mg/kg IV or IM.
Special Considerations:
Onset of action for IV, IO administration occurs within 5 minutes and will peak within 30 minutes. Furosemide is a diuretic, so the patient will likely have urinary urgency. Be prepared to help the patient void.
Pregnancy class C.

MORPHINE SULFATE

Classification: Opiate agonist, Schedule C-II.
Action: Binds with opioid receptors. Morphine is capable of inducing hypotension by depression of the vasomotor centers of the brain, as well as release of the chemical histamine. In the management of angina, morphine reduces stimulation of the sympathetic nervous system caused by pain and anxiety. Reduction of sympathetic stimulation reduces heart rate, cardiac work, and myocardial oxygen consumption.

Indications: Moderate to severe pain, including chest pain associated with acute coronary syndrome (ACS), CHF, pulmonary edema.

Adverse Effects: Respiratory depression, hypotension, nausea/vomiting, dizziness, lightheadedness, sedation, diaphoresis, euphoria, dysphoria, worsening of bradycardia and heart block in some patients with acute inferior wall MI, seizures, cardiac arrest, anaphylactoid reactions.

Contraindications: Respiratory depression, shock, known sensitivity. Use with caution in hypotension, acute bronchial asthma, respiratory insufficiency, head trauma.

Dosage:

Pain:

- **Adult:** 2.5 to 15 mg IV, IO, IM, or subcutaneous administered slowly over a period of several minutes. The dose is the same whether administered IV, IO, IM, or subcutaneous.
- **Pediatric:**
  - **6 months to 12 years:** 0.05 to 0.2 mg/kg IV, IO, IM, or subcutaneous.
  - **Younger than 6 months:** 0.03 to 0.05 mg/kg IV, IO, IM, or subcutaneous.

Chest Pain Associated with Acute Coronary Syndromes, Congestive Heart Failure, and Pulmonary Edema:

Administer small doses and reevaluate the patient. Large doses may lead to respiratory depression and worsen the patient's hypoxia.

- **Adult:** 2 to 4 mg slow IV, IO over a 1- to 5-minute period with increments of 2 to 8 mg repeated every 5 to 15 minutes until patient relieved of chest pain.
- **Pediatric:** 0.1 to 0.2 mg/kg per dose IV, IO.

Special Considerations:

Monitor vital signs and pulse oximetry closely. Be prepared to support patient's airway and ventilations.

Overdose should be treated with naloxone.

Pregnancy class C.

NITROGLYCERIN (NITROLINGUAL, NITROQUICK, NITRO-DUR)

© Sue Heaton/Alamy Stock Photo.

© Allik Camazine/Alamy Stock Photo.

Classification: Antianginal agent.

Action: Relaxes vascular smooth muscle, thereby dilating peripheral arteries and veins. This causes pooling of venous blood and decreased venous return to the heart, which decreases preload. Nitroglycerin also reduces left ventricular systolic wall tension, which decreases afterload.

Indications: Angina, ongoing ischemic chest discomfort, hypertension, myocardial ischemia associated with cocaine intoxication.

(continues)

NITROGLYCERIN (NITROLINGUAL, NITROQUICK, NITRO-DUR) *(continued)*

Adverse Effects: Headache, hypotension, bradycardia, lightheadedness, flushing, cardiovascular collapse, methemoglobinemia.

Contraindications: Hypotension, severe bradycardia or tachycardia, increased intracranial pressure, intracranial bleeding, patients taking any medications for erectile dysfunction (such as sildenafil [Viagra], tadalafil [Cialis], or vardenafil [Levitra]), known sensitivity to nitrates. Use with caution in anemia, closed-angle glaucoma, hypotension, postural hypotension, uncorrected hypovolemia.

Dosage:
- **Adult:**
  - **Sublingual tablets:** One tablet (0.3 to 0.4 mg) at 5-minute intervals to a maximum of 3 doses.
  - **Translingual spray:** One (0.4 mg) spray at 5-minute intervals to a maximum of three sprays.
  - **Ointment:** 2% topical (Nitro-Bid ointment): Apply 1 to 2 inches (3 to 5 cm) of paste over the chest wall, cover with transparent wrap, and secure with tape.
  - **IV infusion:** 5 mcg/min; may increase rate by 5 to 10 mcg/min every 5 to 10 minutes as needed. End points of dose titration for nitroglycerin include a drop in the blood pressure of 10%, relief of chest pain, and return of ST segment to normal on a 12-lead electrocardiogram (ECG).
- **Pediatric IV infusion:** The initial pediatric infusion is 0.25 to 0.5 mcg/kg per minute IV, IO titrated by 0.5 to 1 mcg/kg per minute. Usual required dose is 1 to 3 mcg/kg per minute to a maximum dose of 5 mcg/kg per minute.

Special Considerations:
Administration of nitroglycerin to a patient with right ventricular MI can result in hypotension. Pregnancy class C.

Drugs Used for Long-Term Management

Common medications used for the long-term management of patients with CHF include digoxin, ACE inhibitors, angiotensin II receptor blockers, and beta blockers. Although these medications are not likely to be administered by prehospital providers in this setting, many patients with heart disease take some or all of them. Paramedics must be familiar with these medications because patients can experience ill effects from them that the paramedic may need to recognize and treat.

Digoxin is used in patients with CHF to increase myocardial contractility and often to slow the heart rate. Digoxin may also be used in patients with chronic atrial fibrillation. Simply put, digoxin helps the heart beat stronger and slower. When the heart beats fast, less time is available for the ventricle to fill with blood, which means less blood can fill the ventricle; therefore, cardiac output is decreased. When the heart rate is slowed, the ventricles are given more time to fill, and cardiac output is increased.

Blood delivering oxygen to the cells of the heart travels through the coronary arteries. When the heart contracts (systole), the coronary arteries are also squeezed; that action prevents oxygen-rich blood from moving forward. The only time that blood can carry oxygen to the heart is between contractions (diastole). By slowing the heart rate, cardiac consumption of oxygen is reduced, and blood flow to the heart is increased. In summary, the benefits of a drug-induced reduction of heart rate include the following:

- Decreased myocardial oxygen consumption
- Improved stroke volume, increasing cardiac output
- Prolonged diastolic coronary blood flow

A rapid heart rate (especially atrial fibrillation) reduces the filling of the heart, leading to decreased cardiac output and blood pressure.

Lisinopril is an ACE inhibitor. When angiotensin is inhibited, production of the most powerful vasoconstrictor in the body halts. As a result, the patient will have a decrease in blood pressure and mild diuresis. ACE inhibitors also reduce cardiac ischemic events, mortality rate, and hospital admissions for people with CHF.

A new class of medications known as angiotensin II receptor blockers (ARBs) are used in CHF patients when they are unable to tolerate an ACE inhibitor medication. These medications are not considered a primary treatment for CHF, but they are prescribed as an alternative to ACE inhibitor medications. ARB medications are also used outside of CHF to treat hypertension and kidney dysfunction.

Metoprolol, a beta blocker, binds to beta adrenergic receptors and decreases blood pressure and heart rate, which are beneficial to the diseased heart. Metoprolol is a **cardioselective beta blocker** used to control hypertension and decrease cardiac workload in the patient with CHF. Adding a beta blocker to an ACE inhibitor has been shown to decrease mortality rate and hospital admissions in symptomatic patients with heart failure.

DIGOXIN (LANOXIN)

Classification: Cardiac glycoside.
Action: Inhibits sodium-potassium-adenosine triphosphatase membrane pump, resulting in an increase in calcium inside the heart muscle cell, which causes an increase in the force of the heart's contraction.
Indications: CHF, to control the ventricular rate in chronic AF and atrial flutter, narrow-complex paroxysmal supraventricular tachycardia.
Adverse Effects: Headache, weakness, GI disturbances, arrhythmias, nausea/vomiting, diarrhea, vision disturbances.
Contraindications: Digitalis allergy, VT and VF, heart block, sick sinus syndrome, tachycardia without heart failure, pulse lower than 50 to 60 beats/min, MI, ischemic heart disease, patients with preexcitation AF or atrial flutter (i.e., a delta wave, characteristic of Wolff-Parkinson-White syndrome, visible during normal sinus rhythm).
Dosage: Dosage is individualized.
Special Considerations:
Low levels of serum potassium can lead to digoxin toxicity and bradycardia.
  Conditions such as administration of steroids or diuretics or vomiting and
  diarrhea can produce low levels of potassium and subsequent digoxin toxicity.
Pregnancy class C.

NDC 12345-678-90

Digoxin Injection
Pediatric
100 mcg (0.1 mg) in 1 mL
10 ampuls 1 mL each
Protect from light. **Rx only**

Angiotensin-Converting Enzyme Inhibitors, Beta Blockers, and Calcium Channel Blockers

Angiotensin-Converting Enzyme Inhibitors

Many patients with CHF are prescribed ACE inhibitors. This class of drugs blocks, or antagonizes, the enzyme responsible for the production of the hormone **angiotensin II**. Angiotensin II is a vasoconstrictor that is 40 times more powerful than norepinephrine. In addition to being a vasoconstrictor, angiotensin II also has positive inotropic and chronotropic properties. Therefore, drugs that block the production of angiotensin II (ACE inhibitors) reduce blood pressure, decrease cardiac afterload, reduce heart rate, and reduce the force of contraction of the heart. ACE inhibitors reduce the mortality rate in patients with moderate and severe CHF.

ANGIOTENSIN-CONVERTING ENZYME (ACE) INHIBITORS: CAPTOPRIL (CAPOTEN), ENALAPRIL (VASOTEC), LISINOPRIL (PRINIVIL, ZESTRIL), RAMIPRIL (ALTACE)

Classification: ACE inhibitors.
Action: Blocks the enzyme responsible for the production of angiotensin II, resulting in a decrease in blood pressure.
Indications: Congestive heart failure, hypertension, post-MI.
Adverse Effects: Headache, dizziness, fatigue, depression, chest pain, hypotension, palpitations, cough, dyspnea, upper respiratory infection, nausea/vomiting, rash, pruritus, angioedema, renal failure.
Contraindications: Angioedema related to previous treatment with an ACE inhibitor, known sensitivity. Use with caution in aortic stenosis, bilateral renal artery stenosis, hypertrophic obstructive cardiomyopathy, pericardial tamponade, elevated serum potassium levels, acute kidney failure.
Dosage:
- **Adult:** Medication is administered orally. Dosage is individualized.
- **Pediatric:** Medication is administered orally. Dosage is individualized.

Special Considerations:
Pregnancy class D.

Beta Blockers

Beta blockers are helpful in the long-term management of patients with CHF; however, beta blockers should be avoided in patients who are unstable or have decompensated CHF. In the management of a patient with chronic heart failure, the dose of beta blockers is slowly and progressively increased over a prolonged period.

METOPROLOL (LOPRESSOR, TOPROL XL)

Classification: Beta adrenergic antagonist, antianginal, antihypertensive, Class II antiarrhythmic.
Action: Inhibits the strength of the heart's contractions, as well as heart rate. This results in a decrease in cardiac oxygen consumption. Metoprolol is a selective beta$_1$ type blocker.
Indications: ACS, hypertension, SVT, atrial flutter, AF, thyrotoxicosis.
Adverse Effects: Tiredness, dizziness, diarrhea, heart block, bradycardia, bronchospasm, hypotension.
Contraindications: Cardiogenic shock, AV block, bradycardia, known sensitivity. Use with caution in hypotension, chronic lung disease (asthma and COPD).
Dosage:
Cardiac Indications:
- **Adult:** 5 mg slow IV, IO over a 2-minute period; repeat at 5-minute intervals up to a total of three infusions totaling 15 mg IV, IO.
- **Pediatric:** Oral dosing only.

Special Considerations:
Blood pressure, heart rate, and ECG should be monitored carefully.
Use with caution in patients with asthma.
Pregnancy class C.

Calcium Channel Blockers

Certain calcium channel blockers such as verapamil, diltiazem, and nifedipine should be avoided in patients with CHF because they have been shown to increase morbidity and mortality rates in patients with left ventricular systolic dysfunction from heart failure.[5]

▶ Review Questions

1. What are some medical conditions that may predispose a patient to develop CHF?
2. What is the function of a diuretic?
3. How is morphine beneficial in the treatment of heart failure?
4. What are the benefits to the heart of preventing tachycardia when treating someone with heart disease?
5. What is the role of digoxin in the treatment of CHF?
6. Explain the effects of ACE inhibitors on the heart.
7. What precautions should be followed in administering beta blockers to a patient with CHF?

References

1. Bui AL, Horwich TB, Fonarow GC. Epidemiology and risk profile of heart failure. *Nat Rev Cardiol.* 2011;8(1):30–41.
2. Goldberg RJ, Spencer FA, Szklo-Coxe M, et al. Symptom presentation in patients hospitalized with acute heart failure. *Clinical Cardiol.* 2010;33(6):E73–E80. http://doi: 10.1002/clc.20627.
3. Vasan RS, Wilson PW. Epidemiology and causes of heart failure. UpToDate. https://www.uptodate.com/contents/epidemiology-and-causes-of-heart-failure?search=Congestive%20Heart%20Failure&source=search_result&selectedTitle=3~150&usage_type=default&display_rank=3. Updated March 20, 2018. Accessed July 20, 2018.
4. Colucci WS. Treatment of acute decompensated heart failure: components of therapy. UpToDate. https://www.uptodate.com/contents/treatment-of-acute-decompensated-heart-failure-components-of-therapy?source=see_link. Updated August 25, 2017. Accessed July 20, 2018.
5. O'Conner CM, Carson PE, Miller AB, et al. Effect of amlodipine on mode of death among patients with advanced heart failure in the PRAISE trial. Prospective Randomized Amlodipine Survival Evaluation. *Am J Cardiol.* 1998;82:881887.

CHAPTER 11

Endocrine Emergencies

▶ Introduction

This chapter describes pharmacologic treatment of the most common endocrine emergencies, including diabetic emergencies such as hypoglycemia, hyperglycemia, and diabetic ketoacidosis. Adrenal emergencies, including adrenal insufficiency, and thyroid emergencies, including thyrotoxicosis and myxedema coma, are also addressed.

CASE STUDY

You are called to a local supermarket in response to a 63-year-old man who was found unconscious. He has a history of heart disease and type 2 diabetes. He takes a beta blocker and glyburide, an oral hypoglycemic medication. The patient's wife states that he has not eaten much today. On arrival, you find him on the floor, and his mental status is depressed. His airway is patent, and he is breathing with no obstruction. His blood pressure is 120/95 mm Hg, and his heart rate is 120 beats/min. He appears pale and feels clammy to the touch. A glucometer reveals a blood sugar level of 52 mg/dL. Intravenous (IV) access is obtained, and IV 50% dextrose is administered. He begins to awaken and a maintenance IV line with D_5W is begun. Ten minutes after the bolus of dextrose, the patient's repeat blood sugar is 138 mg/dL. His heart rate is improving at 90 beats/min, and his blood pressure is stable.

▶ Overview of Diabetes

Diabetes is a disease manifested by a dysfunctional pancreas. Insulin is required to convert sugars into energy for use by the body. Diabetes takes two different forms, **type 1 diabetes** and **type 2 diabetes**. Patients with type 1 diabetes do not produce insulin. Without insulin, the cells of the body are not able to take sugar into the cell to be used for energy by that cell. Sugar is the main fuel of the cells, and like a car without gasoline, the cells of the body are not able to run without sugar. Patients with type 2 diabetes are capable of making insulin; however, the insulin is not used properly by the body, a condition known as *insulin resistance*. The majority of people with diabetes have type 2.

Insulin is used in patients with type 1 diabetes and some patients with type 2 diabetes. Insulin stimulates the uptake of **glucose** by the cells of the body and lowers the level of sugar in the blood (**FIGURE 11-1**). Insulin allows glucose to enter cells, and potassium follows in turn. Oral hypoglycemic medications are used to manage most patients with type 2 diabetes. These agents act at a receptor on the insulin-producing cells of the pancreas. Some oral hypoglycemic agents also act by improving insulin's action on cells around the body. Oral hypoglycemic medications have a tendency to contribute to hypoglycemia, especially in certain groups of patients such as older adults and people with liver and kidney disease.

Diabetes is a common disease, and paramedics routinely will encounter patients who take various forms of insulin. These various forms differ in their onset and duration of action. Although prehospital providers are exposed to several different forms of insulin, if a paramedic administers insulin to a patient, it will most likely be regular insulin. Several types of insulin are on the market. What distinguishes these different types are the time of onset and the duration of action. Some forms of insulin have a fast onset of action that may last only a few hours. In contrast, other, longer-acting insulins may have a slower onset but last as long as 24 hours. A patient's blood sugar level changes throughout the day. It may be lower between meals or overnight. After a meal or a snack, blood sugar increases (**FIGURE 11-2**). To provide reasonable control of blood sugar, a patient may be taking several different forms of insulin.

Diabetes is an increasingly common disease process. Diabetic emergencies, in particular, are commonly encountered by paramedics. These emergencies typically represent complications of a blood sugar level that is too high (hyperglycemia, potentially resulting in ketoacidosis) or too low (hypoglycemia, resulting in seizure or coma).

Hypoglycemia

Hypoglycemia (low blood sugar) is the most common complication experienced by patients with diabetes and is a life-threatening emergency.[1] It is often referred to as *insulin shock*.

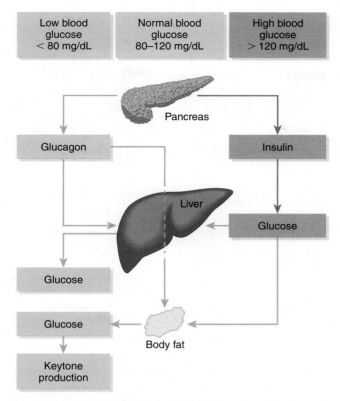

| Low blood glucose < 80 mg/dL | Normal blood glucose 80–120 mg/dL | High blood glucose > 120 mg/dL |

Pancreas

Glucagon

Insulin

Liver

Glucose

Glucose

Glucose

Body fat

Glucose

Keytone production

FIGURE 11-1   The interaction of the hormones insulin and glucagon in the body in relation to blood glucose levels. A rise in blood glucose levels stimulates insulin release from the pancreas. Insulin allows glucose to enter the liver and allows t of amino acids into muscle and free fatty acids into fat tissue. A low glucose level in the blood stimulates glucagon production in the pancreas. When glucagon is present, glucose is released from its stored form in the liver to make it available for the body's cells.

Research has shown that diabetic patients have fewer long-term complications when they maintain tight control of their blood sugar.[2] However, with the increased effort toward improved blood glucose control can come an increased risk of hypoglycemia. A careful analysis that balances the potential benefits of tight blood glucose control and decreased long-term complications of diabetes against the risk of iatrogenic hypoglycemia and its potentially lethal consequences is essential.[3]

Mild hypoglycemia commonly occurs in patients with diabetes and can simply be treated with oral glucose. However, moderate hypoglycemia can lead to serious hypoglycemia—that is, low blood sugar that requires intervention by someone other than the patient. The cause of hypoglycemia is not always recognized, and the patient can have little warning to intervene and prevent worsening of the situation. This is particularly true for patients who have had diabetes for several years because they can lose the ability to recognize symptoms of hypoglycemia, such as tachycardia, pallor, sweating, and anxiety. This condition is referred to as **hypoglycemic unawareness**. In certain populations, 40 to 50% of hypoglycemic episodes go unrecognized.[3] Normally the body has a robust defense system to protect the brain against a significant drop in available blood glucose. When blood glucose drops, a variety of body chemicals, including catecholamines, glucagon, and cortisol, are released to either increase blood glucose levels or shift blood glucose toward the brain.[4]

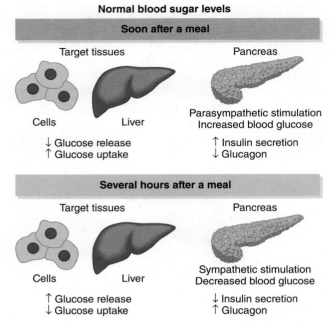

Normal blood sugar levels

Soon after a meal

Target tissues

Cells   Liver

↓ Glucose release
↑ Glucose uptake

Pancreas

Parasympathetic stimulation
Increased blood glucose

↑ Insulin secretion
↓ Glucagon

Several hours after a meal

Target tissues

Cells   Liver

↑ Glucose release
↓ Glucose uptake

Pancreas

Sympathetic stimulation
Decreased blood glucose

↓ Insulin secretion
↑ Glucagon

FIGURE 11-2 Diagram of the counterregulatory mechanisms of glucose metabolism with insulin and glucagon. Several hours after a meal, decreased blood glucose levels will inhibit insulin and stimulate glucagon, as well as the sympathetic nervous system. These changes allow glycogen to release glucose from the liver and decrease glucose uptake by the muscles, making glucose rise in the bloodstream. Immediately after a meal, blood glucose levels rise, stimulating insulin release, decreasing glucagon, and stimulating parasympathetic signals. These changes allow the formation of glycogen and storage of glucose into the liver and peripheral tissues.

These chemicals cause clinical signs and symptoms such as hunger, anxiety, and sweating, which normally alert the person that his or her blood sugar has dropped. When hypoglycemic unawareness occurs, patients do not develop or recognize these signs and symptoms before neurologic impairment occurs. In these situations, patients are unable to take steps to correct the hypoglycemia themselves and become largely dependent on assistance or rescue by others.

Hypoglycemia is often caused by the insufficient intake of sugar from inadequacies in the diet or by excessive insulin from inaccurate dosing or excessive action of the medication. Both factors typically contribute to hypoglycemia. Increased use of glucose by the body, such as occurs during and after exercise or strenuous physical activity, can cause blood sugar to drop rapidly, resulting in hypoglycemia.

The patient in the previous scenario had a hypoglycemic episode, most likely from the oral hypoglycemic medication used to treat his type 2 diabetes. Remember, oral hypoglycemic medications work by increasing insulin secretion. This increased insulin release, combined with the fact that the patient had not eaten much that day, likely resulted in the patient's episode of hypoglycemia.

During hypoglycemia, the body's defenses include secretion of certain hormones and activation of the sympathetic nervous system in an attempt to increase blood sugar. **Glucagon** is secreted by the pancreas in response to low blood sugar. Glucagon mobilizes glucose stored in the liver and muscle in the form of **glycogen**. Glycogen is a molecule that acts as a storage form of glucose. When the body needs additional glucose, such as in exercise or stress, the pancreas releases glucagon. Glucagon stimulates the breakdown of glycogen, producing glucose. Epinephrine, a catecholamine from the adrenal gland, ultimately stimulates an increase in blood sugar. The release of epinephrine also produces an increase in blood pressure, tachycardia, diaphoresis, and anxiety. Recall that the patient in our scenario had all these symptoms.

In the scenario, beta blockers may have prevented a rise in heart rate and blood pressure. For diabetic patients, beta blockers can mask the symptoms of hypoglycemia, and these patients can be more prone to blunted hypoglycemic unawareness.

Management

Hypoglycemia requires prompt treatment. When possible, the treatment of choice is oral glucose. If the patient is conscious, oral glucose can result in an immediate improvement. Oral glucose is available as either a glucose gel or tablet. Glucose gel is easier to tolerate and can prevent the risk of choking in the event of an altered level of consciousness.

ADMINISTRATION OF ORAL GLUCOSE

Equipment Needed:
Medicine, gloves, tongue depressor or other appropriate applicator, PPE
Procedure:
1. Observe standard precautions.
2. Verify the drug order.
3. Confirm right patient, right medication, right dose, right route, and right time.
4. Confirm with the patient that he or she has no allergies to the medication, and document allergies to any other medication.
5. When possible, explain to the patient what medication you are going to administer and why.
6. Ensure the patient is responsive and able to swallow.
7. Place the glucose on a tongue depressor and administer the full tube between the patient's cheek and gum.
8. Record the time of drug administration in the patient care record.
9. Evaluate the patient for desired effects of the medication, as well as any adverse effects.

If the patient has an altered or depressed level of consciousness, as in the previous scenario, or if an adequate airway is not established, parenteral administration of glucose is more appropriate. This is achieved by using IV dextrose. Dextrose is available as 50% dextrose solution. That means that 100 mL of a solution has 50 g of dextrose. The preloaded syringe of 50% dextrose used in most emergency situations is a 50-mL syringe (25 g dextrose in 50 mL solution). Twenty-five percent dextrose has 25 g of dextrose in 100 mL of solution, and 10% dextrose has 10 g of dextrose in 100 mL of solution. Ten percent dextrose is prepared by diluting 50% dextrose 1:4 with IV fluid.

Dextrose solutions that are more concentrated than 5% solutions are considered hypertonic and can cause irritation and pain when injected too rapidly. To avoid this irritation to the vein, any dextrose solution more concentrated than 5% should be slowly injected into a large vein. *Concentrated dextrose solutions should not be administered intramuscularly (IM) or subcutaneously.*

Treatment of hypoglycemia depends on the patient's level of consciousness. If IV access were not possible in the patient in the scenario, the next step would be to administer IM glucagon. This would mobilize glycogen stores from the liver and elevate blood glucose levels rather rapidly. However, a common side effect is vomiting because glucagon delays gastric emptying. Patients who have been fasting for days may not show a pronounced effect because of low glycogen levels in the liver.

Patients with hypoglycemia require close monitoring of the airway, and blood glucose should be checked every 30 minutes. In the previous scenario, even though the first repeat blood sugar was elevated, the glucose should not be lowered too aggressively with insulin because the patient has been using an oral agent whose action can last for several hours. The patient's glucose can potentially be lowered to hypoglycemic levels. In addition, if he is not able to take an oral form of glucose, the use of IV glucose may need to be continued until he can be stabilized.

Patients with depressed mental status who are alcoholics or malnourished may have a deficiency of thiamine. If given dextrose before thiamine administration, such patients can develop a brain condition (**Wernicke-Korsakoff syndrome**) that manifests itself by amnesia, confabulation, attention deficit, disorientation, and vision impairment. To prevent Wernicke-Korsakoff syndrome, administer thiamine before dextrose in malnourished or alcoholic patients.

DEXTROSE (50%, 25%, 10%)

Classification: Antihypoglycemic.
Action: Increases blood glucose concentrations.
Indications: Hypoglycemia.
Adverse Effects: Hyperglycemia, warmth, burning from IV infusion. Concentrated solutions may cause pain and thrombosis of the peripheral veins.
Contraindications: Intracranial and intraspinal hemorrhage, delirium tremens, solution that is not clear, seals that are not intact.
Dosage:
Hyperkalemia:
- **Adult:** 25 g of dextrose 50% IV, intraosseous (IO).
- **Pediatric:** 0.5 to 1 g/kg IV, IO.

Hypoglycemia:
- **Adult:** 10 to 25 g of dextrose 50% IV (20 to 50 mL of dextrose solution).
- **Pediatric:**
   ◦ **Older than 2 years:** 2 mL/kg of dextrose 50%.
   ◦ **Younger than 2 years:** 2 to 4 mL/kg of dextrose 10%.

Special Considerations:
Pregnancy class C.

GLUCAGON

Classification: Hormone.
Action: Converts glycogen to glucose.
Indications: Hypoglycemia, beta-blocker overdose.
Adverse Effects: Nausea/vomiting, rebound hyperglycemia, hypotension, sinus tachycardia.
Contraindications: Pheochromocytoma, insulinoma, known sensitivity.
Dosage:
Hypoglycemia:

- **Adult:** 1 mg IM, IV, IO, or subcutaneous.
- **Pediatric (<44 pounds [20 kg]):** 0.5 mg IM, IV, IO, or subcutaneous.

Beta-Blocker Overdose:

- **Adult:** 3 to 10 mg IV, IO over a 1-minute period, followed by a second dose of 10 mg IV (or IV infusion 3 to 5 mg/hour) if the symptoms of bradycardia and hypotension recur. (Note that this dose is much higher than the dose required to treat hypoglycemia; avoid using the supplied glycerin-based reconstitution solution when larger doses of glucagon are being administered.)
- **Pediatric:** For patients weighing <44 pounds (20 kg), the dose is 0.5 mg.

Special Considerations:
Pregnancy class B.

THIAMINE (VITAMIN B₁)

Classification: Vitamin B_1.
Action: Thiamine combines with adenosine triphosphate to produce thiamine diphosphate, which acts as a coenzyme in carbohydrate metabolism.
Indications: Wernicke-Korsakoff syndrome, beriberi, nutritional supplementation.
Adverse Effects: Itching, rash, pain at injection site.
Contraindications: Known sensitivity.
Dosage:
Wernicke-Korsakoff Syndrome:

- **Adult:** 100 mg IV, IO.
- **Pediatric:** Not recommended for pediatric patients.

Special Considerations:
Pregnancy class A.

Diabetic Ketoacidosis

CASE STUDY

You are called to respond to a 10-year-old girl who has had vomiting and intermittent diarrhea for the past 6 days. The child's parents state that she has lost 15 pounds (7 kg) in 3 weeks. She is thin, with tachypnea and a fruity odor to her breath. Her heart rate is 180 beats/min, and her blood pressure is 90/60 mm Hg. Her weight is estimated at 50 pounds (23 kg). IV access is obtained, and Ringer's lactate solution is begun at a maintenance rate (approximately 65 mL/hr). The glucometer reading is 560 mg/dL. Her pulse oximetry reading is 99% on room air despite rapid breathing. Her airway is patent and she is stable, although she continues to breathe rapidly. You start the patient on some oxygen by nasal cannula and place her on a cardiac monitor.

Diabetic ketoacidosis (DKA) occurs most commonly in patients with type 1 diabetes, although it can also occur in patients with type 2 diabetes. The key problem in DKA is a lack of insulin. In diabetic patients, too little insulin prevents the cells of the body from using glucose and, consequently, blood glucose rises. The cells cannot use the glucose but still require a source of fuel. Therefore, the glucose-starved cells start to break down fat, producing acid and chemicals known as **ketone bodies**.

Patients with DKA have metabolic acidosis, dehydration, and electrolyte abnormalities. The type of acidosis that these patients have is known as **ketoacidosis**, which is distinct from lactic acidosis. Ketoacidosis occurs when the body uses alternative fuel sources for energy production because of the inability to burn glucose from the lack of insulin. Conversely, **lactic acidosis** occurs in shock states when oxygen is lacking; the cellular machinery uses an inefficient energy-generating process known as *anaerobic metabolism*. The product of anaerobic metabolism is lactate; hence, patients generate lactic acidosis. These two forms of acidosis are not related.

> The purpose of a car's fuel pump is to deliver fuel from the tank to the injectors of the engine. In the absence of a functional fuel pump, the car's engine can be starved of fuel despite having a tank full of gasoline. In the case of DKA, insulin can be thought of as the fuel pump, and glucose as the fuel. Despite there being plenty of glucose (the fuel), the lack of insulin (the bad fuel pump) is preventing the glucose from being delivered to the cellular machinery.

High blood glucose levels often result in loss of glucose in the urine, and patients can become dehydrated due to electrolyte imbalances as the body uses water as a carrier to move electrolytes or remove various electrolytes from the body. Within the kidney, glucose is filtered into the tubules that collect the urine produced. As the fluid passes through the tubules of the kidney, the glucose is reabsorbed. In cases in which the concentration of the blood glucose is elevated, the amount of glucose passed into the kidney tubules exceeds the kidney's ability to reabsorb the glucose back into the bloodstream, and glucose is spilled into the urine. The spilling of glucose into the urine typically occurs at a serum blood glucose of approximately 300 mg/dL. In Chapter 5, the concept of osmosis was discussed. The glucose molecule in the urine also decreases the reabsorption of water by the kidney and the patient rapidly becomes dehydrated. In this situation, patients have symptoms of increased thirst, increased urination, racing of the heart, and vomiting. The breath of a patient in DKA is often described as "fruity" because of the presence of the ketone bodies.

The preceding scenario illustrates a case of new-onset DKA in a pediatric patient. A similar scenario can present in a known diabetic patient who has become ill or perhaps has not received adequate insulin treatment.

Management

Treatment of DKA includes correction of dehydration and acidosis with IV fluids and insulin. *However, fluid replacement needs to be undertaken slowly.* Remember that the patient in the case lost weight and deteriorated over a 3-week period. As such, IV fluid administration should not be too rapid or aggressive unless the patient has cardiovascular instability. The patient is demonstrating tachycardia (heart rate of 180 beats/min), so an initial bolus of 10 mL/kg would be reasonable. If a fluid bolus is anticipated, place a large-bore IV catheter if possible. Remember, conditions that quickly develop should be quickly corrected, and situations that slowly develop should be slowly corrected. The recommendation for adults is a 15- to 20-mL/kg initial normal saline fluid bolus.[5]

> (*continued*) After starting an IV line, you prepare to administer a fluid bolus. You determine that with her magnitude of hypovolemia, the patient should receive some intravascular fluid resuscitation. The patient weighs approximately 50 pounds (22 kg). You plan to administer a fluid bolus of approximately 10 mL/kg (22 kg × 10 mL/kg = 220 mL). You start a 250-mL fluid bolus of normal saline solution. Next, you calculate her maintenance IV fluid rate at 62 mL/hr. After the fluid bolus, you plan to run the IV fluids at a maintenance rate of 1.5 times, or approximately 93 mL/hr (maintenance rate × 1.5 = 62 mL/hr × 1.5 = 93 mL/hr).

BOX 11-1 Pediatric Maintenance Fluids

To determine the appropriate rate of maintenance fluid, the provider must know or estimate the child's weight in kilograms. Remember that 1 kg equals approximately 2.2 pounds.

For the first 10 kg of weight, the IV fluid rate is 4 mL/hr per kilogram.

- A 5-kg child has an IV rate of 20 mL/hr (4 mL/hr per kilogram × 5 kg).
- A 10-kg child has an IV rate of 40 mL/hr (4 mL/hr per kilogram × 10 kg).
- For the second 10 kg of weight (10 to 20 kg of body weight), add 2 mL/kg for each additional kilogram.
- For a 12-kg child, start with an IV rate of 40 mL/hr for the first 10 kg of body weight and then add 4 mL/hr for the remaining 2 kg. The IV rate then is 44 mL/hr.
  - 10 kg × 4 mL/kg per hour = 40 mL/hr
  - 2 kg × 2 mL/kg per hour = 4 mL/hr
  - Total maintenance rate = 44 mL/hr

To calculate the IV maintenance rate for children larger than 20 kg, add an additional 1 mL/hr per kilogram.

- A 25-kg child will have an IV maintenance rate of:
  - First 10 kg = 40 mL/hr
  - Second 10 kg = 20 mL/hr
  - Remaining 5 kg = 1 mL/kg per hour × 5 kg = 5 mL/hr

Therefore, the total maintenance rate is 65 mL/hr.

Often IV fluids administered at maintenance to 1.5 times the maintenance rate are adequate for initial stabilization with the initial fluid bolus. (See **BOX 11-1** for pediatric maintenance rates.) The IV fluid of choice initially should not include potassium replacement because the presence of ketoacidosis suggests an elevated potassium level. (Once urine output is ensured and electrolyte status can be determined at a hospital, potassium replacement becomes increasingly important.) Treatment of DKA with insulin, as well as correction of the acidosis, moves potassium into cells and rapidly lowers blood potassium levels. Prehospital treatment should include an isotonic solution such as normal saline or Ringer's lactate. The use of bicarbonate is controversial and should be avoided except when ordered by medical direction in extreme situations.[6]

In the preceding scenario, the patient's rapid breathing is the result of **ketonemia** (the presence of recognizable concentrations of ketone bodies in the plasma), acidosis, and the body's attempt to relieve itself of carbon dioxide. The fruity odor to her breath is also consistent with the presence of ketones. Her elevated heart rate is the result of a combination of responses to the body's detection of low plasma volume from dehydration, as well as the release of catecholamines such as epinephrine and norepinephrine. Patients with hyperkalemia need to be monitored for peaked T waves on the electrocardiogram (ECG). Compared with adults, children are less likely to have cardiovascular complications as potassium levels rise; however, monitoring cardiovascular status in all patients with DKA is still necessary.

Aggressive hydration, particularly with hypotonic fluids, has been shown to contribute to complications of therapy, such as cerebral edema or swelling of the brain. Conservative fluid management is therefore key!

If a patient's cardiovascular condition requires an IV fluid bolus, volume resuscitation should be conservative. In pediatric patients, boluses should be limited to 10 mL/kg at a time with fluids such as normal saline and Ringer's lactate and not repeated unless significant instability exists. Vital signs (blood pressure, heart rate, and respiratory rate) should be closely monitored, and neurologic status should be assessed. If a hypovolemic patient with DKA is resuscitated too quickly, the patient can develop cerebral edema (swelling of the brain). Therefore, patients should be monitored for changes in their neurologic status.[7] A classic mistake made when caring for these patients is the addition of dextrose-containing solutions (D_5W, D_5NS, D_5 Ringer's lactate) to IV fluids. Once the patient with DKA is admitted to intensive care and the blood sugar level approaches 250 to 300 mg/dL, he or she will be switched to fluids that contain low concentrations of dextrose, such as D_5 Ringer's lactate solution. The reason to start glucose at this level of blood sugar (250 to 300 mg/dL) is to prevent the development of hypoglycemia while the blood sugar is lowered with insulin and to protect against the development of cerebral edema.

Insulin. Many EMS agencies do not carry insulin; simple IV fluid administration is often sufficient to improve hyperglycemia and help correct the metabolic acidosis until the patient can be transported and treated at a medical facility. If insulin is available and appropriate, it can be given as a bolus or drip.[8] The use of IV bolus insulin has been debated and remains a less-desirable method of treating hyperglycemia in DKA than an insulin infusion.

IV insulin has been shown to be significantly more effective than IM or subcutaneous administration, at least in the initial treatment of DKA.[7] In a patient with poor perfusion from hypovolemia or shock, subcutaneous insulin may not absorb appropriately, leading to a slow onset of action. Blood sugar should be monitored every 30 to 60 minutes while the patient is on an insulin drip or after a subcutaneous injection of insulin. The desired response should be a decrease in blood sugar by 10% per hour, or no faster than approximately 50 mg/dL per hour. Conversely, if the rate of decrease exceeds 50 mg/dL per hour, the insulin infusion may need to be decreased to prevent hypoglycemia. Acidosis often persists for several hours and can require up to 24 hours to resolve once the hyperglycemia has been corrected. Hydration and reestablishment of renal function are also critical.

INSULIN, REGULAR (HUMULIN R, NOVOLIN R)

Classification: Hormone.
Action: Binds to a receptor on the membrane of cells and facilitates the transport of glucose into cells.
Indications: Hyperglycemia, insulin-dependent diabetes mellitus, hyperkalemia.
Adverse Effects: Hypoglycemia, tachycardia, palpitations, diaphoresis, anxiety, confusion, blurred vision, weakness, depression, seizures, coma, insulin shock, hypokalemia.
Contraindications: Hypoglycemia, known sensitivity.
Dosage:
Diabetic Ketoacidosis:

- **Adult:** 0.1 U/kg IV, IO, or subcutaneous. Because of poor perfusion of the peripheral tissues, subcutaneous administration is much less effective than the IV, IO route. IV, IO insulin has a very short half-life; therefore IV, IO insulin without an infusion is not that effective. The rate for an insulin infusion is 0.05 to 0.1 U/kg per hour IV, IO. When dosing insulin, use a U-100 insulin syringe to measure and deliver the insulin. The time from administration to action, as well as the duration of action, varies greatly among different people, as well as at different times in the same person.

Hyperkalemia:

- **Adult:** 10 U IV, IO of regular insulin (Insulin R), coadministered with 50 mL of $D_{50}W$ over 5 minutes.
- **Pediatric:** 0.1 U/kg Insulin R IV, IO.

Special Considerations:
Only regular insulin can be given IV, IO. *Insulin is a high-risk medication and should be verified with another appropriately trained provider whenever possible.*
Pregnancy class B.

RAPID-ACTING INSULINS

Although paramedics will likely not use insulin analogs in the field, an understanding of the newer forms of rapid-acting insulins is important because many patients take these products.

Insulin lispro (Humalog), insulin aspart (NovoLog), and insulin glulisine (Apidra) are three forms of synthetic insulin whose molecular structure makes them optimal for use in the treatment of type 1 diabetes. Onset of action occurs within 10 minutes, and peak action is 90 minutes, with a duration of action of 2 to 4 hours in some patients.

These insulin products do not require a 30-minute wait when administered subcutaneously before a meal. They can even be administered immediately after a meal in some patients. This is desirable in the pediatric patient in particular, whose eating habits are variable; often their insulin doses are based on their carbohydrate intake.

▶ Overview of Acute Adrenal Insufficiency

CASE STUDY

You are called to the home of a 54-year-old man who was found unconscious on his bathroom floor. According to his wife, he had a pituitary tumor resection 6 months ago. His medications include levothyroxine (Levothroid) and hydrocortisone (Cortef). He has had the flu for the past 4 days, with a fever of 101°F (38.6°C), vomiting, and diarrhea. He has not eaten much in the past few days and has had no oral intake today according to his wife. Assessment reveals a weak-appearing man lying on his side. No evidence of acute trauma is visible. He is pale and his eyes appear sunken. He is breathing rapidly but without audible wheezes. His blood pressure is 100/60 mm Hg, heart rate is 140 beats/min, and respiratory rate is 30 breaths/min. He weighs approximately 154 pounds (70 kg), and his blood glucose is 48 mg/dL. You obtain peripheral IV access immediately and administer 50% dextrose at 2 mL/kg (approximately 140 mL in this patient). A repeat blood sugar reading after the dextrose bolus is 95 mg/dL. A bolus of normal saline is then begun at 1 L over a 1-hour period, and blood sugar is monitored every 15 to 30 minutes. The next blood sugar reading is 90 mg/dL, and the fluid is changed to D_5W. IV hydrocortisone is given at a dose of 100 mg. The patient arrives at the local emergency department approximately 55 minutes later by your ambulance. His blood pressure has increased to 110/70 mm Hg, heart rate is now 100 beats/min, and respiratory rate is 20 breaths/min. A repeat blood glucose reading is 120 mg/dL.

Acute adrenal insufficiency is a life-threatening emergency that is often underdiagnosed and undertreated. However, treatment cannot be delayed because the patient's cardiovascular and metabolic status will rapidly deteriorate. The adrenal glands are located on top of each of the kidneys and are responsible for the production and secretion of several important hormones. The **adrenal medulla** produces catecholamines such as epinephrine and norepinephrine, which help the body respond during times of stress. The adrenal cortex, or outer layer of the gland, produces **steroid hormones**, including those responsible for electrolyte stability (called **mineralocorticoids**), and anti-inflammatory stress hormones (called **glucocorticoids** or **cortisol**). In addition to its anti-inflammatory function, cortisol contributes to the body's stress response, particularly during times of severe illness, surgery, and trauma. Blood pressure, heart rate, and blood glucose all increase in response to cortisol action.

In some patients, adrenal insufficiency results from the lack of an enzyme, which renders them unable to produce cortisol sufficiently, such as in **congenital adrenal hyperplasia (CAH)**. Adrenal insufficiency can also result from infection, injury, and an autoimmune reaction of the gland (such as the result of tuberculosis, trauma, or Addison disease). Sometimes the adrenal glands are unable to produce adequate stress hormones because of a lack of central input from the pituitary gland. The pituitary gland secretes a hormone called **adrenocorticotropin (ACTH)**, which in turn stimulates the necessary signaling at the adrenal gland and results in the production and release of cortisol and other adrenal hormones. Patients who are treated with steroids for chronic conditions (e.g., chronic obstructive pulmonary disease [COPD], asthma, and connective tissue diseases) may develop acute adrenal insufficiency when their steroids are interrupted or during periods of illness or injury.

Management

Patients with adrenal insufficiency usually are treated regularly with the physiologic replacement of cortisone (Cortone). Solu-Cortef is the parenteral form of hydrocortisone, and Cortef is the enteral form. Patients are typically instructed how to increase their dosage at times of illness or surgery to achieve the normal stress levels that the body naturally would produce during these situations. Many patients have access to an "emergency kit" of IM hydrocortisone (Cortef, Solu-Cortef) to administer the necessary medication when oral tablets cannot be taken.

In the previous scenario, the patient has adrenal insufficiency. Despite having functioning adrenal glands, he does not have the correct input from the pituitary gland to stimulate adrenal production and release cortisol during stressful times, such as fever and illness. In patients without adrenal insufficiency, cortisol is secreted at three to four times the normal levels during periods of stress. This patient has a history of hydrocortisone (Cortef, Solu-Cortef) replacement, which should have been increased during illness or in conjunction with surgery to simulate the body's increased needs. The oral increase in medication is limited during periods of vomiting. In addition, intravascular volume is depleted, contributing to the patient's hypotension. If IV access cannot be obtained, IM hydrocortisone can be administered.

HYDROCORTISONE SODIUM SUCCINATE (CORTEF, SOLU-CORTEF)

Classification: Corticosteroid.
Action: Reduces inflammation by multiple mechanisms. As a steroid, it replaces the steroids that are lacking in adrenal insufficiency.
Indications: Adrenal insufficiency, allergic reactions, anaphylaxis, asthma, COPD.
Adverse Effects: Leukocytosis, hyperglycemia, increased infection, decreased wound healing, increased rate of death from sepsis.
Contraindications: Cushing syndrome, known sensitivity to benzyl alcohol. Use with caution in diabetes, hypertension, heart failure, known systemic fungal infection, renal disease, idiopathic thrombocytopenia, psychosis, seizure disorder, gastrointestinal disease, glaucoma, known sensitivity.

Dosage:
Anaphylactic Shock and Adrenal Insufficiency:
- **Adult:** 100 to 500 mg IV, IO, or IM.
- **Pediatric:** 2 to 4 mg/kg per day IV, IO, or IM (max: 500 mg).

Asthma and COPD:
- **Adult:** 100 to 500 mg IV, IO, IM.
- **Pediatric:** 1 mg/kg IV, IO. The dose may be reduced for infants and children, but it is governed more by the severity of the condition and response of the patient than by age or body weight. Dose should not be less than 25 mg daily.

Special Considerations:
Pregnancy class C.

▶ Overview of Thyroid Disorders

Thyrotoxicosis

CASE STUDY

You are called to the scene of a 64-year-old woman who is having a panic attack. She has a history of increased appetite, diarrhea, itching, irritability, and 10-pound (5-kg) weight loss over the past month. She has had insomnia for the past 2 to 3 weeks. Her husband states that she has always been healthy and is currently taking no medications. She has no history of substance abuse and no allergies. The patient appears nervous and fidgety. Her heart rate is 145 beats/min, blood pressure is 140/80 mm Hg, and respiratory rate is 30 breaths/min. Her face is reddened, and she has swelling in her neck that appears to be a goiter. Her upper eyelids are slightly swollen and retracted. She is breathing rapidly but without effort, and her lung sounds are clear. The ECG shows sinus tachycardia. IV access is obtained.

The thyroid gland is a small gland found in the neck over the voice box. The thyroid produces hormones commonly called *thyroid hormones*. Thyroid hormones are important in regulating the body's metabolic rate. When the body produces excessive amounts of thyroid hormone, the metabolic rate is increased. Elevated blood levels of thyroid hormone can result in a state known as **thyrotoxicosis**. Thyrotoxicosis is caused by autoimmune disease, infections, and cancer. Patients with thyrotoxicosis commonly experience tachycardia, tremor, diaphoresis, weight loss, and intolerance for warm rooms and environments. A life-threatening manifestation of thyrotoxicosis is called a **thyroid storm**.

Management

Treatment of thyrotoxicosis is aimed at protecting the various organ systems from the action of excessive thyroid hormone. Antithyroid agents are used for long-term management of thyroid disorders. These medications act within the thyroid gland to prevent production of thyroid hormone. **Thionamide agents** (propylthiouracil and methimazole) are oral antithyroid medications commonly used for the long-term management of hyperthyroidism. However, these agents inhibit the synthesis—not the release—of thyroid hormone. Therefore, other medications should be used for the short-term treatment of thyrotoxicosis.

Thyroid hormone affects the cardiovascular system by sensitizing it to catecholamines, resulting in significant elevations of blood pressure and heart rate. Beta blockers can be used to treat hypertension, tachycardia, and other symptoms experienced by a patient with thyroid toxicity.[8] Beta blockers work by inhibiting the binding of catecholamines to the receptor site. Symptoms such as tremulousness, anxiety, palpitations, sweating, eyelid retraction, and tachycardia are improved with this treatment. Examples of beta blockers used to treat thyrotoxicosis include esmolol (Brevibloc), labetalol (Trandate, Normodyne), and metoprolol (Lopressor).

ESMOLOL (BREVIBLOC)

Classification: Beta-adrenergic antagonist, Class II antiarrhythmic.
Action: Inhibits the strength of the heart's contractions, as well as heart rate, resulting in a decrease in cardiac oxygen consumption.
Indications: Acute coronary syndrome (ACS), myocardial infarction, acute hypertension, supraventricular tachyarrhythmias, thyrotoxicosis.
Adverse Effects: Hypotension, sinus bradycardia, atrioventricular (AV) block, cardiac arrest, nausea/vomiting, hypoglycemia, injection site reaction.
Contraindications: Acute bronchospasm, COPD, second- or third-degree heart block, bradycardia, cardiogenic shock, pulmonary edema, sick sinus syndrome, known sensitivity. Use with caution in patients with

(continues)

ESMOLOL (BREVIBLOC) *(continued)*

pheochromocytoma, Prinzmetal's angina, cerebrovascular disease, stroke, poorly controlled diabetes mellitus, hyperthyroidism, thyrotoxicosis, renal disease.

Dosage:

- **Adult:** 0.5 to 1 mg/kg IV, IO over a 1-minute period, followed by a 50-mcg/kg per minute (0.05 mg/kg) infusion over a 4-minute period (maximum total: 200 mcg/kg). If patient response is inadequate, administer a second bolus of 500 mcg/kg (0.5 mg/kg) over a 1-minute period, and then increase infusion to 100 mcg/kg per minute. Maximum infusion rate: 300 mcg/kg per minute.

Special Considerations:

Half-life 5 to 9 minutes.

Any adverse effects caused by administration of esmolol are brief because of the drug's short half-life. Resolution of effects usually within 10 to 20 minutes.

Pregnancy class C.

LABETALOL (NORMODYNE, TRANDATE)

Classification: Beta-adrenergic antagonist, antianginal, antihypertensive.

Action: Binds with both the beta$_1$ and beta$_2$ receptors and alpha$_1$ receptors in vascular smooth muscle. Inhibits the strength of the heart's contractions, as well as heart rate. This results in a decrease in cardiac oxygen consumption.

Indications: ACS, supraventricular tachycardia (SVT), severe hypertension.

Adverse Effects: Usually mild and transient; hypotensive symptoms, nausea/vomiting, bronchospasm, arrhythmia, bradycardia, AV block.

Contraindications: Hypotension, cardiogenic shock, acute pulmonary edema, heart failure, severe bradycardia, sick sinus syndrome, second- or third-degree heart block, asthma or acute bronchospasm, cocaine-induced ACS, known sensitivity. Use caution in pheochromocytoma, cerebrovascular disease or stroke, poorly controlled diabetes, with hepatic disease. Use with caution at lowest effective dose in chronic lung disease.

Dosage:

Cardiac Indications:

Note: Monitor blood pressure and heart rate closely during administration.

- **Adult:** 10 mg IV, IO over a 1- to 2-minute period. May repeat every 10 minutes to a maximum dose of 150 mg or give initial bolus and then follow with infusion at 2 to 8 mg/min.
- **Pediatric:** 0.2 to 1 mg/kg to a maximum dosage of 3 mg/kg per hour; may also administer 0.25 to 3 mg/kg per hour as an infusion.

Severe Hypertension:

- **Adult:** Initial dose is 20 mg IV, IO slow infusion over a 2-minute period. After the initial dose, blood pressure should be checked every 5 minutes. Repeat doses can be given at 10-minute intervals. The second dose should be 40 mg IV, IO, and subsequent doses should be 80 mg IV, IO, to a maximum total dose of 300 mg. The effect on blood pressure typically will occur within 5 minutes from the time of administration. Alternatively, may be administered via IV infusion at 2 mg/min to a total maximum dose of 300 mg.
- **Pediatric:** 0.25 to 3 mg/kg per hour IV, IO infusion with a maximum dose of 3 mg/kg per hour.

Special Considerations:

Pregnancy class C.

METOPROLOL (LOPRESSOR, TOPROL XL)

Classification: Beta-adrenergic antagonist, antianginal, antihypertensive, Class II antiarrhythmic.

Action: Inhibits the strength of the heart's contractions, as well as heart rate. This results in a decrease in cardiac oxygen consumption.

Indications: ACS, hypertension, SVT, atrial flutter, atrial fibrillation, thyrotoxicosis.

Adverse Effects: Tiredness, dizziness, diarrhea, heart block, bradycardia, bronchospasm, drop in blood pressure.

Contraindications: Cardiogenic shock, AV block, bradycardia, known sensitivity. Use with caution in hypotension, chronic lung disease (asthma and COPD).

Dosage:

Cardiac Indications:

- **Adult:** 5 mg slow IV, IO over a 2-minute period; repeat at 5-minute intervals up to a total of three infusions totaling 15 mg IV, IO.
- **Pediatric:** Oral dosing only.

Special Considerations:

Blood pressure, heart rate, and ECG should be monitored carefully.
Use with caution in patients with asthma.
Pregnancy class C.

Overview of Myxedema Coma

Patients may similarly suffer from a deficit in available thyroid hormones. When thyroid hormone levels are low (a condition known as **hypothyroidism**), patients are placed on long-term synthetic thyroid hormone replacement. If hypothyroidism is severe, patients may develop **myxedema coma**, a life-threatening medical emergency with a high mortality rate. Symptoms of myxedema coma include decreased mental status and hypothermia.[9] Patients may manifest other signs such as hypotension, bradycardia, decreased respiratory effort, and a number of electrolyte abnormalities. There is often swelling (myxedema) of the hands or face. The treatment of myxedema coma is primarily supportive care in the prehospital setting until the patients reach definitive care. EMS treatment may include airway management, mechanical ventilation, fluid boluses, or other cardiovascular support. Hospital treatment includes continued supportive treatment and IV replacement of various thyroid hormones. Glucocorticoid hormones may be administered if the medical control physician suspects concurrent adrenal insufficiency.

▶ Review Questions

1. Explain the difference between patients with type 1 diabetes and type 2 diabetes in regard to their ability to produce insulin.
2. What is the risk of beta blockers in patients with diabetes?
3. What adverse effects will a patient likely experience after the administration of glucagon for hypoglycemia?
4. When treating a patient with DKA, what is the complication of aggressive fluid resuscitation with hypotonic fluids?
5. Can a prehospital provider treat DKA without the administration of insulin?
6. In times of stress, what are some of cortisol's actions?
7. What are the manifestations of the increased metabolic rate during thyrotoxicosis?

References

1. Kumar JG, Abhilash KPP, Saya RP, Tadipaneni N, Bose JM. A retrospective study on epidemiology of hypoglycemia in Emergency Department. *Indian J Endocrinol Metab*. 2007;21(1):119–124.
2. Nathan DM. The diabetes control and complications trial/epidemiology of diabetes interventions and complications study at 30 years: overview. *Diabetes Care*. 2014;37(1):9–16.
3. Cryer PE. Minimizing hypoglycemia in diabetes. *Diabetes Care*. 2015;38(8):1583–1591.
4. Martín-Timón I, del Cañizo-Gómez FJ. Mechanisms of hypoglycemia unawareness and implications in diabetic patients. *World J Diabetes*. 2015;6(7):912–926.
5. Hirsch IB, Emmett M. Diabetic ketoacidosis and hyperosmolar hyperglycemic state in adults: treatment. UpToDate. https://www.uptodate.com/contents/diabetic-ketoacidosis-and-hyperosmolar-hyperglycemic-state-in-adults-treatment. Updated January 13, 2017. Accessed August 17, 2018.
6. Morris L, Murphy M, Kitabchi A. Bicarbonate therapy in severe diabetic ketoacidosis. *Ann Intern Med*. 1986;105:836.
7. Harris G, Fiordalisi I, Harris WL, Mosovich LL, Finberg L. Minimizing the risk of brain herniation during treatment of diabetic ketoacidemia: a retrospective and prospective study. *J Pediatr*. 1990;117:22–31.
8. Kitabchi A, Wall B. Diabetic ketoacidosis. *Med Clin North Am*. 1995;79:9.
9. Ross DS. Myxedema coma. UpToDate. https://www.uptodate.com/contents/myxedema-coma. Updated May 22, 2017. Accessed August 17, 2018.

CHAPTER 12

Hypertensive Emergencies

OBJECTIVES

1. Define *hypertensive urgency* and *hypertensive emergency*.
2. Describe the use of the following medications for the treatment of hypertensive encephalopathy, hypertensive intracranial hemorrhage, and pulmonary edema with hypertension: esmolol (Brevibloc), nicardipine (Cardene), furosemide (Lasix), sodium nitroprusside (Nipride), and labetalol (Trandate, Normodyne).
3. Describe the use of aspirin and nitroglycerin (Nitrolingual, NitroQuick, Nitro-Dur) in the treatment of myocardial ischemia with hypertension.
4. Discuss medications used in the treatment of preeclampsia and eclampsia: magnesium sulfate and hydralazine (Apresoline).
5. Discuss medications used in the treatment of hypertension with seizure: diazepam (Valium) and phentolamine (Regitine).

MEDICATIONS THAT APPEAR IN CHAPTER 12

Esmolol (Brevibloc)
Nicardipine (Cardene)
Furosemide (Lasix)
Sodium nitroprusside (Nipride, Nitropress)

Labetalol (Normodyne, Trandate)
Aspirin, ASA
Nitroglycerin (Nitrolingual, NitroQuick, Nitro-Dur)

Magnesium sulfate
Hydralazine (Apresoline)
Diazepam (Valium)
Phentolamine (Regitine)

▶ Introduction

Approximately 75 million people in the United States have hypertension.[1] This disease is often called "the silent killer" because its victims may have no symptoms until the condition advances to the point of damaging organs and threatening the patient's life. Hypertensive emergencies require rapid identification and management by prehospital care providers. Specific emergencies often respond better to certain antihypertensive medications, which this chapter will explain.

You are called to the home of a 52-year-old man who is unresponsive. His wife states that he has had high blood pressure for 3 years and diabetes since his 20s. He has been diagnosed with hypertension, for which he takes clonidine (Catapres). He stopped taking his other blood pressure medications a few months ago. She came home from shopping and found him unresponsive on the floor of their kitchen. His vital signs are blood pressure, 240/140 mm Hg; pulse, 128 beats/min; and respirations, 32 breaths/min. He is drooling. You note bilateral rales in his posterior lung fields. His right pupil is fixed and dilated.

In most cases, **hypertension**, or high blood pressure, has no identifiable cause, which is referred to as **essential hypertension**. Ninety percent of people with hypertension have essential hypertension.[2] Other identifiable causes of hypertension include kidney disease, arterial disease, steroids, and some endocrine tumors.

The systolic and diastolic pressures that have defined chronic hypertension have varied over the years. Historically, more emphasis was placed on systolic blood pressure, but diastolic hypertension has been determined to perhaps be more damaging in the long term. Systolic hypertension is dangerous for older adults because it can lead to the development of strokes. For most patients with hypertension, treatment is long term and requires multiple drug therapies.

When hypertension is not diagnosed or treatment recommendations are not followed, hypertensive emergencies can arise. These cases can present as hypertensive urgency or hypertensive emergency. **Hypertensive urgency** is a severe elevation of the blood pressure without evidence of organ damage. **Hypertensive emergency**, also known as **malignant hypertension**, is a severe elevation in blood pressure complicated by evidence of end-organ damage. End-organ damage can occur in the kidneys (kidney failure), heart (heart failure), and brain (intracranial bleed or altered level of consciousness). Patients experiencing hypertensive emergencies can present with reports of headache, visual changes, altered level of consciousness, or heart failure. Specific hypertensive emergencies include the following:

- Hypertensive encephalopathy
- Hypertensive intracranial hemorrhage
- Pulmonary edema with hypertension
- Myocardial ischemia with hypertension
- Preeclampsia and eclampsia (hypertension with proteinuria in pregnancy)

Precipitating factors for hypertensive emergencies are listed in **BOX 12-1**.

BOX 12-1 Precipitating Factors for Hypertensive Emergencies

Renal vascular hypertension
Renal disease
Connective tissue diseases (e.g., scleroderma)
Drug abuse (sympathomimetics, cocaine, PCP)
Withdrawal from antihypertensives
Tyramine ingestion while taking a monoamine oxidase inhibitor (MAOI)
Preeclampsia, eclampsia
Pheochromocytoma
Head injury
Tumor-secreting vasoconstricting hormones

▶ Overview of Hypertensive Encephalopathy, Hypertensive Intracranial Hemorrhage, and Pulmonary Edema with Hypertension

The patient in the previous scenario is experiencing a hypertensive emergency, most likely hypertensive encephalopathy or possibly intracranial hemorrhage. This is an absolute emergency that, if not rapidly treated, can result in coma and death. Hypertensive encephalopathy is acute in onset and reversible. Patients often have severe headache, vomiting, and altered mental status. Intracranial bleeds are caused by a rupture of a blood vessel from elevated blood pressure. This diagnosis is confirmed by both physical examination and history. Findings include history of hypertension and possible abrupt cessation of antihypertensive medication. Physical findings include elevated blood pressure, pulmonary rales, and an altered mental status.

When determining which pharmacologic agent to use in the treatment of this emergency, the cause should be considered. This patient has risk factors for hypertensive encephalopathy and an intracranial bleed.

Management

Patients in a hypertensive emergency require a decrease in their blood pressure. However, do not reduce a patient's blood pressure to normal levels (e.g., 120/80 mm Hg). A too-rapid reduction of blood pressure or one at too great of a magnitude can result in ischemia of the brain or retina, leading to a stroke or blindness. Capillaries adapt to a higher "normal" blood pressure and are unable to rapidly compensate to maintain perfusion when blood pressure decreases too rapidly. The objective of the treatment of a hypertensive emergency is to reduce the mean arterial blood pressure by 10% to 20% over the first hour.[3] Continued reduction should then occur gradually, by no more than 25% total over the first day.

The drugs chosen to treat a particular hypertensive emergency vary by the cause of the rise in blood pressure. The patient in the previous scenario has either an intracranial hemorrhage or hypertensive encephalopathy. Many providers mistakenly think that nitroglycerin is a good drug to use in hypertensive emergencies. Nitroglycerin is a potent venodilator. Only at high doses does nitroglycerin act as an arterial dilator. Nitroglycerin decreases blood pressure by venodilation, which decreases the blood returning to the right side of the heart, which decreases the cardiac preload, which in turn decreases the patient's cardiac output. If a patient is having a hypertensive emergency resulting in decreased blood flow to the brain, a decrease in cardiac output would be undesirable. In patients having a hypertensive emergency in which the affected end organ is the brain with a possible cerebral vascular accident (stroke), the best choice of drug therapy is usually a beta blocker (often labetalol) or nicardipine (Cardene).[4]

Esmolol (Brevibloc) is a rapid, short-acting beta$_1$ blocker. A unique property of esmolol is that it has little effect on the blood pressure of people who are not hypertensive. Esmolol also has a very short half-life of 9 minutes. If, after administration of esmolol, a patient's blood pressure is too low, the effect will not be prolonged. This drug is an excellent choice for the patient in the preceding scenario. Labetalol (Trandate, Normodyne) would be another potential choice of a beta blocker to use in this scenario. Labetalol has a half-life of 5 to 8 hours. Therefore, if labetalol causes an adverse effect, the duration will be much longer.

Nicardipine (Cardene) is another example of a calcium channel blocker with a number of desirable properties, including rapid onset of action, lack of toxic metabolites, and ease of titration to desired effect. Thus, nicardipine effects resemble those of nitroprusside in terms of onset, duration, and offset of action. Nicardipine is a good option in the management of severe hypertension with or without target-organ damage.

Furosemide (Lasix) is a potent **diuretic**. Commonly referred to as "water pills," diuretics are medications that help reduce circulating intravascular volume by promoting an increase in urine production by the kidney. Furosemide's mechanism of action is to block salt and fluid reabsorption in the kidney, which results in a significant increase in urine output. This process is referred to as **diuresis**.

(*continued*) This patient with a hypertensive emergency has two organs that are affected: the brain and the lungs. Given the depressed mental status and dilated pupil, you are suspicious that he has suffered an intracranial hemorrhage. The rales or crackles in his lungs indicate that he also has some degree of pulmonary edema. The patient is protecting his airway adequately and has spontaneous respirations. You place the patient on supplemental oxygen, start an intravenous (IV) line, and place him on a cardiac monitor. You discuss the patient with medical direction and receive orders to administer furosemide 40 mg IV push and to give a bolus and start an infusion of esmolol.

Sodium nitroprusside (Nipride) is a common medication used for patients in a hypertensive emergency. Nipride is a potent drug, and the onset of action is within 1 minute of administration. Its action is quickly terminated when the infusion is discontinued. Nitroprusside works by dilating both the arteries and veins. The pressure receptors (**baroreceptors**) located in the walls of some blood vessels sense the drop in blood pressure and compensate for the decrease by increasing the heart rate. An increase in heart rate can be quite damaging for a patient with coronary artery disease. Remember that the patient in this scenario has a heart rate of 128 beats/min.

This drug can increase a patient's intracranial pressure (ICP). In this scenario, the patient has an altered mental status and a right pupil that is fixed and dilated. Given the history and physical findings, the patient may have had an intracranial hemorrhage. Because nitroprusside could increase the ICP and worsen the patient's brain injury, it would not be an appropriate drug choice for this patient. Additionally, assess whether the cause for the hypertension is an acute myocardial infarction (AMI); if the patient has had a myocardial infarction, nitroglycerin is the preferred drug.

When using sodium nitroprusside, exercise great caution not to drop the blood pressure too rapidly or by too great of a magnitude.

Labetalol (Trandate, Normodyne) is a selective alpha$_1$ blocker and nonselective beta blocker. As an alpha-blocking agent, labetalol decreases blood pressure by blocking alpha-mediated contraction of vascular smooth muscle. As a drug with beta$_1$-blocking properties, it also acts on the heart to decrease heart rate, contractility, and blood pressure. Labetalol is often a first choice for treating intracranial bleeds because it does not negatively affect cerebral perfusion pressure. The use of labetalol for hypertension is perhaps more safe than nitroprusside because labetalol does not cause a rapid and uncontrolled drop in blood pressure. However, the patient in this scenario has rales that are audible in both lung fields. Labetalol should be used with caution in this patient. Hypertension and rales indicating pulmonary edema are signs of impending congestive heart failure. In that case, using furosemide (Lasix) to help control the pulmonary edema with a beta blocker would be an effective alternative. (Lasix is also discussed in Chapter 10.)

ESMOLOL (BREVIBLOC)

Classification: Beta adrenergic antagonist, Class II antiarrhythmic.

Action: Inhibits the strength of the heart's contractions, as well as heart rate, resulting in a decrease in cardiac oxygen consumption.

Indications: Acute coronary syndrome (ACS), MI, acute hypertension, supraventricular tachycardia (SVT), thyrotoxicosis.

Adverse Effects: Hypotension, sinus bradycardia, atrioventricular (AV) block, cardiac arrest, nausea/vomiting, hypoglycemia, injection site reaction.

Contraindications: Acute bronchospasm, chronic obstructive pulmonary disease (COPD), second- or third-degree heart block, bradycardia, cardiogenic shock, pulmonary edema, sick sinus syndrome, known sensitivity. Use with caution in patients with pheochromocytoma, Prinzmetal's angina, cerebrovascular disease, stroke, poorly controlled diabetes mellitus, hyperthyroidism, thyrotoxicosis, renal disease.

Dosage:

- **Adult:** 0.5 to 1 mg/kg IV, intraosseous (IO) over a 1-minute period, followed by a 50-mcg/kg per minute (0.05 mg/kg) infusion over a 4-minute period (maximum total: 200 mcg/kg). If patient response is inadequate, administer a second bolus of 500 mcg/kg (0.5 mg/kg) over a 1-minute period, and then increase infusion to 100 mcg/kg per minute. Maximum infusion rate: 300 mcg/kg per minute.

Special Considerations:

Half-life 5 to 9 minutes.

Any adverse effects caused by administration of esmolol are brief because of the drug's short half-life.

Resolution of effects usually within 10 to 20 minutes.

Pregnancy class C.

NICARDIPINE (CARDENE)

Classification: Calcium channel blocker.

Action: Blocks calcium movement into the smooth muscle of the blood vessel walls, causing vasodilation.

Indications: Hypertension, angina

Adverse Effects: Edema, headaches, flushing, sinus tachycardia, hypotension.

Contraindications: Aortic stenosis, hypotension, known sensitivity. Use with caution in heart failure, cardiac conduction abnormalities, cerebrovascular disease, depressed AV node conduction.

Dosage:

- **Adult:** 5 mg/hr IV, IO; may increase by 2.5 mg/hr every 5 to 15 minutes (max dose: 15 mg/hr). Once the patient has achieved the desired blood pressure, decrease infusion to a maintenance dose of 3 mg/hr.
- **Pediatric:** 0.5 to 5 mcg/kg per minute IV, IO infusion.

Special Considerations:

Pregnancy class C.

FUROSEMIDE (LASIX)

Classification: Loop diuretic.

Action: Inhibits the absorption of the sodium and chloride ions and water in the loop of Henle, as well as the convoluted tubule of the nephron. This results in decreased absorption of water and increased production of urine.

Indications: Pulmonary edema, congestive heart failure (CHF), hypertensive emergency.

Adverse Effects: Vertigo, dizziness, weakness, orthostatic hypotension, hypokalemia, thrombophlebitis. Patients with anuria, severe renal failure, untreated hepatic coma, increasing azotemia, and electrolyte depletion can develop life-threatening consequences.

Contraindications: Known sensitivity to sulfonamides or furosemide.

Dosage:

Congestive Heart Failure and Pulmonary Edema:

- **Adult:** 20 to 40 mg IV, IO administered slowly over a 1- to 2-minute period. Begin with 40 mg in emergent situations. If a satisfactory response is not achieved within 1 hour, an additional dose of 80 mg can be given. A maximum single IV dose is 160 to 200 mg.
- **Pediatric:** 1 mg/kg IV, IO, or intramuscularly (IM). If the response is not satisfactory, an additional dose of 2 mg/kg may be administered no sooner than 2 hours after the first dose.

Hypertensive Emergency:

- **Adult:** 40 mg IV, IO.
- **Pediatric:** 1 mg/kg IV or IM.

Special Considerations:

Onset of action for IV, IO administration occurs within 5 minutes and will peak within 30 minutes. Furosemide is a diuretic, so the patient will likely have urinary urgency. Be prepared to help the patient void.

Pregnancy class C.

SODIUM NITROPRUSSIDE (NIPRIDE, NITROPRESS)

© Jones & Bartlett Learning.

Classification: Antihypertensive agent.

Action: Causes direct relaxation of both arteries and veins.

Indications: Hypertensive emergencies.

Adverse Effects: Cyanide or thiocyanate toxicity, nausea/vomiting, dizziness, headache, restlessness, abdominal pain, methemoglobinemia.

Contraindications: Hypotension, increased ICP, cerebrovascular disease, coronary artery disease, hepatic disease, renal disease, pulmonary disease.

Dosage:
- **Adult:** 0.3 to 10 mcg/kg per minute IV, IO. Titrate to desired blood pressure.
- **Pediatric:** 0.5 to 10 mcg/kg per minute IV, IO. Titrate to desired blood pressure.

Special Considerations:

Nitroprusside will break down when exposed to ultraviolet light. Therefore, the infusion should be shielded from light by wrapping the bag with aluminum foil. Doses less than 2 mcg/kg per minute are less likely to cause toxicity.

Pregnancy class C.

LABETALOL (NORMODYNE, TRANDATE)

Classification: Beta-adrenergic antagonist, antianginal, antihypertensive.

Action: Binds with both the beta$_1$ and beta$_2$ receptors and alpha$_1$ receptors in vascular smooth muscle. Inhibits the strength of the heart's contractions, as well as heart rate. This effect results in a decrease in cardiac oxygen consumption.

Indications: ACS, SVT, severe hypertension.

Adverse Effects: Usually mild and transient; hypotensive symptoms, nausea/vomiting, bronchospasm, arrhythmia, bradycardia, AV block.

Contraindications: Hypotension, cardiogenic shock, acute pulmonary edema, heart failure, severe bradycardia, sick sinus syndrome, second- or third-degree heart block, asthma or acute bronchospasm, cocaine-induced ACS, known sensitivity. Use caution in pheochromocytoma, cerebrovascular disease or stroke, poorly controlled diabetes, with hepatic disease. Use with caution at lowest effective dose in chronic lung disease.

Dosage:

Cardiac Indications:

Note: Monitor blood pressure and heart rate closely during administration.
- **Adult:** 10 mg IV, IO over a 1- to 2-minute period. May repeat every 10 minutes to a maximum dose of 150 mg or give initial bolus and then follow with infusion at 2 to 8 mg/min.
- **Pediatric:** 0.2 to 1 mg/kg to a maximum dosage of 3 mg/kg per hour; may also administer 0.25 to 3 mg/kg per hour as an infusion.

Severe Hypertension:
- **Adult:** Initial dose is 20 mg IV, IO slow infusion over a 2-minute period. After the initial dose, blood pressure should be checked every 5 minutes. Repeat doses can be given at 10-minute intervals. The second dose should be 40 mg IV, IO, and subsequent doses should be 80 mg IV, IO, to a maximum total dose of 300 mg. The effect on blood pressure typically will occur within 5 minutes from the time of administration. Alternatively, may be administered via IV infusion at 2 mg/min to a total maximum dose of 300 mg.
- **Pediatric:** 0.25 to 3 mg/kg per hour IV, IO infusion with a maximum dose of 3 mg/kg per hour.

Special Considerations:

Pregnancy class C.

▶ Overview of Myocardial Ischemia with Hypertension

CASE STUDY

You are dispatched to a 63-year-old man with chest pain. The patient describes the discomfort as a pressure on the left side of his chest, with some radiation to the jaw and left arm. He also reports feeling short of breath. You observe that the patient appears to be quite anxious and is sweating profusely. The patient's daughter tells you that he had a heart attack approximately 1 month ago. When he was in the hospital, he had a cardiac catheterization, with a stent placed in one of his coronary arteries. Shortly after being discharged from the hospital, the patient lost his insurance coverage and stopped taking his "heart pills." At this point, the patient protests and reports that he is still taking aspirin every day. You learn that he has a history of urinary retention, diabetes, hypertension, and hyperlipidemia, and he has smoked for more than 40 years. On physical examination, his pulse is 110 beats/min, blood pressure is 200/148 mm Hg, respirations are 24 breaths/min with bilateral rales, and his skin is moist. The pulse oximeter is reading 93%.

This patient's history is classic for acute myocardial ischemia and infarction (see Chapter 6). However, he has the added complication of experiencing a hypertensive emergency and thus requires immediate treatment. The patient's significant risk factors for AMI include diabetes, hypertension with abrupt cessation of medications, hyperlipidemia (high cholesterol), and a significant smoking history. He also recently had an AMI with stent placement, which is significant because coronary stents can reocclude.

Management

This patient needs to be treated for his AMI, but this chapter focuses on blood pressure management in the face of ischemia and infarction.

After initial management of this patient with oxygen, initiation of an IV line, and placement of a cardiac monitor, one 325-mg nonenteric coated aspirin should be administered, followed by nitroglycerin.

Aspirin is most commonly used to reduce pain, fever, and inflammation. Another benefit of aspirin is that it prohibits platelets from adhering to one another. Inhibiting platelet aggregation with the use of aspirin has been proven to reduce the mortality rate of patients having an AMI. In the scenario presented, aspirin will not treat the hypertension, but it will limit growth of a clot in the coronary artery stent if it is occluded and possibly preserve cardiac muscle.

Nitroglycerin is a vasodilating agent that dilates venules to a greater degree than it does arterioles. Dilation of veins reduces blood return to the heart, which decreases cardiac preload. Reduced preload reduces cardiac output, which lowers blood pressure. In addition, reducing preload decreases the actual tension of the myocardial wall. The amount of work (energy input) required by the heart muscle is also decreased; therefore, the demand for oxygen is less, which helps balance oxygen supply and demand. Arterial dilation is significantly less than venous dilation. When the arterioles dilate, the coronary vessels increase in diameter; subsequently, the heart muscle receives more oxygen-enriched blood flow. These properties make nitroglycerin a desirable choice for AMI or myocardial ischemia.

After aspirin and nitroglycerin, beta blockers such as labetalol and esmolol are excellent choices. The benefits of beta blockers are that they reduce the stress to the injured heart by reducing the heart rate and force of contraction. Beta blockers improve survival in patients with myocardial ischemia. Metoprolol is a beta blocker commonly used in scenarios such as that presented previously.

ASPIRIN, ASA

Classification: Antiplatelet, nonnarcotic analgesic, antipyretic.

Action: Prevents the formation of a chemical known as thromboxane A2, which causes platelets to clump together, or aggregate, and form plugs that cause obstruction or constriction of small coronary arteries.

Indications: Fever, inflammation, angina, AMI, and patients complaining of pain, pressure, squeezing, or crushing in the chest that may be cardiac in origin.

Adverse Effects: Anaphylaxis, angioedema, bronchospasm, bleeding, stomach irritation, nausea/vomiting.

© ClassicStock/S. FELD/Medical Images.

Contraindications: Gastrointestinal bleeding, active ulcer disease, hemorrhagic stroke, bleeding disorders, children with chickenpox or flulike symptoms, known sensitivity.

Dosage:

Note: Chewable "baby" aspirin 81 mg, standard adult aspirin dose 325 mg.

Myocardial Infarction:

- **Adult:** 160 to 325 mg orally (alternatively, four 81-mg chewable aspirin are often given), 300-mg rectal suppository.
- **Pediatric:** 3 to 5 mg/kg per day to 5 to 10 mg/kg per day given as a single dose.

Pain or Fever:

- **Adult:** 325 to 650 mg orally (1 to 2 adult tablets) every 4 to 6 hours.
- **Pediatric:** 60 to 90 mg/kg per day in divided doses every 4 to 6 hours.

Special Considerations:

Pregnancy class C except the last 3 months of pregnancy, when aspirin is considered pregnancy class D.

NITROGLYCERIN (NITROLINGUAL, NITROQUICK, NITRO-DUR)

© Sue Heaton/Alamy Stock Photo.

© Allik Camazine/Alamy Stock Photo.

(continues)

NITROGLYCERIN (NITROLINGUAL, NITROQUICK, NITRO-DUR) *(continued)*

Classification: Antianginal agent.

Action: Relaxes vascular smooth muscle, thereby dilating peripheral arteries and veins. This causes pooling of venous blood and decreased venous return to the heart, which decreases preload. Nitroglycerin also reduces left ventricular systolic wall tension, which decreases afterload.

Indications: Angina, ongoing ischemic chest discomfort, hypertension, myocardial ischemia associated with cocaine intoxication.

Adverse Effects: Headache, hypotension, bradycardia, lightheadedness, flushing, cardiovascular collapse, methemoglobinemia.

Contraindications: Hypotension, severe bradycardia or tachycardia, right-sided myocardial infarction, increased ICP, intracranial bleeding, patients taking any medications for erectile dysfunction (such as sildenafil [Viagra], tadalafil [Cialis], or vardenafil [Levitra]), known sensitivity to nitrates. Use with caution in anemia, closed-angle glaucoma, hypotension, postural hypotension, uncorrected hypovolemia.

Dosage:

- **Adult:**
  - **Sublingual tablets:** 1 tablet (0.3 to 0.4 mg) at 5-minute intervals to a maximum of three doses.
  - **Translingual spray:** 1 (0.4 mg) spray at 5-minute intervals to a maximum of three sprays.
  - **Ointment:** 2% topical (Nitro-Bid ointment): Apply 1 to 2 inches of paste over the chest wall, cover with transparent wrap, and secure with tape.
  - **IV infusion:** 5 mcg/min; may increase rate by 5 to 10 mcg/min every 5 to 10 minutes as needed. End points of dose titration for nitroglycerin include a drop in the blood pressure of 10%, relief of chest pain, and return of ST segment to normal on a 12-lead electrocardiogram.
- **Pediatric IV infusion:** The initial pediatric infusion is 0.25 to 0.5 mcg/kg per minute IV, IO titrated by 0.5 to 1 mcg/kg per minute. Usual required dose is 1 to 3 mcg/kg per minute to a maximum dose of 5 mcg/kg per minute.

Special Considerations:

Administration of nitroglycerin to a patient with right ventricular MI can result in hypotension. Pregnancy class C.

(continued) You place the patient on oxygen, start an IV line, and place him on a cardiac monitor. Given the patient's history, you are concerned that he has myocardial ischemia with resultant hypertension. You give the patient a 325-mg nonenteric coated aspirin and tell him to bite and swallow the tablet. You then administer a 0.3-mg nitroglycerin tablet. The first nitroglycerin tablet does little to reduce his blood pressure or relieve the chest pain. Therefore, 5 minutes later you administer a second 0.3-mg tablet of nitroglycerin, which improves the blood pressure.

▶ Overview of Preeclampsia and Eclampsia

CASE STUDY

You are called to attend to a 34-year-old woman who is 36 weeks pregnant. She is actively seizing. On arrival, you see an obviously gravid female in a tonic-clonic seizure. Her husband states that she had been complaining of a headache and blurry vision. She was seizing for 5 minutes before your arrival. The patient's vital signs are blood pressure, 220/158 mm Hg; pulse, 124 beats/min; respirations, labored; and skin, warm and moist.

The patient in this scenario has an obstetric emergency known as **eclampsia**. The cause of this vasospastic form of hypertension is unique to pregnant women, and the cause is not known. Without appropriate treatment, the risk of death to the mother and fetus is significant. (Note in this scenario that the ultimate treatment is delivery of the baby.) Preeclampsia (also known as *toxemia* and *pregnancy-induced hypertension*) consists of high blood pressure, protein in the urine, and edema (swelling) of the extremities. This condition can rapidly become severe, with very high blood pressure, visual disturbances, failing kidneys, and liver damage. In rare cases, preeclampsia develops into eclampsia, in which potentially fatal convulsions occur. It also can become **HELLP syndrome**, which consists of *h*emolysis, or the breaking down of red blood cells; *el*evated liver enzymes; and *l*ow *p*latelet count. HELLP is potentially fatal to both the mother and her unborn child or children.

Management

Benzodiazepines typically have been used for seizure control. However, eclampsia warrants a different approach for seizure control, including administration of magnesium sulfate and hydralazine.

Magnesium sulfate acts as a membrane stabilizer and cerebral vasodilator. These effects are believed to reduce the chance of ischemia to brain tissue. With adequate dosing of magnesium, many patients with eclampsia have relief from the seizure and hypertension. Magnesium sulfate is the drug of choice for seizure control in eclampsia.

Hydralazine (Apresoline) is a vasodilating agent that selectively dilates the arteries. It can be used in the treatment of any hypertensive crisis and is often used for the treatment of preeclampsia and eclampsia. Administration of hydralazine produces a decrease in arterial pressure, so blood pressure is lowered. Additionally, a reflex tachycardia occurs once the baroreceptors sense this drop in pressure, and thus heart rate increases. Therefore, this drug would not be a good choice in a person with heart disease because of the associated increase in heart rate. Hydralazine is the drug of choice for hypertension in eclampsia if magnesium fails. Nitroprusside and labetalol have been used and determined to be safe.

MAGNESIUM SULFATE

Classification: Electrolyte, tocolytic, mineral.
Action: Required for normal physiologic functioning. Magnesium is a cofactor in neurochemical transmission and muscular excitability. Magnesium sulfate controls seizures by blocking peripheral neuromuscular transmission. Magnesium is also a peripheral vasodilator and an inhibitor of platelet function.
Indications: Torsades de pointes, cardiac arrhythmias associated with hypomagnesemia, eclampsia and seizure prophylaxis in preeclampsia, status asthmaticus.
Adverse Effects: Magnesium toxicity (signs include flushing, diaphoresis, hypotension, muscle paralysis, weakness, hypothermia, and cardiac, central nervous system [CNS], or respiratory depression).
Contraindications: AV block, gastrointestinal obstruction. Use with caution in renal impairment.
Dosage:
Pulseless Ventricular Fibrillation/Ventricular Tachycardia with Torsades de Pointes or Hypomagnesemia:
- **Adult:** 1 to 2 g in 10 mL D$_5$W IV, IO administered over 15 minutes or faster with cardiac arrest.
- **Pediatric:** 25 to 50 mg/kg IV, IO over 10 to 20 minutes; may administer faster for torsades de pointes (max single dose: 2 g).

(continues)

MAGNESIUM SULFATE *(continued)*

Torsades de Pointes with a Pulse or Cardiac Arrhythmias with Hypomagnesemia:
- **Adult:** 1 to 2 g in 50 to 100 mL D$_5$W IV, IO administered over 5 to 60 minutes. Follow with 0.5 to 1 g/hr IV, IO titrated to control torsades de pointes.
- **Pediatric:** 25 to 50 mg/kg IV, IO over 10 to 20 minutes (max single dose: 2 g).

Eclampsia and Seizure Prophylaxis in Preeclampsia:
- **Adult:** 4 to 6 g IV, IO over 20 to 30 minutes, followed by an infusion of 1 to 2 g/hr.

Status Asthmaticus:
- **Adult:** 1.2 to 2 g slow IV, IO (over 20 minutes).
- **Pediatric:** 25 to 50 mg/kg (diluted in D$_5$W) slow IV, IO (over 10 to 20 minutes).

Special Considerations:
Pregnancy class A.

HYDRALAZINE (APRESOLINE)

Classification: Antihypertensive agent, vasodilator.
Action: Directly dilates the peripheral blood vessels.
Indications: Hypertension associated with preeclampsia and eclampsia, hypertensive crisis.
Adverse Effects: Headache, angina, flushing, palpitations, reflex tachycardia, anorexia, nausea/vomiting, diarrhea, hypotension, syncope, peripheral vasodilation, peripheral edema, fluid retention, paresthesias.
Contraindications: Patients taking diazoxide or MAOIs, coronary artery disease, stroke, angina, dissecting aortic aneurysm, mitral valve and rheumatic heart diseases.
Dosage:

Preeclampsia and Eclampsia:
- **Adult:** 5 to 10 mg IV. Repeat every 20 to 30 minutes until systolic blood pressure of 90 to 105 mm Hg is attained.

Acute Hypertension Not Associated with Preeclampsia:
- **Adult:** 10 to 20 mg IV, or IM.
- **Pediatric:**
  - **1 month to 12 years:** 0.1 to 0.2 mg/kg IV or IM every 4 to 6 hours as needed (max: 20 mg/dose).

Special Considerations:
Pregnancy class C.

▶ Overview of Hypertension with Seizure

CASE STUDY

You are called to the scene of a 24-year-old man who is unresponsive. You arrive to find a young man who is seizing and still unresponsive. His wife indicates that he has just started regularly using cocaine. On examination, you find that the patient's blood pressure is 260/168 mm Hg; pulse is 124 beats/min; respirations are 24 breaths/min; and skin is red, hot, and moist. The patient's pupils are dilated, and he is drooling.

Cocaine is a sympathomimetic drug that stimulates the adrenergic nervous system. People who use cocaine can present with an overstimulation of the nervous system and potentially end-organ damage. They are prone to cardiac arrhythmias, hypertensive emergencies, and chest pain. In this scenario, the patient has a significantly elevated blood pressure with seizure activity. This indicates end-organ damage and a severe hypertensive emergency.

Management

Hypertensive emergencies caused by a drug such as cocaine are treated differently from other hypertensive emergencies. Beta blockers are contraindicated in such scenarios because they can worsen coronary vasoconstriction. When a beta blocker is used, unopposed stimulation of the peripheral alpha receptors occurs from the catecholamine (cocaine), which can lead to an increase in blood pressure and make symptoms worse.

Diazepam (Valium) is a benzodiazepine used to help induce sleep, relieve anxiety, and relax muscle spasm. This drug is quite effective in the treatment of seizures and is indicated for use in seizures caused by cocaine. Lorazepam (Ativan) is another benzodiazepine that may be used in these situations.[5]

Diazepam works in a number of ways. It promotes relaxation of muscle, actually restoring tone to the peripheral nervous system that had been inhibited by the cocaine, limiting myocardial oxygen demand, and causing peripheral vasodilation and a drop in blood pressure.

Phentolamine (Regitine) is both an $alpha_1$ and $alpha_2$ blocker. It blocks the receptors of the adrenergic sympathetic nervous system. It is most commonly used in pheochromocytoma and states of excessive catecholamines (e.g., increased levels of epinephrine and norepinephrine). It is the drug of choice for cocaine-induced hypertension. Nitroglycerin and sodium nitroprusside are also options for treating hypertension that is refractory to phentolamine in these patients.[5]

DIAZEPAM (VALIUM)

Classification: Benzodiazepine, Schedule C-IV.
Action: Binds to the benzodiazepine receptor and enhances the effects of GABA. Benzodiazepines act at the level of the limbic, thalamic, and hypothalamic regions of the CNS and can produce any level of CNS depression required (including sedation, skeletal muscle relaxation, and anticonvulsant activity).
Indications: Anxiety, skeletal muscle relaxation, alcohol withdrawal, seizures.
Adverse Effects: Respiratory depression, drowsiness, fatigue, headache, pain at the injection site, confusion, nausea, hypotension, oversedation.
Contraindications: Children younger than 6 months, acute-angle glaucoma, CNS depression, alcohol intoxication, known sensitivity.
Dosage:
Anxiety:
- **Adult:**
  - **Moderate:** 2 to 5 mg slow IV, IM.
  - **Severe:** 5 to 10 mg slow IV, IM (administer no faster than 5 mg/min).
  - **Low:** Low dosages are often required for older adults or debilitated patients.
- **Pediatric:** 0.2 to 0.3 mg/kg per dose IV, IM every 4 hours to a maximum dose of 0.6 mg/kg.

Delirium Tremens from Acute Alcohol Withdrawal:
- **Adult:** 10 mg IV

Seizure:
- **Adult:** 5 to 10 mg slow IV, IO every 10 to 15 minutes; maximum total dose 30 mg.
- **Pediatric:**
  - **IV, IO:**

(continues)

DIAZEPAM (VALIUM) *(continued)*

- **5 years and older:** 1 mg over a 3-minute period every 2 to 5 minutes to a maximum total dose of 10 mg.
- **Older than 30 days to younger than 5 years:** 0.2 to 0.5 mg over a 3-minute period; may repeat every 2 to 5 minutes to a maximum total dose of 5 mg.
- **Neonate:** 0.1 to 0.3 mg/kg per dose given over a 3- to 5-minute period; may repeat every 15 to 30 minutes to a maximum total dose of 2 mg. (Not a first-line agent due to sodium benzoic acid in the injection.)
  - **Rectal administration:** If vascular access is not obtained, diazepam may be administered rectally to children.
    - **12 years and older:** 0.2 mg/kg.
    - **6 to 11 years:** 0.3 mg/kg.
    - **2 to 5 years:** 0.5 mg/kg.
    - **Younger than 2 years:** Not recommended.

Special Considerations:
Make sure that IV, IO lines are well secured. Extravasation of diazepam causes tissue necrosis. Diazepam is insoluble in water and must be dissolved in propylene glycol. This produces a viscous solution; give slowly to prevent pain on injection.
Pregnancy class D.

PHENTOLAMINE (REGITINE)

Classification: Alpha antagonist, antihypertensive.
Action: Blocks alpha adrenergic receptors, causing vasodilation.
Indications: Hypertensive emergencies and hypertension caused by pheochromocytoma, cocaine-induced vasospasm of the coronary arteries.
Adverse Effects: Sinus tachycardia, angina, dizziness, orthostatic hypotension, prolonged hypotensive episodes, nausea/vomiting, diarrhea, weakness, flushing, nasal congestion.
Contraindications: Known sensitivity. Use with caution in AMI, angina, coronary insufficiency, evidence suggestive of coronary artery disease, peptic ulcer disease.

Dosage:
Hypertensive Crisis:
- **Adult:** 5 to 15 mg IV, IO, or IM.
- **Pediatric:** 0.05 to 0.1 mg/kg IV, IO; or 1 mg/dose.

Cocaine-Induced Vasospasm:
- **Adult:** 5 mg IV, IO or IM.
- **Pediatric:** 0.05 to 0.1 mg/kg IV, IO; or 1 mg/dose.

Special Considerations:
Pregnancy class C.

▶ Review Questions

1. List five types of specific hypertensive emergencies.
2. When treating a patient with malignant hypertension, what is the maximal safe amount that a paramedic should attempt to decrease the blood pressure?
3. List contraindications for the use of nitroprusside.
4. Which antihypertensive medication needs to be protected from light? Why?
5. By what mechanism does labetalol decrease blood pressure?

6. For what drug intoxication is the use of labetalol contraindicated? Why?
7. What is the preferred drug to reduce blood pressure in a patient having an AMI?
8. What is the drug of choice when treating seizures from eclampsia?
9. How does hydralazine affect a patient's heart rate?
10. List three contraindications for the use of beta blockers.

References

1. National Center for Chronic Disease Prevention and Health Promotion, Division for Heart Disease and Stroke Prevention. High blood pressure fact sheet. Centers for Disease Control and Prevention. https://www.cdc.gov/dhdsp/data_statistics/fact_sheets/fs_bloodpressure.htm. Updated June 16, 2016. Accessed August 17, 2018.
2. Bolívar JJ. Essential hypertension: an approach to its etiology and neurogenic pathophysiology. *Int J Hypertens.* 2013;547809. doi:10.1155/2013/547809.
3. Elliott WJ, Varon J. Evaluation and treatment of hypertensive emergencies in adults. UpToDate. https://www.uptodate.com/contents/evaluation-and-treatment-of-hypertensive-emergencies-in-adults. Updated December 18, 2017. Accessed August 17, 2018.
4. Filho JO, Mullen MT. Initial assessment and management of acute stroke. UpToDate. https://www.uptodate.com/contents/initial-assessment-and-management-of-acute-stroke?sectionName=BLOOD%20PRESSURE%20MANAGEMENT&topicRef=3837&anchor=H14&source=see_link#H19. Updated June 8, 2018. Accessed August 17, 2018.
5. Nelson L, Odujebe O. Cocaine: acute intoxication. UpToDate. https://www.uptodate.com/contents/cocaine-acute-intoxication. Updated February 26, 2018. Accessed August 17, 2018.

CHAPTER 13

Poisonings, Overdoses, and Intoxications

OBJECTIVES

1. Discuss the use of activated charcoal in the treatment of poisonings.
2. List treatment options for acetaminophen overdose.
3. List clinical manifestations of cyclic antidepressant overdose.
4. Discuss medications used in the treatment of cyclic antidepressant overdose: sodium bicarbonate, magnesium sulfate, phenylephrine (Neo-Synephrine), norepinephrine (Levophed), diazepam (Valium), and phenytoin (Dilantin).
5. Discuss medications used in the treatment of beta-blocker overdose: atropine sulfate and glucagon.
6. Discuss the use of benzodiazepines and haloperidol (Haldol) in the treatment of amphetamine and methamphetamine intoxication.
7. Discuss medications used in the treatment of cocaine intoxication: benzodiazepines, nitroglycerin (Nitrolingual, NitroQuick, Nitro-Dur), aspirin, morphine sulfate, and phentolamine (Regitine).
8. Discuss the use of naloxone (Narcan) in the treatment of a narcotic overdose.
9. Discuss medications used in the treatment of organophosphate and nerve agent exposure: atropine sulfate and pralidoxime (2-PAM).

MEDICATIONS THAT APPEAR IN CHAPTER 13

Activated charcoal	Phenytoin (Dilantin)	Nitroglycerin (Nitrolingual, NitroQuick, Nitro-Dur)
Sodium bicarbonate	Fosphenytoin (Cerebyx)	Aspirin, ASA
Magnesium sulfate	Atropine sulfate	Morphine sulfate
Phenylephrine (Neo-Synephrine)	Glucagon	Phentolamine (Regitine)
Norepinephrine (Levophed)	Midazolam (Versed)	Naloxone (Narcan)
Diazepam (Valium)	Lorazepam (Ativan)	Pralidoxime (2-PAM, Protopam)
	Haloperidol (Haldol)	

▶ Introduction

Poisonings and overdoses account for a significant percentage of EMS responses. In 2010, more than 42,000 people died from overdose or poisoning. In that same year, unintentional poisoning was second only to motor vehicle crashes as a leading cause of unintentional death for people ages 25 to 64 years.[1] EMS providers see certain types of overdoses, such as ethanol (alcohol) or opioids on a frequent basis and should be intimately familiar with presentation and appropriate treatment strategies. Other types of poisonings or overdoses may be seen only on rare occasions, requiring EMS providers to recall distant information or consult a reliable reference to provide optimal treatment. Poisoning and overdose situations may be associated with trauma, suicide attempts, psychiatric illness, or other types of medical emergencies. In adults, poisonings are usually the result of a psychiatric disorder or recreational drug use. Children younger than 6 years are another group commonly treated for intoxications or poisonings. A third group of patients with toxin exposure are victims of biologic or chemical terrorism.

This chapter addresses the following poisonings, overdoses, and intoxications:

- Acetaminophen overdose
- Cyclic antidepressant overdose
- Beta-blocker overdose
- Amphetamine and methamphetamine intoxication
- Cocaine intoxication
- Narcotic overdose
- Organophosphate and nerve agent exposure

▶ Syrup of Ipecac and Activated Charcoal

Syrup of Ipecac

The objectives of any emergency provider caring for a poisoning victim are simple and straightforward. The initial priorities are the same as those in all emergencies: patency of the airway, adequate ventilation, and sufficient perfusion of blood to the critical organs. The next goal is to prevent or reduce absorption of the toxin, which can require removal of any particulate matter in the case of skin absorption, removal of the patient to a safe environment when dealing with toxic fumes, and possible administration of **activated charcoal** for ingested poisons.

For decades, administration of **syrup of ipecac** was advocated for the home and prehospital treatment of poisoning. The objective of giving ipecac is to reduce absorption of the ingested poison by inducing the patient to vomit the toxin. Ipecac induces vomiting in approximately 90% of people 10 to 20 minutes after administration.[2,3] Syrup of ipecac is no longer recommended for use in poisoned patients in either homes or healthcare facilities. Ipecac is no longer manufactured in the United States, but it is possible that EMS providers may encounter patients who have received ipecac at home. Ipecac may predispose patients to aspiration, exacerbation of injury following a caustic ingestion, and a variety of other concerns.[4]

Activated Charcoal

The first pharmacologic intervention in poisoning cases is the administration of activated charcoal. Activated charcoal reduces the absorption of the ingested poison by providing a large surface area to which the ingested poison can bind. A 1-g dose of activated charcoal provides approximately 300 to 2,000 square meters (m^2) of surface area to which the toxin can adhere, limiting absorption.[5]

A careful risk-versus-benefit analysis should be performed before administering activated charcoal. Activated charcoal causes patients to have nausea and vomiting. More frequent, smaller doses of activated charcoal can decrease the frequency of vomiting associated with charcoal administration. Before administration, the provider should evaluate the patient's level of consciousness and ability to cooperate with the therapy. In many overdose scenarios, known ingested substances may be minimally toxic. Depending on the timing, it may also be minimally beneficial to administer activated charcoal, as the ingested substance may already be fully absorbed by the gastrointestinal (GI) tract. Activated charcoal is typically administered only when it can be given within *one hour* of ingestion; however, there are certain specific indications for using activated charcoal much later.[6]

Despite widespread support for its use, evidence that activated charcoal reduces the rate of complications or deaths in patients who have been poisoned is lacking.[6,7] Activated charcoal is not recommended in all ingestions. Some ingested substances are not absorbed by activated charcoal, such as iron, lithium, alcohols, ethylene glycol, organophosphates, acids and bases, and cyanide. See **BOX 13-1** for a list of agents that are not well bound to activated charcoal and those drugs cleared by hemoperfusion and hemodialysis.

BOX 13-1 Methods of Removal for Various Drugs

Agents Not Well Bound to Activated Charcoal	Agents Cleared by Hemodialysis
Bromides	Ammonium chloride
Caustics	Amphetamine
Cyanide	Atenolol
Ethylene glycol	Phenobarbital
Iron	Procainamide
Isopropyl alcohol	Sotalol
Lithium	Ethanol
Methanol	Methanol
Agents Cleared by Hemoperfusion	Ethylene glycol
Acetaminophen	Isopropanol
Theophylline	Aspirin
Methotrexate	Lithium
Phenylbutazone	Arsenic
Procainamide	
Quinidine	

ACTIVATED CHARCOAL

Classification: Antidote, adsorbent.
Action: When certain chemicals and toxins are in proximity to the activated charcoal, the chemical will attach to the surface of the charcoal and become trapped.
Indications: Toxic ingestion.
Adverse Effects: Nausea/vomiting, constipation, or diarrhea. If aspirated into the lungs, charcoal can induce a potentially fatal form of pneumonitis.
Contraindications: Ingestion of acids, alkalis, ethanol, methanol, cyanide, ferrous sulfate or other iron salts, lithium; coma; GI obstruction, known minimally toxic ingestion.
Dosage:
- **Adult:** 50 to 100 g/dose.
- **Pediatric:** 1 to 2 g/kg.

Special Considerations:
Pregnancy class C.

▶ Acetaminophen Overdose

CASE STUDY

You are called to provide assistance to a distraught young woman who has recently broken up with her boyfriend. When you arrive, her mother tells you that she thinks her daughter ingested approximately 40 tablets (500 mg/tablet) of acetaminophen. You find a 16-year-old girl who is crying and reporting cramping abdominal pain. Her vital signs are stable.

Acetaminophen (Tylenol) is one of the most commonly used drugs in intentional overdoses. In children, the typical presentation of an acetaminophen overdose is abdominal pain, nausea, and vomiting. These symptoms are often absent in adults, even after large ingestions. The clinical symptoms of such an overdose can be absent for days before deterioration of liver function.

Management

Although acetaminophen overdose is a common intoxication, prehospital care is only supportive. The initial care for this patient after a poisoning or overdose is the same as for any other critically ill or injured patient. The airway may require assistance or intervention to stay open. Patients may have an altered mental status and not be able to maintain a patent airway, or the airway may be obstructed with emesis. Supplemental oxygen should be administered if the patient demonstrates significant hypoxia. An intravenous (IV) line should be placed as an access point for medications or IV fluid if needed. Hypotension should be treated with a bolus of dextrose-free IV fluids. If the patient requires emergency administration of phenytoin, an IV line containing dextrose will result in precipitation of the phenytoin. *N*-acetylcysteine (Mucomyst) is a very effective antidote for acetaminophen if administered within 16 hours of the ingestion. Its effectiveness declines significantly if treatment is delayed for greater than 24 hours.

When treating overdoses, avoid IV fluids such as 5% dextrose in normal saline or 5% dextrose in Ringer's lactate solution. If the patient has a seizure, the administration of phenytoin will result in precipitation of the drug.

▶ Cyclic Antidepressant Overdose

CASE STUDY

You are called to the apartment of a 25-year-old woman who was found by her roommate to have a depressed level of consciousness. The roommate is concerned that the patient overdosed on her antidepressant medication. You assess the patient and find that her heart rate is 134 beats/min. Her skin is dry, and she responds by groaning and turning away from you. You place her on oxygen and the cardiac monitor, and your partner starts an IV of normal saline.

Overdose from antidepressants is a common cause of overdose deaths.[8] The clinical manifestations of cyclic antidepressant overdose include the following:

- Depressed level of consciousness
- Wide-complex cardiac arrhythmias
- Hypotension
- Seizures

Management

After the provision of initial supportive care, the first step is administration of activated charcoal if no contraindications exist. In this scenario, the patient's decreased level of consciousness would contraindicate the administration of activated charcoal.

Cardiac arrhythmias are the most life-threatening manifestation of the symptoms of cyclic antidepressant overdose. Widening of the QRS complex to greater than 100 ms and progression to frank ventricular tachycardia are likely to occur early after ingestion. If the patient has a wide-complex QRS rhythm, treatment with sodium bicarbonate is appropriate. Some patients develop the cardiac rhythm torsades de pointes, which is treated with magnesium sulfate injection. Other antiarrhythmics are not indicated and may be harmful due to QT prolongation and/or additive effects on sodium channels.

SODIUM BICARBONATE

Classification: Electrolyte replacement.
Action: Counteracts existing acidosis.
Indications: Acidosis, drug intoxications (e.g., barbiturates, salicylates, methyl alcohol).
Adverse Effects: Metabolic alkalosis, hypernatremia, injection site reaction, sodium and fluid retention, peripheral edema.
Contraindications: Metabolic alkalosis, hypocalcemia.
Dosage:
Metabolic Acidosis During Cardiac Arrest:
- **Adult:** 1 mEq/kg slow IV, intraosseous (IO); may repeat at 0.5 mEq/kg in 10 minutes.
- **Pediatric:** Same as adult dosing.
Metabolic Acidosis Not Associated with Cardiac Arrest:
- **Adult:** Dosage should be individualized.
- **Pediatric:** Dosage should be individualized.
Special Considerations:
Do not administer into an IV, IO line in which another medication is being given.
Because of the high concentration of sodium within each ampule of sodium bicarbonate, use with caution in patients with heart failure and renal disease.
Pregnancy class C.

MAGNESIUM SULFATE

Classification: Electrolyte, tocolytic, mineral.

Action: Required for normal physiologic functioning. Magnesium is a cofactor in neurochemical transmission and muscular excitability. Magnesium sulfate controls seizures by blocking peripheral neuromuscular transmission. Magnesium is also a peripheral vasodilator and an inhibitor of platelet function.

Indications: Torsades de pointes, cardiac arrhythmias associated with hypomagnesemia, eclampsia and seizure prophylaxis in preeclampsia, status asthmaticus.

Adverse Effects: Magnesium toxicity (signs include flushing, diaphoresis, hypotension, muscle paralysis, weakness, hypothermia, and cardiac, CNS, or respiratory depression).

Contraindications: Atrioventricular (AV) block, GI obstruction. Use with caution in renal impairment.

Dosage:

Pulseless Ventricular Fibrillation/Ventricular Tachycardia with Torsades de Pointes or Hypomagnesemia:
- **Adult:** 1 to 2 g in 10 mL D$_5$W IV, IO administered over 15 minutes or faster with cardiac arrest.
- **Pediatric:** 25 to 50 mg/kg IV, IO over 10 to 20 minutes; may administer faster for torsades de pointes (max single dose: 2 g).

Torsades de Pointes with a Pulse or Cardiac Arrhythmias with Hypomagnesemia:
- **Adult:** 1 to 2 g in 50 to 100 mL D$_5$W IV, IO administered over 5 to 60 minutes. Follow with 0.5 to 1 g/hr IV, IO titrated to control torsades de pointes.
- **Pediatric:** 25 to 50 mg/kg IV, IO over 10 to 20 minutes (max single dose: 2 g).

Eclampsia and Seizure Prophylaxis in Preeclampsia:
- **Adult:** 4 to 6 g IV, IO over 20 to 30 minutes, followed by an infusion of 1 to 2 g/hr.

Status Asthmaticus:
- **Adult:** 1.2 to 2 g slow IV, IO (over 20 minutes).
- **Pediatric:** 25 to 50 mg/kg (diluted in D$_5$W) slow IV, IO (over 10–20 minutes).

Special Considerations:
Pregnancy class A.

Many patients who have overdosed on cyclic antidepressants have hypotension that does not respond to aggressive administration of IV fluids. This hypotension is best treated with phenylephrine or norepinephrine.

PHENYLEPHRINE (NEO-SYNEPHRINE)

Classification: Adrenergic agonist.

Action: Stimulates the alpha receptors, causing vasoconstriction, which results in increased blood pressure.

Indications: Neurogenic shock, spinal shock, cases of shock in which the patient's heart rate does not need to be increased, drug-induced hypotension.

Adverse Effects: Hypertension, ventricular tachycardia (VT), headache, excitability, tremor, myocardial infarction (MI), exacerbation of asthma, cardiac arrhythmias, reflex bradycardia, soft tissue necrosis.

Contraindications: Acute MI, angina, cardiac arrhythmias, severe hypertension, coronary artery disease, pheochromocytoma, narrow-angle glaucoma, cardiomyopathy, MAOI therapy, known sensitivity to phenylephrine or sulfites.

Dosage:
- **Adult:** 100 to 180 mcg/min IV, IO. Once the blood pressure has been stabilized, the dose can be reduced to 40 to 60 mcg/min.
- **Pediatric (2 to 12 years):** 5 to 20 mcg/kg IV, IO followed by 0.1 to 0.5 mcg/kg per minute IV, IO (max dose: 3 mcg/kg per minute IV, IO).

Special Considerations:
Pregnancy class C.

NOREPINEPHRINE (LEVOPHED)

Classification: Adrenergic agonist, inotropic, vasopressor.

Action: Norepinephrine is an alpha$_1$, alpha$_2$, and beta$_1$ agonist. Alpha-mediated peripheral vasoconstriction is the predominant clinical result of administration, resulting in increasing blood pressure and coronary blood flow. Beta-adrenergic action produces inotropic stimulation of the heart and dilates the coronary arteries.

Indications: Cardiogenic shock, septic shock, severe hypotension.

Adverse Effects: Dizziness, anxiety, cardiac arrhythmias, dyspnea, exacerbation of asthma.

Contraindications: Patients taking monoamine oxidase inhibitors (MAOIs), known sensitivity. Use with caution in hypovolemia.

Dosage:
- **Adult:** Add 4 mg to 250 mL of D$_5$W or D$_5$NS, but not normal saline alone. 0.1 to 0.5 mcg/kg per minute as IV, IO, titrated to maintain blood pressure >80 mm Hg. Many settings still use non-weight-based dosing of 2 to 4 mcg/minute titrated upward for the desired clinical effect. Refractory shock may require doses as high as 30 mcg/min.
- **Pediatric:** 0.05 to 2 mcg/kg per minute IV, IO infusion, to a maximum dose of 2 mcg/kg per minute.

Special Considerations:
Do not administer in same IV line as alkaline solutions.
Half-life 1 minute.
Pregnancy class C.

Seizures are also a common manifestation of a cyclic antidepressant overdose. Seizure activity can run the spectrum from brief and self-limiting to intractable. In some cases, seizure activity can precede ventricular tachycardia.[9] The seizures can be treated with diazepam (Valium) or another benzodiazepine. Diazepam is usually effective, and these seizures are often of short duration. Fosphenytoin (Cerebyx), phenytoin (Dilantin), and barbiturate medications can also be used for seizures that persist despite initial treatment with benzodiazepines.

(*continued*) After obtaining the patient's vital signs, you attempt to gain some additional history from her. While answering the questions, she stops speaking midsentence, stares, and then does not respond to your questioning. She then begins to exhibit generalized tonic-clonic seizure activity. Your partner grabs the patient's head to prevent her from banging her head and harming herself. Her airway is patent, and respirations are spontaneous and nonlabored. You administer diazepam 5 mg IV. Shortly after administration the seizures stop. The patient is groggy and disoriented. While repeating your assessment and vital signs, you note that she has widening of her QRS complex. You notify medical direction about the seizure and the electrocardiogram

(ECG) findings. You request to administer sodium bicarbonate. You receive an order to administer 50 mEq sodium bicarbonate IV push. Through the remainder of the transport to the hospital, the patient remains somnolent but answers all your questions and follows all commands. Her vital signs are stable, and her QRS duration seems to have returned to normal.

DIAZEPAM (VALIUM)

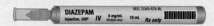

Classification: Benzodiazepine, Schedule C-IV.

Action: Binds to the benzodiazepine receptor and enhances the effects of gamma-aminobutyric acid (GABA). Benzodiazepines act at the level of the limbic, thalamic, and hypothalamic regions of the CNS and can produce any level of CNS depression required (including sedation, skeletal muscle relaxation, and anticonvulsant activity).

Indications: Anxiety, skeletal muscle relaxation, alcohol withdrawal, seizures.

Adverse Effects: Respiratory depression, drowsiness, fatigue, headache, pain at the injection site, confusion, nausea, hypotension, oversedation.

Contraindications: Children younger than 6 months, acute-angle glaucoma, CNS depression, alcohol intoxication, known sensitivity.

Dosage:

Anxiety:

- **Adult:**
  - **Moderate:** 2 to 5 mg slow IV, intramuscularly (IM).
  - **Severe:** 5 to 10 mg slow IV, IM (administer no faster than 5 mg/min).
  - **Low:** Low dosages are often required for elderly or debilitated patients.
- **Pediatric:** 0.2 to 0.3 mg/kg per dose IV, IM every 4 hours to a maximum dose of 0.6 mg/kg.

Delirium Tremens from Acute Alcohol Withdrawal:

- **Adult:** 10 mg IV.

Seizure:

- **Adult:** 5 to 10 mg slow IV, IO every 10 to 15 minutes; maximum total dose 30 mg.
- **Pediatric:**
  - **IV, IO:**
    - **5 years and older:** 1 mg over a 3-minute period every 2 to 5 minutes to a maximum total dose of 10 mg.
    - **Older than 30 days to younger than 5 years:** 0.2 to 0.5 mg over a 3-minute period; may repeat every 2 to 5 minutes to a maximum total dose of 5 mg.
    - **Neonate:** 0.1 to 0.3 mg/kg per dose given over a 3- to 5-minute period; may repeat every 15 to 30 minutes to a maximum total dose of 2 mg. (Not a first-line agent due to sodium benzoic acid in the injection.)
  - **Rectal administration:** If vascular access is not obtained, diazepam may be administered rectally to children.
    - **12 years and older:** 0.2 mg/kg.
    - **6 to 11 years:** 0.3 mg/kg.
    - **2 to 5 years:** 0.5 mg/kg.
    - **Younger than 2 years:** Not recommended.

Special Considerations:

Make sure that IV, IO lines are well secured. Extravasation of diazepam causes tissue necrosis.

Diazepam is insoluble in water and must be dissolved in propylene glycol. This produces a viscous solution; give slowly to prevent pain on injection.

Pregnancy class D.

PHENYTOIN (DILANTIN)

Classification: Anticonvulsant.
Action: Depresses seizures by affecting the movement of sodium and calcium into neural tissue.
Indications: Generalized tonic-clonic seizures.
Adverse Effects: Nausea/vomiting, depression of cardiac conduction, sedation, nystagmus, tremors, ataxia, dysarthria, gingival hypertrophy, hirsutism, facial coarsening, hypotension.
Contraindications: Sinus bradycardia, sinoatrial block, second- and third-degree heart block, Adams-Stokes syndrome, known sensitivity to hydantoins.
Dosage:

- **Adult:** 15 to 20 mg/kg IV, IO should be administered slowly at a rate not exceeding 50 mg/min. (This requires approximately 20 minutes in a 70-kg patient.)
- **Pediatric:** 15 to 20 mg/kg IV, IO, administered at a rate of 1 to 3 mg/kg per minute.

Special Considerations:
Continuously monitor the ECG and blood pressure during administration. Monitor IV site for signs of infiltration.
Pregnancy class D.

FOSPHENYTOIN (CEREBYX)

Classification: Anticonvulsant.
Action: Depresses seizures by affecting the movement of sodium and calcium into neural tissue.
Indications: Generalized tonic-clonic seizures.
Adverse Effects: Depression of cardiac conduction, sedation, nystagmus, delirium, tremors, ataxia, dysarthria, hypertension, hypotension, pain or irritation at injection site.
Contraindications: Sinus bradycardia, sinoatrial block, second- and third-degree heart block, Adams-Stokes syndrome, known sensitivity to hydantoins.
Dosage:

- **Adult and Pediatric:** Dosing is ordered in *milligram phenytoin equivalents* (PE) rather than in milligrams. Administer 15 to 20 mg PE/kg IV, IO, administered at a rate of <150 PE/min.

Special Considerations:
Continuously monitor the ECG and blood pressure during administration. Monitor IV site for signs of infiltration.
Pregnancy class D.

▸ Beta-Blocker Overdose

CASE STUDY

You are called to assist a 78-year-old woman who has been diagnosed with depression after the recent death of her husband of 50 years. The patient's daughter found the patient with an empty bottle of labetalol. The date on the bottle indicates that the prescription of 40 tablets was refilled only 3 days ago. Your assessment of the patient reveals an elderly woman who is minimally responsive. Her heart rate is 42 beats/min, and blood pressure is 74/44 mm Hg. Her skin is cool and dry.

As seen in this scenario, patients who have overdosed on beta blockers usually have bradycardia, heart block, and hypotension.[10,11] Some beta blockers can also cause delirium, seizures, and coma when taken in excessive doses. Patients typically will manifest these symptoms within 6 hours of ingestion.

Management

The initial treatment for bradycardia is administration of atropine and IV fluids. In most cases of beta-blocker overdose, atropine therapy is often inadequate. Administration of atropine after the overdose of beta blockers is only symptomatic therapy. If atropine increases the heart rate, the effect of the atropine is often brief and the bradycardia will recur. The main goal of therapy is to improve the patient's perfusion. This increase in perfusion can occur even when the patient still has some degree of bradycardia.

Atropine is the initial treatment for bradycardia from beta blockers, but glucagon is considered the antidote for beta-blocker overdose. However, glucagon's success is variable. In some cases, it works immediately, but other patients have no response at all. Glucagon, which typically is used to treat diabetic emergencies, can increase the heart rate and blood pressure after beta-blocker overdose. Glucagon works by increasing the concentration of an energy-storing chemical inside the cells known as **cyclic adenosine monophosphate (cAMP)**. The increased concentration of cAMP results in the heart beating stronger (inotropy) and faster (chronotropy).[12]

If a patient reverts to a shock-like state with bradycardia despite repeated dosing of glucagon, physicians at the hospital may elect to place the patient on an infusion or drip of glucagon. Although this is not a prehospital intervention, paramedics may be exposed to this therapy when transporting patients between facilities as a member of a critical care transport or flight service team.

> Drugs commonly used to treat bradycardia and hypotension, such as epinephrine, norepinephrine, and dopamine, are not successful in the treatment of beta-blocker overdose.

ATROPINE SULFATE

Classification: Anticholinergic (antimuscarinic).

Action: Competes reversibly with acetylcholine at the site of the muscarinic receptor. Receptors affected, in order from the most sensitive to the least sensitive, include salivary, bronchial, sweat glands, eye, heart, and GI tract.

Indications: Symptomatic bradycardia, asystole or pulseless electrical activity, nerve agent exposure, organophosphate poisoning.

© Jones & Bartlett Learning.

Adverse Effects: Decreased secretions resulting in dry mouth and hot skin temperature, intense facial flushing, blurred vision or dilation of the pupils with subsequent photophobia, tachycardia, restlessness. Atropine may cause paradoxical bradycardia if the dose administered is too low or if the drug is administered too slowly.

Contraindications: Acute MI; myasthenia gravis; GI obstruction; closed-angle glaucoma; known sensitivity to atropine, belladonna alkaloids, or sulfites. Will not be effective for infranodal (type II) AV block and new third-degree block with wide QRS complex.

Dosage:

Symptomatic Bradycardia:

- **Adult:** 0.5 mg IV, IO every 3 to 5 minutes to a maximum dose of 3 mg.
- **Adolescent:** 0.02 mg/kg (minimum 0.1 mg/dose; maximum 1 mg/dose) IV, IO up to a total dose of 2 mg.
- **Pediatric:** 0.02 mg/kg (minimum 0.1 mg/dose; maximum 0.5 mg/dose) IV, IO, up to a total dose of 1 mg.

Nerve Agent or Organophosphate Poisoning:

- **Adult:** 1 to 6 mg IV, IM; repeat if needed every 5 minutes until symptoms dissipate.
- **Pediatric:** 0.05 mg/kg IV, IM every 10 to 30 minutes as needed until symptoms dissipate.
- **Infants <15 pounds (7 kg):** 0.05 mg/kg IV, IM every 5 to 20 minutes as needed until symptoms dissipate.

Special Considerations:

Severe organophosphate exposures may require *massive* amounts of atropine, well beyond what is carried in most EMS vehicles.

Half-life 2.5 hours.

Pregnancy class C; possibly unsafe in lactating mothers.

Atropine used for the treatment of bradycardia has a maximum dose of 3 mg or 0.04 mg/kg. However, when treating organophosphate poisoning, atropine dosing should be repeated until secretions are dried.

GLUCAGON

Classification: Hormone.
Action: Converts glycogen to glucose.
Indications: Hypoglycemia, beta-blocker overdose.
Adverse Effects: Nausea/vomiting, rebound hyperglycemia, hypotension, sinus tachycardia.
Contraindications: Pheochromocytoma, insulinoma, known sensitivity.
Dosage:

Hypoglycemia:

- **Adult:** 1 mg IM, IV, IO, or subcutaneous.
- **Pediatric (<44 pounds [20 kg]):** 0.5 mg IM, IV, IO, or subcutaneous.

Beta-blocker overdose:

- **Adult:** 3 to 10 mg IV, IO over a 1-minute period, followed by a second dose of 10 mg IV (or IV infusion 3–5 mg/hr) if the symptoms of bradycardia and hypotension recur. (Note that this dose is much higher than the dose required to treat hypoglycemia; avoid using the supplied glycerin-based reconstitution solution when larger doses of glucagon are being administered.)
- **Pediatric:** For patients weighing <44 pounds (20 kg), the dose is 0.5 mg.

Special Considerations:

Pregnancy class B.

The dose of glucagon used to treat beta-blocker overdose is significantly higher than the dose required to treat hypoglycemia.

Most patients will have nausea and vomiting after glucagon administration. Be prepared with a basin and suction to keep the airway patent.

▶ Amphetamine and Methamphetamine Intoxication

CASE STUDY

Y ou are dispatched to the local police department to evaluate a 24-year-old man who is currently in police custody. You arrive to find the patient in an agitated and restless state. He is extremely diaphoretic. His heart rate is 130 beats/min, and blood pressure is 182/110 mm Hg. With some effort you are able to establish an IV line and administer a diazepam 5 mg IV dose. The patient yanks the IV line out and remains agitated and threatening to everyone in the vicinity. Next, you administer haloperidol 10 mg IM. After several minutes, the patient begins to calm down and you are able to get him onto the ambulance stretcher without physical force or restraints.

Drugs such as amphetamines and methamphetamines increase the body's levels of circulating epinephrine and norepinephrine—the "fight-or-flight" hormones. These elevated levels of epinephrine and norepinephrine are responsible for the observed tachycardia, hypertension, hyperthermia, agitation, and mydriasis (pupil dilation). Because of super-normal levels of the catecholamines, patients with amphetamine and methamphetamine overdoses can also have myocardial ischemia, cardiac arrhythmia, seizure, stroke, intracranial hemorrhage, and death.

Management

Neither gastric lavage nor activated charcoal has a role in managing these intoxications, because most of the drug has been absorbed by the time the patient is seen by a prehospital provider. Benzodiazepines (diazepam, midazolam, and lorazepam) can be used to control agitation, and haloperidol can be administered to those who do not respond to benzodiazepine therapy.

Activated charcoal is not used in amphetamine overdose, because most of the drug is absorbed by the time EMS arrives at the hospital.

Benzodiazepines work by binding with a benzodiazepine receptor. GABA, a naturally occurring neurotransmitter in the body, binds to the same receptors. When either a benzodiazepine or GABA binds to this receptor, it allows additional chloride ions to enter the cell that bears the receptor. The net effect is that the influx of chloride causes the cell to be less excitable. Clearly this is a desirable effect when these receptors are on the cells of the brain and nervous tissue and the patient is agitated, anxious, or seizing. Haloperidol (Haldol) is a potent antipsychotic agent often used to treat agitation. This drug has a low incidence of sedation and hypotension.

MIDAZOLAM (VERSED)

© Dr P. Marazzi/Science Source.

Classification: Benzodiazepine, Schedule C-IV.

Action: Binds to the benzodiazepine receptor and enhances the effects of the brain chemical (neurotransmitter) GABA. Benzodiazepines act at the level of the limbic, thalamic, and hypothalamic regions of the CNS to produce short-acting CNS depression (including sedation, skeletal muscle relaxation, and anticonvulsant activity).

Indications: Sedation, anxiety, skeletal muscle relaxation.

Adverse Effects: Respiratory depression, respiratory arrest, hypotension, nausea/vomiting, headache, hiccups, cardiac arrest.

Contraindications: Acute-angle glaucoma, pregnant women, known sensitivity.

Dosage:

Sedation:

Note: The dose of midazolam needs to be individualized. Every dose should be administered slowly over a period of 2 minutes. Allow 2 minutes to evaluate the clinical effect of the dose given.

- **Adult:**
  - **Healthy and younger than 60 years:** *Some patients require as little as 1 mg IV, IO. No more than 2.5 mg should be given over a 2-minute interval.* If additional sedation is required, continue to administer small increments over 2-minute periods (max dose: 5 mg). If the patient also has received a narcotic, he or she will typically require 30% less midazolam than the same patient not given the narcotic.
  - **60 years and older and debilitated or chronically ill patients:** This group of patients has a higher risk of hypoventilation, airway obstruction, and apnea. The peak clinical effect can take longer in these patients; therefore, dose increments should be smaller, and the rate of injection should be slower. *Some patients require a dose as small as 1 mg IV, IO, and no more than 1.5 mg should be given over a 2-minute period.* If additional sedation is required, additional midazolam should be given at a rate of no more than 1 mg over a 2-minute period (max dose: 3.5 mg). If the patient also has received a narcotic, he or she will typically require 50% less midazolam than the same patient not given the narcotic.
  - **Continuous infusion:** Continuous infusions can be required for prolonged transport of intubated, critically ill, and injured patients. After an initial bolus dose, the adult patient will require a maintenance infusion dose of 0.02 to 0.1 mg/kg per hour (1–7 mg/hr).
- **Pediatric (weight-based):** Pediatric patients typically require higher doses of midazolam than do adults on the basis of weight (in mg/kg). Younger pediatric patients (younger than 6 years) require higher doses (in mg/kg) than older pediatric patients. Midazolam takes approximately 3 minutes to reach peak effect; therefore, wait at least 2 minutes to determine effectiveness of drug and need for additional dosing.
  - **12 to 16 years:** Same as adult dosing. Some patients in this age group require a higher dose than that used in adults, but rarely does a patient require more than 10 mg.
  - **6 to 12 years:** 0.025 to 0.05 mg/kg IV, IO up to a total dose of 0.4 mg/kg. Exceeding 10 mg as total dose usually is not necessary.
  - **6 months to 5 years:** 0.05 to 0.1 mg/kg IV, IO up to a total dose of 0.6 mg/kg. Exceeding 6 mg as total dose usually is not necessary.

(continues)

MIDAZOLAM (VERSED)   *(continued)*

- ○ **Younger than 6 months:** Dosing recommendations for this age group is unclear. Because this age group is especially vulnerable to airway obstruction and hypoventilation, use small increments with frequent clinical evaluation. Dose: 0.05 to 0.1 mg/kg IV, IO.

Special Considerations:
Patients receiving midazolam require frequent monitoring of vital signs and pulse oximetry. Be prepared to support the patient's airway and ventilation.
Pregnancy class D.

LORAZEPAM (ATIVAN)

Classification: Benzodiazepine, Schedule C-IV.
Action: Binds to the benzodiazepine receptor and enhances the effects of the brain chemical GABA, an inhibitory transmitter, and may result in a state of sedation, hypnosis, skeletal muscle relaxation, anticonvulsant activity, coma.
Indications: Preprocedure sedation induction, anxiety, status epilepticus.
Adverse Effects: Headache, drowsiness, ataxia, dizziness, amnesia, depression, dysarthria, euphoria, syncope, fatigue, tremor, vertigo, respiratory depression, paradoxical CNS stimulation.
Contraindications: Known sensitivity to lorazepam, benzodiazepines, polyethylene glycol, propylene glycol, or benzyl alcohol; chronic obstructive pulmonary disease; sleep apnea (except while being mechanically ventilated); shock; coma; acute closed-angle glaucoma.
Dosage: Note: IV, IO lorazepam needs to be administered slowly.

© Scott Camazine/Science Source.

Analgesia and Sedation:
- **Adult:** 2 mg or 0.44 mg/kg IV, IO, whichever is smaller. This dosage will provide adequate sedation in most patients and should not be exceeded in patients older than 50 years.
- **Pediatric:** 0.05 mg/kg IV, IO. Each dose should not exceed 2 mg IV, IO.

Seizures:
- **Adult:** 2 to 4 mg IV, IO given over 2 to 5 minutes; may repeat in 10 to 15 minutes (max total dose: 8 mg in a 12-hour period).
- **Pediatric:** 0.1 mg/kg slow IV, IO given over 2 to 5 minutes (max single dose: 4 mg). May repeat at half the original dose in 10 to 15 minutes if seizure activity resumes.

Special Considerations:
Be prepared to support the patient's airway and ventilation.
Pregnancy class D.

HALOPERIDOL (HALDOL)

Classification: Antipsychotic agent.
Action: Selectively blocks postsynaptic dopamine receptors.
Indications: Psychotic disorders, agitation.
Adverse Effects: Extrapyramidal symptoms, drowsiness, **tardive dyskinesia**, hypotension, hypertension, VT, sinus tachycardia, QT prolongation, torsades de pointes.
Contraindications: Depressed mental status, Parkinson disease.
Dosage:

- **Adult:**
  - ○ **Mild agitation:** 0.5 to 2 mg orally (PO) or IM.
  - ○ **Moderate agitation:** 5 to 10 mg PO or IM.
  - ○ **Severe agitation:** 10 mg PO or IM.
- **Pediatric:** 1 to 5 mg IM or PO for acute psychosis or agitation.

Special Considerations:
IV use is considered "off-label" although it is used routinely in many settings. Consult department protocols or state/regional guidelines prior to administering. Monitor ECG if administered IV.
Pregnancy class C.

▶ Cocaine Intoxication

CASE STUDY

You are called to an office tower to assist a 35-year-old man reporting chest pain. You enter an office suite where a party is taking place with caterers and a live band. You and your partner are quickly escorted to a large office in the rear, where you find the patient. He is sitting on the floor and appears extremely agitated. He is rocking back and forth and is covered in sweat. A coworker of the patient tells you that he looks terrible and is reporting chest pain. Upon additional questioning by your partner, she admits that she and the patient were doing cocaine before the patient exhibited these symptoms. On your examination, the patient is warm and diaphoretic. His heart rate is 142 beats/min and blood pressure is 182/108 mm Hg. His lungs are clear. He is alert and oriented to date and place but remains agitated and aggressive. The patient has no motor or sensory deficits, but his pupils are 8 mm and reactive to light.

Management

Intoxication with cocaine results in an adrenergic response, with the resultant clinical findings of tachycardia, hypertension, dilated pupils, hyperthermia, and agitation. The initial treatment for the agitation includes the use of benzodiazepines such as diazepam (Valium), midazolam (Versed), or lorazepam (Ativan). Haloperidol (Haldol) is the second-line drug used in patients who do not respond to the benzodiazepines or who are psychotic.

Cocaine can produce serious cardiovascular complications such as tachycardia, hypertension, chest pain, and myocardial ischemia.[13] The chest pain associated with cocaine intoxication is ischemic in nature. The patient initially should be given a benzodiazepine such as diazepam. Up to this point the treatment for cocaine intoxication is similar to therapy for amphetamine use.

(continued) You administer 5 mg Valium to the patient, and he becomes less agitated. You place him on supplemental oxygen and provide three doses of sublingual nitroglycerin and one aspirin. Despite these drug interventions, the patient still reports chest pain that rates as a 7 on a scale of 1 to 10.

Because the chest pain seen with cocaine intoxication is often ischemic in nature, the drug therapy used in other forms of chest pain is indicated—administration of nitroglycerin.[14,15]

NITROGLYCERIN (NITROLINGUAL, NITROQUICK, NITRO-DUR)

Classification: Antianginal agent.

Action: Relaxes vascular smooth muscle, thereby dilating peripheral arteries and veins. This causes pooling of venous blood and decreased venous return to the heart, which decreases preload. Nitroglycerin also reduces left ventricular systolic wall tension, which decreases afterload.

Indications: Angina, ongoing ischemic chest discomfort, hypertension, myocardial ischemia associated with cocaine intoxication.

Adverse Effects: Headache, hypotension, bradycardia, lightheadedness, flushing, cardiovascular collapse, methemoglobinemia.

© Sue Heaton/Alamy Stock Photo.

Contraindications: Hypotension, severe bradycardia or tachycardia, right-sided myocardial infarction, increased intracranial pressure, intracranial bleeding, patients taking any medications for erectile dysfunction (such as sildenafil [Viagra], tadalafil [Cialis], or vardenafil [Levitra]), known sensitivity to nitrates. Use with caution in anemia, closed-angle glaucoma, hypotension, postural hypotension, uncorrected hypovolemia.

© Allik Camazine/Alamy Stock Photo.

Dosage:

- **Adult:**
  - **Sublingual tablets:** One tablet (0.3–0.4 mg) at 5-minute intervals to a maximum of three doses.
  - **Translingual spray:** One (0.4 mg) spray at 5-minute intervals to a maximum of three sprays.
  - **Ointment:** 2% topical (Nitro-Bid ointment): Apply 1 to 2 inches of paste over the chest wall, cover with transparent wrap, and secure with tape.
  - **IV infusion:** 5 mcg/min; may increase rate by 5 to 10 mcg/min every 5 to 10 minutes as needed. End points of dose titration for nitroglycerin include a drop in the blood pressure of 10%, relief of chest pain, and return of ST segment to normal on a 12-lead ECG.
- **Pediatric IV infusion:** The initial pediatric infusion is 0.25 to 0.5 mcg/kg per minute IV, IO titrated by 0.5 to 1 mcg/kg per minute. Usual required dose is 1 to 3 mcg/kg per minute to a maximum dose of 5 mcg/kg per minute.

Special Considerations:

Administration of nitroglycerin to a patient with right ventricular MI can result in hypotension. Pregnancy class C.

The patient in the preceding scenario has ischemic chest pain. Therefore, the administration of aspirin should be considered. Aspirin reduces the effectiveness of platelets to form clots. Platelets are formed elements of the blood that, when activated, are responsible for the formation of small plugs that seal blood vessels, such as in the case of a laceration. In the case of ischemic chest pain, the activated platelets form small plugs that occlude the flow of blood vessels in the heart. The spasm of the coronary arteries and occlusion with platelet plugs result in the heart muscle not receiving the critical amount of oxygen. Administering aspirin inhibits the enzyme cyclooxygenase and impairs platelet function for the life of the platelet, which is 7 days.

If the patient's chest pain persists after treatment with benzodiazepines, nitroglycerin, and aspirin, the paramedic should consider administration of morphine, fentanyl, or other opioid medication. Phentolamine (Regitine) is another medication that may be used in this situation. Phentolamine is an alpha adrenergic blocker aimed at reducing systemic blood pressure and vasoconstriction of the coronary arteries.[16] Adrenergic receptors, when stimulated, produce the clinical responses of hypertension, tachycardia, dilated pupils, agitation, and hyperthermia. Alpha receptors result in vasoconstriction and hypertension. When the patient is given phentolamine, the drug binds to the alpha receptor, preventing the cocaine molecule from producing its clinical effects of vasoconstriction and hypertension. Alpha receptors do not produce an increase in heart rate (chronotropy) or forcefulness of heart contraction (inotropy). Those effects are mediated by beta receptors.

Hypertension from cocaine should not be treated with beta blockers because they can exacerbate the coronary artery vasoconstriction and result in an increased chance of death.[17]

> Treatment of cocaine-induced hypertension can constrict coronary arteries and produce cardiac complications and even death.

Some patients with cocaine intoxication have seizures. The best method of stopping these seizures is administrating a benzodiazepine, such as diazepam, followed by a loading dose of phenytoin.

ASPIRIN, ASA

Classification: Antiplatelet, nonnarcotic analgesic, antipyretic.

Action: Prevents the formation of a chemical known as thromboxane A2, which causes platelets to clump together, or aggregate, and form plugs that cause obstruction or constriction of small coronary arteries.

Indications: Fever, inflammation, angina, acute MI, and patients complaining of pain, pressure, squeezing, or crushing in the chest that may be cardiac in origin.

Adverse Effects: Anaphylaxis, angioedema, bronchospasm, bleeding, stomach irritation, nausea/vomiting.

© ClassicStock/S. FELD/Medical Images.

Contraindications: GI bleeding, active ulcer disease, hemorrhagic stroke, bleeding disorders, children with chickenpox or flulike symptoms, known sensitivity.

Dosage: Note: "Baby aspirin" 81 mg, standard adult aspirin dose 325 mg.

Myocardial Infarction:
- **Adult:** 160 to 325 mg PO (alternatively, four 81-mg baby aspirin are often given), 300-mg rectal suppository.
- **Pediatric:** 3 to 5 mg/kg per day to 5 to 10 mg/kg per day given as a single dose.

Pain or Fever:
- **Adult:** 325 to 650 mg PO (1–2 adult tablets) every 4 to 6 hours.
- **Pediatric:** 60 to 90 mg/kg per day in divided doses every 4 to 6 hours.

Special Considerations:
Pregnancy class C except the last 3 months of pregnancy, when aspirin is considered pregnancy class D.

MORPHINE SULFATE

Classification: Opiate agonist, Schedule C-II.

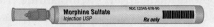

Action: Binds with opioid receptors. Morphine is capable of inducing hypotension by depression of the vasomotor centers of the brain, as well as release of the chemical histamine. In the management of angina, morphine reduces stimulation of the sympathetic nervous system caused by pain and anxiety. Reduction of sympathetic stimulation reduces heart rate, cardiac work, and myocardial oxygen consumption.

Indications: Moderate to severe pain, including chest pain associated with ACS, heart failure, pulmonary edema.

Adverse Effects: Respiratory depression, hypotension, nausea/vomiting, dizziness, lightheadedness, sedation, diaphoresis, euphoria, dysphoria, worsening of bradycardia and heart block in some patients with acute inferior wall MI, seizures, cardiac arrest, anaphylactoid reactions.

Contraindications: Respiratory depression, shock, known sensitivity. Use with caution in hypotension, acute bronchial asthma, respiratory insufficiency, head trauma.

Dosage:

- **Adult:** 2 to 10 mg IV, IO, IM, or subcutaneous administered slowly over a period of several minutes. The dose is the same whether administered IV, IO, IM, or subcutaneous.
- **Pediatric <50 kg:** 0.025 to 0.2 mg/kg IV, IO, IM, or subcutaneous.

Special Considerations:

Monitor vital signs and pulse oximetry closely. Be prepared to support patient's airway and ventilations.

Patients may report a "flushed" or hot feeling immediately following administration. Assess for signs of allergic reaction; however, this is typically a histamine release.

Overdose should be treated with naloxone.

Pregnancy class C.

PHENTOLAMINE (REGITINE)

Classification: Alpha antagonist, antihypertensive.

Action: Blocks alpha-adrenergic receptors, causing vasodilation.

Indications: Hypertensive emergencies and hypertension caused by pheochromocytoma, cocaine-induced vasospasm of the coronary arteries.

Adverse Effects: Sinus tachycardia, angina, dizziness, orthostatic hypotension, prolonged hypotensive episodes, nausea/vomiting, diarrhea, weakness, flushing, nasal congestion.

Contraindications: Known sensitivity. Use with caution in acute MI, angina, coronary insufficiency, evidence suggestive of coronary artery disease, peptic ulcer disease.

Dosage:

Hypertensive Crisis:

- **Adult:** 5 to 15 mg IV, IO, or IM.
- **Pediatric:** 0.05 to 0.1 mg/kg IV, IO; or 1 mg/dose

Cocaine-Induced Vasospasm:

- **Adult:** 5 mg IV, IO, or IM.
- **Pediatric:** 0.05 to 0.1 mg/kg IV, IO; or 1 mg/dose.

Special Considerations:

Pregnancy class C

▶ Overview of Narcotic Overdose

CASE STUDY

Your unit is dispatched to a local rescue mission to evaluate an unconscious man who was found on the street. You arrive to find a 23-year-old man who is well-known to the police as a heroin abuser. On assessment, the patient moans because of deep pain. His blood pressure is 72/52 mm Hg, heart rate is 112 beats/min, and respirations are 12 breaths/min and very shallow. On physical examination, the patient is grossly intoxicated with alcohol. His upper extremities have multiple needle tracks, as well as small, circular scars that appear to be from previous skin abscesses. As you roll the patient to inspect his back, you find a bag that contains drug paraphernalia, needles, and a substance that looks like heroin. He has no obvious external signs of traumatic injury.

Overdose can occur with any type of opiate use, in either medical or abuse settings. Opiates, or narcotics, are commonly abused medications. Heroin, a common drug of abuse and overdose, is classified as an opiate and is responsible for the majority of opiate-related overdoses.[18] Heroin is often abused by injecting the drug intravenously, known as "mainlining," although the most common method of heroin abuse is snorting the drug. In Asian countries, heroin is commonly smoked. Overdose typically occurs with heroin use because the quantity of heroin in any given sample can vary greatly. Heroin is also more soluble in fat, allowing the drug to reach higher levels in the system more rapidly than other forms of opiates.

Patients with an opiate/narcotic overdose typically have a depressed level of consciousness, hypotension, and respiratory depression. In any patient with a depressed level of consciousness, prehospital care must focus on supporting the ABCs (airway, breathing, circulation). Even when the provider has a strong and well-founded suspicion of the cause of the patient's altered level of consciousness, as in this case, the obligation is to rule out common and easily treated metabolic conditions such as diabetic complications of hypoglycemia or diabetic ketoacidosis. In most cases, the cause of altered level of consciousness is unknown.

Management

Naloxone (Narcan), a drug known as a competitive antagonist, binds to the opiate receptor to prevent the opiate from exerting its effects of altered mental status, hypotension, and respiratory depression. Naloxone should be administered in a dose or manner that is appropriate for the situation. The optimal use of naloxone in most situations is to provide enough opioid reversal to restore breathing, allow the patient to protect his or her airway and improve the patient's overall level of sedation, without completely reversing all the opioid effects or abruptly returning the patient to full consciousness. Too much naloxone may cause a violent narcotic withdrawal syndrome, with agitation, restlessness, vomiting, and other related signs and symptoms. Certain synthetic opioids or potent illicit opioid compounds may require higher doses, repeated administration, or continuous infusions of naloxone to keep the patient breathing. In many multidrug overdose or poisoning situations, it may be advisable to allow opioid effects to predominate, rather than reversing with naloxone. In these instances, the presence of an opioid may be beneficial in mitigating the toxic effects from other substances, particularly those associated with aggression, agitation, and similar behaviors, which might otherwise create a greater risk for the patient or EMS providers.

NALOXONE (NARCAN)

Classification: Opioid antagonist.
Action: Binds the opioid receptor and blocks the effect of narcotics.
Indications: Narcotic overdoses, reversal of narcotics used for procedure-related anesthesia.
Adverse Effects: Nausea/vomiting, restlessness, diaphoresis, tachycardia, hypertension, tremulousness, seizures, cardiac arrest, narcotic withdrawal. Patients who have gone from a state of somnolence from a narcotic overdose to wide awake may become combative.
Contraindications: Known sensitivity to naloxone, nalmefene, or naltrexone. Use with caution in patients with supraventricular arrhythmias or other cardiac disease, head trauma, brain tumor.
Dosage:
- **Adult:** 0.4 to 2 mg IV, IO, endotracheal (ET), IM, or subcutaneous. Alternatively, administer 2 mg intranasally. Higher doses (10–20 mg) may be required for overdoses of synthetic narcotics. A repeat dose of one-third to two-thirds the original dose is often necessary.
- **Pediatric:**
  - **5 years or older or weight >44 pounds (20 kg):** 2 mg IV, IO, ET, IM, or subcutaneous.
  - **Younger than 5 years or weight <44 pounds (20 kg):** 0.1 mg/kg IV, IO, ET, IM, or subcutaneous; may repeat every 2 to 3 minutes.

Special Considerations:
Pregnancy class C

© Tomas Nevesely/Shutterstock.

▶ Organophosphate and Nerve Agent Exposure

CASE STUDY

You are dispatched to the home of a 52-year-old man. The patient's wife tells you that her husband must have caught the flu because he has diarrhea and is vomiting. You assess the patient, who tells you that he is a farmer and was feeling great until he worked the fields that afternoon. Shortly after loading the fertilizer spreader, he began to have nausea, vomiting, and profuse sweating. You perform a physical examination. His heart rate is 144 beats/min, and he is sweating profusely. He seems to be having excessive oral secretions, and his pupils are pinpoint. On auscultation of lung sounds, he has wheezes in all lung fields.

Organophosphates are a class of chemicals found in insecticides and fertilizers and are common in agricultural environments. Organophosphates were originally developed in the 1930s for use as insecticides. Subsequently these chemicals were altered for use as nerve agents. The nerve gases **sarin** and **VX** are potent organophosphates. This class of chemicals can gain access to the body through inhalation, ingestion, and absorption through the skin. Sarin was released in a Tokyo subway by a terrorist group in 1995. Each year, more than 300,000 people globally are poisoned and die from exposure to organophosphates.[19]

Organophosphates poison the body by inhibiting the enzyme **acetylcholinesterase**. Under normal conditions, acetylcholinesterase breaks down and deactivates the neurotransmitter acetylcholine. Without acetylcholinesterase present to break it down, acetylcholine builds up and causes overstimulation of the parasympathetic nervous system. Overstimulation of the parasympathetic nervous system results in both muscarinic and nicotinic effects.

***The effects of muscarinic receptor blockage can be remembered by the mnemonic* DUMBBELS.** *Muscarinic* requires *muscles.* To build muscles, one needs DUMBBELS:

Diarrhea
Urination
Miosis (contraction of pupils)
Bradycardia
Bronchospasm and bronchorrhea
Emesis
Lacrimation
Salivation, secretion, and sweating

The effects of nicotinic receptor blockage can be committed to memory by the mnemonic **MTWHF**. *Nicotinic* is similar to the word *nicotine*, and smokers need nicotine every day of the week (MTWHF):

Mydriasis (dilation of pupils)
Tachycardia
Weakness
Hypertension and hyperglycemia
Fasciculations (involuntary contractions, twitching)

Management

Symptoms of organophosphate intoxication can occur within 5 minutes of exposure. The most dangerous manifestations of organophosphate poisoning are excessive respiratory secretions (bronchorrhea), bronchospasm, and respiratory insufficiency.[20] Excessive respiratory secretions and respiratory failure make securing the airway imperative. Of critical importance is that, if intubation is performed, the rapid depolarizing agent succinylcholine (Anectine) should *not* be used because it cannot be broken down and can result in prolonged paralysis of the patient.[21] The initial drug intervention in patients intoxicated with organophosphates is the administration of atropine.

The most dangerous manifestations of organophosphate poisoning are respiratory complications.

(*continued*) You give the patient a bolus of atropine. His wheezing stops and the secretions decrease. However, the patient remains tachycardic, with a heart rate of 140 beats/min and blood pressure of 184/105 mm Hg. He is extremely weak, as demonstrated by the inability to lift his head or arms.

As demonstrated in this case, atropine reverses the effects of the muscarinic receptors, but the nicotinic effects will persist and the patient will continue to have profound muscle weakness. To reverse the effects of organophosphates on the nicotinic receptors, the provider needs to administer pralidoxime (2-PAM).[22]

PRALIDOXIME (2-PAM, PROTOPAM)

Classification: Cholinergic agonist, antidote.
Action: Reactivates cholinesterase.
Indications: Toxicity from nerve agents (organophosphates) having cholinesterase activity.
Adverse Effects: Dizziness, blurred vision, hypertension, diplopia, hyperventilation, laryngospasm, nausea/vomiting, sinus tachycardia.
Contraindications: Myasthenia gravis, renal failure, inability to control the airway.
Dosage:

- **Adult:** 1 to 2 g (dilute in 100 mL normal saline) over a 15- to 30-minute period. If this is not practical or if pulmonary edema is present, the dose should be given slowly (≥5 minutes) by IV line as a 5% solution in water. Consider IM or subcutaneous administration if IV administration is not possible.
  - **Autoinjector:** Pralidoxime is also available as an autoinjector that delivers 600 mg IM. Repeat doses can be given every 15 minutes to a total of three doses (1,800 mg). Pralidoxime autoinjector is not recommended for pediatric patients.
- **Pediatric:** 15 to 50 mg/kg IV, IO, depending on severity. Consider IM or subcutaneous administration if IV administration is not possible.

Special Considerations:
Pregnancy class C

NDC 12345-678-90
Pralidoxime
(pralidoxime chloride)
for injection, USP   **1 g**
Single Dose Vial
FOR INTRAVENOUS INJECTION:

▶ Review Questions

1. What is the risk of vomiting and aspirating activated charcoal?
2. Activated charcoal is contraindicated in what common overdose?
3. After overdose with a cyclic antidepressant, a patient begins to show a wide-complex tachycardia. What is the initial drug of choice?
4. What is the cardiovascular effect of a too-rapid administration of phenytoin (Dilantin)?
5. What is the pharmacologic antidote for a beta-blocker overdose?
6. What are the effects of methamphetamine on the body?
7. Why are gastric lavage and activated charcoal not effective in treating a methamphetamine overdose?
8. What is the initial drug used for the treatment of agitation in a patient who is intoxicated with cocaine?
9. What are the most dangerous manifestations of organophosphate poisoning?
10. When intubating a victim of organophosphate poisoning, why should you avoid using succinylcholine (Anectine)?

References

1. Kivlehan SM. Understanding overdose. *EMS World.* https://www.emsworld.com/article/10939148/understanding-overdose. Published June 2013. Accessed October 4, 2018.
2. Manoguerra AS, Krenzelok EP. Rapid emesis from high-dose ipecac syrup in adults and children intoxicated with antiemetics and other drugs. *Am J Hosp Pharm.* 1978;35:1360.
3. MacLean WC. A comparison of ipecac syrup and apomorphine in the immediate treatment of ingestion of poisons. *J Pediatr.* 1973;82:121.
4. Höjer J, Troutman WG, Hoppu K, et al. Position paper update: Ipecac syrup for gastrointestinal decontamination. *Clin Toxicol.* 2013;51(3):134–139.
5. American Academy of Clinical Toxicology; European Association of Poison Centres and Clinical Toxicologists. Position statement and practice guidelines on the use of multidose activated charcoal in the treatment of acute poisoning. *J Toxicol Clin Toxicol.* 1999;37:731.

6. Hendrickson RG, Kusin S. Gastrointestinal decontamination of the poisoned patient. UpToDate. https://www.uptodate.com/contents/gastrointestinal-decontamination-of-the-poisoned-patient. Updated January 24, 2017. Accessed October 4, 2018.

7. Menzies DG, Busuttil A, Prescott LF. Fatal pulmonary aspiration of oral activated charcoal. *Br Med J.* 1988; 287:459.

8. Litovitz TL, Klein-Schwartz W, Caravati EM, Youniss J, Crouch B, Lee S. Annual report of the American Association of Poison Control Centers Toxic Exposure Surveillance System. *Am J Emerg Med.* 2001;20:391.

9. Ellison DW, Pentel PR. Clinical features and consequences of seizures due to cyclic overdose. *Am J Emerg Med.* 1989;7:5.

10. Reith DM, Dawson AH, Epid D, Whyte IM, Buckley NA, Sayer GP. Relative toxicity of beta blockers in overdose. *J Clin Pharmacol.* 1996;34:273.

11. Love JN, Howell JM, Litovitz TL, Klein-Schwartz W. Acute beta blocker overdose: factors associated with the development of cardiovascular morbidity. *J Toxicol Clin Toxicol.* 2000;38:275.

12. Taubolet P, Carlou A, Berdeaux A, Bismuth C. Pathophysiology and management of self-poisoning with beta-blockers. *J Toxicol Clin Toxicol.* 1993;31:531.

13. Hollander JE, Hoffman RS. Cocaine-induced myocardial infarction: an analysis and review of the literature. *J Emerg Med.* 1992;10:169.

14. Baumann BM, Perrone J, Hornig SE, Shofer FS, Hollander JE. Randomized, double-blind placebo-controlled trial of diazepam, nitroglycerin, or both for treatment of patients with potential cocaine-associated acute coronary syndromes. *Acad Emerg Med.* 2000;7:878.

15. Honderick T, Williams D, Seaberg D, Wears R. A prospective randomized, controlled trial of benzodiazepines and nitroglycerine or nitroglycerine alone on the treatment of cocaine-associated with acute coronary syndromes. *Am J Emerg Med.* 2003;21:31.

16. Hollander JE, Coates WA, Hoffman RS. Use of phentolamine for cocaine-induced myocardial ischemia. *N Engl J Med.* 1992;327:361.

17. Kloner RA, Hale S. Unraveling the complex effects of cocaine on the heart. *Circulation.* 1993;87:1046.

18. *Results from the 2003 National Survey on Drug Use and Health: National findings,* Washington, DC: United States Department of Health and Human Services; 2004.

19. Bird S. Organophosphate and carbamate poisoning. UpToDate. https://www.uptodate.com/contents/organophosphate-and-carbamate-poisoning. Updated January 23, 2017. Accessed August 18, 2018.

20. Lee P, Tai DYH. Clinical features of patients with acute organophosphate poisoning requiring intensive care. *Intens Care Med.* 2001;27:694.

21. Selden BC, Curry SC. Prolonged succinylcholine-induced paralysis in organophosphate insecticide poisoning. *Ann Emerg Med.* 1987;16:215.

22. Eddleston M, Szinicz L, Eyer P, Buckley N. Oximes in organophosphorus pesticide poisoning: a systemic review of clinical trials. *Q J Med.* 2002;95:275.

© Andrew Brookes/Getty Images

CHAPTER 14

Respiratory Emergencies

OBJECTIVES

1. Define *nasal cannula, rebreather face mask, nonrebreather face mask,* and *Venturi mask.*
2. Discuss the use of oxygen in a respiratory emergency.
3. Describe the two types of bronchodilator agents.
4. Discuss the benefits of the metered-dose inhaler.
5. Demonstrate the proper procedure for administering medication through a metered-dose inhaler.
6. Discuss medications used in the treatment of asthma: albuterol (Proventil, Ventolin), ipratropium bromide (Atrovent), and albuterol/ipratropium (Combivent).
7. Discuss medications used as second-line therapy for acute exacerbation of asthma: dexamethasone (Decadron), methylprednisolone sodium succinate (Solu-Medrol), aminophylline, magnesium sulfate, and racemic epinephrine.
8. Briefly describe the key treatment for patients with chronic obstructive pulmonary disease.

MEDICATIONS THAT APPEAR IN CHAPTER 14

Oxygen
Albuterol (Proventil, Ventolin)
Levalbuterol (Xopenex)
Ipratropium bromide
 (Atrovent)

Albuterol/ipratropium
 (Combivent; DuoNeb)
Dexamethasone (Decadron)
Methylprednisolone sodium
 succinate (Solu-Medrol)

Magnesium sulfate
Racemic epinephrine/
 racepinephrine
 (microNefrin, S_2)

▶ Introduction

Respiratory distress is one of the most common patient presentations encountered by prehospital professionals. Acute respiratory distress affects the young and old, male and female, and people of all ethnicities. Although the underlying pathologic condition causing the respiratory distress may be different, with the exception of acute pulmonary edema most of the prehospital care is aimed at treatment of reversible bronchial constriction, or bronchospasm. Advanced life support (ALS) interventions, including respiratory medication administration, have been shown to significantly reduce mortality in patients with respiratory distress.[1]

▶ Oxygen

Although often overlooked as a drug, oxygen is the most commonly used medication in the prehospital setting. As with any drug, oxygen has associated risks, as well as benefits. Oxygen is used daily by basic and advanced prehospital providers, sometimes with little consideration to its pharmacologic properties. The use of oxygen has become increasingly controversial. In situations such as neonatal resuscitation, **chronic obstructive pulmonary disease (COPD)** exacerbations, and acute coronary syndrome, oxygen use is now carefully titrated to prescribed oxygen saturation ranges, rather than applied indiscriminately.[2-4] EMS providers should anticipate additional changes as ongoing research in this area leads to guideline updates and a significant paradigm shift from traditional approaches to oxygen delivery.

Oxygen is a colorless and odorless gas stored in either green or aluminum cylinders at a pressure of 1,800 to 2,400 pounds per square inch (psi). As the oxygen passes through the attached regulator, the gas pressure is decreased to a working pressure of 60 psi. Oxygen is contained in nine different sizes of cylinders labeled alphabetically (**TABLE 14-1**). An understanding of the capacities of these cylinders is helpful to the prehospital provider in determining the duration of oxygen therapy that a given cylinder can provide (**FIGURE 14-1**).

TABLE 14-1 Oxygen Cylinders: Capacity and Duration of Use

Cylinder	Capacity (L)	Duration of Use at 5 L/min	Duration of Use at 10 L/min
A	76	15 min	8 min
B	196	39 min	20 min
D	396	1.3 hr	40 min
E	659	2.1 hr	1.1 hr
F	2,062	6.8 hr	3.4 hr
M	3,000	10 hr	5.0 hr
G	5,331	17.7 hr	8.8 hr
H	5,570	18.5 hr	9.2 hr
K	7,500	25 hr	12.5 hr

FIGURE 14-1 Different sizes of oxygen cylinders.
© Jones & Bartlett Publishers. Courtesy of MIEMSS.

The quantity of oxygen delivered to a specific patient can be considered in terms of the concentration of inspired oxygen and flow. The atmosphere consists of 78% nitrogen, 21% oxygen, and a variety of other gases that compose the remaining 1%. The concentration of inspired oxygen is referred to as the **fraction of inspired oxygen (FiO$_2$)**. Because the percentage of oxygen in the atmosphere is 21%, the FiO$_2$ in normal room air is 21%. When a patient has shortness of breath, chest pain, or shock, supplemental oxygen is administered to increase the concentration of oxygen breathed by the patient. Increasing the concentration of inspired oxygen increases the content of oxygen in blood and subsequently the amount of oxygen delivered to the heart and peripheral tissues.

Oxygen Delivery Devices

Oxygen delivery devices include the **nasal cannula** and face mask. The basic principle by which these devices work is the creation of a reservoir filled with oxygen-enriched gas. When the patient inhales, he or she breathes from this oxygen-enriched reservoir. Nasal cannulas and nonrebreather face masks typically are the most commonly used noninvasive devices for delivering oxygen in the prehospital setting. However, patients involved in interfacility transfers may use additional devices, as described in this section.

The nasal cannula is a noninvasive means of delivering supplemental oxygen in a low-flow and nonintrusive fashion (**FIGURE 14-2**). Oxygen flows through two nasal prongs into the oropharynx, which acts as an oxygen reservoir, resulting in an increase in the oxygen concentration. A nasal cannula set with a flow rate of 6 L/min is capable of delivering an oxygen concentration between 35 and 45%.

Various oxygen face masks are capable of delivering an oxygen concentration based on the flow rate, reservoir of the mask, presence or absence of a reservoir bag, and side ports in the mask with directional valves. The simple oxygen face mask does not have a reservoir bag or unidirectional side ports. Room gases mix with the oxygen inside the mask. At a flow rate of 6 to 10 L/min, these masks are capable of delivering an FiO$_2$ between 30 and 60%.

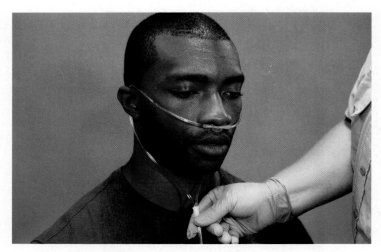

FIGURE 14-2 Nasal cannula.
© Jones & Bartlett Publishers. Courtesy of MIEMSS.

FIGURE 14-3 A. Partial rebreather mask. This mask has an oxygen reservoir bag but no valves over the side ports.
B. Nonrebreather mask. This mask has an oxygen reservoir bag, as well as one-way valves (arrows) over the side ports.
A. © Jones & Bartlett Learning. Courtesy of MIEMSS. **B.** © Jones & Bartlett Learning. Courtesy of MIEMSS.

Rebreather face masks, or **partial rebreather face masks**, have a face mask and a reservoir bag (**FIGURE 14-3A**). Oxygen accumulates in the reservoir bag. During inspiration, the patient inhales oxygen in the reservoir, as well as some room air through the side ports. When the patient exhales, some of the expired breath goes back into the reservoir bag, where it is then rebreathed. Partial rebreather masks are capable of delivering 60% oxygen.

Nonrebreather face masks are similar to rebreather masks in appearance and function, with the exception of having a single one-way exhalation valve on one side of the mask and one on the reservoir bag (**FIGURE 14-3B**). The valve on the side of the mask prevents inhalation of room air during inspiration. One side of the mask is usually missing the one-way valve as a safety precaution to allow ambient air to enter the mask in the event of the loss of oxygen supply from an empty tank or disconnected tubing. The valve on the reservoir prevents any of the exhaled breath from entering the oxygen-rich reservoir. Nonrebreather face masks require a higher flow rate of 12 to 15 L/min and are capable of delivering oxygen concentrations close to 100%.

Emergency departments and hospitals often use the **Venturi mask**. Venturi masks come with a series of small plastic inserts that fit ports on the mask and regulate the concentration of oxygen that the patient can inhale (**FIGURE 14-4**). By changing the plastic insert, the provider can, with a significant degree of precision, alter the oxygen concentration from 24 to 60%. The flow of oxygen depends on the desired FiO$_2$ (**TABLE 14-2**).

FIGURE 14-4 Venturi mask. In the middle are the various plastic inserts that control the concentration of oxygen.
© Jones & Bartlett Publishers. Courtesy of MIEMSS.

TABLE 14-2 Venturi Mask Inserts and Oxygen Flow Rates

Oxygen Delivery (%)	Insert Color	Oxygen Flow Rate (L/min)
24	Blue	2
28	White	4
35	Yellow	6
40	Red	8
60	Green	12

© Jones & Bartlett Learning.

INITIATION OF OXYGEN THERAPY

Equipment Needed:
Oxygen source, oxygen flow meter, mask or cannula
Procedure:
1. Observe standard precautions.
2. When possible, explain to the patient what procedure you are going to perform and why.
3. Ensure the protective seal has been removed from the valve on the tank. Do not lose the washer attached to the seal, because it provides an airtight seal between the regulator and the tank. Turn the valve away from yourself or anyone else.
4. Quickly open and close the valve to blow any dirt or contaminants out of the tank opening.
5. Place the washer over the inlet port on the regulator. Line up the regulator port and pins with the tank opening and holds in the tank valve. Check the flow meter to ensure it is turned off. Tighten the screw by hand.
6. Open the tank to test for an airtight seal. If there is leakage, tighten the screw until the leak stops. Once you have made sure there are no leaks, it must be completely open or completely closed.

7. Adjust the flow meter to the desired setting.
8. When finished, turn off the flow meter and close the tank valve.
9. Open the flow meter momentarily to release the pressure from the regulator.

On occasion, prehospital providers encounter patients with COPD, who require continuous oxygen while at home. Continuous oxygen can require a transtracheal catheter, which is inserted surgically. Transtracheal catheters, like nasal cannulas, are used for long-term oxygen therapy in patients with chronic lung disease. Some patients find that the long-term use of nasal cannulas is irritating to the nose at night; such patients may receive transtracheal catheters, which are held in place by a necklace.

OXYGEN

© Jones & Bartlett Publishers. Courtesy of MIEMSS.

Classification: Elemental gas.
Action: Facilitates cellular energy metabolism.
Indications: Hypoxia, ischemic chest pain, respiratory distress, suspected carbon monoxide poisoning, traumatic injuries, shock.
Adverse Effects: High concentrations can cause decreased level of consciousness and respiratory depression in patients with chronic carbon dioxide retention or chronic lung disease. Oxygen causes systemic and coronary vasoconstriction possibly coronary artery perfusion
Contraindications: Known paraquat poisoning.
Dosage:
Low-Concentration Oxygen:
- A dose of 1 to 4 L/min by a nasal cannula is appropriate.

High-Concentration Oxygen:
- A dose of 10 to 15 L/min via nonrebreather mask is appropriate.

Special Considerations:
Pregnancy class A.

▶ Bronchodilators

CASE STUDY

Your unit has been dispatched to a local high school for a youth having an asthma attack. The dispatcher informs you that the patient is in the gymnasium. You arrive to find a 17-year-old boy sitting in the middle of the basketball court. Several friends are standing around the patient, attempting to assist and calm him. You clear back the crowd and begin your assessment. You find an anxious young man who has rapid and somewhat labored respirations. He is moving air and is able to report that he has a history of asthma and that his current symptoms are consistent with his previous asthma exacerbations. The patient's respiratory rate is 32 breaths/min, heart rate is 110 beats/min, and blood pressure is 142/88 mm Hg.

Patients with **asthma** (an inflammatory disease of the lungs characterized by typically reversible airway obstruction) and COPD have respiratory distress from a functional narrowing of the conducting airways. As a result, these patients report that they feel as though they are breathing through a straw. Spasm of the bronchial smooth muscle, also known as **bronchospasm**, results in a decrease in the airway diameter.

Another factor that contributes to respiratory distress is edema of the mucosa that lines the respiratory tract. This inflammatory edema results in a thickening of the mucosal linings and a resultant decrease in airway diameter. Increased secretions also contribute to the distress of these patients. Any reduction of the radius of the airway, from either broncho-spasm or mucosal edema, can have a profound effect on the flow of gas.

Poiseuille's law is the law of physics that determines the resistance and flow of gas. This law states that the flow of gas through a tube is proportional to the radius of the airway to the fourth power. Therefore, if the radius of an airway decreases from 4 to 3 mm from broncho-spasm or mucosal edema, the potential flow of gas decreases by almost one-third from even this small reduction in the airway.

The first thing the patient in the preceding scenario needs is supplemental oxygen. After oxygen, administration of an inhaled **bronchodilator** would be appropriate.

Bronchodilators can be divided into selective and nonselective agents. Selective agents act preferentially on the bronchial smooth muscle and improve the patient's condition while minimizing side effects. Beta$_2$ agonists are sympathomimetic medications that target the beta$_2$ receptors and cause relaxation of bronchial smooth muscle without stimulating tachycardia or hypertension. Most of these medications are selective for the beta$_2$ receptor; however, para-medics must be cautious because excessive doses can produce the undesirable effects seen with alpha and beta$_1$ stimulation (e.g., tachycardia and hypertension). Use beta$_2$ agonists with caution in patients with a history of heart disease, and always monitor the electrocardiogram during and after treatments. Examples of beta$_2$ agonists include albuterol (Proventil), terbu-taline (Brethine), formoterol (Foradil), and pirbuterol (Maxair).

Nonselective agents act on alpha, beta$_1$, and beta$_2$ adrenergic receptors. Stimulation of the alpha receptors causes constriction of peripheral blood vessels and results in blood pressure elevation. Beta$_1$ receptors, which are predominantly located in cardiac tissue, increase heart rate and cardiac contractility when stimulated. Stimulation of the beta$_2$ receptors results in bronchodilation by relaxation of bronchial smooth muscle. Racemic epinephrine is an exam-ple of a nonselective bronchodilator.

▶ Inhalation Delivery of Medications

The delivery of beta$_2$-specific medications can be accomplished by **nebulization**, parenteral administration, and oral administration. A nebulizer is an instrument that converts a liquid medication into a fine mist to be inhaled. A pneumatic nebulizer uses a gas as the driving force to make this conversion. Ultrasonic nebulizers use ultrasonic sound to convert the liq-uid medication to an inhalable mist. A metered-dose inhaler (MDI) is a pressurized medica-tion chamber that delivers the medication by a propellant spray. The goal of nebulization is to deliver small particles of the medication directly to the receptor sites in the lung by inhalation. To achieve this goal, many variables must be addressed. First, particle size of the nebulized medication is of critical importance. Medication particles that are too large are deposited in the oral pharynx or upper airway, and the medication never makes its way to the lung. Conversely, if the particles of medication are too small, they become suspended in the source gas, inhaled, and exhaled again—without depositing the medication at the target site.

The mechanics of delivering inhaled medications can be accomplished in two basic ways: the MDI and the pneumatically powered nebulizer.

NEBULIZATION THERAPY

Equipment Needed:
Nebulizer unit, tubing, oxygen source, medication
Procedure:
1. Observe standard precautions.
2. Verify the drug order.
3. Confirm right patient, right medication, right dose, right route, and right time.
4. When possible, explain to the patient what medication you are going to administer and why.

5. Prepare all necessary equipment and the medication to be administered.
6. Expose the medication cup by unscrewing the lid. Add the medication to the cup, and reattach the lid.
7. Attach the mouthpiece and the tubing to the nebulizer.
8. Connect the oxygen-connecting hose to the appropriate connector on the nebulizer cup.
9. Attach the other end of the oxygen tubing to an oxygen source, and adjust the flow of oxygen to 6 L/min. A mist should come out of the mouthpiece.
10. Instruct the patient to hold the nebulizer mouthpiece in his or her mouth and breathe as deeply as possible. This process should be continued until the liquid has been used up.
11. Monitor the patient throughout the treatment, and reassess ventilatory adequacy and vital signs after the treatment has been completed. Compare findings with the patient's pretreatment ventilatory adequacy.
12. Repeat the treatment if needed, and provide supplemental oxygen as needed.
13. Record the time of drug administration in the patient care record.
14. Evaluate the patient for desired effects of the medication, as well as any adverse effects. Continued reevaluation should occur throughout transport.

Metered-Dose Inhaler

The MDI delivers a predetermined amount of mediation in the correct particle size propelled by a small amount of gas. The MDI unit comes with two parts: the canister and mouthpiece (**FIGURE 14-5**).

Although they may look as simple as an ordinary spray can, MDIs are more complicated. Remember, particle size is critical. If an MDI is used improperly, the medication will not reach its intended site in the lung.

Imagine driving a car on a curvy mountain road. Experienced drivers know that when approaching a sharp curve they need to slow down to make the curve. If they do not, the car's excessive forward speed will create a momentum that cannot be overcome; the car will hit the guardrail and slide off the road. A similar problem can be encountered with MDIs. Often the propellant in the MDI canister jettisons the medication particles at a rapid speed. The oropharynx, like the mountain road, has several rather sharp curves. If the medication particles move too rapidly, they cannot negotiate the curves of the oropharynx and slam into the walls of the oropharynx. The result is that the medication does not reach the intended site in the lung.

The use of a **spacer device** can facilitate slower movement of the medication particles (**FIGURE 14-6**). The spacer slows the forward movement of the medication particles. When a spacer device is not available, holding the MDI approximately 2 inches (5 cm) from the

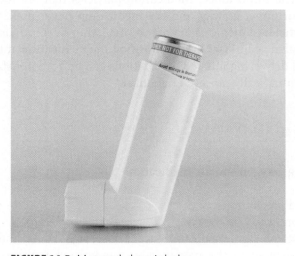

FIGURE 14-5 Metered-dose inhaler.
© Khuntapol/ Getty Images.

FIGURE 14-6 Metered-dose inhaler with spacer.
© Rob Byron/Shutterstock.

mouth also causes the particles to slow before entering the oropharynx, achieving an effect similar to that of the spacer device.

The development of MDIs has allowed patients to carry their rescue medications with them wherever they go. Many EMS systems use MDIs to care for acute bronchospasm. Continuing with the example of driving on a mountain road, a large portion of the medication will not be able to negotiate the many sharp curves of the oropharynx. Much of the medication is deposited on the walls of the oropharynx, resulting in less medication reaching the intended target. If moderate to severe bronchospasm exists, the medication never fully reaches the target sites secondary to the bronchospasm itself. Use of an MDI spacer combined with proper inhalation timing and technique improves medication delivery to receptor sites within the lungs. There is a wide variety of studies and articles that compare the efficacy of nebulizers to MDIs. A larger meta-analysis demonstrated some superiority of an MDI/spacer combination over nebulizers in the setting of asthma.[5]

Determining whether actual medication remains in an MDI can be quite challenging. Counting the number of administered puffs and comparing that number to the capacity on the MDI label is the most accurate method of determining whether medication remains in an MDI. Most patients are not able to keep an accurate count of "puffs" administered, particularly with irregular use of a medication MDI. Methods such as shaking an MDI or performing a "float test" are notoriously inaccurate.[6] Many patients mistakenly believe they are receiving medication from an MDI long after the medication has been exhausted and only propellant remains in the MDI.

METERED-DOSE INHALER

Equipment Needed:
MDI with medication, personal protective equipment (PPE)
Procedure:
 1. Observe standard precautions.
 2. Verify the drug order.
 3. Confirm right patient, right medication, right dose, right route, and right time.
 4. Confirm with the patient that he or she has no allergies to the medication, and document allergies to any other medication.
 5. When possible, explain to the patient what medication you are going to administer and why.
 6. Shake the inhaler for 5 to 10 seconds.
 7. Insert the outlet tube into the patient's mouth.

8. Direct the patient to squeeze the ends of the medication canister to deliver the medication.
9. Instruct the patient to inhale a slow, full, deep breath.
10. Instruct the patient to hold the breath for up to 5 seconds if possible.
11. Repeat if indicated.
12. Record the time of drug administration in the patient care record.
13. Evaluate the patient for desired effects of the medication, as well as any adverse effects. Continued reevaluation should occur throughout transport.

METERED-DOSE INHALER WITH A SPACER

Equipment Needed:
MDI with medication, spacer, PPE
Procedure:
1. Observe standard precautions.
2. Verify the drug order.
3. Confirm right patient, right medication, right dose, right route, and right time.
4. Confirm with the patient that he or she has no allergies to the medication, and document allergies to any other medication.
5. When possible, explain to the patient what medication you are going to administer and why.
6. Shake the inhaler for 5 to 10 seconds.
7. Insert the outlet tube into the spacer.
8. Instruct the patient to place the spacer device into his or her mouth and close the lips over it.
9. Direct the patient to squeeze the ends of the medication canister to deliver the medication.
10. Instruct the patient to inhale a slow, full, deep breath.
11. Instruct the patient to hold the breath for up to 10 seconds if possible.
12. Wait approximately 60 seconds and repeat.
13. Reassess breath sounds, vital signs, and ventilations.
14. Record the time of drug administration in the patient care record.
15. Evaluate the patient for desired effects of the medication, as well as any adverse effects. Continued reevaluation should occur throughout transport.

▶ Overview of Asthma

(*continued*) You determine that the patient is having an asthma attack, likely initiated from exercise. He tells you that he has an inhaler in his gym bag, and you send the gym teacher to retrieve it. The teacher returns minutes later carrying the patient's inhaler. You inspect the label. The name on the label matches that of the patient, and the medication is albuterol. You ask the patient whether he needs your assistance to take the medication. He replies, "I think I need your help." You take the inhaler and shake it 10 times. You then tell the patient that you are going to administer the medication by MDI and instruct him to take a slow, deep breath and hold the breath for 5 seconds if he can. You administer the medication and repeat the process. The patient initially coughs after your administration of the MDI, but his respirations then begin to deepen and slow.

Although many consider asthma to be a relatively mild breathing condition that can be quickly alleviated, more than 3,600 Americans die each year from asthma attacks according to the Centers for Disease Control and Prevention.[7] Over 24 million people in the

United States have been diagnosed with asthma, resulting in over 2 million emergency department visits each year.

Acute asthma attacks can affect patients of all ages. Asthma is caused by a trigger reaction. Triggers can be either **intrinsic** (within the body) or **extrinsic** (outside the body). Examples of intrinsic triggers include exertion, such as an attack triggered by exercise, and anxiety related to stress. Examples of external triggers are reactions to animal dander, dust, insect droppings, pollen, and cleaning chemicals.

Management

A main focus in management of asthma is for the patient to avoid the triggers that initiate attacks whenever possible and mitigate the effects of these triggers. When EMS is called, these goals have not been achieved and patient management is aimed at the reversal of acute bronchospasm. Although parenteral medications can be used to treat patients with asthma, the first line of medications is inhaled beta$_2$-specific drugs. If inhaled bronchodilators fail, intravenous (IV) medications are then administered to reduce bronchospasm and inflammation.

Albuterol (Proventil, Ventolin) is by far the most common inhaled drug used to treat reversible bronchospasm. Albuterol is one of several inhaled bronchodilators that have been developed to target only the beta$_2$ receptor. Prior beta$_2$ agonists had varying degrees of effect on alpha and beta$_1$ receptors, and stimulation of these sites may cause unwanted reactions in already compromised patients (**TABLE 14-3**). For example, stimulation of alpha receptors could cause unwanted vasoconstriction, and stimulation of beta$_1$ receptors could cause increased heart rate. As such, more time between treatments was required to compensate for the unwanted, predominantly beta$_1$, adverse effects. Levalbuterol (Xopenex) is a newer "purified" version of albuterol, which had been believed to cause fewer adverse effects than albuterol. Both appear to be quite effective in acute treatment of asthma exacerbations. Recent studies do not support changing from albuterol to levalbuterol in most situations.[8–10]

The first-generation drugs had significant beta$_1$ effects along with beta$_2$ effects. Second-generation drugs were more beta$_2$ specific but would still increase heart rate and could not be given close together. Finally, third-generation medications predominantly targeted the beta$_2$ receptors. When given by inhalation and specifically targeting the smooth muscle in the airways, they had little or no systemic effect. Without these systemic effects, multiple and continuous treatments could be given for moderate to severe exacerbations.

Ipratropium bromide (Atrovent) is used in more severe exacerbations of asthma or in cases in which the patient has a limited response to treatment with albuterol. Ipratropium

TABLE 14-3 Sympathomimetic Properties of Various Generations of Bronchodilators			
	Alpha	**Beta₁**	**Beta₂**
Generation 1 (Isuprel)	+	+++++	+++++
Generation 2 (Bronkosol)	0	+++	++++
Generation 3 (Albuterol)	0	+	+++++
Epinephrine	++++	++++++	+++++

Plus signs indicate relative efficacy.

© Jones & Bartlett Learning.

bromide is not an adrenergic agent but is considered an anticholinergic. In more severe cases of bronchospasm, additional treatment with ipratropium bromide has provided greater symptomatic relief than albuterol used as a single agent.[11] Adrenergic agents such as albuterol act more centrally in the bronchial tree, whereas cholinergic agents such as ipratropium are more effective in the peripheral airways. Adrenergic agents are more effective in asthma, whereas the peripheral action of ipratropium provides greater benefits in patients with COPD.

Albuterol/ipratropium (Combivent) is a combination product that takes advantage of the different mechanisms of action and anatomic sites of action of albuterol and ipratropium bromide to deliver both medications in a single preparation.

ALBUTEROL (PROVENTIL, VENTOLIN)

Classification: Bronchodilator, beta agonist.
Action: Binds and stimulates beta$_2$ receptors, resulting in relaxation of bronchial smooth muscle.
Indications: Asthma, bronchitis with bronchospasm, and COPD.
Adverse Effects: Hyperglycemia, hypokalemia, palpitations, sinus tachycardia, anxiety, tremor, nausea/vomiting, throat irritation, dry mouth, hypertension, dyspepsia, insomnia, headache, epistaxis, paradoxical bronchospasm.
Contraindications: Angioedema, sensitivity to albuterol or levalbuterol. Use with caution in lactating patients, cardiovascular disorders, cardiac arrhythmias.

© Joseph Gaul/Alamy Stock Photo.

Dosage:
Acute Bronchospasm:
- **Adult:**
  - **MDI:** Four to eight puffs every 1 to 4 hours may be required.
  - **Nebulizer:** 2.5 to 5 mg every 20 minutes for a maximum of three doses. After the initial three doses, escalate the dose or start a continuous nebulization at 10 to 15 mg/hr.
- **Pediatric:**
  - **MDI:**
    - **4 years and older:** Two inhalations every 4 to 6 hours; however, in some patients, one inhalation every 4 hours is sufficient. More frequent administration or more inhalations are not recommended.
    - **Younger than 4 years:** Administer by nebulization.
  - **Nebulizer:**
    - **Older than 12 years:** The dose for a continuous nebulization is 0.5 mg/kg per hour.
    - **Younger than 12 years:** 0.63 to 2.5 mg every 20 minutes for a maximum of three doses. Alternatively, continuous nebulization at 0.5 mg/kg per hour can be delivered to children younger than 12 years.

Asthma in Pregnancy:
- **MDI:** Two inhalations every 4 hours. In acute exacerbation, start with two to four puffs every 20 minutes.
- **Nebulizer:** 2.5 mg (0.5 mL) by 0.5% nebulization solution. Place 0.5 mL of the albuterol solution in 2.5 mL of sterile normal saline. Flow is regulated to deliver the therapy over a 5- to 20-minute period. In refractory cases, some physicians order 10 mg nebulized over a 60-minute period.

Special Considerations:
Pregnancy class C.

LEVALBUTEROL (XOPENEX)

Classification: Beta agonist.
Action: Stimulates beta$_2$ receptors, resulting in relaxation of the smooth muscle in the lungs, uterus, and vasculature that supply skeletal muscle.
Indications: Acute bronchospasm or bronchospasm prophylaxis in patient with asthma.
Adverse Effects: Hyperglycemia, hypokalemia, palpitations, sinus tachycardia, anxiety, tremor, nausea/vomiting, throat irritation, hypertension, dyspepsia, insomnia, headache.

Contraindications: Angioedema, sensitivity to albuterol or levalbuterol. Use with caution in lactating patients, cardiovascular disorders, cardiac arrhythmias. Do not use in patients taking phenothiazines because this may cause prolonged QT interval and cardiac arrhythmias. Also avoid use in patients getting sotalol or other beta blockers because they may decrease bronchodilating effects and cause bronchospasm, prolonged QT interval, and cardiac arrhythmias.
Dosage:
MDI:

- **Adult:** Two inhalations every 4 to 6 hours. In some patients, one inhalation may be sufficient. For acute exacerbations, four to eight inhalations every 20 minutes up to 4 hours, then every 1 to 4 hours as needed (off label).
- **Pediatric:**
  ○ **4 to 12 years:** Two inhalations every 4 to 6 hours. In some patients, one inhalation may be sufficient. For acute exacerbations, four to eight inhalations every 20 minutes for three doses, then two to four inhalations every 1 to 4 hours as needed.
  ○ **Younger than 4 years:** Safe and effective use has not been established. For acute exacerbations, two to four inhalations using a valved holding chamber and face mask every 20 minutes for three doses, then two to four inhalations every 1 to 4 hours as needed.

Nebulizer:

- **Adult:** Usually, 0.63 mg 3 times/day. For acute exacerbations, 1.25 to 2.5 mg every 20 minutes for three doses, then 1.25 to 5 mg every 1 to 4 hours as needed.
- **Pediatric:**
  ○ **6 to 11 years:** Usually, 0.31 mg 3 times/day. For acute exacerbations, 0.075 mg/kg (1.25 mg minimum) every 20 minutes for three doses, then 0.075 to 0.15 mg/kg (5 mg maximum) every 1 to 4 hours as needed.
  ○ **Younger than 6 years:** Safe and effective use has not been established. For acute exacerbations, 1.25 to 2.5 mg every 20 minutes for three doses, then 1.25 to 5 mg every 1 to 4 hours as needed.

Special Considerations:
Pregnancy class C.

IPRATROPIUM BROMIDE (ATROVENT)

Classification: Bronchodilator, anticholinergic.
Action: Antagonizes the acetylcholine receptor on bronchial smooth muscle, producing bronchodilation.
Indications: Asthma, bronchospasm associated with COPD.
Adverse Effects: Paradoxical acute bronchospasm, cough, throat irritation, headache, dizziness, dry mouth, palpitations.
Contraindications: Closed-angle glaucoma, bladder neck obstruction, prostatic hypertrophy, known sensitivity including peanuts or soybeans and atropine or atropine derivatives.

(continues)

IPRATROPIUM BROMIDE (ATROVENT) *(continued)*

Dosage:
MDI:

- **Adult:** Eight inhalations every 20 minutes for up to 3 hours.
- **Pediatric: <12 years:** Four to eight inhalations every 20 minutes for up to 3 hours.

Nebulization:

- **Adult:** 0.5 mg every 20 minutes for three doses, then as needed.
- **Pediatric: 5 to 14 years:** 0.25 to 0.5 mg every 20 minutes for three doses as needed.

Special Considerations:
Ipratropium bromide is not typically used as a sole medication in the treatment of acute exacerbation of asthma. Ipratropium bromide is commonly administered after a beta agonist. Care should be taken to not allow the aerosol spray (especially in the MDI) to come into contact with the eyes. This can cause temporary blurring of vision that resolves without intervention within 4 hours.
Pregnancy class B.

ALBUTEROL/IPRATROPIUM (COMBIVENT; DUONEB)

Classification: Combination bronchodilator.
Action: Binds and stimulates beta$_2$ receptors, resulting in relaxation of bronchial smooth muscle, and antagonizes the acetylcholine receptor, producing bronchodilation.
Indications: Second-line treatment (if bronchodilator is ineffective) in COPD or severe acute asthma exacerbations during medical transport.
Adverse Effects: Headache, cough, nausea, arrhythmias, paradoxical acute bronchospasm.
Contraindications: Allergy to soybeans or peanuts; known sensitivity to atropine, albuterol, or their respective derivatives. Used with caution in patients with asthma, hypertension, angina, cardiac arrhythmias, tachycardia, cardiovascular disease, congenital long QT syndrome, closed-angle glaucoma.
Dosage:
MDI:

- **Adult:** Eight inhalations every 20 minutes for up to 3 hours.

Nebulization:

- **Adult:** 3 mL every 20 minutes for three doses, then as needed.

Special Considerations:
Pregnancy class C.

Second-Line Therapy for Acute Exacerbation of Asthma

The clinical picture of a patient having an asthma attack or exacerbation of COPD is that of a patient gasping for breath, using accessory muscles of respiration, and wheezing. In asthma and COPD, bronchodilators provide symptomatic therapy but do not directly treat the underlying and initiating lung condition. In cases in which a prolonged transport time is likely, consider corticosteroids to treat the inflammatory processes involved in both asthma and COPD. The most commonly used corticosteroids are methylprednisolone and dexamethasone. Both appear to be equally effective in managing moderate or severe asthma symptoms.[12] If there are concerns regarding patient compliance, providers may choose to administer a single dose of dexamethasone over a longer oral course of another corticosteroid.

Peak expiratory flow rate (PEFR) is an objective assessment that can guide a provider's determination of the severity of an exacerbation; the patient's response to therapy; and the indication for therapy, such as the start of steroids. When the initial PEFR is less than 50% of predicted, corticosteroids should be administered after ipratropium bromide administration. Corticosteroids should also be considered when the PEFR does not improve by at least 10% after bronchodilator therapy or when the PEFR is less than 70% after 1 hour of therapy.

Aminophylline and other methylxanthines work to reduce the smooth muscle bronchospasm associated with acute respiratory distress. These medications were once routinely administered as second-line agents for severe asthma exacerbations. Their role has greatly diminished and they are no longer recommended as routine therapies.[13]

Magnesium sulfate has been demonstrated to decrease bronchospasm in a subset of asthmatic patients. Patients who do not show an adequate response to beta$_2$ agonist medications can have a favorable response to magnesium sulfate. Magnesium sulfate should not be used in all patients having an asthmatic attack; however, consider using magnesium in patients who do not improve after beta agonist therapy.

For years, epinephrine administered subcutaneously was the treatment of choice for young patients with asthma. Epinephrine does have strong and desirable beta$_2$ effects; however, it also has strong and undesirable alpha and beta$_1$ effects. Rebound bronchospasm can be a secondary problem with the administration of epinephrine in the management of an asthma attack. Although epinephrine is effective when initially administered, its effects are short-lived. If considering epinephrine for use in adults with asthma, do not underestimate beta$_1$-mediated cardiac complications such as tachycardia and hypertension. For these reasons, epinephrine should be used with caution, if at all, in the treatment of the patient with asthma. Epinephrine may still be indicated if an anaphylactic reaction is suspected.[13]

DEXAMETHASONE (DECADRON)

Classification: Corticosteroid.
Action: Reduces inflammation by multiple mechanisms.
Indications: Anti-inflammatory agent for a wide variety of medical conditions, including asthma, airway edema, acute mountain sickness, cerebral edema, etc.
Adverse Effects: Depression, euphoria, headache, restlessness, hypertension, bradycardia, nausea/vomiting, swelling, diarrhea, weakness, fluid retention, paresthesias.
Contraindications: Fungal infection, known sensitivity (including sulfites). Use with caution in active infections, renal disease, penetrating spinal cord injury.
Dosage:
Numerous dosing options for a wide variety of adult and pediatric indications, including asthma
Special Considerations:
Parenteral formulation may also be administered orally if needed.
Pregnancy class C.

METHYLPREDNISOLONE SODIUM SUCCINATE (SOLU-MEDROL)

Classification: Corticosteroid.
Action: Reduces inflammation by multiple mechanisms.
Indications: Anaphylaxis, asthma, COPD.
Adverse Effects: Depression, euphoria, headache, restlessness, hypertension, bradycardia, nausea/vomiting, swelling, diarrhea, weakness, fluid retention, paresthesias.
Contraindications: Cushing syndrome, fungal infection, measles, varicella, known sensitivity (including sulfites). Use with caution in active infections, renal disease, penetrating spinal cord injury, hypertension, seizures, heart failure.
Dosage:
Asthma and Chronic Obstructive Pulmonary Disease:
- **Adult:** 40 to 80 mg/day IV in divided doses.
- **Pediatric:** 1 mg/kg (up to 60 mg) IV, intraosseous (IO) per day in two divided doses.
Anaphylactic Shock:
- **Adult:** 0.5 to 1 mg/kg IV every 12 hours.
- **Pediatric:** Same as adult dosing.
Special Considerations:
May mask signs and symptoms of infection.
Pregnancy class C.

MAGNESIUM SULFATE

Classification: Electrolyte, tocolytic, mineral.
Action: Required for normal physiologic functioning. Magnesium is a cofactor in neurochemical transmission and muscular excitability. Magnesium sulfate controls seizures by blocking peripheral neuromuscular transmission. Magnesium is also a peripheral vasodilator and an inhibitor of platelet function.
Indications: Torsades de pointes, cardiac arrhythmias associated with hypomagnesemia, eclampsia and seizure prophylaxis in preeclampsia, status asthmaticus.
Adverse Effects: Magnesium toxicity (signs include flushing, diaphoresis, hypotension, muscle paralysis, weakness, hypothermia, and cardiac, central nervous system, or respiratory depression).
Contraindications: Atrioventricular block, gastrointestinal obstruction. Use with caution in renal impairment.
Dosage:
Pulseless Ventricular Fibrillation/Ventricular Tachycardia with Torsades de Pointes or Hypomagnesemia:
- **Adult:** 1 to 2 g in 10 mL D_5W IV, IO administered over 15 minutes or faster with cardiac arrest.
- **Pediatric:** 25 to 50 mg/kg IV, IO over 10 to 20 minutes; may administer faster for torsades de pointes (max single dose: 2 g).
Torsades de Pointes with a Pulse or Cardiac Arrhythmias with Hypomagnesemia:
- **Adult:** 1 to 2 g in 50 to 100 mL D_5W IV, IO administered over 5 to 60 minutes. Follow with 0.5 to 1 g/hr IV, IO titrated to control torsades de pointes.
- **Pediatric:** 25 to 50 mg/kg IV, IO over 10 to 20 minutes (max single dose: 2 g).
Eclampsia and Seizure Prophylaxis in Preeclampsia:
- **Adult:** 4 to 6 g IV, IO over 20 to 30 minutes, followed by an infusion of 1 to 2 g/hr.
Status Asthmaticus:
- **Adult:** 1.2 to 2 g slow IV, IO (over 20 minutes).
- **Pediatric:** 25 to 50 mg/kg (diluted in D_5W) slow IV, IO (over 10–20 minutes).
Special Considerations:
Pregnancy class A.

RACEMIC EPINEPHRINE/RACEPINEPHRINE (MICRONEFRIN, S₂)

Classification: Bronchodilator, adrenergic agent.
Action: Stimulates both alpha and beta receptors, causing vasoconstriction, reduced mucosal edema, and bronchodilation.
Indications: Bronchial asthma, croup.
Adverse Effects: Anxiety, dizziness, headache, tremor, palpitations, tachycardia, cardiac arrhythmias, hypertension, nausea/vomiting.
Contraindications: Glaucoma, elderly, cardiac disease, hypertension, thyroid disease, diabetes, known sensitivity to sulfites.
Dosage:

- 2.25% solution; 0.05 to 0.1 mL/kg (maximum dose 0.5 mL)
- **Adult:** Add 0.5 mL to nebulizer; for hand-bulb nebulizer, administer one to three inhalations; for jet nebulizer, add 3 mL of diluent, swirl the nebulizer, and administer for 15 minutes.

Special Considerations:
Monitor blood pressure, heart rate, and cardiac rhythm for changes. Onset of action is 1 to 5 minutes, effects may persist for 1 to 3 hours. Pregnancy class C.

© Jones & Bartlett Learning.

▶ Chronic Obstructive Pulmonary Disease

COPD is the classification for diseases that cause obstruction in the pulmonary tree. The two most common diseases are emphysema and chronic bronchitis. Both pathologic conditions cause an increase in sputum production and resultant bronchospasm. As the increase in sputum worsens, so can the irritation and the bronchospasm. Initial treatment of mild to moderate COPD exacerbation is aimed at reducing bronchospasm and mobilizing and clearing the sputum from the airways.

Management

In severe exacerbations, treatment is first aimed at oxygenation and ventilation of the patient. Oxygenation needs to be provided with care. Patients with a long-standing history of COPD breathe on what is known as a **hypoxic respiratory drive**. This means that the patient requires a mild degree of hypoxia to continue breathing. If the patient is given too much oxygen, the hypoxic respiratory drive is removed, as well as the patient's stimulus for spontaneous respirations. Therefore, when monitoring these patients, an SaO_2 level in the low 90s as measured by pulse oximetry is considered adequate.

Bronchodilators and steroids are used to manage COPD in a similar fashion as for the treatment of asthma. A detailed discussion of the treatment of pulmonary edema is found in Chapter 10.

▶ Review Questions

1. Explain how FiO_2 is related to the amount of oxygen delivered to the heart and tissues.
2. Explain the difference between a rebreather face mask and a nonrebreather face mask.
3. What class of drugs typically is used in the treatment of bronchospasm, and on what receptors do these drugs act?
4. What are two methods of delivering medications directly to the respiratory bronchioles?
5. What occurs when the particle size of a nebulized medication is too small or too large?
6. What is the purpose of using a spacer device with an MDI?
7. What is the main goal in the management of a patient with asthma?
8. Explain the concept of hypoxic respiratory drive in patients with COPD.

References

1. Stiell IG, Spaite DW, Field B, et al. Advanced life support for out-of-hospital respiratory distress. *N Engl J Med.* 2007;356(21):2156–2164.

2. Lellouche F, Lipes J, L'Her E. Optimal oxygen titration in patients with chronic obstructive pulmonary disease: a role for automated oxygen delivery? *Can Respirat J.* 2013;20(4):259–261.

3. Rawat M, Chandrasekharan PK, Swartz DD, et al. Neonatal resuscitation adhering to oxygen saturation guidelines in asphyxiated lambs with meconium aspiration. *Pediatr Res.* 2016;79(4):583–588.

4. Cornet AD, Kooter AJ, Peters MJ, Smulders YM. The potential harm of oxygen therapy in medical emergencies. *Crit Care.* 2013;17(2):313.

5. Cates CJ, Welsh EJ, Rowe BH. Holding chambers (spacers) versus nebulisers for beta-agonist treatment of acute asthma. *Cochrane Database Syst Rev.* 2013. doi:10.1002/14651858.CD000052.pub3

6. Rubin BK, Durotoye L. How do patients determine that their metered-dose inhaler is empty? *Chest.* 2004;126(4):1134–1137.

7. Centers for Disease Control and Prevention (CDC), National Center for Health Statistics. Asthma. https://www.cdc.gov/nchs/fastats/asthma.htm. Updated March 31, 2017. Accessed August 20, 2018.

8. Brunetti L, Poiani G, Dhanaliwala F, Poppiti K, Kang H, Suh D-C. Clinical outcomes and treatment cost comparison of levalbuterol versus albuterol in hospitalized adults with chronic obstructive pulmonary disease or asthma. *Am J Health-Syst Pharm.* 2015;72(12):1026–1035.

9. Ameredes BT, Calhoun WJ. Levalbuterol versus albuterol. *Curr Allergy Asthma Rep.* 2009;9(5):401–409.

10. Khorfan FM, Smith P, Watt S, Barber KR. Effects of nebulized bronchodilator therapy on hear rate and arrhythmias in critically ill adult patients. *Chest J.* 2011;140(6):1466–1472.

11. Donohue JF, Wise R, Busse W, et al. Efficacy and safety of ipratropium bromide/albuterol compared with albuterol in patients with moderate-to-severe asthma: a randomized controlled trial. *BMC Pulmonary Med.* 2016;16:65.

12. Scarfone RJ. Acute asthma exacerbations in children: emergency department management. UpToDate. https://www.uptodate.com/contents/acute-asthma-exacerbations-in-children-emergency-department-management. Updated February 23, 2018. Accessed October 4, 2018.

13. Fanta CH. Management of acute exacerbations of asthma in adults. UpToDate. https://www.uptodate.com/contents/management-of-acute-exacerbations-of-asthma-in-adults?topicRef=547&source=see_link. Updated April 9, 2018. Accessed August 20, 2018.

CHAPTER 15

Seizures

OBJECTIVES

1. Demonstrate the proper procedure for rectal administration of diazepam, and discuss why rectal administration is sometimes necessary for a patient having a seizure.
2. Discuss benzodiazepines used in the treatment of seizures: diazepam (Valium) and lorazepam (Ativan).
3. Discuss other anticonvulsants (nonbenzodiazepines) used in the treatment of seizures: felbamate (Felbatol), phenytoin (Dilantin), carbamazepine (Tegretol), levetiracetam (Keppra), phenobarbital (Luminal), valproic acid (Depakote), gabapentin (Neurontin), and lamotrigine (Lamictal).

MEDICATIONS THAT APPEAR IN CHAPTER 15

Diazepam (Valium)   Fosphenytoin (Cerebyx)   Valproic acid (Depakote)
Lorazepam (Ativan)   Carbamazepine (Tegretol)   Gabapentin (Neurontin)
Felbamate (Felbatol)   Levetiracetam (Keppra)   Lamotrigine (Lamictal)
Phenytoin (Dilantin)   Phenobarbital (Luminal)

▶ Introduction

Seizure activity is a common emergency that requires prompt management by prehospital professionals. Although most seizures stop without treatment, if a paramedic arrives on the scene of a patient in active seizure, the patient is likely to be in **status epilepticus**.[1] Status epilepticus is defined as a single seizure lasting longer than 5 minutes, continuous seizure activity for longer than 30 minutes, or a series of seizures without full recovery of consciousness between seizures. Status epilepticus affects approximately 60,000 people in the United States each year, with the majority being children. An estimated 5 to 8% of EMS calls involve seizures.[2] Because prolonged seizure activity can lead to brain damage and poor functional status, one of the most important determinants of outcome is duration of seizure activity. Paramedics must know how to manage seizures. Seizure activity is the result of chaotic, abnormal, high-frequency firing of neurons, which can cause an alteration in level of consciousness. On examination, patients having a seizure can display jerking movements referred to as **tonic-clonic seizures**. These patients often have an altered mental status, abnormal eye movement, and incontinence of bowel or bladder. Other types of seizures include "absence" episodes, in which the person appears conscious yet demonstrates pauses in interaction and awareness. Patients may have a "focal" seizure, affecting only a small portion of the brain, with symptoms such as an unusual taste or transient confusion.

CASE STUDY

You receive a call that a 13-year-old boy was found to be unresponsive by his mother at home. According to the mother, the child has had seizures in the past but they have been controlled for the last 12 years with medication. On arrival, the boy is lying supine on the floor and making tonic-clonic, jerking movements. His eyes are rolled back in his head, and he does not respond to stimulation. His pants are wet and you smell urine.

▶ Management

The initial management of seizure activity in both children and adults hinges on maintaining an adequate airway and providing supplemental oxygen, as well as continually assessing that the patient is breathing adequately. Additionally, paramedics should take action to protect the patient from injury by removing the patient from an environment in which he or she is at risk for injury during convulsions. Once a patent airway has been established and adequate oxygenation and ventilation are ensured, the paramedic should attempt to secure venous access for the administration of medication to stop seizure activity.[3]

In this scenario, the initial management of this patient in the midst of active seizure activity includes turning the patient on his side to clear the airway. The next steps would be to quickly ensure that the patient is breathing adequately, administer supplemental oxygen, and obtain an initial set of vital signs. Finally, while attempting to secure vascular access to treat the seizure with intravenous (IV) diazepam (Valium), the provider should take a brief history from the mother to identify any significant medical history, such as diabetes with hypoglycemia; previous seizure history; known medications, including **anticonvulsants**; possible intoxicants; and recreational drugs. The management of hypoglycemia, which is a common cause of seizures, is addressed in Chapter 11.

Benzodiazepines

The mainstay of management for seizure activity and status epilepticus is the administration of anticonvulsant agents. The most common class of agents used in the initial management of seizure activity, particularly in the prehospital setting, are the benzodiazepines.[4] Benzodiazepines are used as the initial class of drugs to stop seizure activity because their principal pharmacologic effects are mitigated through **gamma-aminobutyric acid (GABA)**, an inhibitory neurotransmitter in the central nervous system (CNS).[5] The concept of a receptor was introduced in Chapter 1. GABA is a type of receptor in the CNS. When a drug like benzodiazepine binds with the GABA receptor, the result is inhibition or a decrease in the activity of the CNS. The inhibition of the nervous system is manifested as sedation or the cessation of seizures. Two benzodiazepines commonly used to treat seizure activity are diazepam and lorazepam (Ativan). Both medications have similar efficacy and safety characteristics.[6]

Midazolam (Versed) can also be used to stop an active seizure. Intranasal administration of midazolam has shown to be both safe and effective, causing cessation of seizure activity quicker than rectal diazepam. Midazolam has a shorter duration of action than other benzodiazepines, which may require repeat doses and closer monitoring.

The short half-life of midazolam makes this drug a poor choice when treating seizures.

Starting an IV line in a patient who is actively seizing is a difficult task. Administration of diazepam rectally allows easy access to obtain a rapid blood level of this medication.

RECTAL ADMINISTRATION OF DIAZEPAM

Equipment Needed:
Two 3-mL syringes, 5F feeding tube, saline flush, water-soluble lubricant
Procedure:
1. Observe standard precautions.
2. Verify the drug order.
3. Confirm right patient, right medication, right dose, right route, and right time.
4. Confirm with the patient that he or she has no allergies to the medication, and document allergies to any other medication.
5. When possible, explain to the patient what medication you are going to administer and why.
6. Draw the desired dose of the medication into a 3-mL syringe.
7. Attach a 5F feeding tube to the 3-mL syringe.
8. Into a second 3-mL syringe, draw 1 mL of normal saline to be used as a flush.
9. Ensure that the airway is controlled and patent.
10. Place the patient on his or her side with knees bent toward the chest. Alternatively, with the patient in the supine position, have someone help spread the patient's legs.
11. Apply a water-soluble lubricant (e.g., K-Y Jelly, Johnson & Johnson, New Brunswick, New Jersey) to the tip of the catheter.
12. Introduce the lubricated catheter into the rectum and advance approximately 1 inch (2.5 cm).
13. Inject the diazepam through the catheter, and then flush the feeding catheter with the saline flush.
14. Withdraw the catheter and dispose of it properly.
15. Record the time of drug administration in the patient care record.
16. Evaluate the patient for desired effects of the medication, as well as any adverse effects. Continued reevaluation should occur throughout transport.

DIAZEPAM (VALIUM)

Classification: Benzodiazepine, Schedule C-IV.
Action: Binds to the benzodiazepine receptor and enhances the effects of GABA. Benzodiazepines act at the level of the limbic, thalamic, and hypothalamic regions of the CNS and can produce any level of CNS depression required (including sedation, skeletal muscle relaxation, and anticonvulsant activity).
Indications: Anxiety, skeletal muscle relaxation, alcohol withdrawal, seizures.
Adverse Effects: Respiratory depression, drowsiness, fatigue, headache, pain at the injection site, confusion, nausea, hypotension, oversedation.

(continues)

DIAZEPAM (VALIUM) *(continued)*

Contraindications: Children younger than 6 months, acute-angle glaucoma, CNS depression, alcohol intoxication, known sensitivity.

Dosage:

Anxiety:

- **Adult:**
  - **Moderate:** 2 to 5 mg slow IV, intramuscular (IM).
  - **Severe:** 5 to 10 mg slow IV, IM (administer no faster than 5 mg/min).
  - **Low:** Low dosages are often required for elderly or debilitated patients.
- **Pediatric:** 0.2 to 0.3 mg/kg per dose IV, IM every 4 hours to a maximum dose of 0.6 mg/kg.

Delirium Tremens from Acute Alcohol Withdrawal:

- **Adult:** 10 mg IV.

Seizure:

- **Adult:** 5 to 10 mg slow IV, intraosseous (IO) every 10 to 15 minutes; maximum total dose 30 mg.
- **Pediatric:**
  - **IV, IO:**
    - **5 years and older:** 1 mg over a 3-minute period every 2 to 5 minutes to a maximum total dose of 10 mg.
    - **Older than 30 days to younger than 5 years:** 0.2 to 0.5 mg over a 3-minute period; may repeat every 2 to 5 minutes to a maximum total dose of 5 mg.
    - **Neonate:** 0.1 to 0.3 mg/kg per dose given over a 3- to 5-minute period; may repeat every 15 to 30 minutes to a maximum total dose of 2 mg. (Not a first-line agent due to sodium benzoic acid in the injection.)
  - **Rectal administration:** If vascular access is not obtained, diazepam may be administered rectally to children.
    - **12 years and older:** 0.2 mg/kg.
    - **6 to 11 years:** 0.3 mg/kg.
    - **2 to 5 years:** 0.5 mg/kg.
    - **Younger than 2 years:** Not recommended.

Special Considerations:

Make sure that IV, IO lines are well secured. Extravasation of diazepam causes tissue necrosis. Diazepam is insoluble in water and must be dissolved in propylene glycol. This produces a viscous solution; give slowly to prevent pain on injection.

Pregnancy class D.

(continued) The patient's mother states that he has had seizures since he was quite young and they have been difficult to control. He has been on several medications since his seizures began. Two weeks ago, his neurologist started him on felbamate and valproic acid. The patient slowly begins to awaken and seems confused. You are able to get a set of baseline vitals and start a peripheral IV line. As you get the patient moved to the cot, he begins to have another seizure. Your partner protects the boy's head and airway while you administer diazepam 5 mg IV. The patient's seizures stop. You speak with medical direction about the boy's medical history and medications. They recommend transporting without loading with phenytoin because he is already taking felbamate and valproic acid. The remainder of the transport is without any additional events.

LORAZEPAM (ATIVAN)

Classification: Benzodiazepine, Schedule C-IV.
Action: Binds to the benzodiazepine receptor and enhances the effects of the brain chemical GABA, an inhibitory transmitter, and may result in a state of sedation, hypnosis, skeletal muscle relaxation, anticonvulsant activity, coma.
Indications: Preprocedure sedation induction, anxiety, status epilepticus.
Adverse Effects: Headache, drowsiness, ataxia, dizziness, amnesia, depression, dysarthria, euphoria, syncope, fatigue, tremor, vertigo, respiratory depression, paradoxical CNS stimulation.
Contraindications: Known sensitivity to lorazepam, benzodiazepines, polyethylene glycol, propylene glycol, or benzyl alcohol; chronic obstructive pulmonary disease (COPD); sleep apnea (except while being mechanically ventilated); shock; coma; acute closed-angle glaucoma.
Dosage: Note: IV, IO lorazepam needs to be administered slowly.
Analgesia and Sedation:

© Scott Camazine/Science Source.

- **Adult:** 2 mg or 0.44 mg/kg IV, IO, whichever is smaller. This dosage will provide adequate sedation in most patients and should not be exceeded in patients older than 50 years.
- **Pediatric:** 0.05 mg/kg IV, IO. Each dose should not exceed 2 mg IV, IO.

Seizures:

- **Adult:** 2 to 4 mg IV, IO given over 2 to 5 minutes; may repeat in 10 to 15 minutes (max total dose: 8 mg in a 12-hour period).
- **Pediatric:** 0.1 mg/kg slow IV, IO given over 2 to 5 minutes (max single dose: 4 mg). May repeat at half the original dose in 10 to 15 minutes if seizure activity resumes.

Special Considerations:
Be prepared to support the patient's airway and ventilation.
Pregnancy class D.

Other Anticonvulsants

One major reason patients develop recurrent seizures is a failure to achieve an appropriate blood plasma concentration with their prescribed medication(s). Often this is attributable to noncompliance on the part of patients in adhering to their medical regimen. For this reason, paramedics must acquire a medication history and be familiar with common anticonvulsant medications, including common adverse reactions, even though they may not administer them.

A common cause of seizures is a patient's noncompliance with his or her prescribed medications.

Phenytoin (Dilantin) is an anticonvulsant used to control partial and generalized seizures. As with many anticonvulsant medications, drug levels are monitored to ensure that patients remain within a therapeutic range to control seizures while minimizing side effects. Because phenytoin produces some adverse effects when administered to patients, **prodrug** preparations of phenytoin can be administered. A prodrug is an inactive or less-active form of a drug that, once administered, is converted to the active form of a drug in the body. Prodrugs often have fewer adverse effects than the drug to which they are eventually converted. For example, a prodrug preparation of phenytoin is fosphenytoin (Cerebyx), which is converted to phenytoin after administration. The advantage of fosphenytoin in emergency situations is that the drug can be administered at a more rapid rate than phenytoin. Fosphenytoin can be given either IV or IM.[7,8]

Carbamazepine (Tegretol) is used to treat partial and generalized tonic-clonic seizures. Its action on the brain is similar to that of many of the other anticonvulsants in that it stabilizes the nerve membranes to decrease abnormal nerve cell firing.[9]

Phenobarbital (Luminal) belongs to the class of anticonvulsants referred to as *barbiturates*. Phenobarbital is considered a second-line therapy because of the troublesome side effects it causes, such as sedation, depression, and agitation. As with phenytoin, the liver metabolizes phenobarbital, where it induces some of the hepatic enzymes that can cause accelerated metabolism of several other medications.

Levetiracetam (Keppra) is a newer anticonvulsant, which is seeing increasing use in a variety of settings. It may be used for seizure prophylaxis (off-label), refractory status epilepticus (off-label), and long-term seizure control.

Valproic acid (Depakote) is another drug commonly used to treat seizures, as well as mood disorders. Although generally well tolerated, valproic acid does require regular monitoring of blood levels to ensure maintenance of therapeutic levels and minimize adverse drug reactions.

FELBAMATE (FELBATOL)

Classification: Anticonvulsant.
Action: Although the mechanism of action is not known, it increases the seizure threshold in absence seizures, and prevents the spread of generalized tonic-clonic and partial seizures. It appears to affect both *N*-methyl-D-aspartate (NMDA) and gamma-aminobutyric acid (GABA) function.[10]
Indications: Partial seizures with and without generalization in epileptic adults; partial and generalized seizures associated with Lennox-Gastaut syndrome in children.
Adverse Effects: Nausea/vomiting, suicidal ideation and behavior, depression, insomnia, dyspepsia, upper respiratory tract infection, fatigue, headache, constipation, diarrhea, rhinitis, anxiety, (occasionally fatal) aplastic anemia, photosensitivity.
Contraindications: Blood dyscrasias, hepatic disease, known sensitivity to carbomates.
Dosage: Should be individualized based on condition.
Special Considerations:
Use should be limited to very particular situations. The manufacturer recommends written informed consent prior to initiating therapy.[10]
Pregnancy class C.

PHENYTOIN (DILANTIN)

Classification: Anticonvulsant.
Action: Depresses seizures by affecting the movement of sodium and calcium into neural tissue.
Indications: Generalized tonic-clonic seizures.
Adverse Effects: Nausea/vomiting, depression of cardiac conduction, sedation, nystagmus, tremors, ataxia, dysarthria, gingival hypertrophy, hirsutism, facial coarsening, hypotension.
Contraindications: Sinus bradycardia, sinoatrial block, second and third-degree heart block, Adams-Stokes syndrome, known sensitivity to hydantoins.

Dosage:

- **Adult:** 15 to 20 mg/kg IV, IO should be administered slowly at a rate not exceeding 50 mg/min. (This requires approximately 20 minutes in a 70-kg patient.)
- **Pediatric:** 15 to 20 mg/kg IV, IO, administered at a rate of 1 to 3 mg/kg per minute.

Special Considerations:

Continuously monitor the electrocardiogram (ECG) and blood pressure during administration. Monitor IV site for signs of infiltration.

Pregnancy class D.

FOSPHENYTOIN (CEREBYX)

Classification: Anticonvulsant.

Action: Depresses seizures by affecting the movement of sodium and calcium into neural tissue.

Indications: Generalized tonic-clonic seizures.

Adverse Effects: Depression of cardiac conduction, sedation, nystagmus, delirium, tremors, ataxia, dysarthria, hypertension, hypotension, pain or irritation at injection site.

Contraindications: Sinus bradycardia, sinoatrial block, second and third-degree heart block, Adams-Stokes syndrome, known sensitivity to hydantoins.

Dosage:

- **Adult and Pediatric:** Dosing is ordered in *milligram phenytoin equivalents* (PE) rather than in milligrams. Administer 15 to 20 mg PE/kg IV, IO, administered at a rate of <150 PE/minute.

Special Considerations:

Continuously monitor the ECG and blood pressure during administration. Monitor IV site for signs of infiltration.

Pregnancy class D.

CARBAMAZEPINE (TEGRETOL)

Classification: Anticonvulsant, also possesses antidepressant, antimanic, anticholinergic, antiarrhythmic and muscle relaxant properties. It may be prescribed for a wide variety of indications not related to a seizure disorder.

Action: Decreases the spread of the seizure.

Indications: Partial and generalized tonic-clonic seizures.

Adverse Effects: Dizziness, drowsiness, ataxia, nausea/vomiting, blurred vision, confusion, headache, transient diplopia, visual hallucinations, life-threatening rashes.

Contraindications: AV block, bundle branch block, agranulocytosis, bone marrow suppression, monoamine oxidase inhibitor therapy, hypersensitivity to carbamazepine or tricyclic antidepressants. Use with caution in petit mal, atonic, or myoclonic seizures; liver disease; patients with blood dyscrasia caused by drug therapies or blood disorders; patients with a history of cardiac disease; or patients with a history of alcoholism.

Dosage:

- **Adult:** 200 mg orally (PO) every 12 hours.
- **Pediatric:**
  - **6 to 12 years:** 100 mg PO twice daily.
  - **Younger than 6 years:** 10 to 20 mg/kg per day PO 2 or 3 times per day.

Special Considerations:

Pregnancy class D.

LEVETIRACETAM (KEPPRA)

Classification: Anticonvulsant.
Action: Unknown mechanism, appears to regulate GABA transmission.
Indications: Partial and generalized tonic-clonic seizures.
Adverse Effects: Behavior changes (frequent reason for discontinuation), ataxia, confusion, drowsiness, anorexia, constipation, diarrhea
Contraindications: Hypersensitivity; use in caution in patients prone to emotional or behavioral disorders.
Dosage:
- **Adult:**
  - Status epilepticus: 1,000 to 3,000 mg IV, IO administered over 15 minutes.
  - Oral maintenance: Up to 3,000 mg/day in divided doses.
- **Pediatric:**
  - Status epilepticus: 20 to 60 mg/kg IV/IO, infused at 2 to 5 mg/kg per minute.
  - Oral maintenance: 7 to 10 mg/kg per dose.
Special Considerations:
Pregnancy class C. Monitor emotional and behavioral changes while patients are receiving levetiracetam. Known to cause toxic epidermal necrosis and Stevens-Johnson syndrome.

PHENOBARBITAL (LUMINAL)

Classification: Anticonvulsant, barbiturate, Schedule C-IV.
Action: Depresses seizure activity in the cortex, thalamus, and limbic system; increases threshold for electrical stimulation of motor cortex; produces state of sedation.
Indications: Seizures, may also be used for severe alcohol withdrawal or withdrawal from sedative hypnotic medications (off-label).
Adverse Effects: Depression, agitation, respiratory depression, accelerated metabolism of several other medications.
Contraindications: Liver dysfunction, porphyria, agranulocytosis, known sensitivity to barbiturates. Use with caution with respiratory dysfunction.
Dosage:
- **Adult:** 20 mg/kg IV, IO; infuse at a rate not faster than 50 to 100 mg/min.
- **Pediatric:** 20 mg/kg IV, IO; infuse over 10 minutes.
Special Considerations:
Be prepared to manage the patient's airway.
Pregnancy class D.

VALPROIC ACID (DEPAKOTE)

Classification: Anticonvulsant, antimanic.
Action: It is suggested that valproic acid increases brain concentrations of GABA.
Indications: Seizures, mood disorders.
Adverse Effects: Tremor, confusion, sedation, hypotension, hypertension, tachycardia, transient hair loss, weight gain, weight loss, fatal hepatic failure.
Contraindications: Liver disease.
Dosage: Dosing is individualized.
Special Considerations:
Although generally well tolerated, valproic acid does require regular monitoring of blood levels to ensure maintenance of therapeutic levels while minimizing adverse drug reactions.
Pregnancy class D.

In recent years, several new anticonvulsants have been designed to manage seizures. As these drugs become more commonly used in patients with seizures that are difficult to control, paramedics will see them more frequently and therefore should have a general understanding of their potential side effects and toxicities. Two of these newer anticonvulsant agents are gabapentin (Neurontin) and lamotrigine (Lamictal).

Since gabapentin (Neurontin) was approved as an adjunctive medication for seizure disorders, it has become widely used for many other indications, as well. Unlike many of the other anticonvulsants, gabapentin is well absorbed orally. Gabapentin also has recently been approved for the treatment of many different neuropathic pain syndromes.[11] Gabapentin is useful for the treatment of pain because it acts on nerve cells to stabilize the cell membrane.

Lamotrigine (Lamictal) is another of the newer anticonvulsants approved for therapy for partial and generalized seizures.

GABAPENTIN (NEURONTIN)

Classification: Anticonvulsant.
Action: The exact mechanism of action has not been determined.
Indications: Seizures, neuropathic pain syndromes.
Adverse Effects: Dizziness, ataxia, sleepiness, gait disturbances, upset stomach, peripheral edema.
Contraindications: Known sensitivity. Use with caution in elderly patients, renal impairment.
Dosage:

© Christine Whitehead/Alamy Stock Photo.

- **Adult:** 300 to 1,800 mg PO daily.
- **Pediatric:**
  - **5 to 12 years:** Up to 35 mg/kg per day PO divided in three divided doses daily.
  - **3 to 4 years:** 10 to 15 mg/kg per day PO divided in three divided doses daily.

Special Considerations:
Pregnancy class C.

LAMOTRIGINE (LAMICTAL)

Classification: Anticonvulsant, antimanic agent.

Action: The exact mechanism of action has not been determined. Studies suggest lamotrigine stabilizes neuronal membranes by acting at voltage-sensitive sodium channels, thereby decreasing presynaptic release of glutamate and aspartate, resulting in decreased seizure activity.

Indications: Seizures, bipolar disorders.

Adverse Effects: Headache, dizziness, nausea/vomiting, ataxia, diplopia, severe skin rash, amnesia, abnormal thoughts, speech and depression.

Contraindications: Known sensitivity.

Dosage:
- **Adult:** Medication is administered orally. Dosage is individualized.
- **Pediatric:** Medication is administered orally. Dosage is individualized.

Special Considerations:
Pregnancy class C.

	NDC 12345-678-90
Lamotrigine	Rx only
Tablets USP	**100 mg**

Each uncoated tablet contains: Lamotrigine USP 100 mg — **30 Tablets**
Dispense in a tight container as defined in the USP.
Store at 20°–25°C (68°–77°F); excursion permitted to 15°–30°C (59°–86°F) [see USP Controlled Room Temperature].
PHARMACIST: Dispense the accompanying Medication Guide to each patient.
LOT / EXP — See package outsert for Dosage & Administration.

▶ Review Questions

1. Define *status epilepticus*.
2. Why would rectal administration of a medication be necessary in a patient having a seizure?
3. What class of drugs is used in the initial management of seizures?
4. What eye condition is a contraindication for administration of benzodiazepines?
5. Explain a prodrug and give an example.

References

1. Rainbow J, Browne GJ, Lam LT. Controlling seizures in the prehospital setting: diazepam or midazolam? *J Paediatr Child Health*. 2002;38:582.
2. Silverman EC, Sporer KA, Lemieux JM, et al. Prehospital care for the adult and pediatric seizure patient: current evidence-based recommendations. *West J Emerg Med*. 2017;18(3):419–436.
3. Alldredge BK, Gelb AM, Isaacs SM, et al. A comparison of lorazepam, diazepam, and placebo for the treatment of out-of-hospital status epilepticus. *N Engl J Med*. 2001;345:631.
4. Goodchild CS. GABA receptors and benzodiazepines. *Br J Anaesth*. 1993;71:127.
5. Barsan WG, Ward JT, Otten EJ. Blood levels of diazepam after endotracheal administration in dogs. *Ann Emerg Med*. 1982;11:242.
6. Chamberlain JM, Okada P, Holsti M. Lorazepam vs diazepam for pediatric status epilepticus: a randomized clinical trial. *J Am Med Assoc*. 2014;311(6):1652–1660.
7. Boucher BA, Feler CA, Dean JC, et al. The safety, tolerability, and pharmacokinetics of fosphenytoin after intramuscular and intravenous administration in neurosurgery patients. *Pharmacotherapy*. 1996;16:638.
8. Boucher BA, Feler CA, Dean JC, et al. Fosphenytoin: a novel phenytoin prodrug. *Pharmacotherapy*. 1996;16:777.
9. Sobotka JL, Alexander B, Cook BL. A review of carbamazepine's hematologic reactions and monitoring recommendations. *DICP*. 1990;24:1214.
10. Schachter SC. Antiseizure drugs: mechanism of action, pharmacology, and adverse effects. UpToDate. https://www.uptodate.com/contents/antiseizure-drugs-mechanism-of-action-pharmacology-and-adverse-effects?search=Felbamate&source=search_result&selectedTitle=1~14&usage_type=default&display_rank=1#H20. Updated August 2, 2018. Accessed August 20, 2018.
11. Spina E, Perugi G. Antiepileptic drugs: indications other than epilepsy. *Epileptic Disord*. 2004;6:57.

CHAPTER 16

Shock

MEDICATIONS THAT APPEAR IN CHAPTER 16

Tranexamic acid (TXA; Cyklokapron)
Dobutamine (Dobutrex)

Dopamine (Intropin)
Norepinephrine (Levophed)
Milrinone (Primacor)

Phenylephrine (Neo-Synephrine)

▶ Introduction

To treat shock appropriately, the prehospital professional must understand what shock is, its various causes, and the treatments for each particular type. The treatment for one type of shock may be a vasopressor, but treatment for a second type of shock may be fluid resuscitation. Refractory conditions may require a combination of interventions if the initial approach fails to stabilize the patient's condition. This grows increasingly complicated when more than one category or type of shock is present and the preferred treatment for one will adversely impact another. Failure to identify the various types of shock and match the appropriate treatment with the type of shock can cause the patient significant peril. In regard to therapy of other conditions, the provider must recognize a condition (e.g., ventricular tachycardia) and know the appropriate drug intervention (e.g., amiodarone) for that condition. When treating shock, the provider must recognize the presence of the condition and determine its cause (e.g., hypovolemia) to select the most appropriate intervention. This chapter describes five causes of shock and their appropriate pharmacologic management.

CASE STUDY

Your unit is called to the scene of a multiple motor vehicle crash. The patient you are directed to care for is a 19-year-old man who is the driver of a car that has run off the road and come to rest in a ravine. The patient is trapped in the car by his legs. The vehicle has been stabilized from shifting, and no fuel or electrical hazards are present. The patient is awake and answering questions. His airway is patent. Respirations are rapid and shallow. His heart rate is 132 beats/min, and blood pressure is 100/84 mm Hg. He is alert and oriented. The patient has a large laceration to the forehead, and bleeding is controlled with some direct pressure. The lungs are clear, but the patient is very tender when you palpate the ribs on the left. The abdomen is tender. The patient has an obvious open left femur fracture.

▶ Overview of Shock

Shock is an abnormality of the circulatory system that results in inadequate tissue perfusion and oxygen delivery. Shock can be classified into one of four broad categories.[1] Many patient conditions may result in shock states that are a combination of more than one of these categories (**TABLE 16-1**).

It is extremely important for EMS providers to identify the correct etiology when a patient presents in shock. Table 16-1 describes common clinical conditions associated with each of the four categories of shock. Within a given category or type of shock, such as cardiogenic shock, the definitive intervention or treatment strategy may still vary greatly depending on

TABLE 16-1 Shock Etiology Categories		
Shock Etiology Category	**Mechanism**	**Examples**
Distributive	Adequate fluid volume and cardiac function are present. Reduced vascular tone and/or increased vascular permeability impair blood circulation and systemic tissue perfusion.	Sepsis (septic shock) Burns Anaphylaxis (anaphylactic shock) Spinal cord injury (neurogenic shock) Endocrine emergencies (such as myxedema coma) Poisoning or overdose
Hypovolemic	Loss of circulating blood volume results in decreased cardiac output and decreased systemic tissue perfusion.	Trauma Hemorrhage Reduced fluid intake with ongoing fluid loss (dehydration) Excessive excretion (diuretic medication, sodium imbalances, etc.) Gastrointestinal losses (vomiting, diarrhea)

Shock Etiology Category	Mechanism	Examples
Cardiogenic	Decreased cardiac function causes impaired systemic circulation and decreased tissue perfusion. *Cardiogenic shock may occur even when there is increased cardiac output, such as when the heart is unable to increase cardiac output to meet the massive increases in metabolic demands from conditions such as burns and sepsis.*	Arrhythmia Heart valve or heart muscle dysfunction (myocardial infarction, septal defects, hypoxia) Direct injury to the heart (blunt or penetrating) Cardiotoxic medications, poisoning, or overdose Pericardial tamponade (excessive fluid/pressure within pericardial sac causing decreased cardiac output) *This is considered both a cardiogenic and obstructive cause of shock.*
Obstructive	An obstruction outside of the heart causes reduced cardiac output.	Pulmonary embolism (increased pulmonary vascular resistance causing right-sided heart failure) Tension pneumothorax (vascular flow is compromised, causing reduced blood return to the heart; reduced cardiac preload) Pericardial tamponade (excessive fluid/pressure within pericardial sac causing decreased cardiac output) Aortic stenosis (reduced blood flow out of the heart into systemic circulation)
Combination conditions	More than one shock category is present in a particular condition.	Chest trauma: may cause hypoxia and direct cardiac injury (cardiogenic); pericardial tamponade and tension pneumothorax (obstructive); severe hemorrhage (hypovolemic) Sepsis: loss of vascular tone causing inadequate blood return to the heart (distributive); myocardial depressant substances released during inflammatory response (cardiogenic); increased volume loss from fever and hypermetabolic state (hypovolemic) Burns: loss of vascular tone (distributive); increased fluid losses through skin and exposed tissues along with underlying hypermetabolic state (hypovolemic) Organophosphate poisoning: hypoxia and bradycardia, causing reduced cardiac output (cardiogenic); fluid losses from urination, emesis, bronchorrhea, etc. (hypovolemic)

Original table by Andrew Bartkus. Based on information from: Gaieski DF, Mikkelsen ME. Definition, classification, etiology and pathophysiology of shock in adults. UpToDate. https://www.uptodate.com/contents/definition-classification-etiology-and-pathophysiology-of-shock-in-adults/print. Updated February 18, 2018. Accessed August 29, 2018; and Hochman JS, Reyentovich A. Clinical manifestations and diagnosis of cardiogenic shock in acute myocardial infarction. UpToDate. https://www.uptodate.com/contents/clinical-manifestations-and-diagnosis-of-cardiogenic-shock-in-acute-myocardial-infarction. Updated December 18, 2017. Accessed August 29, 2018

TABLE 16-2 Phases of Shock

	Signs and Symptoms		
Vital Signs	**Compensated Shock**	**Uncompensated Shock**	**Irreversible Shock**
Heart rate	Mild tachycardia	Moderate tachycardia	Bradycardia, severe dysrhythmias
Level of consciousness	Lethargy, confusion, combativeness	Confusion, unconsciousness	Coma
Skin	Delayed capillary refill, cool skin	Delayed capillary refill, cold extremities, cyanosis	Pale, cold, clammy skin
Blood pressure	Normal or slightly elevated measurement	Decreased systolic and diastolic pressure	Frank hypotension

© Jones & Bartlett Learning.

the underlying condition. Unfortunately, a preferred intervention for one category or type of shock often has the potential to worsen symptoms associated with another type of shock. Selecting the appropriate prehospital intervention is essential.

Shock remains reversible for a limited time. Prompt intervention and definitive care can halt the progression of shock. If interventions are delayed, or definitive care cannot be accomplished, shock will progress to multiorgan failure. With each additional failing organ or body system, death becomes significantly more likely. Up to 98% of patients with three or more organ or organ system failures will die.[2] EMS providers are in the optimal position to initiate critical interventions that may halt or slow the progression from shock to death.

Shock may be further described as **compensated shock** or **decompensated shock** (**TABLE 16-2**). These terms indicate whether the body's intrinsic responses and early treatment interventions are effective. As the underlying condition persists, patients lose the ability to compensate, and more dramatic signs begin to appear. A provider should not assume that only hypotensive patients can be in shock. Shock may be present even when the patient's blood pressure appears normal. Impaired oxygen delivery and tissue perfusion can occur in the presence of low, normal, and even elevated blood pressure. Decompensated shock is identified when the patient develops hypotension.[3] Tachycardia may be present or absent, depending on the particular circumstances of the patient's condition. Shock can certainly be present in patients demonstrating a normal heart rate or even bradycardia.

Shock can occur in the presence of low, normal, and even elevated blood pressure.

Regardless of the cause of shock, before becoming unstable a patient's physiologic functioning alters to compensate. Such compensations can involve the shunting of blood from less-critical to more-critical areas, elevation of cardiac output (when possible) with an increase in heart rate or stroke volume, and vasoconstriction. During such periods of compensation, the patient can exhibit normal mentation and only slight alterations in vital signs. As such, these patients can appear stable. However, in reality, these patients are in compensated shock.

The term *stable* is often used to describe patients with normal blood pressure. Shock-related alterations in blood pressure are typically late findings in the patient in shock. The early clinical findings of shock include skin perfusion, respiratory rate, and altered mental status. Patients can have delayed capillary refill, and their skin is often cold and clammy.

Hypotension is a late finding of shock.

In shock, a patient's respiratory rate can increase to improve minute ventilation to compensate for metabolic acidosis. Additionally, increased respiratory rate improves blood return to the heart because the respiratory apparatus serves as a bellows. Improved cardiac return results in improved cardiac output. Conversely, positive pressure ventilation may adversely impact cardiac output. Because the early signs of decompensated shock can be subtle and even misleading, prehospital providers need to maintain a high index of suspicion for shock. Terms such as *stable* and *unstable* can be incorrectly interpreted as *not sick* or *sick*. Therefore patients in shock should more accurately be considered as being either compensated or decompensated. Radial pulse quality (normal/strong versus weak versus absent) has been used to estimate a patient's systolic blood pressure.[4] However, this evaluation does not replace the role of actual blood pressure measurement to identify hypotension. A patient's mental status can be used as a rapid method to infer cerebral perfusion. A normal mental status is reassuring for adequate cerebral perfusion. As cerebral perfusion declines, thought clarity also declines.

▶ Causes of Shock

Shock is not a disease process; rather, it is the *symptom* of an underlying disease process. Treatment of hypotension is often relatively simple, and blood pressure can return to normal after the administration of fluids and a single vasopressor. However, if the cause of hypotension is blood loss from a gastrointestinal bleed or myocardial infarction (MI), the blood flow to vital organs can actually decrease (i.e., worsening of the shock) despite a normal blood pressure. If the patient is in septic shock from a perforated colon, intravenous (IV) fluids and vasopressors do nothing to control the fecal contamination of the abdominal cavity. A patient with a tension **pneumothorax** requires only rapid decompression of the chest; fluids and drugs are not required and can delay definitive therapy (**FIGURE 16-1**).

FIGURE 16-1 Tension pneumothorax. If the amount of air trapped in the pleural space continues to increase, not only is the lung on the affected side collapsed, but the mediastinum is also shifted to the opposite side. The mediastinal shift kinks the inferior vena cava, thus decreasing blood return to the heart and affecting cardiac output while at the same time compressing the opposite lung.

These examples illustrate the importance of understanding the causes of the various forms of shock to provide effective treatment. Four types of shock are hypovolemic, cardiogenic, obstructive, and distributive. Distributive shock can be further divided into three important subcategories. Neurogenic shock, anaphylactic shock, and septic shock, each discussed later, are types of distributive shock when tissue perfusion becomes impaired due to a loss of blood vessel tone or integrity. Other conditions with names such as *respiratory shock*, *spinal shock*, and *psychogenic shock* add an element of confusion, as these conditions do not involve on-going impaired tissue perfusion; as such, they are not discussed in this chapter.

When encountering a patient with suspected hypoperfusion, determine which one of the five causes is the mostly likely source of the patient's hypoperfusion. In some cases the cause is obvious. For example, the patient with a gunshot wound to the abdomen with no radial pulse and a weak, rapid carotid pulse is more than likely to be in **hypovolemic shock**. It is important to note that hypovolemic shock may also occur from loss of blood plasma (water) volume rather than hemorrhage. Many conditions that result in significantly decreased water intake or excessive water losses can cause hypovolemic shock. A 65-year-old man with a blood pressure of 84/58 mm Hg who described chest pain before becoming disoriented is likely in cardiogenic shock, although EMS providers should be careful not to overlook other potential causes of noncardiac chest pain that can be associated with hypotension.

In other cases, the source of the hypotension requires critical thought. Such clinical dilemmas most commonly occur in hypotension after blunt trauma. For example, did hypoperfusion from a cardiac event cause an altered sensorium, which then resulted in a motor vehicle accident or fall?

BOX 16-1 summarizes the treatment for common types of shock states encountered by EMS. Fortunately, one component of therapy is the same for all five causes of shock: IV resuscitation. Significant debate exists regarding the need for and magnitude of IV fluid resuscitation in shock, especially hypovolemic shock from penetrating trauma, which is discussed in greater detail later in the chapter.

The patient in the previous scenario is likely in hypovolemic shock. He has several possible sources of blood loss, including the scalp laceration and the open femur fracture. Other less-obvious sources of blood loss could be from rib fractures or an abdominal injury. The patient has a rapid heart rate, rapid respiration rate, and slight depression of blood pressure. The appropriate therapy for this patient is administration of IV fluids with an isotonic crystalloid solution such as normal saline or Ringer's lactate solution. Controlling ongoing blood loss and administration of fluids will likely improve the vital signs and the delivery of oxygen to peripheral tissues and reverse the shock process. Vasopressor medications may improve his blood pressure; however, they will also likely accelerate any ongoing hemorrhage, dramatically worsening the overall situation.

BOX 16-1 Treatment for the Five Common Causes of Shock

Hypovolemic: Control of hemorrhage, IV fluid, blood products, and perhaps surgery to definitively control any ongoing bleeding.
Cardiogenic: IV fluid, chronotropic drugs, inotropic drugs, vasoconstrictors, and in some cases vasodilators. *Monitor for volume overload (pulmonary edema) when administering IV fluid. Many conditions causing cardiogenic shock require definitive treatment and/or complex monitoring and intervention, well outside the typical realm of EMS.*
Neurogenic: IV fluid and vasoconstrictors.
Septic: IV fluid, vasoconstrictors, inotropic drugs, and eventually control of the infectious source with antibiotics and perhaps surgery.
Anaphylactic: IV fluids, epinephrine, antihistamines, and steroids.

▶ Management

CASE STUDY

You respond to a call at 1:15 a.m. to a bar known to attract a rowdy clientele. Shots have been fired, and initial reports indicate multiple casualties. A crowd has gathered outside the bar. The interior has been vacated except for the owner and staff. Two injuries are present, and both patients are male and approximately 25 years old. One of the patients is sitting on the floor near the back of the bar. He is obviously intoxicated but is looking around the well-lit bar. His right thigh has a pressure dressing fashioned from towels. The dressing is almost entirely saturated with blood. He is asking about his friend, who is lying on the floor.

The second patient has a dressing applied to the left lower quadrant of the abdomen that shows only a few spots of blood. He moves all four extremities as he attempts to sit upright, although he lacks the strength to sit up. As the bar staff speaks to him, he looks at them but does not seem to understand. Your partner reports a systolic blood pressure of 82 mm Hg and a heart rate of 136 beats/min.

Within moments of surveying the scene, it is apparent which patient most urgently requires your attention. A closer examination of the second patient indicates that he has a rapid, weak radial pulse. His fingers are cool, and capillary refill is 4 seconds. He responds only to questions posed in a loud, commanding voice. The patient can identify himself but does not accurately describe his location.

Hypovolemic Shock

Even without a blood pressure cuff, you know the second patient in the previous scenario is in shock. First, he is tachycardic. Prolonged capillary refill and cool extremities indicate peripheral vasoconstriction. His mental status may be clouded by alcohol or drugs, but his altered sensorium is likely affected by marginal cerebral perfusion. The patient's systolic blood pressure of 82 mm Hg and heart rate of 136 beats/min further confirm that he is in shock.

In this case, the circumstances of a gunshot wound to the abdomen clearly led to shock caused by hypovolemia. Cardiogenic shock can be excluded by the events preceding the shock state. Cardiogenic shock or distributive shock might still also be possible if a bullet or bullet fragment injured the heart or pericardial sac or has caused a tension pneumothorax. Neurogenic and septic shock can be excluded by the evidence of peripheral vasoconstriction. Neurogenic shock can be considered only with interrupted spinal cord function, which limits peripheral sympathetic tone. Neurogenic shock is typically associated with a heart rate slower than expected for the degree of hypotension. Penetrating abdominal injuries can lead to sepsis. However, sepsis from intra-abdominal infection caused by a gunshot wound would require more time to develop.

A drop in blood pressure from acute hemorrhage requires a loss of approximately 30% of the circulating blood volume.[5] As a general guideline, circulating blood volume is 7% of the ideal body weight. For a patient with an ideal body weight of 80 kg, the circulating blood volume is 5,600 mL (80 × 0.07 = 5.6 L or 5,600 mL). The circulating volume lost to cause a drop in blood pressure is 1,680 mL (5,600 × 0.30 = 1,680 mL). More than 4 units of blood (1 unit of blood contains 350 mL) must be lost from the circulation before the blood pressure drops.

A drop in blood pressure caused by acute hemorrhage requires a loss of approximately 30% of the circulating blood volume.

The initial therapy for hypovolemic shock is control of the hemorrhage's source, if possible. As control of hemorrhage is obtained, fluid resuscitation is performed. The optimal IV resuscitation fluid choice remains controversial. The fluid infused at initial resuscitation should be a **crystalloid**. Both normal saline and Ringer's lactate solution are widely available and demonstrate superiority over other IV fluids in hemorrhagic shock.[6] Normal saline is nearly isotonic and is compatible with blood. Ringer's lactate solution is another crystalloid that is commonly used; however, it is not compatible with the infusion of blood. IV lines used for blood administration must be flushed with normal saline before the administration of blood. Emerging evidence suggests that Ringer's lactate is superior to normal saline in large-volume resuscitation situations; however, experts recommend an individualized approach to volume, rate, and resuscitation fluid choices based on the particular clinical situation. Follow your agency or regional guidelines regarding the treatment of hemorrhagic or hypovolemic shock.[6]

Normal saline is compatible to be given with infused blood; Ringer's lactate is not.

The route of fluid administration in the prehospital setting is optimally two large-bore peripheral IV sites. In cases in which peripheral veins are not accessible, intraosseous (IO) routes should be considered (see Chapter 5). In adults, begin with 1 to 2 L of an isotonic crystalloid solution.

Patients who demonstrate improved perfusion, heart rate, or blood pressure with crystalloid infusion can be categorized as rapid responders, transient responders, or nonresponders. Rapid responders do not need further aggressive resuscitation. They have no ongoing hemorrhage; the source of bleeding has been controlled with pressure or the patient's normal hemostatic mechanisms. Transient responders improve as their intravascular volume is replenished. However, with ongoing manifestations of poor perfusion return, transient responders require blood transfusion and hemorrhage control. Nonresponders have uncontrolled hemorrhage and require blood transfusion and control of bleeding.

(*continued*) The patient lying on the floor is given normal saline. (For the sake of discussion, transport is delayed in this scenario, but this patient does require rapid transport to a trauma center.) After 15 minutes of on-scene time, the patient has received 2 L of normal saline, and he appropriately responds to your requests to remain quiet. Blood pressure is 98/60 mm Hg, and heart rate is 100 beats/min. This patient is a responder to fluid administration. Ten minutes later, with an additional 250 mL of normal saline on board, the patient is less lucid, he is more tachycardic, and his radial pulse is weaker. He has become a transient responder.

In this case, the paramedic does not yet have control of the bleeding's source. Should the patient's heart rate and blood pressure be returned to normal? Studies suggest that mortality is improved with conservative, rather than aggressive, IV fluid resuscitation in these situations. This patient may benefit from the use of **hypotensive resuscitation** or **permissive hypotension**. That is, the goal is not to return his vital signs to normal, but to maintain physiologic functioning until the source of the hemorrhage can be controlled. Some may ask, "What can be wrong with normal vital signs? Why not infuse more normal saline because he responded initially?" This issue remains controversial,[7] and you should follow your agency or regional EMS guidelines in these situations. Key considerations in this controversy are explored in the following paragraphs.

Part of the study of pharmacology is appropriate dosing. What is the appropriate dose or volume of IV fluids? Administration of IV fluids in excessive amounts or at an overly rapid rate can cause patients to bleed more rapidly. Controversy exists in the medical literature regarding appropriate IV fluid administration in patients with penetrating torso trauma.[8] Control of hemorrhage for torso trauma requires rapid access to a trauma surgeon. In the operating room, and especially in the field, the best chance for hemostasis is the victim's clotting mechanism—in addition to direct pressure or an extremity tourniquet. Administration of IV fluids does nothing to stop the bleeding.

Although obvious, the emphasis that bleeding patients are losing blood, not saline, is still important. Saline lacks the ability to carry oxygen and the factors capable of producing clots. Aggressive fluid resuscitation to restore normal blood pressure can dislodge the fragile clot and cause bleeding to resume. The platelets and coagulation proteins consumed in clot formation would then be lost, and the ability of the body to affect hemostasis would be limited as platelets and coagulation proteins become diluted with aggressive fluid resuscitation. In addition, large volumes of unwarmed fluids can predispose a patient to hypothermia. Because blood coagulation factors function within a narrow temperature range, the onset of hypothermia can render the blood coagulation system less functional and result in ongoing hemorrhage.

Patients in hypovolemic shock may require a blood transfusion. Because of acute blood loss, the hypotensive patient in the scenario has a deficit of at least 30% of blood volume. Transient responders probably need blood, and nonresponders certainly require a blood transfusion. Because most prehospital care providers do not have the availability to transfuse blood, potential delays incurred by establishing IV lines and administering fluids may benefit the patient little or not at all.

Although most ground-based prehospital providers will not find themselves in circumstances that require them to administer blood, the transfusion of blood is a skill often required of air medical providers, those involved in interhospital transport, and military providers.

Even though patients hemorrhage whole blood, transfusion of whole blood is a relatively rare occurrence, even in the hospital setting. The blood product most often transfused is **packed red blood cells (pRBCs)** (**FIGURE 16-2**). Standard blood-banking practices involve separating donated whole blood into components. Red blood cells (RBCs), platelets, and plasma are all separated. In this manner, a single unit of blood can provide therapy for many patients.

Blood component therapy is administered to patients with specific needs. The overwhelming majority of blood donations are provided to patients who do not need the transfusion of whole blood. Blood component therapy also has a practical component. Platelets require storage at a warmer temperature than RBCs. If platelets were stored with RBCs at 39°F (4°C), the platelets would clump with the RBCs and plasma proteins. Coagulation factors in

FIGURE 16-2 Packed red blood cells.

plasma are also labile at 39°F (4°C). Therefore, storage of whole blood at the temperature required for RBCs causes significant problems.

pRBC transfusion offers two benefits: oxygen-carrying capability and volume. The most significant benefit is oxygen-carrying capacity. The oxygen dissolved in plasma is insignificant compared with the oxygen carried by hemoglobin in pRBCs. The volume of one unit of pRBCs is approximately 350 mL.

As with any therapy, the risks and benefits must be weighed. One risk of transfusion therapy is disease transmission. Even though aggressive testing of donors is performed to minimize the risk of disease transmission, the risk of HIV is one in every 1.5 to 2 million units of blood transfused.[9] Hepatitis C transmission occurs in approximately one case per 1 to 2 million units transfused. The risk of hepatitis B transmission is approximately four cases per 1 million units transfused.[10]

In standard transfusion therapy, the greatest risk is ABO-incompatible blood transfusions. For the prehospital provider, ABO incompatibility is not a concern because only type O blood is typically available. Information on a patient's blood type and the testing to confirm the blood type in the field is not practical. For these reasons, only universal donor blood, type O, is available.

To review, the four blood types are O, A, B, and AB. Type A has A antigen on the RBC surface, type B has B antigen on the RBC surface, and type AB has A and B antigens on the RBC surface. Natural antibodies occur against the cell surface antigen that is not present on the RBC surface. That is, a person with type A blood has naturally occurring antibodies against B antigen. Type B patients have antibodies against A antigen, and type AB patients have no antibodies against A or B antigen. Type O patients have antibodies against both A and B antigens. People with type O blood are universal donors because their RBC surfaces do not contain A or B antigen.

The optimal unit of pRBCs for field administration is type O Rh⁻. The Rh status of pRBCs infused is of minimal consequence to male patients or female patients without the possibility of future pregnancy. However, in women with the possibility of future pregnancy, Rh⁺ blood should be avoided. Rh⁻ patients who receive Rh⁺ blood develop antibodies against the Rh factor in approximately 70% to 80% of cases.[11] The seroconversion that occurs can pose a risk in a subsequent pregnancy if the Rh⁻ mother becomes pregnant with an Rh⁺ fetus. The fetus can develop chronic hemolytic disease of the newborn.[12]

CASE STUDY

You are a flight medic on an air ambulance who has been called to transport a gunshot victim (the second patient described in the previous scenario). After you receive the report, you decide that the patient could benefit from transfusion of pRBCs while being transported to the regional trauma center.

ADMINISTERING A BLOOD TRANSFUSION

Equipment Needed:
1 unit pRBCs, blood tubing, normal saline, personal protective equipment
Procedure:
1. Observe standard precautions.
2. Confirm it is the right patient.
3. When possible, explain to the patient what procedure you are going to perform and why. Obtain informed consent if possible.
4. Examine the refrigeration record to ensure the proper pRBC temperature has been maintained.
5. Examine the expiration date on the units. Check the pack number on the transfusion record and compare it with the pack number on the label on the blood product.

6. Confirm the blood is type O.
7. Examine the blood for evidence of leakage, clumps, or abnormal color.
8. Confirm the blood is Rh⁻ if the patient is a woman younger than 50 years. In life-threatening situations, this may be disregarded.
9. Record vital signs of the patient before transfusion and at least every 15 minutes during the transfusion.
10. Ensure all tags and labels remain attached to the unit of blood.
11. Ensure the tubing to the unit of blood is filtered.
12. Confirm the pRBCs will be infused through a line flushed with normal saline.
13. Attach the unit of pRBCs to the tubing and the open valve to begin the transfusion.
14. Closely observe the transfusion during the first 15 mL of transfusion. An acute hemolytic reaction can occur with infusion of even a small volume. If any sign of a transfusion reaction occurs, stop the transfusion immediately. Do not discard the unit; save it for further analysis on arrival to definitive care. Continue monitoring the patient during the remainder of the transfusion, including vital signs with temperature measurements whenever possible.
15. Document identifying numbers of the unit infused, infusion times, and vital signs.

Tranexamic Acid

Tranexamic acid (TXA; Cyklokapron) is an antifibrinolytic agent that is gaining widespread use in the management of surgical and trauma-related hemorrhage. Two large studies showed significant mortality reduction when TXA was given to severe trauma patients.[13] TXA inhibits the body's natural process to break down blood clots, promoting more robust clot formation and ultimately decreasing the severity of hemorrhage. A single 1,000-mg IV dose of TXA should ideally be administered within 3 hours of the traumatic event, although certain healthcare facilities may be using alternate protocols[14] as the research and evidence continue to evolve.

TRANEXAMIC ACID (TXA; CYKLOKAPRON)

Classification: Antifibrinolytic agent, hemostatic agent.
Action: Inhibits intrinsic fibrinolysis, promoting blood clot formation.
Indications: Severe traumatic hemorrhage (off-label), surgical hemorrhage, hyphema (off-label), severe menstrual bleeding, dental bleeding.
Adverse Effects: Visual changes, anxiety, tachycardia, rash, hives.
Contraindications: Hypersensitivity, subarachnoid hemorrhage, thromboembolism.
Dosage:
Acute Traumatic Hemorrhage:
- **Adult:** 1,000 mg IV over 10 minutes, followed by 1,000 mg IV over 8 hours.

Special Considerations:
Pregnancy class B.

CASE STUDY

You are dispatched at 5:30 a.m. to a residence in response to a 65-year-old man with chest pain. You are met at the door by the patient's wife, who reports that her husband has a history of angina beginning 5 years ago. At that time he underwent cardiac catheterization and was found to have a critical narrowing of one of his coronary arteries. He was managed with stent placement and has been free of symptoms since that time. His wife reports that he had been feeling well until this morning. He has been faithful in taking atorvastatin (Lipitor) 20 mg orally every day for hyperlipidemia.

Your patient is found lying on the couch with his right arm hanging limply off the side. He has two pillows under his head and neck. He rouses when addressed. He tells you he has chest pressure like he has never previously had. He also reports feeling short of breath. The discomfort and sense of uneasiness woke him approximately 90 minutes ago, when he left his bedroom for the living room. His extremities are cool. His radial pulse is present. You notice prominent external jugular veins. His heart rate is 104 beats/min, blood pressure is 86/58 mm Hg, and respiratory rate is 22 breaths/min. Rales are present in the lung bases bilaterally.

Cardiogenic Shock

It is evident that the patient in this scenario is in shock, and the task of the prehospital professional is to determine rapidly the type of shock before beginning therapy. With no suggestion of trauma or gastrointestinal blood loss, a hypovolemic source of shock can most likely be excluded. One possible source of hypovolemia would be a leaking aneurysm, but with no abdominal or back pain, blood loss from an abdominal aortic aneurysm is unlikely. The chest pain could be a manifestation of a leaking thoracic aortic aneurysm; however, hypovolemia is effectively excluded by the presence of the full neck veins. A neurogenic source can be excluded by the patient's ability to maintain lower extremity function, as confirmed by his movement to the couch from the bedroom after the onset of the chest discomfort. Sepsis as a cause of his hypotension is also unlikely. The distended neck veins and cool extremities suggest peripheral vasoconstriction and ineffectiveness of the cardiac cycle (signs seen only late in septic shock). The patient is experiencing cardiogenic shock on the basis of presumed myocardial ischemia.

Cardiogenic shock is inadequate tissue perfusion caused by pump failure, most commonly from acute MI.[15] In such cases, the myocardium loses its ability to contract effectively. Factors other than pump failure can result in cardiogenic shock. For example, mechanical factors that result in inadequate filling of the right or left atrium can prevent effective cardiac function. **Pericardial tamponade** is an example of a mechanical source of cardiogenic shock. Other mechanical factors, such as severe cardiac valve dysfunction, can cause cardiogenic shock. In these circumstances, blood does not maintain an effective, unidirectional flow through the heart. Rather, the blood "sloshes" back and forth during the cardiac cycle across the dysfunctional valve. Tissue perfusion is negatively affected by such inefficient flow.

The major clinical feature of cardiogenic shock is evidence of inadequate tissue perfusion manifested by peripheral vasoconstriction, delayed capillary refill, and decreased mental capacity. An additional feature is pulmonary congestion or pulmonary edema. In cases of acute left ventricular dysfunction, the heart is unable to propel blood to the systemic peripheral circulation. The lower pressure right ventricle and pulmonary circulation typically are less affected by pump failure, and blood flow through the right side of the heart to the lungs continues. In the left side of the heart, cardiac emptying to the peripheral circulation is compromised. Left atrial filling pressures increase, resulting in congestion of the pulmonary vascular bed. As a consequence, oxygenation can be impaired. Tachypnea, shortness of breath, and rales are observed. In cases of acute valvular dysfunction, cardiac murmurs can be heard.

The mortality rate for cardiogenic shock is between 48% and 90%.[15,16] Risk factors for death from cardiogenic shock complicating MI include age, previous MI, cold and clammy skin, and oliguria (scanty urine production).[17] The best outcomes are achieved in patients in whom the cause of the cardiac dysfunction can be quickly reversed. For patients with acute MI, reversal is achieved by myocardial revascularization.

For patients with cardiogenic shock caused by cardiac ischemia, nitroglycerin is not indicated because hypotension can be exacerbated by its vasodilatory effects. The use of beta-adrenergic blockers should also be limited. These products should be initiated only after resolution of the state of hypoperfusion.[18]

Heart rate (**chronotropism**), force of cardiac contraction (**inotropism**), and systemic vascular resistance can all be manipulated by adrenergic agonists. The manipulation of these receptors by drugs that bind to them allows the provider to alter cardiac performance. As stated in Chapter 1, adrenergic receptors are categorized into four major groups: alpha$_1$, alpha$_2$, beta$_1$, and beta$_2$. Stimulation of each type of adrenergic receptor results in predominant effects. A patient whose heart would benefit from positive inotropic and chronotropic effects would be well served by a medication that stimulates the beta$_1$-adrenergic receptors. The use of many inotropic agents, including the drugs discussed next, is associated with increased patient mortality.[19] A careful risk–benefit analysis and/or consultation with online medical control is essential.

Two adrenergic agonists are most commonly used in cardiogenic shock: dobutamine and dopamine. Dobutamine is the agent of choice to improve cardiac output in cardiogenic shock for patients with systolic blood pressure greater than 80 mm Hg.[18] Dobutamine's major effect is to increase cardiac contractility and cardiac output. Although it has some beta$_1$ stimulatory effects, dobutamine does not significantly increase heart rate. Tachycardia should be avoided in cardiogenic shock to minimize the heart's oxygen demand. Dobutamine also does not raise systemic vascular resistance. Patients receiving this medication should be closely observed for tachycardia and hypotension. Specifically, dobutamine should be used with caution in atrial fibrillation.

Dopamine is another effective medication for patients in cardiogenic shock.[18] A beta$_1$-mediated increase in contractility and heart rate can improve cardiac output, but the downside of this effect is an increase in myocardial oxygen consumption. Because dopamine causes some alpha-mediated vasoconstriction, it is a good choice for the treatment of cardiogenic shock associated with hypotension (systolic blood pressure less than 80 mm Hg). As the dose of dopamine is increased, a predominantly alpha-mediated vasoconstriction occurs.

Dopamine has beta$_1$ effects, as well as alpha$_1$ effects. The alpha$_1$ stimulation produces vasoconstriction, which increases blood pressure. Dopamine can exacerbate myocardial ischemia from tachycardia and increased systemic vascular resistance.

In patients with cardiogenic shock refractory to dopamine, norepinephrine (Levophed) should be administered.[18] Norepinephrine is an alpha$_1$, alpha$_2$, and beta$_1$ agonist. Alpha-mediated peripheral vasoconstriction is the predominant clinical result of administration. Providers may recommend norepinephrine as the initial vasopressor for hypotensive patients in cardiogenic shock. If used, the lowest possible dose should be administered.

Milrinone (Primacor) is another drug used to treat cardiogenic shock by stimulating the heart to increase cardiac output. The drugs previously discussed in this chapter are medications that treat cardiogenic shock by binding various adrenergic receptors. Milrinone, however, is a member of the class of drugs known as **phosphodiesterase inhibitors**, which ultimately increase the concentration of calcium inside the cardiac cell. As such, milrinone is able to improve cardiac output independently of adrenergic receptors. Because milrinone works by a different mechanism, it can be effective in patients who do not respond to therapy with the adrenergic stimulating agents (dopamine, dobutamine, and norepinephrine).

Milrinone has a positive inotropic effect and peripheral vasodilatory action, but it has no significant chronotropic or arrhythmogenic action. Because of the vasodilatory effect, patients should be closely observed for hypotension.[18]

Special caution is required when infusing vasoactive medications, and monitoring is absolutely critical. Hypoperfusion, cardiac arrhythmias, and exacerbation of myocardial ischemia are real possibilities. Reliable venous access must be maintained. When administering vasoactive drugs, be sure that venous access is reliably secured. Sudden loss of the therapeutic benefits of inotropic or vasopressor medication infusions may be catastrophic for the patient. If an IV line becomes dislodged and the vasoactive drug infiltrates into the soft tissue, the patient may incur extensive soft tissue necrosis at the site of the drug infiltration. The risk of soft tissue damage with subcutaneous infusion of adrenergic agonists from an infiltrated IV site is great. If subcutaneous infiltration does occur, infiltration of 10 mg phentolamine mixed in 5 to 10 mL of normal saline can prevent tissue loss.[20]

DOBUTAMINE (DOBUTREX)

Classification: Adrenergic agent, inotropic.

Action: Acts primarily as an agonist at $beta_1$-adrenergic receptors with minor $beta_2$ and $alpha_1$ effects. Consequently, dobutamine increases myocardial contractility and stroke volume with minor chronotropic effects, resulting in increased cardiac output.

Indications: Heart failure, cardiogenic shock.

Adverse Effects: Tachycardia, premature ventricular contractions, hypertension, hypotension, palpitations, arrhythmias.

Contraindications: Suspected or known poisoning/drug-induced shock, systolic blood pressure <100 mm Hg with signs of shock, idiopathic hypertrophic subaortic stenosis, known sensitivity (including sulfites). Use with caution in hypertension, recent MI, arrhythmias, hypovolemia.

Dosage:

- **Adult:** Initial 0.5 to 1 mcg/kg per minute IV, IO. Maintenance infusions are typically 2 to 20 mcg/kg per minute. At doses >20 mcg/kg per minute, increases of heart rate of >10% may induce or exacerbate myocardial ischemia.
- **Pediatric:** Same as adult dosing.

Special Considerations:

Half-life 2 minutes.

Pregnancy class C.

DOPAMINE (INTROPIN)

Classification: Adrenergic agonist, inotropic, vasopressor.

Action: Stimulates alpha- and beta-adrenergic receptors. At moderate doses (2 to 10 mcg/kg per minute), dopamine stimulates $beta_1$ receptors, resulting in inotropy and increased cardiac output while maintaining dopaminergic-induced vasodilatory effects. At high doses (>10 mcg/kg per minute), alpha-adrenergic agonism predominates, and increased peripheral vascular resistance and vasoconstriction result.

Indications: Hypotension and decreased cardiac output associated with cardiogenic shock and septic shock, hypotension after return of spontaneous circulation following cardiac arrest, symptomatic bradycardia unresponsive to atropine.

Adverse Effects: Tachycardia, arrhythmias, skin and soft tissue necrosis, severe hypertension from excessive vasoconstriction, angina, dyspnea, headache, nausea/vomiting.

© Jones & Bartlett Learning.

Contraindications: Pheochromocytoma, ventricular fibrillation, ventricular tachycardia, or other ventricular arrhythmias, known sensitivity (including sulfites). Correct any hypovolemia with volume fluid replacement before administering dopamine.

Dosage:

- **Adult:** 2 to 20 mcg/kg per minute IV, IO infusion. Starting dose 5 mcg/kg per minute; may gradually increase the infusion by 5 to 10 mcg/kg per minute to desired effect. Cardiac dose is usually 5 to 10 mcg/kg per minute; vasopressor dose is usually 10 to 20 mcg/kg per minute. Little benefit is gained beyond 20 mcg/kg per minute.
- **Pediatric:** Same as adult dosing.

Special Considerations:

Half-life 2 minutes.

Pregnancy class C.

NOREPINEPHRINE (LEVOPHED)

Classification: Adrenergic agonist, inotropic, vasopressor.
Action: Norepinephrine is an alpha$_1$, alpha$_2$, and beta$_1$ agonist. Alpha-mediated peripheral vasoconstriction is the predominant clinical result of administration, resulting in increasing blood pressure and coronary blood flow. Beta-adrenergic action produces inotropic stimulation of the heart and dilates the coronary arteries.
Indications: Cardiogenic shock, septic shock, severe hypotension.
Adverse Effects: Dizziness, anxiety, cardiac arrhythmias, dyspnea, exacerbation of asthma.
Contraindications: Patients taking monoamine oxidase inhibitors (MAOIs), known sensitivity. Use with caution in hypovolemia.
Dosage:
- **Adult:** Add 4 mg to 250 mL of D$_5$W or D$_5$NS, but not normal saline alone. 0.1 to 0.5 mcg/kg per minute as IV, IO, titrated to maintain blood pressure >80 mm Hg. Many settings still use non-weight-based dosing of 2 to 4 mcg/min titrated upward for the desired clinical effect. Refractory shock may require doses as high as 30 mcg/min.
- **Pediatric:** 0.05 to 2 mcg/kg per minute IV, IO infusion, to a maximum dose of 2 mcg/kg per minute.

Special Considerations:
Do not administer in the same IV line as alkaline solutions.
Half-life 1 minute.
Pregnancy class C.

MILRINONE (PRIMACOR)

Classification: Inotropic.
Action: Milrinone is a positive inotropic drug and vasodilator with minimal chronotropic effect. Milrinone inhibits an enzyme, cAMP phosphodiesterase, which results in an increase in the concentration of calcium inside the cardiac cell. The result is improvement in diastolic function and myocardial contractility.
Indications: Cardiogenic shock, heart failure.
Adverse Effects: Cardiac arrhythmias, nausea/vomiting, hypotension.
Contraindications: Valvular heart disease, known sensitivity.
Dosage:
- **Adult:** 50 mcg/kg IV, IO over a period of 10 minutes, followed by an infusion of 0.375 to 0.5 mcg/kg per minute (max dose: 0.75 mcg/kg per minute).
- **Pediatric:** Same as adult dosing.

Special Considerations:
Pregnancy class C.

Neurogenic Shock

CASE STUDY

You are a flight medic and your aircraft is dispatched to a motor vehicle crash in which one person is reported to be entrapped. You arrive to find the patient, a 17-year-old girl, trapped by her legs in the driver's seat. First responders have placed her in a cervical collar and started oxygen. The patient is talking but appears to be somewhat lethargic. Your assessment shows that her airway is clearly patent. Your partner reports a pulse oximeter reading of 93%. Her breath sounds are clear bilaterally, and she appears to be moving her chest wall equally. You note that her respirations appear to be somewhat rapid and shallow and estimate that her respiratory rate is approximately 32 breaths/min. You reach over to take her pulse and note that it is palpable but weak. Her heart rate is only 52 beats/min, and her blood pressure is 90/56 mm Hg. She tells you that she cannot move her legs and that she cannot feel anything below her nipple line.

Once her legs have been freed, you place the patient in full spinal immobilization and extricate her from the vehicle.

Prehospital professionals encounter **neurogenic shock** in patients who have had a spinal cord injury. When the sympathetic pathways from the spinal cord are interrupted by an injury, blood vessels dilate. When all the blood vessels of the affected area dilate, the volume of the vascular tree has enlarged, but the amount of the blood filling the vasculature has remained the same, which results in relative hypovolemia. These patients may appear similar to those with hypovolemic shock, even when they have not lost blood. Complicating matters, if the lesion to the spinal cord involves the sympathetic innervation of the heart, the patient may also have bradycardia, meaning the heart will slow and aggravate the hypotension.

Patients with neurogenic shock may also have bradycardia in addition to hypotension.

Patients with neurogenic shock lose input to the blood vessels from the nervous system. Without this input, the blood vessels dilate. Without losing a single drop of blood, the patient is initially hypovolemic.

Imagine having a car with a 10-gallon tank. In that tank are 10 gallons of gasoline. If for some unexplained reason the tank expands to a 20-gallon capacity with the same 10 gallons of gasoline, the tank is suddenly half full. To maintain the tank's full status, the action would be twofold: try to fill the now-larger tank, and try to reduce the size of the tank.

Fluid infusion to improve preload is the initial therapy for neurogenic shock. Neurogenic shock mainly involves managing a bigger vascular container, and fluid administration simply refills that vascular container. Of note, fluids, not vasopressors, are the initial treatment for neurogenic shock. Prehospital providers encounter multiple-trauma patients who are hypotensive, with the origin being hemorrhage, spinal cord injury, or perhaps both. Do not assume that hypotension is from spinal shock and then rush to use a vasopressor. As previously mentioned, vasopressors used in hemorrhagic shock improve blood pressure but decrease tissue perfusion and oxygen delivery. The net effect is that the shock is worse.

IV fluids, not vasopressors, are the initial treatment for neurogenic shock.

The treatment for the patient with hypotensive trauma is the same whether the cause is hemorrhage or spinal shock: IV fluid therapy. Remember, exercise moderation when providing IV fluids to a hypotensive patient with trauma. Patients with hypotension from neurogenic shock may not exhibit the expected tachycardia and may even have bradycardia because of a loss of cardiac sympathetic tone.

Once the volume status of the patient is adequate, consideration should be given to the use of vasopressor agents. If the patient has a low heart rate, dopamine would be the recommended vasopressor. Dopamine possesses alpha effects, which stimulate the adrenergic receptors on the blood vessels and reestablish the vascular tone lost from the interruption of sympathetic innervation. Dopamine also has $beta_1$ properties that increase the heart rate. Many patients have an adequate heart rate and require only the benefit of an agent capable of providing alpha stimulation. Phenylephrine (Neo-Synephrine) stimulates only the alpha receptor and is the most common choice for patients in neurogenic shock.

PHENYLEPHRINE (NEO-SYNEPHRINE)

Classification: Adrenergic agonist.
Action: Stimulates the alpha receptors, causing vasoconstriction, which results in increased blood pressure.
Indications: Neurogenic shock, spinal shock, cases of shock in which the patient's heart rate does not need to be increased, drug-induced hypotension.
Adverse Effects: Hypertension, ventricular tachycardia, headache, excitability, tremor, MI, exacerbation of asthma, cardiac arrhythmias, reflex bradycardia, soft tissue necrosis.
Contraindications: Acute MI, angina, cardiac arrhythmias, severe hypertension, coronary artery disease, pheochromocytoma, narrow-angle glaucoma, cardiomyopathy, MAOI therapy, known sensitivity to phenylephrine or sulfites.
Dosage:

- **Adult:** 100 to 180 mcg/min IV, IO. Once the blood pressure has been stabilized, the dose can be reduced to 40 to 60 mcg/min.
- **Pediatric (2 to 12 years):** 5 to 20 mcg/kg IV, IO followed by 0.1 to 0.5 mcg/kg per minute IV, IO (max dose: 3 mcg/kg per minute IV, IO).

Special Considerations:
Pregnancy class C.

(*continued*) Once the patient is safely on a cot, immobilized, and placed in the helicopter, you repeat an assessment. Her airway is patent; respirations are shallow and rapid at 28 breaths/min. Heart rate is slow at 54 beats/min, and when you palpate her pulse you note that her skin is warm. Blood pressure is 88/60 mm Hg. Her neurologic status is unchanged, with no motor or sensory function below the nipple line. Your assessment is that the patient has a spinal cord injury and is in spinal shock. Because she is a multiple-trauma victim from a motor vehicle crash, you are also worried that the patient could have blood loss from injuries to internal organs such as the liver and spleen. Therefore the patient could also have an element of hypovolemic shock. You know that the initial treatment for neurogenic shock is the same as for hypovolemic shock: intravascular volume expansion. You administer a bolus of 1 L Ringer's lactate solution, and the vital signs are essentially unchanged. You administer a second liter of Ringer's lactate. She still has some bradycardia (heart rate 60 beats/min), and her blood pressure after the second liter of fluid is 92/58 mm Hg. Her skin is still warm. You consult medical direction and report your neurologic examination of no motor or sensory function below the nipple line, low blood pressure, slow heart rate, and warm skin. She has only minimal response after 2 L of fluid boluses and no obvious signs of external or internal blood loss. Your estimated time to landing at the trauma center is approximately 25 minutes. Because the patient already has bradycardia, you request to start dopamine to avoid increasing the bradycardia as a complication from the phenylephrine. You start the dopamine at 5 mcg/kg per minute. Within approximately 5 minutes the blood pressure increases to 100/64 mm Hg and the heart rate increases to 66 beats/min.

Septic Shock

Septic shock is a state of shock or poor blood perfusion from the systemic effects of an infection. The infection can be localized to the blood, the lungs, urine, or an abscess. The body responds to the infection by a defensive inflammatory response that is exaggerated. The exaggerated response, not the infection, creates the shock state, but the infection initiates the exaggerated response. A common expression states that when falling off a cliff, it is not the fall that kills you, but the sudden stop. This is illustrative of septic shock. In most cases of septic shock, the infection is not what kills the patient; the body's response to the infection does. This simple concept is not understood by many clinicians who encounter septic shock.

In septic shock, the patient has a source of infection that initiates the complex sequence of events in the body known as a *systemic inflammatory response*. This is a massive inflammatory reaction that produces chaos in several of the body's vital organ systems. The inflammatory reaction produces toxins within the body that result in dilation of the blood vessels. Another effect of the produced toxins is that the blood vessels become "leaky," and the patient can become hypovolemic as he or she loses intravascular fluid to the extravascular space. Therefore these patients have vasodilation, such as that seen in neurogenic shock, and decreased intravascular volume, such as that seen in hypovolemic shock. As in neurogenic shock, supportive drug therapy includes intravascular volume expansion with IV fluids and the use of vasopressors after appropriate fluid resuscitation. Patients in severe sepsis or septic shock require an initial fluid bolus of 30 cc/kg (of actual body weight) within the first 3 hours of resuscitation.[21] Vasopressors such as norepinephrine can be used to provide vasopressor support while the underlying source of infection is treated.

A prehospital provider has a limited ability to have a significant effect on the actual infection. The use of IV fluids and vasopressors is supportive care until the source of the infection can eventually be identified and treated. The commonly used vasopressors (norepinephrine and dopamine) have already been discussed.

> Remember the concept introduced at the beginning of the chapter: Shock is a symptom, not a disease, and the ultimate treatment of septic shock is rapid control of the infection. This can entail antibiotics or even surgery.

Anaphylactic Shock

The prehospital management of anaphylaxis and anaphylactic shock is described in Chapter 8.

▶ Review Questions

1. List the early signs of shock.
2. What are the five types of shock?
3. What is a common treatment for all types of shock?
4. What is the initial therapy for hypovolemic shock?
5. What type of IV fluid used in the treatment of hypovolemic shock is compatible with the infusion of blood?
6. Differentiate rapid responders from transient responders and nonresponders.
7. List the benefits of pRBC transfusions as opposed to whole blood.
8. Why should Rh$^+$ blood transfusions be avoided in female patients who may become pregnant?
9. What drug might be a good choice for the treatment of cardiogenic shock in a patient who is not responding to adrenergic agents?
10. Explain why IV fluids, not vasopressors, are the initial therapy for neurogenic shock.
11. For a patient in septic shock, explain why the exaggerated response, not the infection, creates the shock state.

References

1. Gaieski DF, Mikkelsen ME. Definition, classification, etiology and pathophysiology of shock in adults. UpTo-Date. https://www.uptodate.com/contents/definition-classification-etiology-and-pathophysiology-of-shock-in-adults/print. Updated February 18, 2018. Accessed August 29, 2018.

2. Nickson C. Multi-organ dysfunction syndrome. Critical Care Compendium. https://lifeinthefastlane.com/ccc/multi-organ-dysfunction-syndrome-mods/. Updated November 15, 2016. Accessed August 30, 2018.

3. Bonanno FG. Clinical pathology of the shock syndromes. *J Emerg Trauma Shock*. 2011;4(2):233–243.

4. McManus J, Yershov A, Ludwig D, et al. Radial pulse character relationships to systolic blood pressure and trauma outcomes. *Prehosp Emerg Care*. 2005;9(4):423–428.

5. Hooper N, Armstrong TJ. Shock, hemorrhagic. *StatPearls [Internet]*. https://www.ncbi.nlm.nih.gov/books/NBK470382/. Updated November 27, 2017. Accessed August 30, 2018.

6. Mandel J, Palevsky P. Treatment of hypovolemia or hypovolemic shock in adults. UpToDate. https://www.uptodate.com/contents/treatment-of-hypovolemia-or-hypovolemic-shock-in-adults. Updated March 12, 2018. Accessed August 30, 2018.

7. Kudo D, Yoshida, Kushimoto S. Permissive hypotension/hypotensive resuscitation and restricted/controlled resuscitation in patients with severe trauma. *J Intens Care*. 2017;5(11). doi:10.1186/s40560-016-0202-z.

8. Tischerman SA, Barie P, Bokhari F, et al. Clinical practice guidelines: endpoints of resuscitation. *J Trauma*. 2004;57(4):898–912.

9. Kleinman S. Risk of HIV from blood transfusion. UpToDate. https://www.uptodate.com/contents/risk-of-hiv-from-blood-transfusion. Updated October 19, 2017. Accessed August 30, 2018.

10. Kleinman S. Blood donor screening: laboratory testing. UpToDate. https://www.uptodate.com/contents/blood-donor-screening-laboratory-testing?search=Risk%20of%20hepatitis%20from%20blood%20transfusion&source=search_result&selectedTitle=3~150&usage_type=default&display_rank=3. Updated July 27, 2018. Accessed August 30, 2018.

11. Maya E, Buntugu KA, Pobee F, Srofenyoh E. Rhesus negative woman transfused with rhesus positive blood: subsequent normal pregnancy without anti D production. *Ghana Med J*. 2015;49(1):60–63.

12. United States Department of Defense. *Emergency War Surgery*. 4th ed. Washington, DC: United States Department of Defense; 2013.

13. Reed H. The role of tranexamic acid in EMS and preoperative trauma management. *J Emerg Med Serv*. https://www.jems.com/articles/print/volume-38/issue-4/patient-care/role-tranexamic-acid-ems-preoperative-tr.html. Published March 27, 2013. Accessed October 5, 2018.

14. Napolitano LM. Prehospital tranexamic acid: what is the current evidence? *Trauma Surg Acute Care Open*. 2017;2:e000056. doi:10.1136/tsaco-2016-000056.

15. Hochman JS, Reyentovich A. Clinical manifestations and diagnosis of cardiogenic shock in acute myocardial infarction. UpToDate. https://www.uptodate.com/contents/clinical-manifestations-and-diagnosis-of-cardiogenic-shock-in-acute-myocardial-infarction. Updated December 18, 2017. Accessed August 29, 2018.

16. Malik TS, Hausenloy DJ. Cardiogenic shock and the ICU patient. *J Intens Care Soc*. 2013;4(3):235–243.

17. Hasdal D, Holmes DR Jr, Califf RM, et al. Cardiac shock complicating acute myocardial infarction: predictors of death. *Am Heart J*. 1999;138(1 pt 10):21.

18. Hollenberg S, Kavinsky C, Parrillo J. Cardiogenic shock. *Ann Intern Med*. 1999;131:47.

19. Tariq S, Aronow WS. Use of inotropic agents in treatment of systolic heart failure. *Int J Molecul Sci*. 2015;16(12):29060–29068.

20. Peters JI, Utset OM. Vasopressors in shock management: choosing and using wisely. *J Crit Illness*. 1989;4:62.

21. Schmidt G, Mandel J. Evaluation and management of suspected sepsis and septic shock in adults. UpToDate. https://www.uptodate.com/contents/evaluation-and-management-of-suspected-sepsis-and-septic-shock-in-adults. Updated July 27, 2018. Accessed August 30, 2018.

© Andrew Brookes/Getty Images

CHAPTER 17

Traumatic Brain Injury

▶ Introduction

Head injury, also known as **traumatic brain injury (TBI)**, is one of the leading causes of death and disability after trauma. Every year in the United States, approximately 2.5 million people incur a TBI that is severe enough to require an emergency department visit.[1] Roughly 56,000 people die each year from either isolated TBI or a TBI associated with other injuries, and 282,000 are hospitalized.[2] The role of the prehospital professional in improving outcomes in this group of patients is monumental. Simple interventions initiated in the field have profound effects on the patient in the hours and weeks to follow.

CASE STUDY

Your unit is dispatched to the scene of a gunshot wound. Police have already arrived and secured the scene. On your arrival, law enforcement reports that the victim appears to have been cleaning his handgun when the weapon discharged, shooting the man in the head. You find a 58-year-old man lying supine on the floor, holding a bath towel over the bleeding wound on his forehead. You immediately evaluate his ABCs. His airway is patent, he is breathing spontaneously, and he is perfusing well. He is conscious, answers questions, and moves all four extremities on command. You do not identify any motor or sensory deficits. His heart rate is 88 beats/min, blood pressure is 148/92 mm Hg, respiratory rate is 16 breaths/min, and pulse oximeter reading is 94%. You place the patient on oxygen by a nonrebreather face mask, apply a sterile dressing to the wound, and ask your partner to hold pressure on the wound while you start an intravenous (IV) line.

▶ Traumatic Brain Injury

Any type of head injury involves one of two types of trauma to the brain. **Primary brain injury** occurs directly to the brain from mechanical forces at the time of the initial insult. **Secondary brain injury** occurs hours after the time of the injury. In a significant number of head-injured patients, secondary brain injury leads to delayed death and disability.

The brain is contained in a bony, boxlike structure—the skull. With secondary brain injury, the brain swells, resulting in a decrease in blood flow to the injured brain (**FIGURE 17-1A**). Therefore, the brain experiences additional swelling, resulting in even less blood flow. And so continues the cycle of increased swelling, reduced blood flow, and increased secondary brain injury. As the brain swells, the pressure inside the skull increases; this is known as intracerebral hypertension or **intracranial pressure (ICP)** (**FIGURE 17-1B**). **Hypotension** and **hypoxia** have been noted to double the death rate after head trauma from secondary brain injury.[3]

CASE STUDY

You and your partner are dispatched to a motor vehicle crash in which the driver is reported to be entrapped. You arrive to find a 19-year-old woman trapped in the driver's seat. She appears to be unconscious and has sonorous respirations. A first responder has gained access to the rear seat of the vehicle and has immobilized the patient's cervical spine. The extrication crew informs you that they should have the patient out of the vehicle in a few minutes. You evaluate the patient and find that she does have spontaneous respirations, but they appear to be somewhat labored. Her chest rise and breath sounds are equal. She has a weak radial pulse of approximately 120 beats/min by palpation. On your secondary examination, you discover that the patient has a significant number of facial fractures, a large laceration on her posterior scalp, and unequal pupils. You determine that her other injuries include a right femur fracture.

No specific interventions can prevent primary brain injury, but secondary brain injury is preventable and somewhat treatable. The two most important interventions to avoid secondary brain injury are to prevent hypoxia and hypotension. Therefore the prehospital provider's priorities for patient treatment in a scenario such as the previous one are to ensure patency of the airway, deliver high-flow oxygen, monitor oxygen saturation, apply pressure to the wound to preserve blood volume, and maintain adequate blood pressure with IV fluids.

Management

The treatment of severe TBI has two goals. The initial treatment approach is to correct and prevent hypoxia and hypotension. This is accomplished by ensuring a patent airway, providing supplemental oxygen as necessary, controlling hemorrhage, and providing fluid volume resuscitation as appropriate. Secondary brain injury results in swelling of the brain, which increases the ICP, which reduces blood flow to the brain and oxygen delivery to the brain tissue. Often the swelling of the brain (secondary brain injury) is more lethal than the primary brain injury. As the patient arrives at the hospital, the next priority is to assess for the need for

| ■ CSF | ■ Mass | ■ Brain | ■ Arterial volume | ■ Venous volume |

FIGURE 17-1 A. Severe traumatic brain injury with epidural hematoma and cerebral edema.
B. Monro-Kellie doctrine. *Normal conditions:* The skull contains the brain, arterial blood, venous blood, and cerebrospinal fluid (CSF). *Compensated state, intracranial pressure (ICP) normal:* With an intracranial mass from an intracranial hematoma, the body compensates by decreasing the volume of CSF. *Decompensated state, ICP elevated:* With ongoing expansion of the mass or swelling of the brain, the volumes of venous or arterial blood decrease. The result is an elevation of ICP.

A. © Living Art Enterprises, LLC/Science Source.

emergent surgical intervention. Surgery is typically indicated for penetrating injuries. Blunt injuries such as **epidural hematomas**, **subdural hematomas**, and intracerebral hemorrhages require either surgical intervention or careful monitoring depending on the volume, impact to surrounding structures, or clinical status of the patient.[4] Ongoing management includes continued prevention of hypoxia and hypotension, control of elevated ICP, and ongoing monitoring and supportive treatment.

Good prehospital care may reduce the mortality rate and improve the outcome in head-injured patients in the days to weeks after the injury.

The primary brain injury occurs before any EMS responder arrives on the scene of an emergency. The early care that the head-injured patient receives before arrival at a trauma center or evaluation by a neurosurgeon often determines whether a patient survives and the magnitude of impairment.

The pharmacologic management of TBIs is focused on reducing the magnitude of the secondary brain swelling, decreasing the ICP, and improving the blood flow to the brain.

Mannitol (Osmitrol) is an **osmotic diuretic** that principally works in the injured brain by dehydrating the brain and thereby decreasing swelling. Osmotic diuretics pull fluid out of tissues and cells and move it into the vascular space, where excessive fluids can be filtered out in urine. Mannitol expands the intravascular volume and reduces the viscosity of blood, improving blood flow in the injured brain. Administration of mannitol requires ongoing monitoring of the patient's kidney function, electrolyte levels and serum osmolality.

Hypertonic saline works in a similar fashion as mannitol to decrease brain swelling and ICP by dehydrating the brain. Hypertonic saline has a significantly greater concentration of sodium than normal or physiologic saline (0.9%). (The concentration of hypertonic saline can vary in different regions.) The effect of increased sodium concentration is that water is pulled from brain tissue toward the elevated sodium concentration in the vascular space. This movement of water toward a high sodium concentration is an example of osmosis. The result is dehydration of the brain and a reduction of ICP. It has been shown to decrease brain swelling in patients with TBI who demonstrate secondary brain injury.[5] Despite a growing body of research, the use of hypertonic saline for resuscitation of severe trauma and TBI patients remains controversial.[6] Follow agency or regional protocols in these situations. Patients may experience severe increases in ICP if osmotic/hypertonic fluids are suddenly discontinued.[5]

Sedative medications such as diazepam, lorazepam, and others discussed earlier in this text can also reduce cerebral metabolic demands and ultimately lower ICP.[4] Many of these medications have the added benefit of preventing or controlling seizure activity, which frequently occurs following a TBI. When administering these medications, it is extremely important to monitor the patient's blood pressure. The patient's level of consciousness must also be monitored closely if he or she does not have a definitive airway, such as an endotracheal tube, in place.

(*continued*) The patient is extricated, her spine is immobilized, and she is intubated. You are en route to the hospital. The patient's left pupil is enlarged and nonreactive to light, and she exhibits flexion posturing. You are concerned that the patient has elevated ICP. Your transport time is 35 minutes to the local trauma center, and the weather does not permit helicopter transport. You communicate your concerns to medical direction and obtain permission to administer mannitol.

MANNITOL (OSMITROL)

Classification: Osmotic diuretic.
Action: Facilitates the flow of fluid out of tissues (including the brain) and into interstitial fluid and blood, thereby dehydrating the brain and reducing swelling. Reabsorption by the kidney is minimal, consequently increasing urine output.
Indications: Increased ICP.

Adverse Effects: Pulmonary edema, headache, blurred vision, dizziness, seizures, hypovolemia, nausea/vomiting, diarrhea, electrolyte imbalances, hypotension, hypertension, sinus tachycardia, premature ventricular contractions, angina, phlebitis.

Contraindications: Active intracranial bleeding, heart failure, pulmonary edema, severe dehydration. Use with caution in hypovolemia, renal failure.

Dosage:
- **Adult:** 0.25 to 1 g/kg IV, intraosseous (IO) followed by 0.25 to 1 g/kg infused over 20 to 30 minutes, administered every 4 hours.
- **Pediatric:** 0.25 to 1 g/kg IV, IO followed by 0.25 to 0.5 g/kg infused over 20 to 30 minutes every 4 hours.

Special Considerations:
Mannitol should not be given in the same IV, IO line as blood.
Pregnancy class C.

HYPERTONIC SALINE (3% SALINE)

Classification: Volume expander, electrolyte solution.

Action: The hypertonic nature of this fluid pulls extravascular fluid into the vascular space. Hypertonic saline may, therefore, be used as a volume expander in cases of hypovolemia or to reduce the edema of the swollen brain. Three percent saline has an electrolyte concentration of 513 mEq/L sodium.[7]

Indications: Reduction of increased ICP resulting from TBI, hypovolemic shock.

Contraindications: Pulmonary congestion, pulmonary edema, known sensitivity. Hypertonic saline should not be administered by the IO route.

Dosage: Note: Hypertonic saline is available in several concentrations from 3 to 5%.
- **Adult:** 300-mL bag (3% solution) of hypertonic saline infused IV slowly over 20 minutes.
- **Pediatric:** 0.1 to 1 mL/kg per hour continuous infusion.

Special Considerations:
Hypertonic saline can cause damage to the vein in which it is administered. Use a larger or central vein whenever possible. Monitor carefully for extravasation.
Pregnancy class C.

▶ Review Questions

1. Differentiate primary brain injury and secondary brain injury.
2. What are the effects of hypotension and hypoxia on survival from brain injury?
3. List two goals of the treatment of severe TBI.
4. How does mannitol decrease brain swelling?
5. When administrating hypertonic saline, should the infusion be administered rapidly or slowly, and why?

References

1. Centers for Disease Control and Prevention. *Report to Congress on Traumatic Brain Injury in the United States: Epidemiology and Rehabilitation.* Atlanta, GA: National Center for Injury Prevention and Control; Division of Unintentional Injury Prevention; 2015.
2. Rajajee V. Traumatic brain injury: epidemiology, classification and pathophysiology. UpToDate. https://www.uptodate.com/contents/traumatic-brain-injury-epidemiology-classification-and-pathophysiology. Updated July 18, 2018. Accessed August 30, 2018.
3. Spaite DW, Chengcheng H, Bobrwo BJ, et al. The effect of combined out-of-hospital hypotension and hypoxia on mortality in major traumatic brain injury. *Ann Emerg Med.* 2017;69(1):62–72. doi:10.1016/j.annemergmed.2016.08.007.
4. Rajajee V. Management of acute severe traumatic brain injury. UpToDate. https://www.uptodate.com/contents/management-of-acute-severe-traumatic-brain-injury. Updated July 13, 2018. Accessed August 30, 2018.
5. Boone MD, Oren-Grinberg A, Robinson TM, Chen CC, Kasper EM. Mannitol or hypertonic saline in the setting of traumatic brain injury: what have we learned? *Surg Neurol Int.* 2015;6:177. doi:10.4103/2152-7806.170248.
6. Dubick MA, Shek P, Wade CE. ROC trials update on prehospital hypertonic saline resuscitation in the aftermath of the US-Canadian trials. *Clinics.* 2013;68(6):883–886. doi:10.6061/clinics/2013(06)25.
7. Hyponatremia correction infusate rate. Medscape. https://reference.medscape.com/calculator/hyponatremia-correction-infusate-rate. Accessed August 30, 2018.

PART III

Special Considerations and Procedures

PART III

Special
Considerations and
Procedures

© Andrew Brookes/Getty Images

CHAPTER 18

Critical Care Transport

OBJECTIVES

1. Define the following transport equipment: *intravenous lines, flow controllers, pressure bags, infusion sets, intravenous pumps, drug calculators,* and *fluid warmers.*
2. Discuss medications used in transport for the treatment of HELLP syndrome: magnesium sulfate, phenytoin (Dilantin), hydralazine (Apresoline), and labetalol (Trandate, Normodyne).
3. Discuss the signs and preferred treatment for magnesium sulfate toxicity.
4. Discuss medications used in transport for treatment after cardiac arrest or myocardial infarction: vecuronium (Norcuron), amiodarone (Cordarone), midazolam (Versed), and eptifibatide (Integrilin).
5. Discuss medications used in transport for the treatment of a closed-head injury: propofol (Diprivan), fentanyl citrate (Sublimaze), and mannitol (Osmitrol).
6. Describe the Parkland formula, the Wallace rule of nines, and the rule of palms in treating patients with a burn injury.
7. List signs and symptoms of a blood transfusion reaction.

MEDICATIONS THAT APPEAR IN CHAPTER 18

Magnesium sulfate
Phenytoin (Dilantin)
Fosphenytoin (Cerebyx)
Hydralazine (Apresoline)
Labetalol (Normodyne, Trandate)
Calcium gluconate

Midazolam (Versed)
Amiodarone (Cordarone)
Eptifibatide (Integrilin)
Vecuronium (Norcuron)
Insulin, regular (Humulin R, Novolin R)
Propofol (Diprivan)

Mannitol (Osmitrol)
Fentanyl citrate (Sublimaze)

▶ Introduction

Critical care transport (CCT) can include air medical transport from the scene, as well as ground and air transport from one facility to another. Paramedics typically are quite familiar with the transport of patients from the scene to the hospital. However, interfacility transport involves different patient management strategies, multiple medications, and advanced procedures. Although paramedics are not expected to know every drug used in the medical field, familiarity with commonly used critical care drugs encountered during transport is beneficial. This chapter pulls together the challenges of prolonged transport of critically ill patients and incorporates concepts of drug therapy, safety of administration, medication math, and medication administration equipment.

▶ Transport Equipment

Familiarity with equipment is an important aspect of CCT. This includes intravenous (IV) lines, flow controllers, pressure bags, infusion sets, and IV pumps. (Although some of this equipment may also be presented elsewhere in this text, its inclusion here is specific to the discussion of CCT.)

Intravenous Lines

IV lines are available in several forms. A **peripheral line** is a 14- to 24-gauge catheter inserted into a peripheral vein. A **central venous catheter (CVC)** (also known as a central line) is a special IV catheter inserted into a central vein to allow the quick administration of medications and large volumes of fluid.

The most common central line is a **triple-lumen catheter (TLC)** (**FIGURE 18-1**). It has three ports that are typically color coded: distal, medial, and proximal. Because these catheters are made by several manufacturers, the ends of the catheters must be read to determine their placement. The distal port is the end of the catheter. This port can be used for central venous pressure monitoring, as well. The medial port is between the distal and proximal ports. The proximal port is at the end of the catheter closest to the exit from the patient. TLCs have internal catheter lumens ranging from 14 gauge down to 22 gauge or smaller, depending on the particular port or catheter used.[1,2]

Other types of CVCs may be a better choice in situations where massive amounts of blood products and IV fluids are being administered. Large single-lumen CVCs are capable of delivering much larger fluid volume than TLCs can.[3] CVCs may also be used to monitor blood oxygen levels, perform transvenous cardiac pacing, obtain blood samples, determine patient cardiac output, and perform other specialized functions. EMS providers who transport patients with these devices in place should obtain appropriate training in order to avoid or appropriately manage complications related to the use of these various devices. Careful monitoring is needed with these devices during transport. Inadvertent CVC dislodgement or tubing disconnect may allow large amounts of blood loss directly from central circulation. Catheter migration further into central circulation has the potential to cause other serious complications. Infection is also a serious risk, so EMS providers must use strict aseptic technique when handling CVCs.

Peripherally inserted central catheter (PICC) lines are also common (**FIGURE 18-2**). This catheter's entry point usually is an upper extremity, with the end of the catheter in a central vein. PICC lines must be regularly flushed to prevent clotting. Some patients have implantable devices, such as MediPorts (Bard Access Systems, Salt Lake City, Utah) or PORT-A-CATHs (Smiths Medical, Colonial Way, Watford [UK]). These types of catheters typically are inserted in patients with a chronic medical condition that requires frequent administration of IV medications. A common indication would be a patient with a malignancy needing chemotherapy. A **Huber needle** is a special needle that must be used to access these ports (**FIGURE 18-3**).

Patients occasionally have an **arterial line** in place, which is an invasive line used for continuous blood pressure monitoring. The set includes pressurized tubing, a transducer, and a bag of normal saline inside a **pressure bag**. The pressure bag is required to prevent the backflow of blood into the tubing from the arterial system. If you need to transport a patient with an arterial line but your monitor does not have the capability to monitor invasive blood pressure, meticulous observation is necessary. The pressure bag needs to remain properly inflated in order to keep arterial blood from flowing into the fluid bag. Additionally, the entire length

FIGURE 18-1 Triple-lumen catheter.

FIGURE 18-2 **A.** Peripherally inserted central catheter (PICC) line. **B.** Placement of a PICC line.
A. © Rob Byron/Shutterstock.

of arterial line tubing should remain exposed and visible to transport personnel. Inadvertent tubing disconnection or stopcock opening may lead to massive blood loss if not recognized promptly. Large volumes of patient blood may otherwise go undetected as it pools in patient clothing or linen, or on the EMS stretcher. Arterial lines are used only for monitoring and arterial blood sampling. Do not administer any medications or fluids into these lines.

Flow Controllers

Flow controllers that are not part of a traditional infusion pump are sometimes used during CCT. A commonly used flow controller is the Dial-A-Flo (Hospira, Lake Forest, Illinois) (**FIGURE 18-4**), which can be connected to the IV tubing as an extension set, allowing the paramedic to adjust a dial and ultimately deliver a set volume of fluid.

FIGURE 18-3 Two Huber needles used to enter an implanted part, such as MediPorts and PORT-A-CATHs.

Flow dial

FIGURE 18-4 Dial-A-Flo flow controller. (Flow regulator set distributed by Hospira, Lake Forest, Illinois.)

Pressure Bags

A pressure bag can be used in several different ways. By inflating a pressure bag over IV fluids, the paramedic can increase the amount of volume delivered to the patient at any given time. For example, when transporting a burn victim who needs increased fluids to maintain a normotensive blood pressure, the fluids can be placed in a pressure bag. Pressure bags are used to increase the rate of IV administration beyond what is possible with simply placing the IV bag to wide-open flow with only gravity. When high IV flow rates are required, a pressure bag is often necessary. A patient need not be hypotensive to require a pressure bag.

Two types of pressure bags allow the paramedic to accommodate either 500- or 1,000-mL bags of fluid. The setup of both bags is the same: a slot for placement of the IV fluid, a connector from the bag to a balloon pump, a valve regulator, and an attached stopcock (**FIGURE 18-5**). The stopcock must be in the lateral (perpendicular to the tubing) position to inflate the bag. Once the bag is inflated to the desired pressure of 300 mm Hg, a green regulator valve appears. If the bag is overinflated, a red regulator valve appears, prompting a decrease in pressure. The stopcock must be turned upward to maintain the pressure in the bag. When the bag is ready to be deflated, simply turn it downward.

FIGURE 18-5 A 1,000-mL pressure bag.

When administering IV fluids with a pressure bag, aspirate any air from the IV fluid bag to avoid an air embolism.

Infusion Sets

Paramedics must be familiar with the different types of **infusion sets** that may be used in an interfacility transport. Infusion sets are used in the administration of IV fluids through peripheral or CVCs. The four main types of infusion sets are **macrodrip**, **microdrip**, **blood tubing sets**, and **volume-control chamber** sets. Each of these infusion sets can also be packaged for use as an infusion pump. In addition, infusion sets can be vented or nonvented. **Multidrip infusion sets** are widely used.

Macrodrip Infusion Sets

Macrodrip infusion sets allow the administration of 1 mL of fluid in 10 to 15 drops, depending on the set (**FIGURE 18-6A**). They are used to administer rapid infusions and basic maintenance fluids such as normal saline and Ringer's lactate solution.

Microdrip Infusion Sets

Microdrip infusion sets can administer 1 mL of fluid in 60 drops, which makes drug calculations easier for administration without the use of a pump (**FIGURE 18-6B**). For example, 1 mL/min equals 60 drops in 1 minute (or 1 drop every second). For use in practice, determine the number of milliliters needed per minute to determine the drip rate.

When you grab an infusion set during an emergency, remember this: A needle in the middle of the drip chamber means it is a *micro* set (which makes calculations easier). No needle means it is a *macro* set.

FIGURE 18-6 **A.** Macrodrip infusion set. **B.** Microdrip infusion set.

Blood Tubing Sets

Blood tubing sets are usually found as Y-type blood sets. They deliver approximately 10 drops/mL with an integrated blood filter. The Y-type set allows the administration of an infusion of both normal saline and blood at the same time.

> Normal saline is the only IV fluid compatible with the administration of blood.

Volume-Control Chamber Sets

Volume-control chamber sets are used to prevent fluid overloading in patients (**FIGURE 18-7**). For example, a volume-control chamber set can be used when transporting a pediatric patient to prevent the administration of excessive amounts of fluids. To use a volume-control chamber set properly, first fill it with the desired amount of fluid. Then, set the clamp between the IV fluid and the volume-control chamber for the remainder of the administration. The clamp between the volume-control chamber and the patient can now be opened for safe administration of fluids or medications. IV infusions can be injected in the volume-control chamber and diluted with the IV fluids to be administered over a specific period.

Vented and Nonvented Infusion Sets

Vented infusion sets are necessary for the administration of fluids packaged in glass containers, such as nitroglycerin, eptifibatide (Integrilin), propofol (Diprivan), and albumin. To distinguish vented and nonvented sets, look at the tubing itself. Vented sets have a side port at the drip chamber that can be opened to allow air to flow into the closed fluid container. **Nonvented infusion sets** do not have a port for air to flow into the closed fluid container. Nonvented sets are used for fluids not packaged in glass containers, such as crystalloid solutions. Medications packaged in glass containers must be administered with a vented set so that the tubing line can be primed with the medication because of the vacuum created from the fluid.

> You just grabbed a nonvented set and are hanging mannitol. What should you do? Insert an 18- to 20-gauge needle into the spike insertion port on the glass bottle, allowing air into the bottle so that the fluid can flow with gravity.

Multidrip Infusion Sets

A new infusion set being widely used is the multidrip infusion set (**FIGURE 18-8**). The most widely used set is the Selec-3 system (Biomedix Inc., St. Paul, Minnesota). This system allows the paramedic to alternate among a 10-, 15-, and 60-drop set on one system. It is a quick, easy,

FIGURE 18-7 The volume-control chamber provides an additional level of safety to avoid inadvertent infusion of fluids to a pediatric patient or other volume-sensitive patient.
© Jones & Bartlett Learning.

FIGURE 18-8 Biomedix Selec-3 IV system multidrip infusion set.

and cost-effective way to make changes to the infusion rate without changing drip sets. The drop number can be changed by twisting the drip chamber to the desired drip set.

Intravenous Pumps

A commonly used **IV pump** for CCT is a three-channel pump, which allows the administration of three separate drugs. Multichannel pumps are lightweight devices that are easier to transport (**FIGURE 18-9**). They are equipped with technology that integrates a drug calculator

FIGURE 18-9 Multichannel infusion system.
© Rudy Umans/Shutterstock.

into the system. The MiniMed system, which typically is used with a three-channel pump, can be used with two types of infusion sets. The first is a traditional spike set with a pump chamber, known as a *whole set*. The second set has a pump chamber without a spike set, known as a *half set*. Half sets can be used with a 60-mL syringe and attached to the carrying case for the infusion pump.

> When using a syringe for the administration of medications, an alarm may sound. The pump will ask for confirmation that the pulling pressures are appropriate. Once the pulling pressures are adequate, a checkmark appears on the display screen for the malfunctioned channel.

A syringe system is helpful to decrease bulk when transporting a patient. A syringe system uses a large syringe containing the medication. The entire syringe is placed in a pump calibrated to compress the plunger of the syringe slowly and deliver the medication at the desired infusion rate. The syringe decreases the risk involved with transporting a patient on multiple drips supplied in glass bottles. However, when using the syringe with the half set, note the time of transport. If necessary, draw up an additional syringe while at the transferring facility to ensure enough of the desired medication is available during transport—or revert to the spike set. The half set with syringe helps decrease the number of air bubbles in the tubing by gently pushing the fluid through the system.

If problems arise while using any pump system, most systems provide on-screen, step-by-step instructions to resolve the problem. Infusion pumps are quite sensitive to air, so all air must be removed from the IV tubing before inserting the pump chamber on the tubing in the system. This is most commonly avoided with syringes so that the fluid is pushed through the tubing to clear the line. Because each infusion pump is different, knowledge of the infusion sets, setup procedures, and maintenance of your particular system is vital.

A wide variety of pumps and infusion sets used in the hospital setting are not frequently seen in EMS. EMS systems and other healthcare agencies use both non-needle and needle administration infusion sets. Paramedics in CCT must be prepared for both types of injection ports. As detailed in this chapter, filter needles are necessary for the safe administration of certain medications. A filter needle looks like a conventional needle but has the added ability to filter out solid material that may be floating in the fluids. Filter needles can be used when inline IV tubing filters are not available. They are also used to draw medications from glass ampules.

USE OF A VOLUMETRIC SYRINGE

Equipment needed:
Volumetric pump, syringe, IV tubing, sharps, personal protective equipment (PPE), medication, gloves

Procedure:
1. Observe standard precautions.
2. Verify the drug order.
3. Confirm right patient, right medication, right dose, right route, and right time.
4. Confirm with the patient that he or she has no allergies to the medication, and document allergies to any other medication.
5. When possible, explain to the patient what medication you are going to administer and why.
6. Turn the pump on, and calculate the required amount of fluid to be infused during transport. For a portable unit, turn on the pump and check its battery life before beginning the medication administration. If the battery is low, plug in the pump.
7. Draw the medication into the syringe, expelling all the air.
8. Attach the syringe to a port on the tubing that does not have a drip set.
9. Place the syringe into the pump you are using, and administer the medication.
10. Record the time of drug administration in the patient care record.
11. Evaluate the patient for desired effects of the medication, as well as any adverse effects. Continued reevaluation should occur throughout transport.

USE OF A VOLUMETRIC PUMP

Equipment needed:
Volumetric pump, medication, gloves, IV tubing

Procedure:
1. Observe standard precautions.
2. Verify the drug order.
3. Confirm right patient, right medication, right dose, right route, and right time.
4. Confirm with the patient that he or she has no allergies to the medication, and document allergies to any other medication.
5. When possible, explain to the patient what medication you are going to administer and why.
6. Turn the pump on, and prime the medication tubing to ensure all air is out of the system so that no alarms sound. For a portable unit, turn on the pump and check its battery life before beginning medication administration. If the battery is low, plug in the pump.
7. Select the channel to administer the medication. Then, insert the cassette into the channel on the pump.
8. Close the channel door, and then select the channel from the main menu.
9. Choose the infusion type, either drug calculator or rate, and volume to be infused.
10. Select the rate, and program that number into the pump. Select the volume to be infused, and program that number into the pump.
11. Attach the tubing to the patient, and begin the infusion.
12. Record the time of drug administration in the patient care record.
13. Evaluate the patient for desired effects of the medication, as well as any adverse effects. Continued reevaluation should occur throughout transport.

Drug Calculators

Because most infusion systems integrate drug calculators, knowledge of how to access the calculators and configure the pump for transport is important. Although the drug calculator includes information on only a limited number of medications, it can be quite advantageous.

The drug calculator can make titration of critical medication quicker and easier, which also helps prevent medication administration errors.

Fluid Warmers

Patients who require rapid fluid resuscitation or large amounts of transfused blood are at risk for developing hypothermia. A **fluid warmer** can help prevent hypothermia in such situations (**FIGURE 18-10**). IV fluids that are warmed in microwaves or "blanket warmers" are frequently above the recommended 104 to 107.6°F (40 to 42°C). Newer in-line fluid warmers heat fluid within IV tubing, just prior to it entering the patient's body, without significant ambient temperature loss (**FIGURE 18-11**).[4] Temperatures greater than 109.4°F (43°C) are associated with red blood cell hemolysis.[5]

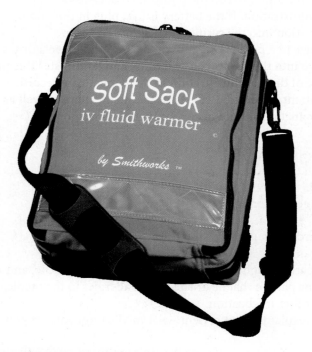

FIGURE 18-10 Fluid warmer.
Courtesy of Smithwork Medical Inc.

FIGURE 18-11 In-line fluid warmer.
© Barry Slaven/Medical Images.

▶ Common CCT Scenarios

Several common scenarios exist in which a paramedic can be called to assist in the care of critical patients during transport between hospitals. These scenarios include HELLP syndrome or **preeclampsia**, status following cardiac arrest or myocardial infarction, diabetic ketoacidosis, closed-head injury, burn injury, and blood administration.

HELLP Syndrome, Preeclampsia, and Eclampsia

HELLP syndrome is an acronym for a pregnancy condition characterized by *h*emolysis, *e*levated *l*iver enzymes, and *l*ow *p*latelets. The syndrome occurs during the second half of pregnancy. The cause of HELLP syndrome is not well understood. It may be an inflammatory condition that is somehow related to preeclampsia and eclampsia; however, consensus regarding its etiology is limited.[6] Preeclampsia is a pregnancy condition with hypertension and proteinuria occurring after 20 weeks' gestation in women without a prior history of hypertension.[7] Eclampsia occurs when a patient with preeclampsia develops seizure activity, not associated with another identifiable cause. HELLP syndrome and preeclampsia/eclampsia may be present in the same patient, or exist as isolated conditions.

Management

Treatment of these considerations is primarily geared toward correcting a significantly low platelet count, managing hypertension, and preventing seizures. The treatment that the paramedic provides during transport likely is based on laboratory findings identified at the referring hospital. Drugs often used in this treatment include magnesium sulfate, phenytoin, hydralazine, and labetalol.

Seizures are commonly associated with the development of HELLP syndrome and represent the conversion of preeclampsia into eclampsia. The treatment of choice for seizures is IV magnesium sulfate. Magnesium sulfate is administered for the prophylactic treatment of seizures in these patients at significantly higher doses than when it is given for other indications. Magnesium can cause toxicity in patients, and certain aspects must be monitored during transport, such as urine output, deep tendon reflexes, and respiratory depression. Magnesium is superior to phenytoin for the prevention and treatment of eclampsia and associated seizures.[8] *Magnesium is also often used to slow or suspend preterm labor; however, this indication remains controversial.*[9]

MAGNESIUM SULFATE

Classification: Electrolyte, tocolytic, mineral.
Action: Required for normal physiologic functioning. Magnesium is a cofactor in neurochemical transmission and muscular excitability. Magnesium sulfate controls seizures by blocking peripheral neuromuscular transmission. Magnesium is also a peripheral vasodilator and an inhibitor of platelet function.
Indications: Torsades de pointes, cardiac arrhythmias associated with hypomagnesemia, eclampsia and seizure prophylaxis in preeclampsia, status asthmaticus.
Adverse Effects: Magnesium toxicity (signs include flushing, diaphoresis, hypotension, muscle paralysis, weakness, hypothermia, and cardiac, central nervous system [CNS], or respiratory depression).
Contraindications: Atrioventricular (AV) block, gastrointestinal (GI) obstruction. Use with caution in renal impairment.

(continues)

MAGNESIUM SULFATE

(continued)

Dosage:
Pulseless Ventricular Fibrillation/Ventricular Tachycardia with Torsades de Pointes or Hypomagnesemia:
- **Adult:** 1 to 2 g in 10 mL D_5W IV, intraosseous (IO) administered over 15 minutes or faster with cardiac arrest.
- **Pediatric:** 25 to 50 mg/kg IV, IO over 10 to 20 minutes; may administer faster for torsades de pointes (max single dose: 2 g).

Torsades de Pointes with a Pulse or Cardiac Arrhythmias with Hypomagnesemia:
- **Adult:** 1 to 2 g in 50 to 100 mL D_5W IV, IO administered over 5 to 60 minutes. Follow with 0.5 to 1 g/hr IV, IO titrated to control torsades de pointes.
- **Pediatric:** 25 to 50 mg/kg IV, IO over 10 to 20 minutes (max single dose: 2 g).

Eclampsia and Seizure Prophylaxis in Preeclampsia:
- **Adult:** 4 to 6 g IV, IO over 20 to 30 minutes, followed by an infusion of 1 to 2 g/hr.

Status Asthmaticus:
- **Adult:** 1.2 to 2 g slow IV, IO (over 20 minutes).
- **Pediatric:** 25 to 50 mg/kg (diluted in D_5W) slow IV, IO (over 10 to 20 minutes).

Special Considerations:
Pregnancy class A.

PHENYTOIN (DILANTIN)

Classification: Anticonvulsant.
Action: Depresses seizures by affecting the movement of sodium and calcium into neural tissue.
Indications: Generalized tonic-clonic seizures.
Adverse Effects: Nausea/vomiting, depression of cardiac conduction, sedation, nystagmus, tremors, ataxia, dysarthria, gingival hypertrophy, hirsutism, facial coarsening, hypotension.
Contraindications: Sinus bradycardia, sinoatrial block, second-and third-degree heart block, Adams-Stokes syndrome, known sensitivity to hydantoins.
Dosage:
- **Adult:** 15 to 20 mg/kg IV, IO should be administered slowly at a rate not exceeding 50 mg/min. (This requires approximately 20 minutes in a 70-kg patient.)
- **Pediatric:** 15 to 20 mg/kg IV, IO, administered at a rate of 1 to 3 mg/kg per minute.

Special Considerations:
Continuously monitor the ECG and blood pressure during administration. Monitor the IV site for signs of infiltration.
Pregnancy class D.

The hypertension associated with HELLP syndrome and preeclampsia must be treated to improve the prognosis of both mother and baby. A decrease in blood pressure reduces the risk of placental abruption, seizure activity, and maternal cerebral hemorrhage. Hydralazine (Apresoline) is a commonly used medication for the treatment of maternal hypertension. It should be initiated with a systolic blood pressure greater than 160 mm Hg or a diastolic pressure greater than 105 mm Hg.[10] Labetalol is an alternative medication that can cause less maternal hypotension than hydralazine. A detailed discussion of hydralazine and other medications used in pregnancy-related hypertension is found in Chapter 19.

FOSPHENYTOIN (CEREBYX)

Classification: Anticonvulsant.

Action: Depresses seizures by affecting the movement of sodium and calcium into neural tissue.

Indications: Generalized tonic-clonic seizures.

Adverse Effects: Depression of cardiac conduction, sedation, nystagmus, delirium, tremors, ataxia, dysarthria, hypertension, hypotension, and pain or irritation at injection site.

Contraindications: Sinus bradycardia, sinoatrial block, second- and third-degree heart block, Adams-Stokes syndrome, known sensitivity to hydantoins.

Dosage:

- **Adult and Pediatric:** Dosing is ordered in *milligram phenytoin equivalents* (PE) rather than in milligrams. Administer 15 to 20 mg PE/kg IV, IO, administered at a rate of <150 PE/minute.

Special Considerations:

Continuously monitor the ECG and blood pressure during administration. Monitor the IV site for signs of infiltration.

Pregnancy class D.

HYDRALAZINE (APRESOLINE)

Classification: Antihypertensive agent, vasodilator.

Action: Directly dilates the peripheral blood vessels.

Indications: Hypertension associated with preeclampsia and eclampsia, hypertensive crisis.

Adverse Effects: Headache, angina, flushing, palpitations, reflex tachycardia, anorexia, nausea/vomiting, diarrhea, hypotension, syncope, peripheral vasodilation, peripheral edema, fluid retention, paresthesias.

Contraindications: Patients taking diazoxide or monoamine oxidase inhibitors (MAOIs), coronary artery disease, stroke, angina, dissecting aortic aneurysm, mitral valve and rheumatic heart diseases.

Dosage:

Preeclampsia and Eclampsia:

- **Adult:** 5 to 10 mg IV. Repeat every 20 to 30 minutes until systolic blood pressure of 90 to 105 mm Hg is attained.

Acute Hypertension Not Associated with Preeclampsia:

- **Adult:** 10 to 20 mg IV, or intramuscular (IM) administration.
- **Pediatric: 1 month to 12 years:** 0.1 to 0.2 mg/kg IV or IM every 4 to 6 hours as needed (max: 20 mg/dose).

Special Considerations:

Pregnancy class C.

LABETALOL (NORMODYNE, TRANDATE)

Labetalol Hydrochloride
Injection, USP
20 mL Multi-Dose vial
100 mg/20 mL (5 mg/mL)
For Intravenous Injection Only
Sterile   NDC 12345-678-90
Rx only

Classification: Beta adrenergic antagonist, antianginal, antihypertensive.

Action: Binds with both the beta$_1$ and beta$_2$ receptors and alpha$_1$ receptors in vascular smooth muscle. Inhibits the strength of the heart's contractions, as well as heart rate. This results in a decrease in cardiac oxygen consumption.

Indications: Acute coronary syndrome (ACS), supraventricular tachycardia, severe hypertension.

Adverse Effects: Usually mild and transient; hypotensive symptoms, nausea/vomiting, bronchospasm, arrhythmia, bradycardia, AV block.

Contraindications: Hypotension, cardiogenic shock, acute pulmonary edema, heart failure, severe bradycardia, sick sinus syndrome, second- or third-degree heart block, asthma or acute bronchospasm, cocaine-induced ACS, known sensitivity. Use caution in pheochromocytoma, cerebrovascular disease or stroke, poorly controlled diabetes, with hepatic disease. Use with caution at lowest effective dose in chronic lung disease.

Dosage:

Cardiac Indications:

Note: Monitor blood pressure and heart rate closely during administration.

- **Adult:** 10 mg IV, IO over a 1- to 2-minute period. May repeat every 10 minutes to a maximum dose of 150 mg or give initial bolus and then follow with infusion at 2 to 8 mg/min.
- **Pediatric:** 0.2 to 1 mg/kg to a maximum dosage of 3 mg/kg per hour; may also administer 0.25 to 3 mg/kg per hour as an infusion.

Severe Hypertension:

- **Adult:** Initial dose is 20 mg IV, IO slow infusion over a 2-minute period. After the initial dose, blood pressure should be checked every 5 minutes. Repeat doses can be given at 10-minute intervals. The second dose should be 40 mg IV, IO, and subsequent doses should be 80 mg IV, IO, to a maximum total dose of 300 mg. The effect on blood pressure typically will occur within 5 minutes from the time of administration. Alternatively, may be administered via IV infusion at 2 mg/min to a total maximum dose of 300 mg.
- **Pediatric:** 0.25 to 3 mg/kg per hour IV, IO infusion with a maximum dose of 3 mg/kg per hour.

Special Considerations:

Pregnancy class C.

CASE STUDY

You arrive at a small community hospital to transport a 22-year-old woman who is 8 months pregnant and has been diagnosed with HELLP syndrome. The patient is receiving an infusion of magnesium sulfate, and intermittent doses of hydralazine. You have a multichannel infusion pump. The patient has a 20-gauge IV in her right hand with the magnesium infusing.

Two questions arise from the previous scenario: Are those medications compatible? Does the paramedic need additional access?

Magnesium sulfate is not compatible with hydralazine. When administering multiple medications, paramedics should consult a drug compatibility reference. Additional access is needed. After the initiation of an 18-gauge IV in the left antecubital fossa, the paramedic would be ready to transfer the medications to the infusion pump. A syringe and half set could be used. The paramedic would label the syringe with the medication and concentration to calculate a drip rate in the event of a pump failure.

(*continued*) During transport, the patient has decreased level of consciousness with decreased respiratory rate, decreased urine output by Foley catheter, and absent deep tendon reflexes.

Magnesium sulfate toxicity is the likely culprit in the previous scenario. The treatment for magnesium toxicity includes the administration of 10 to 20 mL of 10% calcium gluconate IV push. Calcium gluconate should be on board when an interfacility patient being infused with magnesium is transported. When transporting a patient receiving a specific medication, be familiar with the adverse effects and how to reverse them.

CALCIUM GLUCONATE

Classification: Electrolyte solution.
Action: Counteracts the toxicity of hyperkalemia by stabilizing the membranes of the cardiac cells, reducing the likelihood of fibrillation.
Indications: Hyperkalemia, hypocalcemia, hypermagnesemia.
Adverse Effects: Soft tissue necrosis, hypotension, bradycardia (if administered too rapidly).
Contraindications: Ventricular fibrillation, digitalis toxicity, hypercalcemia.
Dosage: Supplied as 10% solution; therefore, each milliliter contains 100 mg of calcium gluconate.

- **Adult:** 500 to 1,000 mg IV, IO administered slowly at a rate of approximately 1 to 1.5 mL/min; maximum dose 3 g IV, IO. It may also be ordered as 60 mg/kg per dose.
- **Pediatric:** 60 to 100 mg/kg IV, IO slowly over a 5- to 10-minute period; maximum dose 3 g IV, IO.

Special Considerations:
Do not administer by IM or subcutaneous routes, which causes significant tissue necrosis. Pregnancy class C.

Treatment After Cardiac Arrest or Inferior Myocardial Infarction

CASE STUDY

Your helicopter has been dispatched for the interfacility transport of a 55-year-old man who sustained an inferior myocardial infarction with a ventricular fibrillation arrest approximately 1 hour ago. The patient has been resuscitated. You arrive to find the patient intubated, chemically sedated, and paralyzed. The following infusions are running: vecuronium (Norcuron), midazolam (Versed), amiodarone (Cordarone), and eptifibatide (Integrilin). You are transporting the patient to a tertiary care center 30 minutes away by air for an immediate cardiac catheterization. The patient weighs 220 pounds (100 kg).

Management

Because this patient has myocardial ischemia and a dangerous cardiac arrhythmia, the goals of the paramedic during transport are to prevent additional cardiac ischemia with eptifibatide (Integrilin), prevent additional cardiac arrhythmias with amiodarone (Cordarone), and continue appropriate sedation with a midazolam (Versed) infusion and neuromuscular paralysis with vecuronium (Norcuron).

The patient is currently receiving four drug infusions; when multichannel pumps are used, only three medications can be connected to the electronic pump. Ideally, a second infusion pump should be available for when more than three medication infusions are needed, or as backup in the event of battery or mechanical failure of the primary infusion pump. If an additional infusion pump is not available, CCT providers must carefully weigh the risks and benefits associated with the various medications involved. In the preceding scenario, one of the medications should be put on a Dial-A-Flo or converted to an IV bolus. During air transport, a Dial-A-Flo works only with the addition of pressure to the system because of the decrease in atmospheric pressure and the close proximity of the bag to the patient.

An aircraft has no room for IV poles; both rotor and fixed-wing aircraft have profound space limitations. Therefore, the IV bag may rest directly on the patient or be elevated only inches above the patient. However, when in an ambulance, hang the IV bag several feet above the patient.

> Next time you start an IV line on a patient, watch how the drip rate increases when you elevate the bag and how it decreases when you lower the IV bag. This concept is the same one that led cities to build water towers on hills.

In the previous case study, the paramedic could use a pressure bag. Continuing the scenario, you administer midazolam (Versed), amiodarone (Cordarone), and eptifibatide (Integrilin) by electronic pump. The vecuronium (Norcuron) infusion will run without a pump. To maintain the vecuronium infusion, you place the medication bag into a pressure bag and add a Dial-A-Flo. A vecuronium infusion traditionally is mixed in a 100-mL bag of fluid, which would make the use of a pressure bag quite difficult. One dose of vecuronium as a bolus is easier to administer than the use of additional equipment. Vecuronium has a duration of action of approximately 25 to 40 minutes. Because this will last the duration of the flight, giving the paralytic medication as a bolus rather than an infusion would be more beneficial.

Other transport considerations include the use of half versus full administration sets. Because eptifibatide (Integrilin) is packaged in a glass container, syringes would be beneficial.

MIDAZOLAM (VERSED)

Classification: Benzodiazepine, Schedule C-IV

Action: Binds to the benzodiazepine receptor and enhances the effects of the brain chemical (neurotransmitter) gamma-aminobutyric acid (GABA). Benzodiazepines act at the level of the limbic, thalamic, and hypothalamic regions of the CNS to produce short-acting CNS depression (including sedation, skeletal muscle relaxation, and anticonvulsant activity).

Indications: Sedation, anxiety, skeletal muscle relaxation.

© Dr P. Marazzi/Science Source

Adverse Effects: Respiratory depression, respiratory arrest, hypotension, nausea/vomiting, headache, hiccups, cardiac arrest.

Contraindications: Acute-angle glaucoma, pregnant women, known sensitivity.

Dosage:

Sedation:

Note: The dose of midazolam needs to be individualized. Every dose should be administered slowly over a period of 2 minutes. Allow 2 minutes to evaluate the clinical effect of the dose given.

- **Adult:**
  - **Healthy and younger than 60 years:** *Some patients require as little as 1 mg IV, IO. No more than 2.5 mg should be given over a 2-minute interval.* If additional sedation is

required, continue to administer small increments over 2-minute periods (max dose: 5 mg). If the patient also has received a narcotic, he or she will typically require 30% less midazolam than the same patient not given the narcotic.

- ○ **60 years and older and debilitated or chronically ill patients:** This group of patients has a higher risk of hypoventilation, airway obstruction, and apnea. The peak clinical effect can take longer in these patients; therefore, dose increments should be smaller, and the rate of injection should be slower. *Some patients require a dose as small as 1 mg IV, IO, and no more than 1.5 mg should be given over a 2-minute period.* If additional sedation is required, additional midazolam should be given at a rate of no more than 1 mg over a 2-minute period (max dose: 3.5 mg). If the patient also has received a narcotic, he or she will typically require 50% less midazolam than the same patient not given the narcotic.
- ○ **Continuous infusion:** Continuous infusions can be required for prolonged transport of intubated, critically ill, and injured patients. After an initial bolus dose, the adult patient will require a maintenance infusion dose of 0.02 to 0.1 mg/kg per hour (1 to 7 mg/hr).

- **Pediatric**
  - ○ **Weight-based:** Pediatric patients typically require higher doses of midazolam than do adults on the basis of weight (in mg/kg). Younger pediatric patients (younger than 6 years) require higher doses (in mg/kg) than older pediatric patients. Midazolam takes approximately 3 minutes to reach peak effect; therefore wait at least 2 minutes to determine the drug's effectiveness and the need for additional dosing.
  - ○ **12 to 16 years:** Same as adult dosing. Some patients in this age group require a higher dose than that used in adults, but rarely does a patient require more than 10 mg.
  - ○ **6 to 12 years:** 0.025 to 0.05 mg/kg IV, IO up to a total dose of 0.4 mg/kg. Exceeding 10 mg as a total dose usually is not necessary.
  - ○ **6 months to 5 years:** 0.05 to 0.1 mg/kg IV, IO up to a total dose of 0.6 mg/kg. Exceeding 6 mg as a total dose usually is not necessary.
  - ○ **Younger than 6 months:** Dosing recommendations for this age group is unclear. Because this age group is especially vulnerable to airway obstruction and hypoventilation, use small increments with frequent clinical evaluation. Dose: 0.05 to 0.1 mg/kg IV, IO.

Special Considerations:
Patients receiving midazolam require frequent monitoring of vital signs and pulse oximetry. Be prepared to support the patient's airway and ventilation.
Pregnancy class D.

AMIODARONE (CORDARONE)

Classification: Antiarrhythmic, Class III
Action: Acts directly on the myocardium to delay repolarization and increase the duration of the action potential.
Indications: Ventricular arrhythmias; second-line agent for atrial arrhythmias.
Adverse Effects: Burning at the IV site, hypotension, bradycardia.
Contraindications: Sick sinus syndrome, second- and third-degree heart block, cardiogenic shock, when episodes of bradycardia have caused syncope, sensitivity to benzyl alcohol and iodine.

© Jones & Bartlett Learning.

(continues)

AMIODARONE (CORDARONE)

(continued)

Dosage:
Ventricular Fibrillation and Pulseless Ventricular Tachycardia:
- **Adult:** 300 mg IV, IO. May be followed by one dose of 150 mg in 3 to 5 minutes.
- **Pediatric:** 5 mg/kg (max dose: 300 mg); may repeat 5 mg/kg IV, IO up to 15 mg/kg.

Relatively Stable Patients with Arrhythmias Such as Premature Ventricular Contractions or Wide-Complex Tachycardias with a Strong Pulse:
- **Adult:** 150 mg in 100 mL D$_5$W IV, IO over a 10-minute period; may repeat in 10 minutes; once ROSC is accomplished, begin an infusion of 1 mg/min for 6 hours then decrease to 0.5 mg/min; up to a maximum dose of 2.2 g over 24 hours.
- **Pediatric:** 5 mg/kg very slow IV, IO (over 20 to 60 minutes); may repeat in 5-mg/kg doses up to 15 mg/kg (max dose: 300 mg).

Special Considerations:
Pregnancy class D.

EPTIFIBATIDE (INTEGRILIN)

Classification: Glycoprotein IIb/IIIa inhibitor
Action: Prevents the aggregation of platelets by binding to the glycoprotein IIb/IIIa receptor.
Indications: Unstable angina or non-ST-segment elevation myocardial infarction—to manage medically and for those undergoing percutaneous coronary intervention.
Adverse Effects: Bleeding from the GI tract, internal bleeding, intracranial hemorrhage, hypotension, stroke, anaphylactic shock.
Contraindications: Bleeding from any source, severe uncontrolled hypertension, surgery or trauma within the previous 6 weeks, stroke within the previous 30 days, renal failure, thrombocytopenia.

Dosage:
- **Adult:** Loading dose: 180 mcg/kg IV, IO (max dose: 22.6 mg) over 1 to 2 minutes, then 2 mcg/kg per minute IV, IO infusion (max dose: 15 mg/hr).
- **Pediatric:** No current dosing recommendations exist for pediatric patients.

Special Considerations:
Half-life approximately 90 to 150 minutes.
Pregnancy class B.

VECURONIUM (NORCURON)

Classification: Neuromuscular blocker, nondepolarizing
Action: Antagonizes acetylcholine at the motor end plate, producing skeletal muscle paralysis.
Indications: To induce neuromuscular blockade for the facilitation of endotracheal intubation.
Adverse Effects: Muscle paralysis, apnea, dyspnea, respiratory depression, sinus tachycardia, urticaria.
Contraindications: Known sensitivity to bromides. Use with caution in heart disease, liver disease.
Dosage:
- **Adult:** 0.08 to 0.1 mg/kg IV, IO. Use an infusion of 0.8 to 1.2 mcg/kg per minute for ongoing chemical paralysis.
- **Pediatric:** 0.1 to 0.15 mg/kg. Use an infusion of 1 to 2.5 mcg/kg per minute for ongoing chemical paralysis.

> **Special Considerations:**
> Pregnancy class C.
> *Carefully monitor and provide adequate sedation and analgesia for patients who are chemically paralyzed with vecuronium. This medication has no sedative or analgesic effects. Patients may appear to be unconscious while having completely intact awareness, hearing, and sensation of pain.*

> *(continued)* You are in the middle of transport when a pump channel failure occurs. You are administering midazolam (Versed), amiodarone (Cordarone), and eptifibatide (Integrilin).

In this situation, the best solution would be to convert the midazolam infusion to intermittent boluses. This would continue accurate dosing of the antiarrhythmic and antiplatelet medications for the duration of the flight. If additional pump failures occur, the appropriate dosage should be calculated with a microdrip set.

Eptifibatide (Integrilin) is packaged as 0.75 mg/mL and 2 mg/mL. For the following example, the 0.75 mg/mL preparation is used. The dose is typically 2 mcg/kg per minute before a coronary catheterization. The infusion pump is running at 16 mL/hr.

Calculate the drip rate. This patient should receive 200 mcg/min, or 12,000 mcg/hr or 12 mg/hr.

$$2 \text{ mcg/kg/min} \times 100 \text{ kg} = 200 \text{ mcg/min}$$

$$200 \text{ mcg/min} \times 60 \text{ min/hr} = 12{,}000 \text{ mcg/hr}$$

Convert units: $12{,}000 \text{ mcg} \times 1 \text{ mg}/1{,}000 \text{ mcg} = 12 \text{ mg}$

Infusion rate:

$$12 \text{ mg/hr} \times 1 \text{ mL}/0.75 \text{ mg} = 16 \text{ mL/hr}$$

Drip rate:

$$200 \text{ mcg/min} \times 60 \text{ gtt}/1 \text{ mL} \times 1 \text{ mL}/750 \text{ mcg} = (200 \times 60)/750 = 16 \text{ gtt/min}$$
(canceling units: gtt/min; remember, 0.75 mg/mL = 750 mcg/mL)

With a microdrip set, you would administer 16 gtt/min.

Diabetic Ketoacidosis

CASE STUDY

You work on a fixed-wing aircraft (airplane) and are called to a small rural hospital in Florida to transfer a 5-year-old girl to Tennessee. The child was on vacation with her parents when she became sick. The only history you have on the patient is that she was diagnosed with type 1 diabetes 6 months ago. Her blood glucose level is currently 450 mg/dL. Her parents have requested that she be transferred to her pediatric endocrinologist in Tennessee. When you arrive at the emergency department (ED), the nurse practitioner notifies you that the patient has been diagnosed with diabetic ketoacidosis (DKA). Her potassium level is 5.0, and pH is 7.28. She is currently on oxygen at 4 L/min by nasal cannula. A left subclavian TLC was placed before your arrival.

In the following section, some of the logistical problems of caring for a child in DKA for several hours are identified and explained. A more detailed discussion of DKA and its pharmacologic treatment is found in Chapter 11.

> (*continued*) The patient weighs 55 pounds (25 kg). The nurse practitioner has given her a 250-mL bolus of normal saline for initial hypotension, started insulin at 5.0 U/hr, and initiated normal saline with 20 mEq potassium chloride (KCl). You realize that you need to administer KCl 40 mEq/L of fluid, but the hospital stocks only normal saline with 20 mEq KCl.

Management

You need to make some decisions on how to manage the fluids during transport. Next, you must decide how to transport the fluids. You typically would use a volume-control chamber, also known as a *buretrol* or *volutrol set*, to administer fluids to a pediatric patient. Therefore, you can use a volume-control chamber set manufactured to fit into an infusion pump or a volume-control chamber that flows strictly to gravity.

Volume-control chamber sets are manufactured in such a way as to provide additional protection against the accidental administration of excessive fluid. In pediatric patients the amount of fluid being administered must be closely monitored to prevent complications of fluid overload. If a volume-control chamber is filled with the desired amount of fluid and clamped off to the bag of fluid, accidental administration of excessive fluid as a result of pump malfunctions is virtually impossible. This type of simple safety device commonly is used to prevent the complication of inadvertent volume overload or drug overdose in children's hospitals and pediatric intensive care units.

Insulin can be drawn into a syringe and infused with a half set through the infusion pump. Insulin is usually mixed at a 1:1 concentration of medication and fluid (e.g., a 100-mL bag of fluids would have 100 U = 1 U/mL). Therefore, consider how long the patient will be traveling so that enough medication is on hand. In the previous scenario, the air and travel time to and from the airport is approximately 4.5 hours. Therefore, if insulin is run at 5 U/hr, at least 23 mL are needed for transport (5 U/hr × 4.5 hours = 22.5 U). Filling the syringe to 50 mL to prevent running out of insulin would be wise.

> (*continued*) You have safely arrived at the aircraft, and the patient is loaded. Forty-five minutes have passed getting from the hospital to the airport, and you have not checked the patient's blood glucose level. A fingerstick test reveals a glucose level of 380 mg/dL. You have exceeded the 10% per hour of reduction in blood glucose that is safe for the patient (450 × 0.10 = 45 and 450 − 45 = 405). You realize that the hospital did not correctly calculate the insulin infusion and set the pump at a higher dose than 0.1 U/kg per hour.

In this situation, the drip must be gradually titrated to reduce the patient's blood glucose level. Based on the patient's weight, the infusion should be delivered at 2.5 U/hr. Suppose you started the pump as a basic infusion, and now you cannot get the pump to use decimals. If the pump has an integrated drug calculator, you should be able to enter the drug calculator, input the appropriate information, and titrate the drip accordingly. If insulin is not integrated into the pump, you can use the dosage calculator. Input your concentration of the drug, weight, and desired dose.

> (*continued*) The remainder of the transport goes smoothly until you check the patient's glucose level and realize that it has dropped below 250 mg/dL.

FIGURE 18-12 Portable laboratory analysis machine.

In this situation, you must add dextrose to the IV fluids. However, if you do not have dextrose on board, you can make D_5NS. D_5 is 5 g dextrose per 100 mL fluid. Therefore, inject a syringe of D_{50} into a 1-L bag of saline and infuse at the maintenance rate.

In this scenario the paramedic should notify the receiving medical team that the transfer took 4.5 hours and that the potassium level before transfer was 5.0 mg/dL. The receiving team will quickly draw a basic metabolic panel and an arterial blood gas reading to determine whether the patient's hyperkalemia and acidosis are resolving. Many air medical agencies use portable laboratory analysis machines (**FIGURE 18-12**). This scenario is an excellent example of situations where these devices are extremely helpful. As the patient's blood glucose and serum pH are corrected, her blood potassium levels will be decreasing as the potassium ions shift back inside various body cells. Over the 4.5-hour transport, it is possible that her serum potassium has become dangerously low.

INSULIN, REGULAR (HUMULIN R, NOVOLIN R)

Classification: Hormone
Action: Binds to a receptor on the membrane of cells and facilitates the transport of glucose into cells.
Indications: Hyperglycemia, insulin-dependent diabetes mellitus, hyperkalemia.
Adverse Effects: Hypoglycemia, tachycardia, palpitations, diaphoresis, anxiety, confusion, blurred vision, weakness, depression, seizures, coma, insulin shock, hypokalemia.
Contraindications: Hypoglycemia, known sensitivity.
Dosage:
Diabetic Ketoacidosis:
- **Adult:** 0.1 U/kg IV, IO, or subcutaneous. Because of poor perfusion of the peripheral tissues, subcutaneous administration is much less effective than the IV, IO route. IV, IO

(continues)

INSULIN, REGULAR (HUMULIN R, NOVOLIN R) *(continued)*

insulin has a very short half-life; therefore, IV, IO insulin without an infusion is not that effective. The rate for an insulin infusion is 0.05 to 0.1 U/kg per hour IV, IO. When dosing insulin, use a U-100 insulin syringe to measure and deliver the insulin. The time from administration to action, as well as the duration of action, varies greatly among different people, as well as at different times in the same person.

Hyperkalemia:
- **Adult:** 10 U IV, IO of regular insulin (Insulin R), coadministered with 50 mL of $D_{50}W$ over 5 minutes.
- **Pediatric:** 0.1 U/kg regular insulin IV, IO.

Special Considerations:
Only regular insulin can be given IV, IO. *Insulin is a high-risk medication and should be verified with another appropriately trained provider whenever possible.*
Pregnancy class B.

Closed-Head Injury

CASE STUDY

You are dispatched to transport a 25-year-old man who was involved in an all-terrain vehicle accident. He was not wearing a helmet. He has a closed-head injury with cerebral edema and a left femur fracture immobilized in a traction splint. The patient must be taken by ground because of icy conditions that prevent air transport. You arrive at the hospital to find the patient intubated and sedated with propofol. Mannitol, fentanyl, and a 1-L bolus of Ringer's lactate are infusing, as well. The patient weighs 220 pounds (100 kg).

Management

Transporting a patient with a traumatic brain injury (TBI) can be complex. The most concerning TBI is the closed-head injury with increased intracranial pressure (ICP). In these patients the goal of treatment is to help decrease swelling while supporting the patient's physiologic status. Increased cerebral edema can result in herniation, but it can also cause a decrease in the amount of perfusion to the brain.

Monitoring blood pressure is essential in the transport of a patient with a closed-head injury. Cerebral blood flow is calculated by the difference between the mean arterial pressure (MAP) and the ICP divided by the cerebral vascular resistance. Cerebral perfusion averages 50 mL of blood per 100 g of brain tissue per minute. Because of the difficulty in calculating the cerebral blood flow clinically, the cerebral perfusion pressure (CPP) is used. CPP is calculated from the MAP and ICP. A goal of 60 to 70 for the CPP is needed to ensure adequate cerebral perfusion.[11] Therefore, increases in ICP and decreases in MAP can result in insufficient blood flow to the brain.[12] A systolic blood pressure of at least 110 mm Hg is needed to ensure minimal blood flow to the brain. In cases in which high ICP is suspected, systolic blood pressure must be higher.

MAP is determined by the following formula:

$$(1/3 \text{ SBP} - \text{DBP}) + \text{DBP} = \text{MAP}$$

where SBP is systolic blood pressure and DBP is diastolic blood pressure. Cerebral perfusion pressure is determined by the following formula:

$$\text{MAP} - \text{ICP} = \text{CPP}$$

MAP can be calculated from the blood pressure or given as a digital readout from an automatic blood pressure machine. ICP is typically measured with an external ventricular drain. Because measuring ICP is impractical during transport, rough estimates can be determined by observing patients for signs and symptoms. Altered mental status, nausea, projectile vomiting, and unequal pupils can be signs of increasing ICP.

A MAP of greater than 80 mm Hg with an ICP of 20 mm Hg results in a CPP of at least 60 mm Hg.[13] If a patient has a systolic blood pressure less than 110 mm Hg, fluid resuscitation is necessary. Sedation and neuromuscular blocking agents may be needed to help control oxygenation and ventilation to ensure an appropriate carbon dioxide level. Continuous oxygen saturation monitoring is recommended, with a desired level of greater than 90%. In an unresponsive patient with extensor posturing and flaccidity, the recommended ventilation rates are 20 breaths/min for adults, 30 breaths/min for children, and 35 to 40 breaths/min for infants. In the absence of signs of herniation, avoid hyperventilation. In patients without posturing or flaccidity, a carbon dioxide level of 35 to 40 mm Hg is desired.[13] Use end-tidal carbon dioxide monitoring to calculate the patient's carbon dioxide level. However, keep in mind that expired carbon dioxide is 3 to 5 mm Hg lower than arterial carbon dioxide.[14]

(continued) The patient's blood pressure is 90/40 mm Hg. This translates into an MAP of 57 mm Hg and a possible CPP of 37 mm Hg. Therefore, the patient is receiving a fluid bolus to improve the blood pressure.

Propofol (Diprivan) is the hypnotic medication of choice for patients with closed-head injuries because it decreases cerebral metabolism, thus decreasing oxygen consumption. It is also easily titrated and has a short half-life, allowing an accurate neurologic examination at the hospital. Propofol is a phenol derivative classified as an anesthetic. It is used for induction and maintenance of anesthesia, as well as sedation in intubated patients in intensive care. The mechanism of action is dose dependent and causes CNS depression resembling that caused by benzodiazepines and barbiturates, with rapid hypnosis and minimal excitation. Onset of action is approximately 10 to 40 seconds, and duration is 3 to 10 minutes. Propofol is a medication with limited application in prehospital care.

PROPOFOL (DIPRIVAN)

Classification: Anesthetic
Action: Produces rapid and brief state of general anesthesia.
Indications: Anesthesia induction.
Adverse Effects: Apnea, cardiac arrhythmias, asystole, hypotension, hypertension, pain at injection site.
Contraindications: Hypovolemia, known sensitivity (including soybean oil, eggs).
Dosage: A general induction dose used to produce a state of unconsciousness rapidly is 1.5 to 3 mg/kg IV, IO.

© Julia Hiebaum/Alamy Stock Photo.

(continues)

PROPOFOL (DIPRIVAN) *(continued)*

Patient Group	Dosage	Rate of Administration (10 mg/mL)
Healthy adults younger than 55 years	2 to 2.5 mg/kg IV, IO	40 mg every 10 seconds
Older or debilitated patients	1 to 1.5 mg/kg IV, IO	20 mg every 10 seconds
Cardiac patients	0.5 to 1.5 mg/kg IV, IO	20 mg every 10 seconds
Patients with head injuries	1 to 2 mg/kg IV, IO	20 mg every 10 seconds
Pediatric (3 to 16 years)	2.5 to 3.5 mg/kg IV, IO	20 mg every 10 seconds

© Jones & Bartlett Learning.

After the induction bolus, the patient must be given intermittent boluses or a maintenance infusion. For an average adult, an intermittent dose is 20 to 50 mg as needed. Alternatively, a propofol infusion may be ordered. Maintenance of anesthesia with a propofol infusion can be achieved by following the following protocols:

- **Adult patients:** 25 to 75 mcg/kg per minute IV, IO. Prolonged infusions begin at 5 mcg/kg per minute and are titrated up to a maximum dose of 50 mcg/kg per minute.
- **Older adult, debilitated, or head-injured patients:** Use approximately 80% of the normal adult dose.
- **Pediatric:** 30 to 300 mcg/kg per minute IV, IO.

Special Considerations:

Propofol should be administered only by personnel trained and equipped to manage the patient's airway and provide mechanical ventilation. Propofol bolus administration may be restricted to only be administered by physicians and licensed-independent providers; consult your state EMS regulations and local protocols. In older adults and debilitated patients, avoid rapid administration to prevent hypotension, apnea, airway obstruction, and/or oxygen desaturation. Continue to monitor the patient's oxygenation and vital signs and try to limit use of propofol to patients who are intubated. Propofol should not be administered through the same IV catheter as blood or plasma. Pain can occur at the site of injection, which can be minimized by the use of larger veins, slower rates of administration, and administration of 1 mL 1% lidocaine before propofol administration.

Propofol is listed as a pregnancy class B; however, propofol should be avoided in pregnant women because it crosses the placenta and can cause neonatal depression.

Because patients with closed-head injuries have undergone a traumatic experience, pain is a serious issue. The use of fentanyl citrate (Sublimaze) can potentiate propofol, with minimal hemodynamic effects. Mannitol (Osmitrol), an osmotic diuretic, is specifically used for cerebral edema. It expands the intravascular volume while decreasing the viscosity of blood. Both mechanisms can help improve cerebral blood flow. Mannitol can crystallize in cold temperatures, which requires special considerations in the field.

MANNITOL (OSMITROL)

Classification: Osmotic diuretic
Action: Facilitates the flow of fluid out of tissues (including the brain) and into interstitial fluid and blood, thereby dehydrating the brain and reducing swelling. Reabsorption by the kidney is minimal, consequently increasing urine output.
Indications: Increased ICP.
Adverse Effects: Pulmonary edema, headache, blurred vision, dizziness, seizures, hypovolemia, nausea/vomiting, diarrhea, electrolyte imbalances, hypotension, hypertension, sinus tachycardia, PVCs, angina, phlebitis.
Contraindications: Active intracranial bleeding, congestive heart failure (CHF), pulmonary edema, severe dehydration. Use with caution in hypovolemia, renal failure.

Dosage:
- **Adult:** 0.25 to 1 g/kg IV, IO followed by 0.25 to 1 g/kg infused over 20 to 30 minutes, administered every 4 hours.
- **Pediatric:** 0.25 to 1 g/kg IV, IO followed by 0.25 to 0.5 g/kg infused over 20 to 30 minutes every 4 hours.

Special Considerations:
Mannitol should not be given in the same IV, IO line as blood.
Pregnancy class C.

FENTANYL CITRATE (SUBLIMAZE)

Classification: Narcotic analgesic, Schedule C-II
Action: Binds to opiate receptors, producing analgesia and euphoria.
Indications: Pain.
Adverse Effects: Respiratory depression, apnea, hypotension, nausea/ vomiting, dizziness, sedation, euphoria, sinus bradycardia, sinus tachycardia, palpitations, hypertension, diaphoresis, syncope, pain at injection site.
Contraindications: Known sensitivity. Use with caution in TBI, respiratory depression.

© Joe Amon/Contributor/Denver Post/Getty Images.

Dosage: Note: Dosage should be individualized.
- **Adult:** 50 to 100 mcg/dose (0.05 to 0.1 mg) IM or slow IV, IO (administered over 1 to 2 minutes).
- **Pediatric:** 1 to 2 mcg/kg IM or slow IV, IO (administered over 1 to 2 minutes).

Special Considerations:
Pregnancy class B.

CASE STUDY

You use a multichannel pump to administer Ringer's lactate, fentanyl, propofol, and mannitol. The Ringer's lactate solution can hang by gravity. Should half or whole sets be used? The first bottle of mannitol is currently hanging, and each bottle will run over a 15-minute period. Based on the patient's weight, he will need four bottles (100 kg × 0.5 g = 50 g). The propofol is infusing at 1.8 mL/hr. The concentration is 100 mg/mL. The nurse tells you that the patient is receiving 30 mcg/kg per minute (30 mcg/100 kg per minute = 3,000 mcg/min, or 180 mg/hour; 180 mg/100 mg per milliliter = 1.8 mL/hr). Both propofol and mannitol are packaged in glass bottles, so you administer them with a half set and syringe. With a ground transport time of 1 hour, the amount of fluids and syringe should be sufficient. The fentanyl infusion is running at 100 mcg/hr. Fentanyl is mixed as 50 mcg/mL, resulting in an infusion of 2 mL/hr.

When administering medication, be sure to label the syringes with the medication and concentration of the drug. This is especially important in the event of pump failure. The pump should have a drug calculator for the propofol so that the drug can be titrated as necessary during transport. In addition, a filter for the administration of mannitol is important. In cold temperatures, crystals in the patient can be avoided by inserting a filter needle where the mannitol enters the IV tubing. Although mannitol is infused by a pump, the medication can still crystallize between the IV pump and the patient.

(*continued*) During transport, you are withdrawing mannitol for administration when you see crystals in the bottle.

With cold ambient temperatures, mannitol crystallization is not uncommon. According to the manufacturer's instructions, mannitol should be warmed to revert the medication to its previous fluid state without precipitation. If a fluid warmer is available, store the mannitol with the fluids until time for administration. If not, activate a disposable heat pack and wrap it around the mannitol. After the fluid is warmed, shake it vigorously to clear the crystals.

Burn Injury

CASE STUDY

You are working as a flight paramedic and have been called to transfer a patient from a rural hospital to a regional burn center. You arrive and learn you are transporting a 47-year-old man who sustained full-thickness burns in a house fire. The ED has placed a 7.5 endotracheal tube, Foley catheter, and left femoral TLC. The patient arrived at the ED approximately 1 hour ago by EMS immediately from the scene. A dose of 500 mL Ringer's lactate has been infused. The patient weighs 175 pounds (79 kg).

Management

Fluid replacement is essential in preventing hypovolemia in critically ill burn patients. Major fluid shifts and losses occur during the first 24 hours of a burn injury. Fluid resuscitation is crucial during this period. Large amounts of crystalloid must be administered to replace the intravascular fluid loss that results from shifts to the interstitial spaces.

Parkland Formula of Burn Resuscitation. The Parkland formula is the most commonly used resuscitative formula.[15] It is a pure crystalloid formula that helps replace fluids within the first 24 hours of a burn. The following formula can be used to calculate fluid needs in a major adult burn patient:

$$\text{2 to 4 mL} \times \text{Weight in kilograms} \times \text{Total body surface area burned}$$

Half the total fluid is administered in the first 8 hours, and the remaining half is administered over the following 16 hours. Therefore, paramedics must know how to calculate the total body surface area (TBSA) burned to provide adequate fluid resuscitation to the patient. Additionally, a maintenance fluid of D_5 Ringer's lactate (D_5LR) is administered to children because of their decreased glycogen stores and needed replacement of glucose.[16]

For example, an 8-year-old child who weighs 42 kg has a TBSA burn of 25%. Time since injury is 1 hour, and the patient has received 500 mL Ringer's lactate. Maintenance fluids of D_5LR and resuscitation fluids of Ringer's lactate for this patient are shown in **TABLES 18-1** and **18-2**.

The total amount of resuscitative fluids administered in the first 24 hours is 3,150 mL. Half this volume (1,575 mL) must be administered in the first 8 hours *from the time of injury*. The second half of the fluid must be given in the remaining 16 hours.

$$\text{Total volume of resuscitation fluids} = \text{3,150 mL}$$

$$\text{First 8 hours: 3,150 mL/2} = \text{1,575 mL}$$

Because the patient has already received 500 mL, subtract 500 from 1,575 mL:

$$\text{1,575 mL} - \text{500 mL} = \text{1,075 mL}$$

This amount must be administered in the first 8 hours from the time of injury, not the first 8 hours of your care. One hour has already passed since the time of injury. Divide the amount of fluids by 7.

$$\text{1,075 mL/7 hours} = \text{154 mL/hr for the next 7 hours}$$

TABLE 18-1 Maintenance Fluids of D_5LR			
Weight (kg)	**mL/kg**	**Calculation**	**Total**
First 10 kg	100 mL	10×100	1,000 mL
Second 10 kg	50 mL	10×50	500 mL
Each kilogram >20 kg	20 mL	22×20	440 mL
			1,940 mL as D_5LR

Hourly infusion of 81 mL/hr of D_5LR for the first 24 hours.

© Jones & Bartlett Learning.

TABLE 18-2 Resuscitation Fluids of Ringer's Lactate		
3 to 4 mL $\times$ **Weight (kg)**	**TBSA**	**Fluid Resuscitation**
$3 \times 42 = 126$	126×25	3,150 mL

To calculate the rate of resuscitation fluids for the remaining 16 hours, take the total 24-hour resuscitative fluid requirements (3,150 mL), divide that number by 2, then divide that number by 16.

Total 24-hour resuscitative fluid requirements = 3,150 mL

Amount of fluids to be given from hours 9 to 24: 3,150 mL/2 = 1,575 mL

Hourly rate for fluids for hours 9 to 24 = 1,575 mL/16 hr = 98 mL/hr

Therefore, total fluids are D_5LR at 81 mL for 24 hours and Ringer's lactate at 154 mL/hr for 7 hours followed by Ringer's lactate at 98 mL/hr for the next 16 hours. Administration with a volume-control chamber set would be appropriate.

Urine output is closely monitored in burn patients to help determine whether patients are receiving an adequate amount of resuscitative fluid. The urine output in adult patients should total 0.5 mL/kg per hour, and the urine output for pediatric patients should be 1 mL/kg per hour if they weigh less than 30 kg. Therefore, the insertion of a Foley catheter and/or strict intake and output recording is recommended if the patient has sustained a burn large enough to require fluid resuscitation.

Wallace Rule of Nines and Rule of Palms. The Wallace rule of nines is the most commonly used method of estimating the TBSA of large burn injuries. The rule of nines divides the patient's body surface area into units divisible by nine. This calculation is accurate for adult patients but not for children because of the disproportion of their body surface area. A modification to the rule of nines has been developed for children. The Wallace rule of nines for adults is shown in **TABLE 18-3** and **FIGURE 18-13**.

The rule of palms is an accurate method of estimating burns that are either scattered or comprise less than 10% TBSA. This estimation is based on the patient's palm as representative of 1% of TBSA. The palm does not include the fingers.

The Lund-Browder chart (**FIGURE 18-14**) is the more accurate calculator of TBSA, but it is not commonly used in the field because the rule of nines and rule of palms are faster and

TABLE 18-3 The Wallace Rule of Nines

Body Part	Adult
Head and neck (front and back)	9%
Each arm (front and back)	9%
Each leg (front and back)	18%
Anterior trunk (chest and abdomen)	18%
Posterior trunk (including the buttocks)	18%
Perineum	1%

© Jones & Bartlett Learning.

FIGURE 18-13 The Wallace rule of nines.

Age (years)	A ($\frac{1}{2}$ of head)	B ($\frac{1}{2}$ of one thigh)	C ($\frac{1}{2}$ of one leg)
0	$9\frac{1}{2}$	$2\frac{3}{4}$	$2\frac{1}{2}$
1	$8\frac{1}{2}$	$3\frac{1}{4}$	$2\frac{1}{2}$
5	$6\frac{1}{2}$	4	$2\frac{3}{4}$
10	$5\frac{1}{2}$	$4\frac{1}{4}$	3
15	$4\frac{1}{2}$	$4\frac{1}{2}$	$3\frac{1}{4}$
Adult	$3\frac{1}{2}$	$4\frac{3}{4}$	3

FIGURE 18-14 Lund-Browder chart.

simpler. When using these methods of estimating TBSA, calculate only the areas of partial and full-thickness burns for TBSA. Do not use superficial areas for estimation.

> (*continued*) You assess the patient and find full-thickness burns to his entire head, anterior trunk, posterior trunk, and bilateral upper extremities circumferentially. You must determine the TBSA of this patient, as well as how much Ringer's lactate is required in the first 8 hours of resuscitation.

The TBSA of this patient is 63% according to the Wallace rule of nines. The patient requires 5,040 mL in the first 8 hours of resuscitation when multiplying by two. Calculate TBSA as follows:

- Entire head = 9%
- Anterior trunk = 18%
- Posterior trunk = 18%
- Bilateral upper extremities circumferentially = 9% × 2 = 18%
- TBSA = 63%

According to the Parkland formula, the amount of fluid resuscitation needed is as follows:

- Amount of fluid needed in 24 hours = 2 to 4 mL × weight in kilograms × TBSA of burn injury
- Amount of fluid needed in 24 hours = 2 mL × 80 kg (convert pounds to kilograms) × 63
- Amount of fluid needed in 24 hours = 10,080 mL

Half the fluid needed in 24 hours is given in the first 8 hours. Therefore, the patient requires 5,040 mL in the first 8 hours. The patient has already received 500 mL before arriving at the hospital. Now, the fluid to be administered is 4,540 mL, and it has been 1 hour since the injury. How much fluid is initially needed must be assessed to help guide the amount needed during transport.

$$4,540/7 = 649 \text{ mL/hr for the next 7 hours}$$

Changes to the formula can be made if urine output decreases or the patient becomes hypovolemic. Simply recalculate the Parkland formula but multiply by three.

> (*continued*) You are ready to transfer the patient to the burn center. You wrap the wounds in sterile sheets or bandages. You do not place sterile water or normal saline on the bandages for transport because the cool solution could cause the patient to become hypothermic. Also, this patient has circumferential burns to his bilateral upper extremities, so you frequently check his peripheral pulses to assess for compartment syndrome and the need for escharotomies.

Blood Administration

CASE STUDY

You are called to transport a victim of multiple trauma from a local hospital to a level 1 trauma center. You arrive on the scene to find a 35-year-old man who was involved in a two-vehicle, head-on collision with ejection and rollover. He has a ruptured spleen, grade III liver laceration, and fractured pelvis. His blood pressure is 84/45 mm Hg, heart rate is 132 beats/min, and respiratory rate is 24 breaths/min. The hospital has initiated two 14-gauge IV lines in the patient's bilateral antecubital fossae. Blood tubing is prepared with normal saline. The hospital has requested 2 U of O⁻ blood. You are expected to prepare the patient and begin administering the blood transporting to the trauma center.

The administration of blood and blood products is an important aspect of CCT. Because paramedics are introduced to blood administration only during CCTs, this procedure is not typically emphasized during EMS education. For this reason, blood administration may seem intimidating. However, blood is no different from other medications administered. Blood also has adverse effects and signs and symptoms to observe. The following section provides an overview of information needed for safe blood administration.

The following factors must be considered when administering blood products: compatible fluids, filtration, time, and transfusion reactions.

The only IV fluid compatible with blood is normal saline. Ringer's lactate, although a more efficient volume expander, cannot be administered with blood because the calcium causes clotting. Any solutions that include dextrose also must not be used with blood because of the risk of hemolysis. No additional medications should be administered into a line with blood because of the risks of hemolysis.

Blood tubing incorporates a filter to allow easy administration of blood products. The filter prevents the administration of cells that have clotted in the tubing. The Y portion of the blood tubing allows a bag of normal saline to be infused after the blood administration to prevent wasting blood in the tubing. When administering blood through smaller-bore IV catheters, such as a 20-gauge catheter, saline may be needed to help dilute the blood and prevent complications in the catheter tip.[17]

In addition to the fluids, degradation of blood components must be prevented. Blood must be administered within 30 minutes of removal from the refrigerator. If a unit of blood reaches 10°C (50°F), the red blood cells degrade and the blood must be discarded. Pooled platelets also require the blood to be discarded.[17]

Monitoring for Transfusion Reactions

Transfusion reactions are the most dangerous aspect of blood administration. The types of transfusion reactions are described as follows:[17]

- *An acute hemolytic transfusion reaction* is caused by ABO incompatibility. Signs and symptoms include fever, chills, low back pain, flushing, tachycardia, hypotension, and cardiac arrest.
- *An acute nonhemolytic transfusion reaction* is caused by a reaction to donor white blood cells, platelets, or plasma proteins. Signs and symptoms include headache, muscle aches, respiratory distress, cardiac arrhythmias, fever, and chills.
- *An anaphylactic transfusion reaction* is caused by an anti-immunoglobulin A reaction to the donor. Signs and symptoms include hives, urticaria, fever, flushing, and itching.
- *Circulatory overload* is caused by rapid blood transfusion. Signs and symptoms include pulmonary congestion, restlessness, cough, shortness of breath, hypertension, and distended neck veins.
- *Bacteremia* is caused by contaminated blood. Signs and symptoms include chills, fever, hypotension, vomiting, diarrhea, and septic shock.

Monitoring vital signs (including temperature), patient symptoms, and respiratory status are vital in patients who receive blood products. If a transfusion reaction is suspected, stop the transfusion, disconnect the blood tubing set, reconnect new IV tubing, and flush the line with saline.

▶ Review Questions

1. Name four types of infusion sets.
2. You are transporting a patient with the infusion pump set at 30 mL/hr. A pump failure occurs. What is the drip rate on a microdrip (60 gtt) set?
3. When transporting a patient on a magnesium drip, what should be available on board? Why?

4. What is the role of amiodarone in transporting a patient with myocardial ischemia?
5. Explain how fast you should decrease the blood glucose level in a patient with DKA and when you should initiate dextrose in the fluids.
6. In a patient with a closed-head injury, how is the CPP calculated?
7. Why is immediate fluid replacement critical in treating patients with burn injuries?
8. Explain the Wallace rule of nines.
9. What should you do if you suspect a patient is having a reaction to a blood transfusion?

References

1. Triple lumen central venous catheter (Seldinger technique). Medikit. http://www.globalmedikit.in/product/triple-lumen-central-venous-catheter-seldinger-technique. Accessed August 30, 2018.
2. Hickman/Broviac/Leonard central venous catheters. C. R. Bard. https://www.crbard.com/Peripheral-Vascular/en-US/Products/HICKMAN-BROVIAC-LEONARD-Central-Venous-Cathete#SpecificationTable. Accessed August 30, 2018.
3. Traylor S, Bastani A, Butris-Daut N, et al. Are three ports better than one? An evaluation of flow rates using all ports of a triple lumen central venous catheter in volume resuscitation. *Am J Emerg Med*. 2018;36(5):739–740.
4. Collins N, Daly S, Johnson P, Smith G. Pre-hospital use of intravenous in-line fluid warmers to reduce morbidity and mortality for major trauma patients: a review of the current literature. *Austral J Paramed*. 2015;12(2). https://ajp.paramedics.org/index.php/ajp/article/view/139/262. Accessed August 30, 2018.
5. Poder TG, Nonkani WG, Tsakeu Leponkouo E. Blood warming and hemolysis: a systematic review with meta-analysis. *Transfusion Med Rev*. 2015;29(3):172–180.
6. Sibai BM. HELLP syndrome. UpToDate. https://www.uptodate.com/contents/hellp-syndrome. Updated February 20, 2018. Accessed August 30, 2018.
7. Lam MTC, Dierking E. Intensive Care Unit issues in eclampsia and HELLP syndrome. *Int J Crit Illness Inj Sci*. 2017;7(3):136–141.
8. Roy J, Mitra JK, Pal A. Magnesium sulphate *versus* phenytoin in eclampsia: Maternal and foetal outcome—a comparative study. *Australasian Med J*. 2013;6(9):483–495.
9. Simhan HN, Caritis S. Inhibition of acute preterm labor. UpToDate. https://www.uptodate.com/contents/inhibition-of-acute-preterm-labor#H549493316. Updated November 3, 2017. Accessed October 5, 2018.
10. Padden MO. HELLP syndrome: Recognition and perinatal management. *Am Fam Physician*. 1999;60:829.
11. Prabhakar H, Sandhu K, Bhagat H, Durga P, Chawla R. Current concepts of optimal cerebral perfusion pressure in traumatic brain injury. *J Anaesthesiol Clin Pharmacol*. 2014;30(3):318–327.
12. Marik PE, Varon J, Trask T. Management of head trauma. *Chest*. 2002;122:699.
13. Haddad SH, Arabi YM. Critical care management of severe traumatic brain injury in adults. *Scand J Trauma Resusc Emerg Med*. 2012;20:12.
14. Gabriel EJ, Ghajar J, Jagoda A. *Guidelines for Prehospital Management of Traumatic Brain Injury*. Washington, DC: Brain Trauma Foundation, US Department of Transportation; 2005.
15. Haberal M, Sakallioglu Abali AE, Karakayali H. Fluid management in major burn injuries. *Indian J Plast Surg*. 2010;43(Suppl):S29–S36.
16. American Burn Association. *Advanced Burn Life Support Course Provider Manual*. Chicago, IL: American Burn Association; 2005.
17. Meyers E, Hopkins T. *Nurse's Clinical Pocket Guide*. 2nd ed. Philadelphia, PA: FA Davis Company; 2008.

© Andrew Brookes/Getty Images

CHAPTER 19

Special Considerations: Pregnancy, Pediatrics, Geriatrics, and Renal Failure

OBJECTIVES

1. Explain how physiologic changes in pregnancy can alter the pharmacologic mechanisms of a drug.
2. Differentiate the five categories in the Pregnancy Safety Category system—A, B, C, D, and X—and explain the pregnancy, lactation, and fertility labeling program that is currently being implemented by the FDA.
3. Discuss medications used for the treatment of asthma during pregnancy: albuterol (Proventil, Ventolin), terbutaline (Brethine), ipratropium bromide (Atrovent), prednisone, methylprednisolone sodium succinate (Solu-Medrol), and hydrocortisone sodium succinate (Solu-Cortef).
4. Explain the difference between chronic hypertension and gestational hypertension.
5. Discuss medications used in the treatment of hypertensive conditions during pregnancy: labetalol (Normodyne, Trandate), hydralazine (Apresoline), and magnesium sulfate.
6. Explain the impact of diabetic ketoacidosis in the pregnant patient.
7. Explain why blood pressure is not a good early indicator of perfusion in pediatric patients in shock.
8. Discuss why intraosseous lines are a beneficial alternative to intravenous lines in gaining vascular access in pediatric patients.
9. Explain why pediatric drug dosages are often determined by weight.
10. Discuss medications used in the treatment of pediatric bradycardia: epinephrine and atropine sulfate.

11. Discuss medications used in the treatment of pediatric tachycardia: adenosine (Adenocard) and amiodarone (Cordarone).
12. Define *polypharmacy* and its impact on the treatment of older adult patients.
13. Explain hemodialysis and peritoneal dialysis in the treatment of patients in end-stage renal disease.

MEDICATIONS THAT APPEAR IN CHAPTER 19

Diphenhydramine hydrochloride (Benadryl)
Albuterol (Proventil, Ventolin)
Terbutaline (Brethine, Brethaire)
Ipratropium bromide (Atrovent)
Prednisone

Methylprednisolone sodium succinate (Solu-Medrol)
Hydrocortisone sodium succinate (Cortef, Solu-Corte)
Labetalol (Normodyne, Trandate)
Hydralazine (Apresoline)
Magnesium sulfate

Insulin, regular (Humulin R, Novolin R)
Epinephrine
Atropine sulfate
Adenosine (Adenocard)
Amiodarone (Cordarone)
Procainamide (Pronestyl)
Lidocaine (Xylocaine)

▶ Introduction

Drug therapy in certain groups of patients requires special considerations regarding route of administration, dosage, adverse effects, and drug metabolism and elimination. When caring for a pregnant woman, the prehospital provider must be mindful that he or she is caring for two patients, the mother and the fetus. Medication administered to the mother is also administered to the fetus. Therefore, medications administered to pregnant women should be known to not adversely affect the physiology or development of the unborn child. Intravenous (IV) access is more difficult to achieve in pediatric patients, who may require different routes of drug administration. In addition, given their smaller body mass, pediatric patients require dose adjustment based on their body weight. Older adults may have a gradual to profound deterioration in function of the heart, lungs, kidneys, and liver. An additional factor in the care of older adults is the number of medications that these patients take on a long-term basis. The daily use of several medications (polypharmacy) can produce several potentially severe drug interactions that may cause or contribute to the initial call to EMS or result from a medication administered by a prehospital provider. Patients with renal failure are unable to excrete drugs that require excretion by the kidneys. Therefore, the patients typically require smaller doses and must be monitored more closely for the development of toxicity from active drug metabolites that cannot be adequately removed by the kidneys.

▶ Special Considerations in Pregnancy

Caring for an ill or injured pregnant patient can evoke a great deal of anxiety and apprehension in a prehospital provider. With pregnant patients, care is being provided to both the mother and her unborn child. An additional pressure is the vulnerability of the fetus to any medication administered to the mother; the administration of an inappropriate medication could lead to harm to or malformation of the fetus.

Physiologic Changes

To properly care for pregnant patients, prehospital providers must understand the normal physiologic changes that occur during pregnancy (**BOX 19-1**). Many of these changes are capable of altering the absorption, distribution, breakdown, and elimination of medications.

BOX 19-1 Normal Physiologic Adaptations to Pregnancy

Cardiovascular
- Decreasing systemic vascular resistance, coupled with increasing cardiac output.
- Increased resting heart rate (approximately 24% over baseline).
- Initial reduction of BP in early pregnancy, then returns to near baseline in the third trimester.
- Circulating blood plasma volume increases by approximately 50% above baseline.
- Cardiac blood return and cardiac output become dependent on patient position. In the supine position, both cardiac output and preload are significantly decreased (approximately 25–30%), coupled with increased heart rate.
- Peripheral edema (combination of cardiac, renal, and hematologic changes).

Hematologic
- Significant increase of circulating plasma volume causing a dilutional anemia and decreased blood viscosity.
- Overall increase in red blood cell mass related to changes in plasma erythropoietin.
- Hypercoagulable state with approximately 20% decrease in prothrombin time and partial thromboplastin time.
- Decreased colloid osmotic pressure caused by decreased serum albumin levels.

Renal
- Increased renal blood flow and increased glomerular filtration rate.
- Hyponatremia.
- Proteinuria. Mild proteinuria is normal; significant proteinuria suggests preeclampsia or other similar condition.

Other
- Increased minute ventilation.
- Respiratory alkalosis.
- Frequent or increased urination.

Data from Foley MR. Maternal adaptations to pregnancy: Cardiovascular and hemodynamic changes. UpToDate. https://www.uptodate.com/contents/maternal-adaptations-to-pregnancy-cardiovascular-and-hemodynamic-changes?topicRef=4788&source=see_link. Updated October 10, 2017. Accessed April 8, 2019; Thadhani RI, Maynard SE. Maternal adaptations to pregnancy: Renal and urinary tract physiology. UpToDate. https://www.uptodate.com/contents/maternal-adaptations-to-pregnancy-renal-and-urinary-tract-physiology. Updated April 27, 2018. Accessed April 8, 2019.

Nausea and vomiting, commonly referred to as *morning sickness*, is caused by a hormone-induced delay in gastric emptying. Although pregnancy does not alter the absorption of a given drug, the delay in gastric emptying results in a delay from the time a patient takes an oral medication to the time the drug is delivered to the intestine, where it is absorbed.

Respiratory drugs are rapidly effective in pregnant women because of increased minute ventilation.

Pregnant women have higher minute ventilation than do nonpregnant women, so inhaled medications result in systemic effects more rapidly than in nonpregnant women. For pregnant women, drugs delivered by inhalation are absorbed at a much more rapid rate than are oral medications.

The weight gain of pregnancy alters the woman's body composition. Pregnancy increases the percentage of body fat, which creates a larger volume of distribution for fat-soluble drugs. The increase in the proportion of body fat also decreases the concentration of albumin in the blood. Serum albumin is a major protein in blood plasma and is important in maintaining colloid osmotic pressure of the blood. A reduction in serum albumin affects drug distribution and plasma levels.

Pregnancy also induces a decrease in liver function and an increase in renal function. As a result, the breakdown of a drug by the liver can be slowed, but the excretion of that drug's by-products can be increased by an improvement in kidney function.

Medication Risks

The **placenta** is the lifeline between the mother and fetus. Oxygen, nutrients, and medications cross from the mother to the fetus via the placenta. An administered medication that has no effect on the mother can have a profound toxic effect on the fetus. The mother's circulatory system delivers medication to the fetus, but the fetus must break down and excrete the drug unassisted by the mother. Because the fetal liver and kidneys are immature, a dose of a given medication can have potentially toxic effects on the fetus.

In general, emergency medical care is complicated by the lack of reliable historical information from patients when they are confused, when they experience altered mental status, or even when they are unconscious. For this reason, providers should assume that all women of reproductive age are potentially pregnant. In addition, some women are not yet aware that they are pregnant. Therefore medication should be given only to a patient who is obviously pregnant or potentially pregnant when the benefit of that medication outweighs the potential risks.

Teratogenic drugs are medications that can result in a characteristic set of malformations in the fetus. The greatest period of vulnerability for the development of malformations is between the 4th and 12th weeks after the last menstrual period. Teratogenic drugs typically affect the development of an organ system at a particular period of vulnerability.

The U.S. Food and Drug Administration (FDA) classifies drugs into several categories based on their risk to the fetus (**TABLE 19-1**). Drugs are categorized as A, B, C, D, or X. A is the safest, and B, C, and D correspond to progressively more dangerous drugs. Category X drugs are the most dangerous to use in pregnancy and should be avoided. The Pregnancy Safety Category system is limited in its usefulness because the majority of research studies conducted to determine a drug's safety have used animals. Furthermore, a large number of medications have not yet been rated. The assignment of a category to a medication is made by the manufacturer and not the government or other regulatory or safety agency. In addition, assignments to the FDA safety categories are made when a drug is new and little is known about its safety. The FDA began changing requirements for medication pregnancy safety information in 2015. Newer medication information requirements include not only pregnancy safety, but also information on lactation and fertility risks (including fertility risk to males). Older medications approved prior to 2001 are not affected. Medications approved after 2001 but before 2015 will gradually transition in the newer pregnancy, lactation, and fertility information.[1,2]

For a drug to affect a fetus, it must cross the placenta and enter the fetal circulation. Generally, the greater the effect of a medication on the mother, the greater the probability that it

TABLE 19-1 FDA Pregnancy Safety Categories	
Category	**Description**
A	Controlled studies show no risk to the fetus.
B	Animal findings show risk to the fetus, although human studies do not; *or*, if no human studies are available, animal studies show no risk.
C	No human studies are available, and animal studies either show fetal risk or are not available.
D	Some investigational evidence shows risk of harm to the fetus, but potential benefits may outweigh the risks.
X	Animal or human studies or post-marketing investigations show fetal risk that outweighs possible benefits.

will cross the placenta and act on the fetus. Drugs that have large molecular weights are less likely to cross the placenta than are drugs with smaller molecular weights. Two common medications with large molecular weights are heparin and insulin. Neither of these medications can be given in an oral form because their large molecular size prevents absorption from the gastrointestinal (GI) tract, and neither of these medications can cross the placenta. However, most medications have a low molecular weight and can readily cross the placenta.

Lipophilic drugs are soluble in fat. Because the placenta is largely composed of fatty tissue, lipophilic medications are more likely to cross the placenta. In contrast, **lipophobic** medications, those that are not fat soluble, have a more difficult time crossing the placenta.

Drugs with short half-lives are also safer for pregnant patients than are those with long half-lives. A drug with a long half-life results in higher maternal serum levels for a longer period. The longer the drug remains in the mother's bloodstream, the greater the opportunity that it will cross the placenta into the fetal bloodstream.

DIPHENHYDRAMINE HYDROCHLORIDE (BENADRYL)

Classification: Antihistamine.
Action: Binds and blocks H_1 histamine receptors.
Indications: Anaphylactic reactions.
Adverse Effects: Drowsiness, dizziness, headache, excitable state (children), wheezing, thickening of bronchial secretions, chest tightness, palpitations, hypotension, blurred vision, dry mouth, nausea/vomiting, diarrhea.
Contraindications: Acute asthma, which thickens secretions; patients with cardiac histories; known sensitivity.
Dosage:
- **Adult:** 25 to 50 mg IV, intraosseous (IO), intramuscular (IM).
- **Pediatric 2 to 12 years:** 1 to 1.25 mg/kg IV, IO, IM.

Special Considerations:
Pregnancy class B.

Asthma

CASE STUDY

Your unit is dispatched to the home of a 28-year-old woman reporting shortness of breath. While en route, the dispatcher informs you that the patient is 32 weeks pregnant and is having an asthma attack. You arrive on the scene, and the husband leads you and your partner into the family room. He tells you that the patient has a history of asthma. She tested herself with a peak flowmeter and found that her peak expiratory flow rate (PEFR) was 45% of her baseline. When you reach the patient, you find an obviously pregnant woman sitting in a chair and appearing to be in respiratory distress. Your partner places the patient on oxygen and a pulse oximeter as you begin the assessment. The patient's respirations are labored with a rate of 32 breaths/min, heart rate of 88 beats/min, blood pressure of 102/76 mm Hg, and pulse oximeter reading of 94%. She is using the accessory muscles of her neck to breathe. On examination, she appears to have rhonchi and wheezes in all lung fields, heart sounds are normal, and her abdomen is remarkable for a gravid uterus. Neurologically she is following all commands and has no detectable motor or sensory deficits. Her skin is warm and moist. You determine that the patient would benefit from pharmacologic intervention for the treatment of her asthma.

Asthma is a reasonably common condition during pregnancy. Women with a long-standing history of asthma may note that the condition is exacerbated by pregnancy, whereas other women have their first occurrence of asthma during pregnancy. As in all conditions encountered during pregnancy, the fetus benefits by the mother's receipt of excellent care. If left untreated, asthma can have significantly negative results for both the mother and fetus. It is safer for a pregnant woman to take medications than to have exacerbations of asthma.

Management

The initial therapy for a pregnant woman having an asthma attack includes oxygen and a bronchodilator. Beta$_2$ agonists commonly used for the treatment of asthma are listed as Category C medications. Research using a large number of pregnant women has demonstrated that the medications typically used for the treatment of asthma can be used without noted perinatal complications.[3]

> Asthma is a common condition of pregnancy, and treatment medications can be used without perinatal complications.

The beta-agonist albuterol (Proventil, Ventolin) is the first-line therapy for treatment of asthma in pregnant women.[4] Pregnant patients who have asthma should be instructed to carry albuterol with them at all times. Albuterol is most commonly administered by a metered-dose inhaler (MDI) with a spacer or as a nebulization therapy. Nebulization is a common method of albuterol administration used by many prehospital providers. Some providers argue that nebulization is inefficient because of the large size of the particles and the loss of medication from the expiratory port of the nebulization system. MDIs with spacers can obtain similar clinical improvement in the asthma with smaller doses of medication. Four to six MDI inhalations with a spacer are roughly equivalent to one nebulization therapy.

An alternative medication to treat asthma in pregnant patients is subcutaneous terbutaline (Brethine). The use of terbutaline is somewhat controversial. The FDA issued a "black box" warning regarding terbutaline use for preterm labor in 2011, requiring additional labeling information regarding the risk to pregnant patients. Other sources suggest that terbutaline is an acceptable alternative in pregnant patients with asthma.[5,6]

ALBUTEROL (PROVENTIL, VENTOLIN)

Classification: Bronchodilator, beta agonist.
Action: Binds and stimulates beta$_2$ receptors, resulting in relaxation of bronchial smooth muscle.
Indications: Asthma, bronchitis with bronchospasm, and chronic obstructive pulmonary disease (COPD).
Adverse Effects: Hyperglycemia, hypokalemia, palpitations, sinus tachycardia, anxiety, tremor, nausea/vomiting, throat irritation, dry mouth, hypertension, dyspepsia, insomnia, headache, epistaxis, paradoxical bronchospasm.
Contraindications: Angioedema, sensitivity to albuterol or levalbuterol. Use with caution in lactating patients, cardiovascular disorders, cardiac arrhythmias.
Dosage:
Acute Bronchospasm:
- **Adult:**
  - **MDI:** 4 to 8 puffs every 1 to 4 hours may be required.
  - **Nebulizer:** 2.5 to 5 mg every 20 minutes for a maximum of three doses. After the initial three doses, escalate the dose or start a continuous nebulization at 10 to 15 mg/hr.

© Joseph Gaul/Alamy Stock Photo.

- **Pediatric:**
  - **MDI:**
    - **4 years and older:** 2 inhalations every 4 to 6 hours; however, in some patients, 1 inhalation every 4 hours is sufficient. More frequent administration or more inhalations are not recommended.
    - **Younger than 4 years:** Administer by nebulization.
  - **Nebulizer:**
    - **Older than 12 years:** The dose for a continuous nebulization is 0.5 mg/kg per hour.
    - **Younger than 12 years:** 0.63 to 2.5 mg every 20 minutes for a maximum of three doses. Alternatively, continuous nebulization at 0.5 mg/kg per hour can be delivered to children younger than 12 years.

Asthma in Pregnancy:
- **MDI:** Two inhalations every 4 hours. In acute exacerbation, start with 2 to 4 puffs every 20 minutes.
- **Nebulizer:** 2.5 mg (0.5 mL) by 0.5% nebulization solution. Place 0.5 mL of the albuterol solution in 2.5 mL of sterile normal saline. Flow is regulated to deliver the therapy over a 5- to 20-minute period. In refractory cases, some physicians order 10 mg nebulized over a 60-minute period.

Special Considerations:
Pregnancy class C.

TERBUTALINE (BRETHINE, BRETHAIRE)

Classification: Adrenergic agonist.
Action: Stimulates the beta$_2$ receptor, producing relaxation of bronchial smooth muscle and bronchodilation.
Indications: Prevention and reversal of bronchospasm.
Adverse Effects: Cardiac arrhythmias, arrhythmia exacerbation, angina, anxiety, headache, tremor, palpitations, dizziness.
Contraindications: Known sensitivity to sympathomimetics. Use with caution in hypertension, cardiac disease, cardiac arrhythmias, diabetes, older adults, monoamine oxidase inhibitor (MAOI) therapy, pheochromocytoma, thyrotoxicosis, seizure disorder.
Dosage:
- **Adult:** 0.25 mg subcutaneous every 20 minutes for 3 doses. The usual site for the subcutaneous injection is the lateral deltoid.
- **Pediatric:** 0.005 to 0.01 mg/kg subcutaneous every 20 minutes for 3 doses.

Special Considerations:
Pregnancy class B.

(*continued*) You administer an albuterol nebulization therapy over a 20-minute period, with a plan to repeat the therapy every 20 minutes if the patient does not demonstrate satisfactory improvement. With an initial PEFR of less than 50%, you determine that the patient is having a severe exacerbation of her asthma and warrants additional drug therapy.

The next drug used to treat a pregnant patient having a severe exacerbation of asthma with a PEFR of less than 50% would be ipratropium bromide (Atrovent). Ipratropium bromide is used in severe exacerbations of asthma and in cases in which the patient has an unsatisfactory response to treatment with albuterol. In more severe cases of asthma, additional treatment with ipratropium bromide has provided greater symptomatic relief than albuterol used as a single agent.

IPRATROPIUM BROMIDE (ATROVENT)

Classification: Bronchodilator, anticholinergic.
Action: Antagonizes the acetylcholine receptor on bronchial smooth muscle, producing bronchodilation.
Indications: Asthma, bronchospasm associated with COPD.
Adverse Effects: Paradoxical acute bronchospasm, cough, throat irritation, headache, dizziness, dry mouth, palpitations.
Contraindications: Closed-angle glaucoma, bladder neck obstruction, prostatic hypertrophy, known sensitivity including peanuts or soybeans and atropine or atropine derivatives.
Dosage:
MDI:
- **Adult:** 8 inhalations every 20 minutes for up to 3 hours.
- **Pediatric <12 years:** 4 to 8 inhalations every 20 minutes for up to 3 hours.

Nebulization:
- **Adult:** 0.5 mg every 20 minutes for 3 doses, then as needed.
- **Pediatric 5 to 14 years:** 0.25 to 0.5 mg every 20 minutes for 3 doses as needed.

Special Considerations:
Ipratropium bromide is not typically used as a sole medication in the treatment of acute exacerbation of asthma. Ipratropium bromide is commonly administered after a beta agonist.
Care should be taken to not allow the aerosol spray (especially in the MDI) to come into contact with the eyes. Contact with the eyes can cause temporary blurring of vision that resolves without intervention within 4 hours.
Pregnancy class B.

NDC 12345-678-90
Ipratropium bromide
Inhalation Aerosol Rx only
(Ipratropium bromide HFA)
Each actuation delivers 17 mcg ipratropium bromide from the mouthpiece.
12.9 grams
200 metered actuations with Dose indicator
LOT
EXP

(*continued*) After administration of ipratropium bromide, the patient shows some improvement in her dyspnea, but she is still wheezing. Given the magnitude of the PEFR reduction and the persistent symptoms, you determine she could potentially benefit from corticosteroid therapy.

Asthma is a condition characterized by bronchospasm and inflammation of the airway. Corticosteroids (also discussed in Chapter 14) are a group of medications that are synthetic versions of glucocorticoid (and mineral corticoid) steroid hormones in the body, produced in the adrenal cortex. These medications should be administered in cases of severe exacerbations and certainly for impending respiratory failure.[7] Prednisone, methylprednisolone (Solu-Medrol), and hydrocortisone (Solu-Cortef) are the steroids most commonly used in the treatment of asthma. Several studies also suggest a single dose of dexamethasone (Decadron) as an alternative to other corticosteroids,[7,8] particularly when patient compliance is a concern following hospital discharge. Systemic corticosteroids (glucocorticoids) are controversial in pregnant patients. Research suggests a relationship between the use of systemic corticosteroids and premature births, congenital malformations, and preeclampsia.[4] The decision to administer corticosteroids can be made by monitoring the PEFR. When the initial PEFR is less than 50% of predicted, corticosteroids should be administered after ipratropium bromide (**BOX 19-2**). Corticosteroids should also be considered when the PEFR does not improve by at least 10% after bronchodilator therapy or if the PEFR is lower than 70% after 1 hour of therapy.[9]

BOX 19-2 Indications for the Use of Steroids in Asthma

PEFR <50% of predicted after ipratropium bromide (Atrovent) administration.
PEFR does not improve by >10% after bronchodilator administration.
PEFR <70% predicted after 1 hour of therapy.

Fanta CH. Management of acute exacerbations of asthma in adults. UpToDate. https://www.uptodate.com/contents/management-of-acute-exacerbations-of
-asthma-in-adults. Updated April 9, 2018. Accessed September 10, 2018.

The beneficial effects of corticosteroids may not become apparent for several hours after administration. An IV preparation of a steroid may be used in an emergency when oral dosing is not practical. Orally administered steroids are rapidly absorbed, with nearly complete bioavailability. More is not necessarily better in the case of systemic corticosteroids, and large doses of corticosteroids have not been demonstrated to be any more beneficial than smaller doses. A review of several published investigations has shown that higher doses of steroids do not provide a benefit in either lung function or preventing respiratory failure.[10] The uses of inhaled steroids have been debated regarding their effectiveness in acute asthma exacerbations.[11]

PREDNISONE

Classification: Corticosteroid.
Action: Reduces inflammation.
Indications: Inflammatory conditions, such as asthma with bronchospasm.
Adverse Effects: Many adverse effects of steroid use are not related to short-term use but typically are seen with long-term use and during withdrawal.
Contraindications: Cushing's syndrome, fungal infections, measles, varicella, known sensitivity.
Dosage:
- **Adult:** Dosage must be individualized.
- **Pediatric:** Dosage must be individualized.

Special Considerations:
Pregnancy class C.

METHYLPREDNISOLONE SODIUM SUCCINATE (SOLU-MEDROL)

Classification: Corticosteroid.
Action: Reduces inflammation by multiple mechanisms.
Indications: Anaphylaxis, asthma, COPD.
Adverse Effects: Depression, euphoria, headache, restlessness, hypertension, bradycardia, nausea/vomiting, swelling, diarrhea, weakness, fluid retention, paresthesias.
Contraindications: Cushing's syndrome, fungal infection, measles, varicella, known sensitivity (including sulfites). Use with caution in active infections, renal disease, penetrating spinal cord injury, hypertension, seizures, heart failure.

Dosage:
Asthma and COPD:
- **Adult:** 40 to 80 mg/day IV in divided doses.
- **Pediatric:** 1 mg/kg (up to 60 mg) IV, IO per day in two divided doses.

Anaphylactic Shock:
- **Adult:** 0.5 to 1 mg/kg IV every 12 hours.
- **Pediatric:** Same as adult dosing.

Special Considerations:
May mask signs and symptoms of infection.
Pregnancy class C.

HYDROCORTISONE SODIUM SUCCINATE (CORTEF, SOLU-CORTEF)

Classification: Corticosteroid.

Action: Reduces inflammation by multiple mechanisms. As a steroid, it replaces the steroids that are lacking in adrenal insufficiency.

Indications: Adrenal insufficiency, allergic reactions, anaphylaxis, asthma, COPD.

Adverse Effects: Leukocytosis, hyperglycemia, increased infection, decreased wound healing, increased rate of death from sepsis.

Contraindications: Cushing's syndrome, known sensitivity to benzyl alcohol. Use with caution in diabetes, hypertension, heart failure, known systemic fungal infection, renal disease, idiopathic thrombocytopenia, psychosis, seizure disorder, GI disease, glaucoma, known sensitivity.

Dosage:

Anaphylactic Shock and Adrenal Insufficiency:

- **Adult:** 100 to 500 mg IV, IO, or IM.
- **Pediatric:** 2 to 10 mg/kg per day IV, IO, or IM (max: 500 mg).

Special Considerations:

Pregnancy class C.

Hypertensive Crisis

CASE STUDY

You work for an EMS agency in a rural area. The closest hospital is a 25-bed facility with a two-bed emergency department (ED). Because of severe storms in the region, you and your partner have had a slow afternoon. You are dispatched to the local hospital to transfer a pregnant woman to a regional university hospital 120 miles away. You arrive at the ED and obtain a report from the emergency physician. She walks you over to the bed, where you meet a 26-year-old woman who is 35 weeks pregnant. The patient arrived at the ED slightly more than 1 hour before your arrival. She reported a headache that lasted all day, and her husband states that she seemed to become more somnolent as the day progressed. When they first admitted the patient to the ED, her blood pressure was 180/112 mm Hg. One week ago the patient was seen by her family physician, who determined her blood pressure was normal at that time. Today, with the report of headache and a significantly elevated blood pressure, the emergency physician obtained blood and urine tests in an attempt to confirm the diagnosis of preeclampsia. The obstetrician at the university hospital who handles high-risk pregnancies has accepted the patient, but because of inclement weather, the patient will need to be transported by ground. You and your partner will care for this patient over the next several hours during transport.

Hypertension is a relatively common condition during pregnancy, with an incidence of approximately 10%.[12] Hypertension in pregnancy is such a serious problem that it accounts for 14% of all pregnancy-related deaths.[13] Several types of hypertension can occur during pregnancy, ranging from benign to life-threatening in their course.

It is extremely important to evaluate for preeclampsia in pregnant patients with hypertension. This is done by evaluating the patient's blood pressure, checking for proteinuria (protein in the urine), and assessing for signs of end-organ dysfunction. Once preeclampsia is diagnosed, expert consultation and aggressive management, with or without antihypertensive medications, are essential. Eclampsia occurs when a woman experiencing preeclampsia has seizures. The only definitive treatment for preeclampsia and eclampsia is the delivery of the fetus; however, it is still possible for eclampsia (seizures) to occur up to 6 weeks after delivery.

Chronic hypertension occurs when the patient has a history of hypertension that precedes the pregnancy. It may be possible to see exacerbations of chronic hypertension during pregnancy, requiring aggressive management. **Gestational hypertension** is elevated blood pressure that first occurs during pregnancy but does not meet the diagnostic criteria of eclampsia.

Management

In the case of severe hypertension, the mother should be treated with antihypertensive agents in an effort to reduce maternal complications. A number of sources use 160/110 mm Hg as the threshold for aggressive antihypertensive management in pregnant patients.[14–16] Clearly the young woman in the scenario exceeds both thresholds.

> (*continued*) You perform an initial evaluation. The patient currently is resting comfortably, and her blood pressure is 140/94 mm Hg. She reports some improvement in her headache but tells you she prefers the lights off to avoid aggravating her headache. You load her into the ambulance and begin the several-hour trip down the highway. Approximately 20 minutes into the trip, the patient states that her head is starting to bother her again. You retake her blood pressure, which is 176/112 mm Hg. You are worried about the severity of her hypertension and the return of her symptoms. You believe her blood pressure should be treated.

Patients should be considered candidates for pharmacologic therapy for hypertension when their systolic blood pressure exceeds 160 mm Hg or diastolic pressure exceeds 110 mm Hg. If the patient's blood pressure exceeds these measurements, the prehospital provider should consult with medical direction or follow standing local protocols. The two drugs often used to treat hypertensive conditions during pregnancy are labetalol (Normodyne, Trandate) and hydralazine (Apresoline).

An excellent medication used for the treatment of hypertensive crisis in pregnancy is the beta blocker labetalol. Hydralazine is another common antihypertensive medication used during pregnancy. Evaluation of research trials that used hydralazine determined that hydralazine can result in a greater likelihood of inducing maternal hypotension, and the drug should not be used as a first-line agent for the acute treatment of hypertension.[11,12] Nitroglycerin is another effective antihypertensive drug. One advantage of nitroglycerin (as previously discussed in Chapter 12) is its short half-life of only 1 to 3 minutes.

The danger in using any antihypertensive agent is dropping the blood pressure to the point at which placental blood flow decreases.

LABETALOL (NORMODYNE, TRANDATE)

Classification: Beta-adrenergic antagonist, antianginal, antihypertensive.
Action: Binds with both the beta$_1$ and beta$_2$ receptors and alpha$_1$ receptors in vascular smooth muscle. Inhibits the strength of the heart's contractions, as well as the heart rate. This results in a decrease in cardiac oxygen consumption.
Indications: Acute coronary syndrome (ACS), supraventricular tachycardia (SVT), severe hypertension.
Adverse Effects: Usually mild and transient; hypotensive symptoms, nausea/vomiting, bronchospasm, arrhythmia, bradycardia, atrioventricular (AV) block.

Labetalol Hydrochloride
Injection, USP
20 mL Multi-Dose vial
100 mg/20 mL (5 mg/mL)
For Intravenous Injection Only
Sterile   NDC 12345-678-90
Rx only

NDC 12345-678-90
20 mL
Multi-Dose vial
Labetalol Hydrochloride
Injection, USP
100 mg/20 mL (5 mg/mL)
For Intravenous Injection Only
Rx only   Sterile

(continues)

LABETALOL (NORMODYNE, TRANDATE)   *(continued)*

Contraindications: Hypotension, cardiogenic shock, acute pulmonary edema, heart failure, severe bradycardia, sick sinus syndrome, second- or third-degree heart block, asthma or acute bronchospasm, cocaine-induced ACS, known sensitivity. Use caution in pheochromocytoma, cerebrovascular disease or stroke, poorly controlled diabetes, with hepatic disease. Use with caution at lowest effective dose in chronic lung disease.

Dosage:

Cardiac Indications:

Note: Monitor blood pressure and heart rate closely during administration.

- **Adult:** 10 mg IV, IO over a 1- to 2-minute period. May repeat every 10 minutes to a maximum dose of 150 mg or give initial bolus and then follow with infusion at 2 to 8 mg/min.
- **Pediatric:** 0.2 to 1 mg/kg to a maximum dosage of 3 mg/kg per hour; may also administer 0.25 to 3 mg/kg per hour as an infusion.

Severe Hypertension:

- **Adult:** Initial dose is 20 mg IV, IO slow infusion over a 2-minute period. After the initial dose, blood pressure should be checked every 5 minutes. Repeat doses can be given at 10-minute intervals. The second dose should be 40 mg IV, IO, and subsequent doses should be 80 mg IV, IO, to a maximum total dose of 300 mg. The effect on blood pressure typically will occur within 5 minutes from the time of administration. Alternatively, may be administered via IV infusion at 2 mg/min to a total maximum dose of 300 mg.
- **Pediatric:** 0.25 to 3 mg/kg per hour IV, IO infusion with a maximum dose of 3 mg/kg per hour.

Special Considerations:

Pregnancy class C.

HYDRALAZINE (APRESOLINE)

Classification: Antihypertensive agent, vasodilator.
Action: Directly dilates the peripheral blood vessels.
Indications: Hypertension associated with preeclampsia and eclampsia, hypertensive crisis.
Adverse Effects: Headache, angina, flushing, palpitations, reflex tachycardia, anorexia, nausea/vomiting, diarrhea, hypotension, syncope, peripheral vasodilation, peripheral edema, fluid retention, paresthesias.
Contraindications: Patients taking diazoxide or MAOIs, coronary artery disease, stroke, angina, dissecting aortic aneurysm, mitral valve and rheumatic heart diseases.

Dosage:

Preeclampsia and Eclampsia:

- **Adult:** 5 to 10 mg IV. Repeat every 20 to 30 minutes until systolic blood pressure of 90 to 105 mm Hg is attained.

Acute Hypertension Not Associated with Preeclampsia:

- **Adult:** 10 to 20 mg IV, or IM.
- **Pediatric: 1 month to 12 years:** 0.1 to 0.2 mg/kg IV or IM every 4 to 6 hours as needed (max: 20 mg/dose).

Special Consideration:

Pregnancy class C.

(*continued*) You repeat the blood pressure measurement to ensure no error occurred. The second blood pressure reading is 180/108 mm Hg. The patient tells you that her headache is 8 on a pain scale of 1 to 10. She asks you to turn off the lights in the compartment because they are aggravating her headache. After consultation with medical direction, you administer labetalol 20 mg IV. After a few minutes, you measure her blood pressure again. No improvement has occurred with the labetalol. After 20 minutes, still no improvement in the patient's blood pressure or symptoms has occurred. You administer labetalol 40 mg IV, wait several minutes, and then retake the blood pressure. The blood pressure has decreased to 146/94 mm Hg, and the patient seems to have some relief from her headache.

The definitive treatment for eclampsia is delivery of the fetus, which is generally avoided in the prehospital setting. Prehospital providers often are required to participate in the inter-hospital transfer to a specialty facility of a woman with eclampsia or preeclampsia. One of the goals of therapy is to prevent or treat the seizures. The agent of choice for prevention and treatment of eclamptic seizures is magnesium sulfate. Magnesium is indicated when the diastolic blood pressure is greater than 100 mm Hg and signs of an impending seizure are present.

MAGNESIUM SULFATE

Classification: Electrolyte, tocolytic, mineral.
Action: Required for normal physiologic functioning. Magnesium is a cofactor in neurochemical transmission and muscular excitability. Magnesium sulfate controls seizures by blocking peripheral neuromuscular transmission. Magnesium is also a peripheral vasodilator and an inhibitor of platelet function.
Indications: Torsades de pointes, cardiac arrhythmias associated with hypomagnesemia, eclampsia and seizure prophylaxis in preeclampsia, status asthmaticus.
Adverse Effects: Magnesium toxicity (signs include flushing, diaphoresis, hypotension, muscle paralysis, weakness, hypothermia, and cardiac, central nervous system, or respiratory depression).
Contraindications: AV block, GI obstruction. Use with caution in renal impairment.
Dosage:
Pulseless Ventricular Fibrillation (VF)/Ventricular Tachycardia (VT) with Torsades de Pointes or Hypomagnesemia:
- **Adult:** 1 to 2 g in 10 mL D_5W IV, IO administered over 15 minutes or faster with cardiac arrest.
- **Pediatric:** 25 to 50 mg/kg IV, IO over 10 to 20 minutes; may administer faster for torsades de pointes (max single dose: 2 g).
Torsades de Pointes with a Pulse or Cardiac Arrhythmias with Hypomagnesemia:
- **Adult:** 1 to 2 g in 50 to 100 mL D_5W IV, IO administered over 5 to 60 minutes. Follow with 0.5 to 1 g/hr IV, IO titrated to control torsades de pointes.
- **Pediatric:** 25 to 50 mg/kg IV, IO over 10 to 20 minutes (max single dose: 2 g).
Eclampsia and Seizure Prophylaxis in Preeclampsia:
- **Adult:** 4 to 6 g IV, IO over 20 to 30 minutes, followed by an infusion of 1 to 2 g/hr.
Status Asthmaticus:
- **Adult:** 1.2 to 2 g slow IV, IO (over 20 minutes).
- **Pediatric:** 25 to 50 mg/kg (diluted in D_5W) slow IV, IO (over 10 to 20 minutes).
Special Considerations:
Pregnancy class A.

Diabetic Ketoacidosis

Despite intensive control of diabetes during pregnancy, pregnant women with diabetes may develop diabetic ketoacidosis (DKA), which is a state of insulin deficiency that produces a condition of hyperglycemia, dehydration, and metabolic acidosis. A detailed discussion is found in Chapter 11. DKA in pregnancy can be fatal for the fetus, with fetal mortality rates approaching 50%. Elevated maternal blood glucose levels result in osmotic diuresis and electrolyte shifts. The loss of circulatory blood volume and electrolyte shifts in the mother result in a drop in placental blood flow and oxygen content.

Management

In addition to the initial treatment priorities of maintaining the airway, breathing, and circulatory status, the paramedic should administer 1 L of an isotonic fluid (0.9% saline or Ringer's lactate) over a 1-hour period. After this initial fluid bolus, the IV infusion should continue at a rate of 250 to 500 mL/hr. This strategy of fluid resuscitation with isotonic fluids should continue until the patient's blood glucose level is approximately 250 mg/dL. Once the blood sugar level is less than 250 mg/dL, the fluid should be changed to an IV fluid that contains 5% dextrose. This addition of 5% dextrose prevents a too-rapid and perhaps dangerous decline in the serum glucose concentration.

Many EMS agencies do not carry insulin because of its need for refrigeration; however, paramedics may see insulin-dependent patients during interhospital transfers. If ordered, an initial insulin bolus of 0.1 U/kg IV should be given. This typically is followed by an insulin infusion running at a dose of 0.05 to 0.1 U/kg per hour. During an insulin infusion, blood glucose measurements are taken hourly or every other hour. If the blood glucose level does not decrease by 25% after 2 hours, the paramedic should double the initial insulin infusion dose. Once the blood glucose level reaches 250 mg/dL, the IV fluid should be changed to one containing 5% dextrose, and the insulin infusion rate should be decreased by one half. Once the blood glucose level has reached 150 mg/dL, the insulin infusion rate should be decreased to 1 to 2 U/hr.

INSULIN, REGULAR (HUMULIN R, NOVOLIN R)

Classification: Hormone.
Action: Binds to a receptor on the membrane of cells and facilitates the transport of glucose into cells.
Indications: Hyperglycemia, insulin-dependent diabetes mellitus, hyperkalemia.
Adverse Effects: Hypoglycemia, tachycardia, palpitations, diaphoresis, anxiety, confusion, blurred vision, weakness, depression, seizures, coma, insulin shock, hypokalemia.
Contraindications: Hypoglycemia, known sensitivity.
Dosage:
Diabetic Ketoacidosis:

- **Adult:** 0.1 U/kg IV, IO, or subcutaneous.
  Because of poor perfusion of the peripheral tissues, subcutaneous administration is much less effective than the IV, IO route. IV, IO insulin has a very short half-life; therefore, IV, IO insulin without an infusion is not that effective. The rate for an insulin infusion is 0.05 to 0.1 U/kg per hour IV, IO. When dosing insulin, use a U-100 insulin syringe to measure and deliver the insulin. The time from administration to action, as well as the duration of action, varies greatly among different people, as well as at different times in the same person.

Hyperkalemia:
- **Adult:** 10 U IV, IO of regular insulin (Insulin R), coadministered with 50 mL of $D_{50}W$ over 5 minutes.
- **Pediatric:** 0.1 U/kg Insulin R IV, IO.

Special Considerations:

Only regular insulin can be given IV, IO. *Insulin is a high-risk medication and should be verified with another appropriately trained provider whenever possible.*

Pregnancy class B.

▶ Special Considerations for Pediatric Patients

The following section discusses the pediatric population and special issues that must be considered in their treatment. It is often said that children are not little adults, and in many ways this is true. Regarding IV access; fluid management; and the treatment of shock, pain, and cardiac and neurologic emergencies, several key differences between pediatric and adult patients are critical to keep in mind when delivering care to children.

Drug Dosing

In addition to being smaller than adults, the body composition of infants and children is dramatically different from that of adults. The various body compartments, as described in Chapter 5, have different relative sizes than those of the adult. In adults, 60% of the body, based on total body mass, is water. The percentage of total body water of an infant is approximately 80%, a proportion that decreases to approximately 60% by adulthood. In the first year of life, the percentage of fat nearly doubles in infants. Infants have a much smaller percentage of muscle mass than adults, but they have much larger brains and livers in relation to their total body weight. Infants and children also have large volumes of distribution and rapid metabolic rates. Because of differences in a child's metabolism during the various stages of development, a simple linear reduction of an adult drug dose is not appropriate.

Information on pediatric drug dosing is usually given on the basis of age, weight, or body surface area of the child. In most cases, drugs for pediatric use usually recommend a particular dose in milligrams per kilogram. For many drugs, the recommended weight-based dose (or weight-normalized dose) is presented for children of different ages or weight groups. For many drugs, the weight-normalized dose increases as the weight of the child decreases. A dose appropriate for an 8-year-old may be too small for a 2-year-old.

The provider must be mindful that the calculated pediatric dose should not exceed the recommended adult dose.

CASE STUDY

You are called to the home of an 18-month-old boy who has had vomiting and diarrhea for 4 days. He has not had urine output since the night before, and the parents state that he has been sleepy and poorly responsive to normal stimuli. When you arrive, you find a pale boy sleeping in his mother's arms. His heart rate is 120 beats/min, and his blood pressure is 90/70 mm Hg. The mother tells you that the child normally weighs approximately 24 pounds (11 kg); she believes he has lost 4 pounds (2 kg) since he became ill. His breathing is shallow, and his eyes appear sunken. You are in a rural area, and the transport time to the nearest hospital is approximately 40 minutes. You examine the patient's extremities and find that his pulses are weak. Few veins are visible, and IV access is critical at this point. You decide that IO access is necessary. Once secured, you administer a bolus of 0.9% normal saline (10 mL/kg, or approximately 100 mL). You reassess vital signs, and his heart rate is now 110 beats/min. Blood pressure remains unchanged. You maintain IV infusion at 60 mL/hr and transport the patient on a monitor.

© Jones & Bartlett Learning.

Hypovolemic Shock

When assessing a child in shock, a critical point to realize is that blood pressure is not the primary vital sign that indicates the patient's status. In most pediatric patients a drop in blood pressure is the last sign of deterioration; therefore, blood pressure is not a good indicator of the child's perfusion. When assessing a child for shock, palpate peripheral pulses and evaluate temperature and capillary refill of the distal extremities.

In hypovolemic pediatric patients, blood pressure is a late sign of deterioration.

Cardiac output (CO) is determined by the stroke volume (SV) of the heart multiplied by the heart rate (HR):

$$CO = HR \times SV$$

Stroke volume is the amount of blood ejected by the heart with each heartbeat. An adult has some variability in stroke volume; however, stroke volume in a child is relatively stable. Therefore the only mechanism that a child has to improve cardiac output in shock is an increased heart rate.

Vascular Access and Management

Vascular access is a challenge in pediatric patients because of the small size of their blood vessels, greater amount of subcutaneous fat, and unwillingness to cooperate with the provider. Vascular access is particularly difficult and time-consuming with children in shock. Each emergency response team should establish a plan for how much time should be spent attempting to obtain access to each IV site and should identify the most appropriately trained personnel to attempt access. If one or two lines are not obtained within 2 to 5 minutes, medications should be given by an alternate method so that resuscitation is not delayed.

The preferred peripheral site for IV placement in a child is the antecubital fossa. In an infant, a scalp vein or a superficial vein of an extremity can be used if larger veins are not accessible (**FIGURE 19-1**). Additional useful equipment includes a tourniquet and 18- to 24-gauge angiocatheters. Disadvantages to a peripheral IV line include risk of the line becoming dislodged, occlusion of the line, and possible tissue injury with extravasation of irritants.

IO lines are an alternative to venous access in children when vascular access is critical but peripheral access is not achievable. A 15- to 18-gauge bone marrow needle with stylet is placed in the marrow cavity of the child's tibia (**FIGURE 19-2**). Placement is directed perpendicular to the flat part of the proximal tibia, and the needle is inserted through the skin 1 to 3 cm (approximately one finger's width) just medial to the tibial tuberosity. The catheter is advanced through the bone into the marrow space, at which point a "pop" is usually felt. Successful placement is confirmed by aspiration of marrow content and easy infusion of fluid.

Alternate sites for IO catheter placement include the distal tibia and distal femur. Most fluids that can be infused through a peripheral IV can also be infused intraosseously, and absorption is rapid from the tibia bone marrow cavity. Once an IO catheter is established

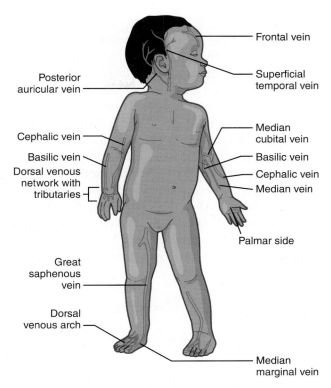

FIGURE 19-1 Various sites for placement of IV catheters in infants.

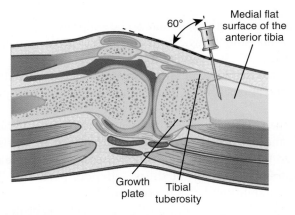

FIGURE 19-2 Anterior tibial placement of an intraosseous infusion.

and fluid boluses have been administered, a peripheral IV line may be more accessible with improved hydration of the child.

Rare but significant complications of IO access include osteomyelitis, cellulitis, infiltration of fluid, anterior compartment syndrome, tibial fracture, and fat embolus. IO lines are not suitable for long-term use, and an increased incidence of leaking at the site of insertion exists. To minimize complications, IO needles should not be placed in fractured bones or at a site that was previously used. They should also not be used for prolonged periods. Additionally, an IO needle should not be placed in patients with a history of osteogenesis imperfecta, a bone condition that makes the bones brittle and susceptible to fracture.

Never place an IO line in a fractured bone.

Once IV access has been obtained, fluid management and treatment of shock can begin. Remember, shock is the collapse of the body's cardiovascular system, which prevents it from providing oxygen and nutrients for the body's vital metabolic needs. Once an airway and adequate oxygenation have been secured and a functioning infusion line has been obtained, fluid resuscitation can begin. Improving the blood volume is best achieved with IV fluids, and if appropriate, blood products may be administered (such as in air medicine or a military setting). If packed red blood cells are required, the provider should transfuse 10 mL/kg of blood.

Volume expansion in children is based on weight rather than the use of a standard bolus, such as in adults. A safe rule of thumb is to give a bolus of no more than 10 to 20 mL/kg at a time, with close reassessment of vital signs between boluses. The bolus is given rapidly over minutes. Appropriate fluids for fluid resuscitation include crystalloids such as 0.9% sodium chloride or Ringer's lactate solution. After each intervention—whether fluid bolus, airway intervention, or cardiac compressions—a full reassessment of the patient's status is critical. Be sure to proceed in the appropriate ABC order so that treatment of shock is most effective. As is true for the care of any injured or ill patient, remember to check and recheck.

> The volume of a fluid bolus for a pediatric patient is 10 to 20 mL/kg.

Arrhythmias

Pediatric cardiac arrhythmias are often referred to in the simple terms of *abnormal heart rate* and rhythms that are either *too fast* or *too slow*. Unlike the complex rhythms more commonly found in adults, children tend to have less history of cardiac disease and symptoms more likely to represent an acute, reversible process. See Chapter 9 for an in-depth discussion of arrhythmias.

The treatment of pediatric arrhythmias can also be simplified. Treatment may consist of only establishing an airway and improving circulation with IV hydration, never underemphasizing the importance of the ABCs in resuscitation.

However, when initial resuscitative measures are not adequate in stabilizing the patient, a sound knowledge of medications for the treatment of arrhythmias in pediatric patients is important.

When approaching the pediatric patient with an arrhythmia, a thorough evaluation should include a history and physical assessment. Children who are at risk for arrhythmias include those with congenital heart disease or other diseases that can lead to heart failure. These patients have symptoms of cardiogenic shock with poor perfusion. They are often pale and short of breath, with irritability and changes in mental status. Remember that blood pressure is a poor indicator of shock in a child. Feel the child. Are his or her feet warm? If not, how far up the arm or leg can you detect the warmness that indicates adequate perfusion? Evaluate capillary refill in the nail beds or over the patella. In the infant or young child who is unable to communicate, the parent or guardian can relay a history of poor feeding or increased somnolence.

Too Slow

Management. The treatment of bradycardia is determined by the stability of the patient. As with all patients, evaluate and establish the airway if required. Evaluate the breathing and determine the adequacy of circulation. If the patient is stable and not hypotensive, oxygen and IV fluids are often adequate treatments until the patient can be transported to a facility for further evaluation. Hypoxia is the most common cause of bradycardia in pediatric patients. Repeated evaluation of the patient's vital signs and ABCs is vital. If the child is in cardiorespiratory distress, he or she may require mechanical compressions and drug therapy. Epinephrine is the first drug used in the treatment of pediatric bradycardia. If the patient remains bradycardic after the epinephrine, move to atropine sulfate.

EPINEPHRINE

Classification: Adrenergic agent, inotropic.
Action: Binds strongly with both alpha and beta receptors, producing increased blood pressure, increased heart rate, bronchodilation.
Indications: Bronchospasm, allergic and anaphylactic reactions, restoration of cardiac activity in cardiac arrest.
Adverse Effects: Anxiety, headache, cardiac arrhythmias, hypertension, nervousness, tremors, chest pain, nausea/vomiting.
Contraindications: Arrhythmias other than VF, asystole, pulseless electrical activity (PEA); cardiovascular disease; hypertension; cerebrovascular disease; shock secondary to causes other than anaphylactic shock; closed-angle glaucoma; diabetes; pregnant women in active labor; known sensitivity to epinephrine or sulfites.

© Jones & Bartlett Learning.

Dosage:
Cardiac Arrest:
- **Adult:** 1 mg (1:10,000 solution) IV, IO; may repeat every 3 to 5 minutes.
- **Pediatric:** 0.01 mg/kg (1:10,000 solution) IV, IO; repeat every 3 to 5 minutes as needed (max dose: 1 mg).

Symptomatic Bradycardia:
- **Adult:** 2 to 10 mcg/min (1:10,000 solution) as a continuous IV infusion; usual dosage range: 2 to 10 mcg/min IV; titrate to effect.
- **Pediatric:** 0.01 mg/kg (1:10,000 solution) IV, IO; may repeat every 3 to 5 minutes (max dose: 1 mg). If giving epinephrine by endotracheal tube, administer 0.1 mg/kg.

Asthma Attacks and Certain Allergic Reactions:
- **Adult:** 0.3 to 0.5 mg (1:1,000 solution) IM or subcutaneous; may repeat every 10 to 15 minutes (max dose: 1 mg).
- **Pediatric:** 0.01 mg/kg (1:1,000 solution) IM or subcutaneous (max dose: 0.5 mg).

Anaphylactic Shock:
- **Adult:** 0.5 mg (1:1,000 solution) IM repeated as needed every 5 to 15 minutes, or transition to IV infusion of 1 to 4 mcg/min, titrated to effect.
- **Pediatric:** 0.01 mg/kg IM, repeated as needed every 5 to 15 minutes, or transitioned to continuous IV infusion rate of 0.1 to 1 mcg/kg per minute (1:10,000 solution); titrate to response.

Special Considerations:
Half-life 1 minute.
Pregnancy class C.

ATROPINE SULFATE

Classification: Anticholinergic (antimuscarinic).
Action: Competes reversibly with acetylcholine at the site of the muscarinic receptor. Receptors affected, in order from the most sensitive to the least sensitive, include salivary, bronchial, sweat glands, eye, heart, and GI tract.
Indications: Symptomatic bradycardia, asystole or PEA, nerve agent exposure, organophosphate poisoning.
Adverse Effects: Decreased secretions resulting in dry mouth and hot skin

© Jones & Bartlett Learning.

(continues)

ATROPINE SULFATE *(continued)*

---

temperature, intense facial flushing, blurred vision or dilation of the pupils with subsequent photophobia, tachycardia, restlessness. Atropine may cause paradoxical bradycardia if the dose administered is too low or if the drug is administered too slowly.

Contraindications: Acute MI; myasthenia gravis; GI obstruction; closed-angle glaucoma; known sensitivity to atropine, belladonna alkaloids, or sulfites. Will not be effective for infranodal (type II) AV block and new third-degree block with wide QRS complex.

Dosage:

Symptomatic Bradycardia:

- **Adult:** 0.5 mg IV, IO every 3 to 5 minutes to a maximum dose of 3 mg.
- **Adolescent:** 0.02 mg/kg (minimum 0.1 mg/dose; maximum 1 mg/dose) IV, IO up to a total dose of 2 mg.
- **Pediatric:** 0.02 mg/kg (minimum 0.1 mg/dose; maximum 0.5 mg/dose) IV, IO, to a total dose of 1 mg.

Nerve Agent or Organophosphate Poisoning:

- **Adult:** 1 to 6 mg IV, IM; repeat if needed every 5 minutes until symptoms dissipate.
- **Pediatric:** 0.05 mg/kg IV, IM every 10 to 30 minutes as needed until symptoms dissipate.
- **Infants <15 lb:** 0.05 mg/kg IV, IM every 5 to 20 minutes as needed until symptoms dissipate.

Special Considerations:

Severe organophosphate exposures may require *massive* amounts of atropine, well beyond what is carried in most EMS vehicles.

Half-life 2.5 hours.

Pregnancy class C; possibly unsafe in lactating mothers.

Too Fast

Management. A heart rhythm that is too fast is also addressed beginning with the sequence of ABCs. Airway is critical because the increased heart rate can indicate respiratory compromise and its associated panic or the body's early response to poor oxygenation. Once the airway is established and oxygenation has been provided, focus attention on evaluation of the circulation. Once IVs have been established, evaluate for dehydration and other disorders that can contribute to the increased heart rate. Fever itself can cause tachycardia; however, fluids help in this situation, as well. Therefore, consider the need for an IV fluid bolus with either 0.9% normal saline or Ringer's lactate at 10 to 20 mL/kg, with rapid and close reassessment of vital signs after each bolus and caution regarding the overzealous administration of fluids, such as in the case of DKA.

Evaluation of the rate, as well as the width of the QRS complex, often helps determine whether the arrhythmia is SVT or VT. In both cases, if the patient is unstable, cardioversion at a dose of 0.5 to 1.0 J/kg is warranted. If the patient is stable but the tachyarrhythmia is presumed to be SVT and is unresponsive to the usual resuscitative measures, consider adenosine (Adenocard) administration.

Adenosine is a drug that slows the heart rate by acting at the AV node to alter the conduction of the electrical stimulation to the pacer. It has an immediate onset, and its half-life is equally as fast, taking effect in 10 seconds or less. An important but concerning fact about the use of adenosine is its ability to cause transient AV block, which can appear to be asystole for the 10-second period. In a child, this is alarming. However, the paramedic must expect and understand this possibility as the rhythm is monitored with administration of adenosine.

In cases of stable VT, amiodarone (Cordarone), procainamide, or lidocaine may be appropriate treatment, followed by cardioversion. However, when a patient has unstable VT, cardioversion should be used appropriately.

ADENOSINE (ADENOCARD)

© Jones & Bartlett Learning.

Classification: Antiarrhythmic.
Action: Slows the conduction of electrical impulses at the AV node.
Indications: Stable reentry SVT. Does not convert atrial fibrillation (AF), atrial flutter, or VT.
Adverse Effects: Common adverse reactions are generally mild and short-lived: sense of impending doom, complaints of flushing, chest pressure, throat tightness, numbness. Patients will have a brief episode of asystole after administration.
Contraindications: Sick sinus syndrome, second- or third-degree heart block, poison-/drug-induced tachycardia, asthma or bronchospasm.
Dosage: Note: Adenosine should be delivered only by rapid IV bolus with a peripheral IV or directly into a vein, in a location as close to the heart as possible, preferably in the antecubital fossa. Administration of adenosine must be immediately followed by a saline flush, and then the extremity should be elevated.

- **Adult:** Initial dose 6 mg rapid IV, IO (over a 1- to 3-second period) immediately followed by a 20-mL rapid saline flush. If the first dose does not eliminate the rhythm in 1 to 2 minutes, administer a second dose of 12 mg rapid IV, IO.
- **Pediatric:**
  - **Children >50 kg**: Same as adult dosing.
  - **Children <50 kg**: Initial dose 0.1 mg/kg IV, IO (max dose: 6 mg) immediately followed by a ≥5-mL rapid saline flush; may repeat at 0.2 mg/kg (max dose: 12 mg).

Special Considerations:
Use with caution in patients with preexisting bronchospasm and those with a history of AF.
Older adults with no history of paroxysmal SVT should be carefully evaluated for dehydration and rapid sinus tachycardia requiring volume fluid replacement rather than simply treated with adenosine.
Pregnancy class C.

AMIODARONE (CORDARONE)

Classification: Antiarrhythmic, Class III.
Action: Acts directly on the myocardium to delay repolarization and increase the duration of the action potential.
Indications: Ventricular arrhythmias; second-line agent for atrial arrhythmias.
Adverse Effects: Burning at the IV site, hypotension, bradycardia.
Contraindications: Sick sinus syndrome, second- and third-degree heart block, cardiogenic shock, when episodes of bradycardia have caused syncope, sensitivity to benzyl alcohol and iodine.

© Jones & Bartlett Learning.

Dosage:
VF and Pulseless VT:
- **Adult:** 300 mg IV, IO. May be followed by one dose of 150 mg in 3 to 5 minutes.
- **Pediatric:** 5 mg/kg (max dose: 300 mg); may repeat 5 mg/kg IV, IO up to 15 mg/kg.

Relatively Stable Patients with Arrhythmias Such as Premature Ventricular Contractions or Wide-Complex Tachycardias with a Strong Pulse:
- **Adult:** 150 mg in 100 mL D_5W IV, IO over a 10-minute period; may repeat in 10 minutes; once return of spontaneous circulation is accomplished, begin an infusion 1 mg/min for 6 hours then decrease to 0.5 mg/min; up to a maximum dose of 2.2 g over 24 hours.
- **Pediatric:** 5 mg/kg very slow IV, IO (over 20 to 60 minutes); may repeat in 5-mg/kg doses up to 15 mg/kg (max dose: 300 mg).

Special Considerations:
Pregnancy class D.

PROCAINAMIDE (PRONESTYL)

Classification: Antiarrhythmic, Class IA.
Action: Blocks influx of sodium through membrane pores, consequently suppresses atrial and ventricular arrhythmias by slowing conduction in myocardial tissue.
Indications: Alternative to amiodarone for stable monomorphic VT with normal QT interval and preserved ventricular function, reentry SVT if uncontrolled by adenosine and vagal maneuvers if blood pressure stable, AF with rapid rate in Wolff-Parkinson-White syndrome.

PROCAINAMIDE
HCl INJECTION, USP

10 mL   Multiple-dose

1 gram/10 mL TOTAL
(100 mg/mL)
NDC 12345-678-90

Rx only

Adverse Effects: Asystole, VF, flushing, hypotension, PR prolongation, QRS widening, QT prolongation.
Contraindications: AV block, QT prolongation, torsades de pointes. Use with caution in hypotension, heart failure.
Dosage:
- **Adult:** 500 to 600 mg over 25 to 3 minutes IV, or 20 to 50 mg/min slow IV, IO (max total dose: 17 mg/kg until one of the following occurs: arrhythmia resolves, hypotension, QRS widens by >50% of original width).
- **Maintenance:** Infusion (after resuscitation from cardiac arrest): mix 1 g in 250 mL solution (4 mg/mL), infuse at 1 to 4 mg/min.
- **Pediatric:** 10 to 15 mg/kg slow IV, IO over 30 to 60 minutes.

Special Considerations:
Pregnancy class C.

LIDOCAINE (XYLOCAINE)

Classification: Antiarrhythmic, Class IB.

Action: Blocks sodium channels, increasing the recovery period after repolarization; suppresses automaticity in the His-Purkinje system and depolarization in the ventricles.

Indications: Ventricular arrhythmias, when amiodarone is not available: cardiac arrest from VF/VT, stable monomorphic VT with preserved ventricular function, stable polymorphic VT with normal baseline QT interval and preserved left ventricular function (when ischemia and electrolyte imbalance are treated), stable polymorphic VT with baseline QT prolongation suggestive of torsades de pointes.

2% Lidocaine HCl Injection, USP 1,000 mg per 50 mL
For Infiltration and Nerve Block.
Methylparaben as preservative
Not for Caudal or Epidural Use. 25 × 50 mL Multiple Dose Vials
(20 mg/mL) Rx only

Adverse Effects: Toxicity (signs may include anxiety, apprehension, euphoria, nervousness, disorientation, dizziness, blurred vision, facial paresthesias, tremors, hearing disturbances, slurred speech, seizures, sinus bradycardia), seizures without warning, cardiac arrhythmias, hypotension, cardiac arrest, pain at injection site.

Contraindications: AV block; bleeding; thrombocytopenia; known sensitivity to lidocaine, sulfite, or paraben. Use with caution in bradycardia, hypovolemia, cardiogenic shock, Adams-Stokes syndrome, Wolff-Parkinson-White syndrome.

Dosage:

Pulseless VT and VF:

- **Adult IV, IO:** 1 to 1.5 mg/kg IV, IO; may repeat at half the original dose (0.5–0.75 mg/kg) every 5 to 10 minutes to a maximum dose of 3 mg/kg. If a maintenance infusion is warranted, the rate is 1 to 4 mg/min.
- **Pediatric IV, IO:** 1 mg/kg IV, IO (maximum: 100 mg). If a maintenance infusion is warranted, the rate is 20 to 50 mcg/kg per minute.

Perfusing Ventricular Rhythms:

- **Adult:** 0.5 to 0.75 mg/kg IV, IO (up to 1 to 1.5 mg/kg may be used). Repeat 0.5 to 0.75 mg/kg every 5 to 10 minutes to a maximum total dose of 3 mg/kg. A maintenance infusion of 1 to 4 mg/min (30 to 50 mcg/kg per minute) is acceptable.
- **Pediatric:** 1 mg/kg IV, IO. May repeat every 5 to 10 minutes to a maximum dose of 3 mg/kg. Maintenance infusion rate is 20 to 50 mcg/kg per minute.

Special Considerations:

Half-life approximately 90 minutes.

Pregnancy class B.

Management of Diabetic Ketoacidosis

Diabetes is a common disease in children. Prehospital providers encounter children with complications of diabetes, which is discussed in Chapter 11. However, a key difference in the treatment of pediatric DKA warrants mention. The child with DKA should not receive a bolus of insulin. However, when possible, the child with DKA should receive an insulin drip in the same fashion as an adult. When treating DKA in adults, physicians and providers are often taught that the first three items are fluids, fluids, and fluids. Do not apply this philosophy to children because aggressive fluid administration in a child with DKA can result in cerebral edema. Cerebral edema has been reported in children receiving fluids in excess of 2.5 times the maintenance rate.

▶ Special Considerations for Older Adults

People continue to live longer with a higher quality of life, largely because of breakthroughs in drug therapy. As a result, an increasing number of older adults take several medications concurrently. These patients are likely to be taking numerous drugs prescribed by several different physicians in addition to over-the-counter medications that are self-prescribed. Sometimes patients are placed on medications without sufficient regard for drug interactions or adverse effects.

Polypharmacy occurs when a patient is taking multiple medications for the treatment of several medical disorders. The danger of polypharmacy is the increased likelihood of an adverse effect or serious drug interaction. Drug interactions are a preventable cause of hospitalization and death among older adults.[17] The risk of an adverse medication reaction increases proportionally with the number of medications a person is taking—13% for two medications, 58% for five medication, up to an 82% chance of adverse reactions when a patient is taking seven or more medications.[17] Medications can interact by altering absorption, distribution, metabolism, or excretion or by directly interfering with the action of another medication.

As the body ages, its ability to respond to various insults decreases. An understanding of age-related changes in anatomy and physiology is necessary to reduce drug-related complications. Older patients often lose muscle mass and total body weight. Therefore, a drug dose acceptable for an adult often should be reduced in an older adult. Certain medications may require weight-based dosing similar to pediatric drug dosing. Despite weighing the same or even less than a large child, many older patients are prescribed standard adult dosages, and the result is drug toxicity.

Age-related physiologic changes in medication response in older adults are attributable to changes in medication absorption, distribution, breakdown, and excretion. Absorption can be reduced by decreased motility of the stomach and reduced production of stomach acid. Breakdown or metabolism of medications from their active to nonactive forms by the liver is less effective with increasing age. Excretion is also affected. With age, the blood flow to the kidneys is often reduced, as is the ability of the kidneys to filtrate and concentrate the urine. After the age of 30 years, adults lose approximately 10% of kidney function per decade due to a variety of structural and physiological changes within the kidney. By age 70 years, a large portion of adults have significantly decreased renal function.[18] Older patients may have a 46% or greater decline in kidney function as a result of normal aging.

The result of these age-related decreases in kidney function is accumulation of drugs or drug by-products. Medications that have the potential of becoming toxic in renal disease include digoxin, antibiotics, antihypertensives, and antiarrhythmics.

Altered drug effects in older adults are also explained by alterations in the way drugs interact with their various receptors. In addition to loss of weight, the body's composition changes with age. A proportional increase in body fat and a decrease in total body water occur. With an increase in body fat, fat-soluble drugs will collect in the fat stores. A decrease in muscle mass leads to a decrease in the volume of distribution of many drugs, which can cause toxic drug levels of water-soluble drugs such as digoxin and theophylline.

In addition, poor nutrition can decrease the body's production of albumin. **Albumin**, a protein produced by the liver, is found in the blood and interstitial space. Many drugs bind to and are transported by albumin. When drugs bind to albumin, a percentage of the drug does not bind to the albumin. The portion of the drug that does not bind to the albumin is the portion that is active. With a decrease in albumin, the total amount of unbound or active drug increases. Therefore, for a given dose, the effectiveness of a drug is increased and potentially toxic.

When caring for older adults, prehospital providers must remember that this group of patients is often taking multiple medications and is clearly at risk for polypharmacy and drug interactions. Any medication that must be administered in an emergency setting can result in an unanticipated interaction and adverse drug effect. Older patients may be at risk for decreased compliance with prescription medications because of problems such as depression, poor memory, dementia, and financial restrictions.

▶ Special Considerations for Patients with Renal Failure

Renal failure is a progressive, rapidly developing, chronic disease that, in its most extreme form, results in permanent loss of kidney function. Patients with renal failure require careful management of their diet, fluid intake, and drug therapy. Acute renal failure is a rapidly developing condition that can occur in up to 10% of patients admitted to an intensive care unit. More than 460,000 people in the United States have chronic kidney failure, and each year more than 47,000 people die from complications of renal failure.[19] The common causes of chronic renal failure include hypertension and diabetes mellitus. Causes of renal failure include trauma, pregnancy, hemorrhage, and complications of drug therapy.

Acute renal failure is a disease that typically occurs in hospitalized patients, but prehospital providers are called to assist or transport patients with chronic renal failure. Many patients with chronic renal failure have a decline in their kidney function managed by medications, vitamins, and special diets.

The most extreme form of chronic renal failure is known as **end-stage renal disease (ESRD)**. Patients with ESRD cannot make urine and require some form of renal replacement therapy or dialysis to stay alive. **Hemodialysis** is the removal of toxic substances from the bloodstream by filtering the patient's blood through a machine and then passing the blood back to the patient. Hemodialysis is an efficient means of cleansing the blood. The principal risks of hemodialysis are hypotension and arrhythmias.

Peritoneal dialysis is the process by which a special solution is delivered to the patient's abdomen through a catheter. The special solution dwells in the abdomen for a period, absorbing many of the toxic substances in the blood. After several hours, the solution is drained and the poisons are removed from the body. Although substantially less efficient than hemodialysis, peritoneal dialysis does not result in hypotension or require anticoagulation. The disadvantage of peritoneal dialysis is the length of time required for dialysis therapy and the risk of infection to the abdominal cavity.

The role of the kidney is largely to remove waste products from the blood and control the internal environment of the body. Therefore, as the kidneys fail, the internal milieu changes the effectiveness of various drugs. One of the normal functions of the kidneys is to produce natural buffers; however, as kidney function declines to less than 20% of normal, patients can develop metabolic acidosis.

The kidney's most obvious function is the creation of urine. With decreasing renal function, the kidneys lose their ability to concentrate urine. Patients usually are able to manage their own fluid balance as long as they control sodium intake. However, patients with renal failure may not be able to tolerate large volumes of IV fluids.

Maintaining potassium balance is another critical function of the kidneys. When kidney function is less than 10% of normal, the potassium balance is impaired and can accumulate to dangerous and critical levels.

In addition to removing toxic waste products, the kidneys have a role in the formation of red blood cells. The kidneys manufacture a protein known as **erythropoietin**, which stimulates the bone marrow to produce red blood cells. Patients with renal failure are not able to make erythropoietin, resulting in a decrease in the number of red blood cells in the bloodstream, or **anemia**. Patients with chronic renal failure often take epoetin alfa (Epogen), a synthetic form of erythropoietin, to increase their blood count and treat the anemia.

When caring for a patient with renal insufficiency or renal failure, prehospital providers should question the need, dosage, and possible interaction of every medication administered. Many drugs are metabolized or excreted by the kidneys, and the dosage of these drugs needs to be reduced in renal failure. Drug dosages often need to be reduced in proportion to the degree of renal impairment.

▶ # Review Questions

1. In what ways do the physiologic changes in pregnancy alter the pharmacologic mechanisms of a drug?
2. What is a teratogenic drug?
3. Name the categories of the Pregnancy Safety Category system.
4. An allergy to what food is a contraindication for the use of ipratropium bromide (Atrovent)?
5. When should you consider the use of corticosteroids for the treatment of asthma?
6. How does gestational hypertension differ from chronic hypertension?
7. At what systolic and diastolic blood pressures should drug therapy be considered for the treatment of hypertension in a pregnant woman?
8. What is diabetic ketoacidosis (DKA), and what is its significance to the fetus?
9. Is blood pressure a reliable sign of pending shock in a pediatric patient?
10. What is stroke volume?
11. List the complications associated with intraosseous infusions.
12. Why are pediatric drug dosages given by weight?
13. What is the most common cause of bradycardia in children?
14. When administering adenosine in the pediatric patient, why should the prehospital care provider monitor for asystole in the first 10 seconds?
15. What is the risk of too-aggressive fluid administration in a child with DKA?
16. Define *polypharmacy,* and describe its danger to older patients.
17. What are the causes of renal failure?
18. What are the causes of chronic renal failure?
19. What classes of drugs can become toxic in patients with kidney disease?
20. Define *hemodialysis.*

References

1. U.S. Food and Drug Administration. *Content and Format of Labeling for Human Prescription Drug and Biological Products; Requirements for Pregnancy and Lactation Labeling.* 21 CFR Part 201. https://s3 .amazonaws.com/public-inspection.federalregister.gov/2014-28241.pdf. Published December 4, 2014. Accessed September 11, 2018.
2. U.S. Food and Drug Administration. FDA Pregnancy Categories. Drugs.com. https://www.drugs.com /pregnancy-categories.html. Accessed September 11, 2018.
3. Schatz M, Zeiger RS, Harden K, Hoffman CC, Chilingar L, Petitti D. The safety of asthma and allergy medications during pregnancy. *J Allergy Clin Immunol.* 1997;100:301.
4. Schatz M, Weinberger SE. Management of asthma during pregnancy. UpToDate. https://www.uptodate.com /contents/management-of-asthma-during-pregnancy. Updated May 7, 2018. Accessed September 11, 2018.
5. Weinberger SE, Schatz M, Dombrowski MP. Patient education: asthma and pregnancy (beyond the basics). UpToDate. https://www.uptodate.com/contents/asthma-and-pregnancy-beyond-the-basics. Updated February 13, 2017. Accessed September 11, 2018.
6. U.S. Food and Drug Administration (2011). FDA Drug Safety Communication: new warnings against use of terbutaline to treat preterm labor. https://www.fda.gov/Drugs/DrugSafety/ucm243539.htm. Accessed September 11, 2018.
7. Alangari AA. Corticosteroids in the treatment of acute asthma. *Annals Thorac Med.* 2014;9(4):187–192.
8. Rehrer MW, Liu B, Rodriguez M, Lam J, Alter HJ. A randomized controlled noninferiority trial of single dose of oral dexamethasone versus 5 days of oral prednisone in acute adult asthma. *Ann Emerg Med.* 2016;68(5):608–613.
9. Murphy S, Sheffer AL, Pauwels RA. *National Asthma Education and Prevention Program: Highlights of the Expert Panel Report II: Guidelines for the Diagnosis and Management of Asthma.* Bethesda, MD; National Heart, Lung, and Blood Institute; 1997.
10. Manser R, Reid D, Abramson M. Corticosteroids for acute severe asthma in hospitalised patients. *Cochrane Database Syst Rev.* 2001;(1):CD001740.
11. Fanta CH. Management of acute exacerbations of asthma in adults. UpToDate. https://www.uptodate .com/contents/management-of-acute-exacerbations-of-asthma-in-adults. Updated April 9, 2018. Accessed September 10, 2018.

12. Muti M, Tshimanga M, Notion GT, Bangure D, Chonzi P. Prevalence of pregnancy induced hypertension and pregnancy outcomes among women seeking maternity services in Harare, Zimbabwe. *BMC Cardiovasc Disord.* 2015;15:111.

13. Filippi V, Chou D, Ronsmans C, et al. Levels and causes of maternal mortality and morbidity. In: Black RE, Laxminarayan R, Temmerman M, et al., eds. *Reproductive, Maternal, Newborn, and Child Health: Disease Control Priorities.* Vol. 2. 3rd ed. Washington, DC: The International Bank for Reconstruction and Development /The World Bank; 2016.

14. Butalia S, Audibert F, Côté AM, et al. Hypertension Canada's 2018 guidelines for the management of hypertension in pregnancy. *Can J Cardiol.* 2018;34(5):526–531.

15. Magloire L, Funai EF. Gestational hypertension. UpToDate. https://www.uptodate.com/contents/gestational-hypertension. Updated May 21, 2018. Accessed September 11, 2018.

16. Scantlebury DC, Schwartz GL, Acquah LA, White WM, Moser M, Garovic VD. The treatment of hypertension during pregnancy: when should blood pressure medications be started? *Curr Cardiol Rep.* 2013;15(11):412.

17. Gujjarlamudi HB. Polytherapy and drug interactions in elderly. *J Mid-Life Health.* 2016;7(3):105–107.

18. Denic A, Glassock RJ, Rule AD. Structural and functional changes with the aging kidney. *Adv Chronic Kidney Dis.* 2016;23(1):19–28.

19. National Institute of Diabetes and Digestive and Kidney Diseases. Kidney disease statistics for the United States. https://www.niddk.nih.gov/health-information/health-statistics/kidney-disease. Accessed September 11, 2018.

© Andrew Brookes/Getty Images

CHAPTER 20

Pharmacology-Assisted Intubation

OBJECTIVES

1. Differentiate the goals of rapid sequence induction from those of rapid sequence intubation.
2. List six questions to ask when preparing for rapid sequence intubation.
3. List three goals of rapid sequence intubation.
4. Differentiate between the goal of rapid sequence intubation and the goal of rapid sequence airway.
5. Discuss the depolarizing chemical paralytic medication used in rapid sequence intubation: succinylcholine (Anectine).
6. Discuss nondepolarizing paralytics used in rapid sequence intubation: rocuronium (Zemuron), vecuronium (Norcuron), atracurium (Tracrium), and pancuronium (Pavulon).
7. Discuss deep sedation medications used in rapid sequence intubation: midazolam (Versed), etomidate (Amidate), ketamine (Ketalar), and the reversal agent flumazenil (Romazicon).
8. List the seven Ps of rapid sequence intubation.

MEDICATIONS THAT APPEAR IN CHAPTER 20

Succinylcholine (Anectine)
Atropine sulfate
Rocuronium (Zemuron)
Vecuronium (Norcuron)

Atracurium (Tracrium)
Pancuronium (Pavulon)
Midazolam (Versed)
Flumazenil (Romazicon)

Etomidate (Amidate)
Ketamine (Ketalar)

▶ Introduction

EMS, emergency department (ED) staff, and other healthcare providers frequently encounter patients who require emergency airway management but are at high risk of aspiration due to full stomachs or other complicating factors. In 1970, Stept and Safar first described a 15-step technique of rapid sequence induction in which patients who had full stomachs

387

could undergo general anesthesia with a lower risk of aspiration.[1] Key components of this technique were the use of short-acting intravenous (IV) barbiturates (the induction) and muscular paralytic drugs (neuromuscular blockade). Despite this approach, aspiration still remains the leading cause of anesthesia-related deaths and should remain a primary concern for EMS providers who use or assist with this procedure.[1] Even in operating room conditions, approximately 1 in every 2,000 to 3,000 patients aspirates during anesthesia.[2] EMS providers perform intubations and rapid sequence induction in uncontrolled settings, on patients with full stomachs and other complicating factors such as positioning/entrapment, facial/airway injuries, and emergent medical conditions. These conditions make emergency airway management particularly challenging for EMS providers.

CASE STUDY

Your unit is called to a local junior high school gymnasium for a woman who is having a seizure. When you arrive, you find the woman lying supine on the floor with several bystanders. You note that there is some vomit on the floor by her head and she is not responding. On examination, you note that she has some vomit around her mouth. You attempt to suction her airway but cannot because her teeth are clenched. You administer oxygen by face mask and place a pulse oximeter. Her oxygen saturation is 82%. You once again try to clear her airway but are not successful. You perform a modified jaw thrust, but this does not improve her oxygen saturation, so you place a nasopharyngeal airway. This maneuver increases her oxygen saturation only slightly to 85%. Her mental status has not improved, but she has not had any additional motor seizure activity. The treatment priority of any emergency is protection or establishment of a patent airway. You cannot be assured that this patient's airway is not obstructed by her tongue or vomit. Jaw thrust maneuvers and nasopharyngeal airways have not rescued the patient from her hypoxia. She will require establishment of an airway with pharmacologic assistance.

Most patients encountered by paramedics present with full stomachs (as well as other obstacles to intubation, such as clenched teeth). The technique of **rapid sequence induction** was adapted for emergency use as **rapid sequence intubation**. Both techniques are known as *RSI*, but the *I* refers to induction or intubation to reflect different goals. For rapid sequence *induction*, the ultimate goal is a patient who is safely anesthetized; for rapid sequence *intubation*, the goal is a patient who is safely endotracheally intubated. In this chapter, *RSI* refers only to rapid sequence *intubation*.

Prehospital RSI and even endotracheal (ET) intubation remain controversial. Changes to the American Heart Association's Advanced Cardiac Life Support curriculum deemphasize the importance of ET intubation during the initial cardiac arrest resuscitation sequence. Other studies demonstrate worse outcomes when ET intubation or RSI is performed in certain subgroups of patients.[3] In general, paramedics and other healthcare providers who frequently perform ET intubation are more successful than those who do not intubate as often. System performance improves when smaller numbers of providers perform a higher volume of procedures, such as in tiered EMS systems with selective ALS dispatch, or in air-medical and critical care transport programs where providers encounter a higher portion of patients needing these procedures. Additionally, energetic educational programs coupled with a robust quality assurance system foster optimal performance of providers in those systems.[3]

EMS providers may witness the transition from the rapid sequence intubation (RSI) approach to a rapid sequence airway (RSA) focus in certain EMS systems and programs. In RSA, rapid sequence induction medications are used to facilitate placement of a supraglottic device rather than an ET tube. Providers may also use a process called pharmacologically assisted laryngeal mask insertion (PALM) where a laryngeal mask airway (LMA) device is placed with the use of an induction agent (sedative), without the use of a neuromuscular blocking medication.[4]

▶ RSI Goals

This chapter describes medications that paramedics can use to facilitate airway management, primarily those that can make ET intubation easier or safer. A major portion of this chapter is dedicated to the discussion of the medications needed to perform RSI. When RSI is performed correctly, the patient is chemically paralyzed, deeply sedated or anesthetized, and endotracheally intubated (**FIGURE 20-1**).

The powerful medications discussed in this chapter allow the paramedic to assume control of the airway and breathing of a critically ill or injured patient. As such, the paramedic must ask himself or herself several questions in preparation for assuming this control, including the following:

- If I administer these drugs, will I be able to intubate the patient if he or she stops breathing?
- If I am unable to intubate the patient, will I be able to ventilate him or her?
- If I am unable to intubate or ventilate this patient, do I have other options?
- Do I have the right equipment on hand? Is the equipment assembled?
- Does the patient have any medical problems or conditions for which these drugs and techniques are contraindicated?
- If I do not act, will this patient die or have permanent brain damage?

RSI has the following three goals:

1. To overcome barriers to intubation (e.g., clenched teeth and combativeness) by establishing a condition of deep sedation and skeletal muscle relaxation while protecting against aspiration of stomach contents into the lungs
2. To provide protection against the body's normal response to intubation, reflexes that can potentially cause cardiac or neurologic deterioration in at-risk patients
3. To provide humane conditions for an unpleasant procedure

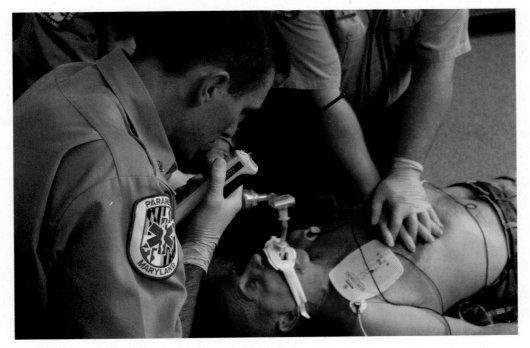

FIGURE 20-1 An endotracheally intubated patient.

CASE STUDY

Y ou are dispatched to the scene of a motor vehicle crash in which a 20-year-old male driver was ejected. You find the patient lying prone on the ground, with snoring respirations. He is unresponsive and bleeding from the nose. His initial blood pressure is 170/90 mm Hg, heart rate is 53 beats/min, respiration rate is 16 breaths/min, and oxygen saturation is 96% on nonrebreather oxygen. The patient is rolled onto and secured to a long spine board with an appropriately sized cervical collar, and a head immobilizer is applied. Your partner establishes an IV line of normal saline while you perform a rapid secondary survey. You estimate the patient's weight to be 190 pounds (86 kg). His left pupil is sluggish and dilated, but the right pupil is normally reactive and 4 mm in diameter. Respirations are adequate with equal breath sounds, the abdomen is mildly distended, and the pelvis is stable.

This patient most likely has a significant closed-head injury, as evidenced by his unresponsiveness and unequal pupils. His relative hypertension and bradycardia may be suggestive of increased intracranial pressure (ICP) and risk for brain herniation. In addition, possible abdominal injuries are a concern given the mild distension. Remember that in every patient who has an altered mental status, a glucose level should be taken at some time during the evaluation (the patient may be a diabetic, and a low glucose level may have caused the accident).

This patient requires ET intubation to protect his airway from aspiration of stomach contents and to prevent hypoxia. When ET intubation is used to prevent or correct hypoxia, there is an obvious benefit to patients with a head injury. In the absence of hypoxia, the benefits of intubation in these patients remain unproven.[5] Other supraglottic airway devices may be equally effective in establishing and maintaining an effective airway in the prehospital setting.

This patient is ideally suited for RSI. Barriers to intubation should be recognized by asking yourself the same series of questions:

1. *Can I intubate?*

Be aware of your own skill limitations. Blood may obscure your view, and the need for cervical immobilization imparts a more limited laryngeal view compared with cases in which neck immobilization is not necessary. Applying front-to-back pressure over the thyroid cartilage can improve visualization of the laryngeal opening.

Providers often confuse the thyroid cartilage (Adam's apple) with the smaller, inferior cricoid cartilage. This distinction is important, as the cricoid cartilage is the only complete cartilage ring around the trachea. In some circumstances, pressure to the cricoid cartilage, also known as the **Sellick maneuver**, is used to prevent regurgitation during bag-mask ventilations.

A modification known as the **BURP maneuver** can provide even better visualization. BURP is a mnemonic for **b**ackward-**u**pward (toward the head), **r**ightward (toward the patient's right), and **p**ressure.

Displacing the jaw anteriorly, as in a jaw or chin thrust airway maneuver, can also improve visualization in these circumstances. This situation is not appropriate for an inexperienced provider to attempt on his or her first RSI.

2. *Can I ventilate?*

Look for anatomic problems that could interfere with your ability to apply a bag-mask device. Such interference can be as simple as a bushy beard that must be quickly trimmed or as complex as massive facial and jaw injuries.

3. *What are my options if I cannot intubate or ventilate?*

You must have a rescue airway. Supraglottic devices such as the LMA, i-gel device, or King Airway provide alternative methods of airway control in situations where the patient cannot be successfully intubated.

4. *Is the equipment on hand? Is it assembled?*

After medication administration is not the time to rummage for equipment. Before administration, ensure a functional suction line, a functional laryngoscope, appropriate sizes of ET tubes, a reliable pulse oximeter reading, a bag-mask with a resuscitation bag attached to an ample supply of oxygen, and an end-tidal carbon dioxide (CO_2) monitor.

5. *Does the patient have any medical contraindications?*

Before you give any drug to any patient for any reason, ask yourself whether any reasons exist why this particular patient should not have a particular medication. As is the case with succinylcholine, certain patients may have lethal reactions. Make a habit of looking for medical identification jewelry on every unconscious patient.

6. *Will this patient die if I do not intubate him or her?*

As with any life-saving maneuver that carries significant risks, you must determine whether the benefits of proceeding outweigh the risks of attempting it. To some extent, the answer depends on your own honest self-assessment of your capabilities. Deferring an airway to the receiving hospital because of a carefully reasoned risk–benefit analysis can be the correct course of action. You may find that the receiving ED team echoes your decision by deferring to the operating room for surgical airway management.

▶ RSI Pharmacology

RSI involves the use of two main classes of drugs, chemical paralytics and sedating agents, in addition to some adjunctive medications.

Chemical Paralysis

The first medical use of chemical paralysis dates back to the use of curare in 1942.[6] Most people are familiar with curare's nonmedical use as the poison used on blow darts (as seen in jungle adventure movies). To understand how chemical paralytics work, a review is helpful of how a muscle gets a stimulus for contraction and, in turn, how that stimulus can be blocked.

For voluntary skeletal contracture, such as the muscles in the arms, legs, chest wall, abdominal wall, neck, pharynx, eyes, diaphragm, and larynx, a nerve impulse is generated in the brain cells (neurons), transmitted to a neuron in the spinal canal, and then transmitted to a nerve that directly communicates with the muscle. At each junction between neurons, called **synapses**, the "hand off" occurs by chemicals called **neurotransmitters** being released on one side of the synapse, diffusing across to the other side, and then initiating an electrochemical impulse along the nerve. The final chemical transmission—between nerve and muscle—is crucial to understanding how chemical paralytics work and how to anticipate problems.

The end of the nerve fiber comes into close contact with the portion of the muscle cell that has receptors for the neurotransmitter sent by the nerve cell. This junction between nerve and muscle cell is known as the **neuromuscular junction**. The nerve side is the presynaptic membrane; the muscle side is the postsynaptic membrane, or **motor end plate**; and the space in between is the **synaptic cleft**. The chemical transmitter used is acetylcholine.

As an electrochemical signal reaches the presynaptic membrane of the neuromuscular junction, acetylcholine is released from storage sites at the end of the nerve cell axon and crosses the synaptic cleft to bind to receptors on the postsynaptic (muscle) side. This occurs quite rapidly because the distance across the cleft is only approximately 0.1 micrometer wide (or 1/10,000 of a millimeter). Once the acetylcholine binds to the postsynaptic membrane at special receptor binding sites, specific **acetylcholine receptors** (which act as special cellular gates) are unlocked and opened, resulting in contraction of the muscle fiber.

Muscle cells contracting in synchrony lead to coordinated muscle contraction. Once depolarization and contraction of the muscle fibers occur, the muscle cell membrane must pump out the ions and reestablish its normal electrical potential in preparation for another contraction. This period needed to restore itself is called the **refractory period**; during this time, the muscle cannot contract again.

Once acetylcholine binds to its receptor site on the postsynaptic membrane, ion flow continues until the acetylcholine molecule disengages. However, if it remains in the synaptic cleft, it can simply bind again. That is prevented by a chemical called acetylcholinesterase, which rapidly breaks the acetylcholine down and prevents continued binding. This breakdown occurs in approximately one tenth of a second. Nerve gas agents and organophosphate pesticides block the cholinesterase (i.e., act as a cholinesterase inhibitor), resulting in exaggerated cholinergic activity and continuous neuromuscular transmission, which explains the twitching and writhing that accompany their exposure. Anticholinergic medications such as atropine are used to treat nerve gas toxicity. Atropine is also used to prevent some of the adverse consequences of succinylcholine.

Paralytic Drugs

Paralytic drugs are divided into two classes: **depolarizing** and **nondepolarizing paralytics**. The characterization of paralytic drugs into these two groups is key to understanding the complications and contraindications that a particular drug can pose to a particular patient.

Depolarizing Paralytics

Succinylcholine (often referred to as *SUX*) is the only depolarizing paralytic in routine medical use. Succinylcholine is chemically similar to acetylcholine; succinylcholine is effectively two molecules of acetylcholine attached head to head. Because of the structural similarity, succinylcholine binds at the same receptor as acetylcholine. However, it does not let go as easily and is not broken down as readily. The result is that the ion gates remain open and, after initial contraction, the muscle cell cannot reestablish its electrical potential (because the gates are still open for ions to flow in) and, therefore, cannot generate further contractions. Succinylcholine acts to depolarize the muscle cell membrane and prevent repolarization; thus it is known as a *depolarizing paralytic drug*.

A baseball pitcher (muscle) is on the mound waiting to receive the ball so that he can throw a pitch. The catcher (nerve) is in a squat, has the ball (acetylcholine) in his glove, and throws it from behind the plate to the pitcher (across the synaptic cleft). The pitcher catches the ball (acetylcholine) in his glove (the receptor binding site), goes into his wind up, and releases the pitch (the contraction).

But wait! If the pitcher's glove is filled with something else, say a football, that stays in the pocket of the glove so that he cannot receive the ball, the pitcher no longer has a baseball to throw. This is what happens with a nondepolarizing paralytic. The receptor site is blocked by a chemical that has a high affinity (attraction) for the binding site but does not initiate a depolarization of the muscle cell (hence a nondepolarizing paralytic) and is not broken down in the synaptic cleft.

If, on the other hand, a baseball is glued to the pitcher's glove, he may make his windup, but no pitch will be thrown. The glued baseball has a high affinity for the receptor site (it is stuck in the glove) and initiates a windup (because it is a baseball, not a football), but no pitch (contraction) results until the pitcher removes the glued baseball and cleans his glove. This reflects a depolarizing paralytic—it is similar in size and shape to the neurotransmitter, but it does not disengage from the receptor and results in *continued* depolarization of the muscle membrane, preventing further contractions.

Succinylcholine is the paralytic agent used most often in both ED and out-of-hospital RSI. Its properties that lend itself well to this use include rapid onset of paralysis (approximately 45 seconds by IV line) and short effective duration (approximately 5 minutes). Unfortunately, it also has detrimental side effects as a consequence of its action to depolarize muscle cell membranes.

The receptors on the postsynaptic motor end plate are relatively few in number. However, when stimulated by acetylcholine in the process of causing muscle cell depolarization, a small amount of potassium is released into the blood. This amount of potassium would be inconsequential in most healthy patients. However, in certain disease states in which the muscle is damaged (e.g., extensive burns) or diseased (e.g., muscular dystrophy) or not receiving nerve stimulation (e.g., neuromuscular disorder), the receptor sites proliferate over the entire muscle cell membrane, not just at the neuromuscular junction. Given the large surface area of the muscle fibers, the increase in the number of receptors is tremendous. Now, instead of an inconsequential release of potassium after succinylcholine-initiated depolarization, a critical and often fatal increase in serum potassium occurs (hyperkalemia), which can lead to sudden cardiac arrest from arrhythmia. Patients who are susceptible to this phenomenon include those with major burns (several days to several months after the burn), neuromuscular disease (e.g., recent stroke, recent cervical spine injury, encephalitis), and myopathic disease (e.g., muscular dystrophy).

Also at risk for lethal hyperkalemia are patients who already have a dangerous but unrecognized elevation in serum potassium, for whom a normally inconsequential increase could push their elevated potassium level beyond a dangerous threshold. These patients include those undergoing kidney dialysis or with kidney failure; those with a significant crush injury or a history of extensive limb entrapment, impairing blood supply for a period; those with certain overdoses such as digoxin or digitalis; and those with overdoses that can cause severe acidosis, such as aspirin, methanol, and ethylene glycol.

> Succinylcholine administration to patients with burns, spinal cord injuries, extensive muscle trauma, renal failure, or muscle disorders can result in life-threatening hyperkalemia.

A major concern for the prehospital use of succinylcholine is that the history of many patients is unknown to the prehospital provider. Even in the more controlled setting of elective surgery, deaths have occurred in patients who underwent preoperative screening but who had unrecognized neuromuscular disease, primarily undiagnosed Duchenne muscular dystrophy in children. For that reason, succinylcholine is no longer used in routine surgery in children. One subtle sign of Duchenne muscular dystrophy is the presence of significantly enlarged lower leg muscles. What this discussion means for the paramedic is that the question "Does this patient have any contraindications to this medication?" must be carefully considered before succinylcholine is given.

Another potentially fatal side effect of succinylcholine administration is a condition known as **malignant hyperthermia**. This is a genetic abnormality in which a patient has exaggerated and sustained muscle contractions in response to certain inhaled general anesthetics and succinylcholine. The increased muscle activity can lead to fatal hyperthermia. If recognized in family members or previously in the patient, such patients may wear medical identification jewelry indicating that they should not receive inhaled anesthetics or succinylcholine.

Other side effects of succinylcholine, again related to its initial depolarizing effects, include increased intragastric pressure (increased risk of vomiting), increased ocular pressure (risk of extrusion of eye contents if an open eye injury exists), increased ICP (concern in head trauma), and masseter spasm (spasm of cheek and jaw muscles that can delay intubation). Finally, succinylcholine can cause severe bradycardia in children because of their increased sensitivity to vagus nerve effects on the heart and the fact that succinylcholine mimics the action of acetylcholine. For that reason, atropine is recommended before succinylcholine in any child younger than approximately 8 years.

Succinylcholine administration in children can produce bradycardia. Pretreat children younger than 8 years old with atropine to avoid bradycardia.

Succinylcholine has a short duration of action because it is completely and rapidly metabolized in the blood by an enzyme called **pseudocholinesterase**. Because breakdown by the liver or kidney is not necessary, succinylcholine dosage does not need to be adjusted for patients with kidney or liver disease. Some people have a genetically determined pseudocholinesterase deficiency and have a significantly prolonged (hours to days) paralysis. This information may be available on medical identification jewelry.

SUCCINYLCHOLINE (ANECTINE)

Classification: Neuromuscular blocker, depolarizing.
Action: Competes with the acetylcholine receptor of the motor end plate on the muscle cell, resulting in muscle paralysis.
Indications: To induce neuromuscular blockade for the facilitation of ET intubation.
Adverse Effects: Anaphylactoid reactions, respiratory depression, apnea, bronchospasm, cardiac arrhythmias, malignant hyperthermia, hypertension, hypotension, muscle fasciculation, post-procedure muscle pain, hypersalivation, rash.
Contraindications: Malignant hyperthermia, burns, trauma. Use with caution in children, cardiac disease, hepatic disease, renal disease, peptic ulcer disease, cholinesterase-inhibitor toxicity, pseudocholinesterase deficiency, digitalis toxicity, glaucoma, hyperkalemia, hypothermia, rhabdomyolysis, myasthenia gravis.
Dosage:
- **Adult:**
  ◦ **IV:** 0.6 mg/kg IV, intraosseous (IO; range 0.3 to 1.1 mg/kg). (Off-label 1 to 1.5 mg/kg for RSI.)
  ◦ **Intramuscular (IM):** 3 to 4 mg/kg (max dose: 150 mg).
- **Pediatric:**
  ◦ **IV:**
    • **Adolescents and older children:** 1 mg/kg IV, IO.
    • **Small children and infants:** 2 mg/kg IV, IO.
  ◦ **IM:** 3 to 4 mg/kg (max dose: 150 mg).
Special Considerations:
IV administration results in neuromuscular blockade in 0.5 to 1 minute. IM administration results in neuromuscular blockade in 2 to 3 minutes.
IV administration in infants and children can potentially result in profound bradycardia and, in some cases, asystole. The incidence of bradycardia is greater after the second dose. The occurrence of bradycardia can be reduced with the pretreatment of atropine.
Succinylcholine can have a significantly prolonged effect in the setting of poisoning with nerve gas agents and organophosphate pesticides.
Pregnancy class C.

ATROPINE SULFATE

Classification: Anticholinergic (antimuscarinic).
Action: Competes reversibly with acetylcholine at the site of the muscarinic receptor. Receptors affected, in order from the most sensitive to the least sensitive, include salivary, bronchial, sweat glands, eye, heart, and gastrointestinal (GI) tract.
Indications: Symptomatic bradycardia, asystole or pulseless electrical activity, nerve agent exposure, organophosphate poisoning.

© Jones & Bartlett Learning.

Adverse Effects: Decreased secretions resulting in dry mouth and hot skin temperature, intense facial flushing, blurred vision or dilation of the pupils with subsequent photophobia, tachycardia, restlessness. Atropine may cause paradoxical bradycardia if the dose administered is too low or if the drug is administered too slowly.
Contraindications: Acute myocardial infarction; myasthenia gravis; GI obstruction; closed-angle glaucoma; known sensitivity to atropine, **belladonna alkaloids**, or sulfites. Will not be effective for infranodal (type II) atrioventricular block and new third-degree block with wide QRS complex.
Dosage:
Symptomatic Bradycardia:
- **Adult:** 0.5 mg IV, IO every 3 to 5 minutes to a maximum dose of 3 mg.
- **Adolescent:** 0.02 mg/kg (minimum 0.1 mg/dose; maximum 1 mg/dose) IV, IO up to a total dose of 2 mg.
- **Pediatric:** 0.02 mg/kg (minimum 0.1 mg/dose; maximum 0.5 mg/dose) IV, IO, to a total dose of 1 mg.

Nerve Agent or Organophosphate Poisoning:
- **Adult:** 1 to 6 mg IV, IM; repeat if needed every 5 minutes until symptoms dissipate.
- **Pediatric:** 0.05 mg/kg IV, IM every 10 to 30 minutes as needed until symptoms dissipate.
- **Infants <15 pounds (7 kg):** 0.05 mg/kg IV, IM every 5 to 20 minutes as needed until symptoms dissipate.

Special Considerations:
Severe organophosphate exposures may require *massive* amounts of atropine, well beyond what is carried in most EMS vehicles.
Half-life 2.5 hours.
Pregnancy class C; possibly unsafe in lactating mothers.

Nondepolarizing Paralytics

Nondepolarizing muscle relaxants act to bind preferentially to the acetylcholine receptor site, preventing binding of acetylcholine (i.e., blocking the key) and ion flow into the cell, thereby preventing muscle contraction. Because the membrane is not allowed to depolarize, these are known as nondepolarizing neuromuscular blocking agents. Curare is a nondepolarizing drug.

Several nondepolarizing muscle relaxants are grouped according to their duration of action: short-, intermediate-, and long-acting agents. Two short-acting agents are mivacurium and rocuronium. Both mivacurium (Mivacron) and rocuronium (Zemuron) have a rapid onset and short duration of action (15 to 30 minutes). Unfortunately, mivacurium (Mivacron) is no longer manufactured and is not available in the United States. Examples of intermediate-acting nondepolarizing agents include vecuronium (Norcuron) and atracurium (Tracrium). Pancuronium (Pavulon) is considered a long-acting agent.

Twelve nondepolarizing agents are currently clinically available for chemical paralysis. They vary in speed of onset, duration of action, mechanism of metabolism, and cost.

Paralytic agents have no effect on consciousness or reduction of pain. Patients must have adequate sedation and analgesia administered in addition to the paralytic agents.

For prehospital and ED use, rocuronium provides a reliable combination of rapid onset, intermediate duration, and reasonable cost. Rocuronium is a rapid-acting, nondepolarizing paralytic that induces muscle paralysis by blocking receptors for acetylcholine and preventing muscle contraction. It has no negative effects on cardiovascular function and does not lower blood pressure or affect heart rate. Rocuronium is primarily metabolized by the liver and, therefore, has an increased duration in patients with liver disease.

Rocuronium has none of the contraindications of succinylcholine and would appear to be an ideal agent. However, the major problem with nondepolarizing agents is that their onset of action is usually slower than that of succinylcholine, and the duration of action is significantly longer. When higher doses of rocuronium are administered during an RSI procedure, the onset time is 1 to 2 minutes, making it a viable alternative to succinylcholine when a rapid onset is needed. Rocuronium maintains effective paralysis for approximately 30 minutes in adults, compared with 5 to 8 minutes for succinylcholine. Those providers who favor succinylcholine over rocuronium usually indicate that it is because of this shorter duration. Even 5 to 8 minutes may seem like an eternity, with major clinical deterioration possible, in "can't intubate/can't ventilate" situations. Careful patient selection, good bag-mask technique, and backup airway devices can mitigate many hazards associated with RSI, making rocuronium the preferred choice in most clinical situations. A variety of nondepolarizing medications, including rocuronium, can be used for ongoing chemical paralysis.

One component of RSI technique is to preoxygenate the patient. This involves applying a tightly fitting nonrebreather mask at 100% oxygen concentration for 5 minutes before the RSI procedure. Alternatively, if the patient is able to cooperate, he or she can take 4 maximal tidal breaths while breathing 100% oxygen. By doing this, the nitrogen that is part of the gas remaining in the alveoli after breathing room air is washed out and replaced by oxygen. This creates a reservoir of oxygen waiting to diffuse from the alveolus into the pulmonary capillaries.

Patients who are properly preoxygenated can sustain up to 6 minutes of complete apnea (as induced by a paralytic) without oxygen saturation dropping below 90%. Note that 6 minutes is ideal; many patients who require intubation require it because of problems with oxygenation in the first place. This illustrates the possible advantage of succinylcholine over rocuronium. It is conceivably possible, although not assured, to administer succinylcholine, have the patient paralyzed for 6 minutes, and emerge from paralysis without the oxygen saturation level falling below 90%, even if you are unable to intubate or successfully ventilate the patient. This is not possible with rocuronium or any of the other nondepolarizing blockers. Therefore, the risk of the vulnerable period of a failed intubation must be weighed against the risk of hyperkalemia and malignant hyperthermia. As stated earlier, it is best not to rely on the shorter duration of succinylcholine as a rescue strategy. *Many harmful clinical conditions, including full cardiac arrest, can occur if you are unable to adequately oxygenate and ventilate an apneic patient following chemical paralysis.*

The use of a technique called apneic oxygenation has emerged as a useful adjunct during RSI procedures. A nasal cannula or specialty catheter is placed onto the patient with oxygen flowing from a second source. This additional oxygen supplementation uses passive diffusion of oxygen from the nasopharynx into the lungs then through the alveoli, reducing the overall risk of hypoxemia during intubation attempts by 30%.[7]

ROCURONIUM (ZEMURON)

Classification: Neuromuscular blocker, nondepolarizing.
Action: Antagonizes acetylcholine at the motor end plate, producing skeletal muscle paralysis.
Indications: To induce neuromuscular blockade for the facilitation of ET intubation.
Adverse Effects: Muscle paralysis, apnea, dyspnea, respiratory depression, sinus tachycardia, urticaria.
Contraindications: Known sensitivity to bromides. Use with caution in heart disease, liver disease.
Dosage:
- **Adult:** 0.6 to 1.2 mg/kg IV, IO (using ideal body weight).
- **Pediatric (older than 3 months):** 0.9 to 1.2 mg/kg IV, IO (off-label).

Special Considerations:
Onset of action is 30 seconds to 2 minutes.
Duration of action is approximately 30 minutes.
Pregnancy class B.

© Dr P. Marazzi/Science Source.

VECURONIUM (NORCURON)

Classification: Neuromuscular blocker, nondepolarizing.
Action: Antagonizes acetylcholine at the motor end plate, producing skeletal muscle paralysis.
Indications: To induce neuromuscular blockade for the facilitation of ET intubation.
Adverse Effects: Muscle paralysis, apnea, dyspnea, respiratory depression, sinus tachycardia, urticaria.
Contraindications: Known sensitivity to bromides. Use with caution in heart disease, liver disease.
Dosage:
- **Adult:** 0.08 to 0.1 mg/kg IV, IO.
- **Pediatric:** 0.1 to 0.15 mg/kg IV, IO.

Special Considerations:
Pregnancy class C.

© Food Collection/ Alamy Stock Photo.

ATRACURIUM (TRACRIUM)

Classification: Nondepolarizing neuromuscular blocker.
Action: Antagonizes acetylcholine receptors at the motor end plate, producing muscle paralysis.
Indications: Neuromuscular blockade to facilitate ET intubation.
Adverse Effects: Flushing, edema, urticaria, pruritus, bronchospasm and/or wheezing, alterations in heart rate, decrease in blood pressure.
Contraindications: Cardiac disease, electrolyte abnormalities, dehydration, known sensitivity.
Dosage:
- **Adult:** 0.4 to 0.5 mg/kg IV, IO; repeat with 0.08 to 0.1 mg/kg every 20 to 45 minutes as needed for prolonged paralysis.
- **Pediatric:**
  - **Older than 2 years:** Same as adult dosing.
  - **Younger than 2 years:** 0.3 to 0.4 mg/kg IV, IO.

Special Considerations:
Do not give by IM injection.
Pregnancy class C.

PANCURONIUM (PAVULON)

Classification: Nondepolarizing neuromuscular blocker.
Action: Antagonizes acetylcholine at the motor end plate, producing skeletal muscle paralysis.
Indications: To induce neuromuscular blockade for the facilitation of ET intubation.
Adverse Effects: Muscle paralysis, apnea, dyspnea, respiratory depression, cutaneous flushing, sinus tachycardia.
Contraindications: Known sensitivity to bromides. Use with caution in heart disease, renal disease.
Dosage:
- **Adult:** 0.06 to 0.1 mg/kg IV, IO; repeat dosing is 0.01 mg/kg every 25 to 60 minutes.
- **Pediatric:** Same as adult dosing.

Special Considerations:
Pregnancy class C.

Deep Sedation Drugs

The second major drug component of RSI is the sedating agent. When used with paralytics, sedation improves the intubation success rate.[8] The purposes of sedation are to protect the brain and heart from dangerous fluctuations in blood pressure and heart rate and prevent the patient from being paralyzed while awake. It would be terrifying for patients to be unable to control their breathing, be fully aware of a painful procedure, and be unable to communicate any discomfort. Therefore, this situation is absolutely to be avoided. Clinical clues that sedation is insufficient include a significant rise in blood pressure, elevation in heart rate, or the presence of tears or unusual sweating.[9,10]

Sedation can be provided on a continuum from light sedation (such as the preanesthesia relaxants given before a patient is taken into surgery) to general anesthesia (during which patients are deeply unconscious without the ability to protect their airway). The sedation level at the drug doses that permit RSI approaches and often reaches general anesthesia levels. The following are common sedation agents: midazolam (Versed), etomidate (Amidate), and ketamine (Ketalar).

Midazolam is a benzodiazepine with anticonvulsant properties, sedative properties, and the ability to induce amnesia for events occurring after administration. Midazolam causes a slight decrease in ICP but does not necessarily blunt the rise in pressure that results from laryngoscopy or intubation.[11] Midazolam causes a decrease in vascular resistance from vascular smooth muscle relaxation; in patients who are hypovolemic or in shock, this can result in a sudden drop in blood pressure and/or a compensatory increase in heart rate. Midazolam should, therefore, be used cautiously in patients with multiple trauma.

Midazolam has no analgesic (pain-killing) effects; do not assume a sedated and paralyzed patient has adequate pain control if only midazolam has been administered. Midazolam can also cause respiratory depression, although this is of clinical concern only if successful intubation is in doubt. When compared with other sedating agents, midazolam has not always engendered the same success as other agents. One reason may be a tendency to underdose because of concerns for hypotension. At 0.2 mg/kg, midazolam has been shown to drop the blood pressure of healthy patients by 10% to 25%.[12] This is more a matter of patient selection than dosing regimen; that is, if potential hypotension is a concern, choose another agent rather than an ineffective dose.

A potential safety feature for midazolam is that its effects can be reversed with flumazenil (Romazicon). Flumazenil is an antagonist to benzodiazepines, just as naloxone (Narcan) is an antagonist to opiates. Flumazenil should be used with caution in people who regularly take benzodiazepine medications because it can produce withdrawal seizures that are difficult to control and complicate airway management efforts. Flumazenil has a variety of other significant contraindications and should be administered in only a small handful of clinical situations, with far greater scrutiny than the decision to administer naloxone.

Etomidate is a unique sedating agent that is not related to narcotics, benzodiazepines, or barbiturates. It was first used in the early 1980s as an alternative to these other classes of medications and has risen rapidly to a preeminent position among the RSI sedation drugs. Etomidate has favorable properties for RSI sedation: It has a very rapid onset (30 seconds), short duration of action (3 to 5 minutes), and minimal effects on the heart and blood vessels. Etomidate lowers ICP and preserves cerebral and heart perfusion; therefore, it does not cause hypotension or worsen shock states. For these reasons, etomidate is the agent of choice for use in RSI for patients with multiple trauma. Etomidate has emerged as the overall sedation method of choice for RSI in the ED and is being used with increasing frequency for RSI in the prehospital setting.[12]

Because of its favorable hemodynamic profile and the fact that it causes less respiratory depression at comparable levels of deep sedation, etomidate is now being used for sedation in EDs for procedures such as major joint and fracture reductions and cardioversion without intubation. Etomidate has also been used to facilitate removal of patients who are painfully entrapped within motor vehicles.

Note that the effective duration of etomidate of 3 to 5 minutes means that patients can wake up before paralysis wears off. Be prepared to either re-sedate (with an agent other than etomidate) or administer a longer-acting sedation agent such as midazolam after successful intubation. That said, if the patient has been properly preoxygenated, the short duration is quite advantageous if intubation cannot be accomplished.

Patients can wake from etomidate before the paralysis wears off. Therefore, patients need to be re-sedated with a longer-acting agent after intubation.

As with midazolam, etomidate has been advocated as a single agent for chemically assisted intubation. However, intubation success rates are not as high as when combined with paralytics. Etomidate causes burning pain on injection.[13]

One additional side effect of etomidate is a dose-related suppression of adrenal function. Because adrenal steroid secretion is one of the mechanisms with which the body responds to stress, a suppression of corticosteroid production can have serious effects on recovery from trauma.

Ketamine is described as a dissociative anesthetic because patients apparently experience a separation of consciousness from the perception of pain. Ketamine is derived from and has some similar properties to a better-known drug, phencyclidine phosphate, known more commonly as *PCP* or *angel dust*. Unfortunately, ketamine has also emerged as a street drug of abuse, often called *Special K*.

Ketamine induces intense sedation, analgesia, and amnesia. Yet protective airway reflexes are generally preserved, even during deep sedation; no significant respiratory depression occurs, and apnea is extremely rare. Ketamine causes a modest increase in blood pressure and heart rate and can increase myocardial oxygen demands. Ketamine should not be used in patients with acute coronary syndromes or myocardial infarction. However, ketamine does offer some protection against arrhythmias precipitated by epinephrine and other stress responses. Therefore, ketamine can work well in patients with hypovolemia. In addition, ketamine has potent bronchodilator properties and may be more advantageous than other agents when patients with severe bronchospasm or status asthmaticus are being intubated.[14] Ketamine does cause a rise in ICP and should not be used if a potential for increased ICP exists (closed-head trauma, brain tumor, stroke or intracranial hemorrhage, or status seizures).

Ketamine has been used extensively for sedation during painful procedures, especially in children, and has an excellent safety record. Ketamine can provide safer conditions for chemically assisting the extrication of patients entrapped within motor vehicles and from collapsed buildings or structures. It has significant potential in natural and manmade disaster situations, particularly those associated with earthquakes and explosions.

Because of the lower incidence of respiratory depression and the maintenance of protective airway reflexes, the intubation and procedural sedation dosages are the same. Ketamine may still cause apnea, so providers should have a bag-mask device, airway devices, and suction readily available when ketamine is being administered.[15] Onset of effect is quite rapid, less than 1 minute. Duration of unconsciousness is 15 to 20 minutes, and analgesia continues for an additional 30 minutes. Ketamine can also be effective when administered intramuscularly. Onset can be delayed to 3 to 5 minutes. Duration of effect is also more prolonged when ketamine is given intramuscularly, lasting approximately 1 hour. Providers are using ketamine for other indications such as adjunctive analgesia when opioid medications are inadequate, and treatment of severe agitation that is refractory to other treatments.

Adverse side effects of ketamine include laryngospasm, increased bronchial secretions, and dysphoric (unpleasant) emergence from sedation. To limit bronchial secretions, an anticholinergic agent such as atropine or glycopyrrolate (Robinul) can be administered. **Emergence phenomena**, such as nightmares and hallucinations, are another adverse effect. In both adults and children, the administration of diazepam can reduce the incidence of unpleasant and sometimes psychologically disturbing dreams on awakening from anesthesia.

MIDAZOLAM (VERSED)

Classification: Benzodiazepine, Schedule C-IV.
Action: Binds to the benzodiazepine receptor and enhances the effects of the brain chemical (neurotransmitter) gamma-aminobutyric acid (GABA). Benzodiazepines act at the level of the limbic, thalamic, and hypothalamic regions of the central nervous system (CNS) to produce short-acting CNS depression (including sedation, skeletal muscle relaxation, and anticonvulsant activity).

© Dr P. Marazzi/Science Source.

Indications: Sedation, anxiety, skeletal muscle relaxation.
Adverse Effects: Respiratory depression, respiratory arrest, hypotension, nausea/vomiting, headache, hiccups, cardiac arrest.
Contraindications: Acute-angle glaucoma, pregnant women, known sensitivity.
Dosage:
Sedation:
Note: The dose of midazolam needs to be individualized. Every dose should be administered slowly over a period of 2 minutes. Allow 2 minutes to evaluate the clinical effect of the dose given.

- **Adult:**
  - **Healthy and younger than 60 years:** *Some patients require as little as 1 mg IV, IO. No more than 2.5 mg should be given over a 2-minute interval.* If additional sedation is required, continue to administer small increments over 2-minute periods (max dose: 5 mg). If the patient also has received a narcotic, he or she will typically require 30% less midazolam than the same patient not given the narcotic.
  - **60 years and older and debilitated or chronically ill patients:** This group of patients has a higher risk of hypoventilation, airway obstruction, and apnea. The peak clinical effect can take longer in these patients; therefore, dose increments should be smaller, and the rate of injection should be slower. *Some patients require a dose as small as 1 mg IV, IO, and no more than 1.5 mg should be given over a 2-minute period.* If additional sedation is required, additional midazolam should be given at a rate of no more than 1 mg over a 2-minute period (max dose: 3.5 mg). If the patient also has received a narcotic, he or she will typically require 50% less midazolam than the same patient not given the narcotic.

- **Continuous infusion:** Continuous infusions can be required for prolonged transport of intubated, critically ill, and injured patients. After an initial bolus dose, the adult patient will require a maintenance infusion dose of 0.02 to 0.1 mg/kg per hour (1 to 7 mg/hr).
- **Pediatric (weight-based):** Pediatric patients typically require higher doses of midazolam than do adults on the basis of weight (in mg/kg). Younger pediatric patients (younger than 6 years) require higher doses (in mg/kg) than older pediatric patients. Midazolam takes approximately 3 minutes to reach peak effect; therefore, wait at least 2 minutes to determine effectiveness of the drug and need for additional dosing.
  - **12 to 16 years:** Same as adult dosing. Some patients in this age group require a higher dose than that used in adults, but rarely does a patient require more than 10 mg.
  - **6 to 12 years:** 0.025 to 0.05 mg/kg IV, IO up to a total dose of 0.4 mg/kg. Exceeding 10 mg as total dose usually is not necessary.
  - **6 months to 5 years:** 0.05 to 0.1 mg/kg IV, IO up to a total dose of 0.6 mg/kg. Exceeding 6 mg as total dose usually is not necessary.
  - **Younger than 6 months:** Dosing recommendations for this age group is unclear. Because this age group is especially vulnerable to airway obstruction and hypoventilation, use small increments with frequent clinical evaluation. Dose: 0.05 to 0.1 mg/kg IV, IO.

Special Considerations:
Patients receiving midazolam require frequent monitoring of vital signs and pulse oximetry. Be prepared to support the patient's airway and ventilation.
Pregnancy class D.

FLUMAZENIL (ROMAZICON)

Classification: Benzodiazepine receptor antagonist, antidote.
Action: Competes with benzodiazepines for binding at the benzodiazepine receptor, reverses the sedative effects of benzodiazepines.
Indication: Benzodiazepine oversedation.
Adverse Effects: Resedation, seizures, dizziness, pain at injection site, nausea/vomiting, diaphoresis, headache, visual impairment.
Contraindications: Cyclic antidepressant overdose; life-threatening conditions that require treatment with benzodiazepines, such as status epilepticus and intracranial hypertension; known sensitivity to flumazenil or benzodiazepines. Use with caution where there is the possibility of unrecognized benzodiazepine dependence and in patients who have a history of substance abuse, who are known substance abusers, or have a history of seizures.

Dosage:
- **Adult:** Initial dose is 0.2 mg IV, IO over a 15-second period. If the desired effect is not observed after 45 seconds, administer a second 0.2-mg dose, again over a 15-second period. Doses can be repeated a total of four times until a total dose of 1 mg has been administered.
- **Pediatric:** Children older than 1 year, 0.01 mg/kg IV, IO given over a 15-second period. May repeat in 45 seconds and then every minute to a maximum cumulative dose of 0.05 mg/kg or 1 mg, whichever is the lower dose.

Special Considerations:
Monitor for signs of hypoventilation and hypoxia for approximately 2 hours.
If the half-life of the benzodiazepine is longer than flumazenil, an additional dose may be needed.
May precipitate withdrawal symptoms in patients dependent on benzodiazepines.
Flumazenil has not been shown to benefit patients who have overdosed on multiple drugs.
Pregnancy class C.

ETOMIDATE (AMIDATE)

Classification: Hypnotic, anesthesia induction agent.

Action: Although the exact mechanism is unknown, etomidate appears to have GABA-like effects.

Indications: Induction for RSI and pharmacologic-assisted intubation, induction of anesthesia.

Adverse Effects: Hypotension, respiratory depression, pain at the site of injection, temporary involuntary muscle movements, frequent nausea/vomiting on emergence, adrenal insufficiency, hyperventilation, hypoventilation, apnea of short duration, hiccups, laryngospasm, snoring, tachypnea, hypertension, cardiac arrhythmias.

Etomidate
Injection, USP

10 mL Single-dose Fliptop Vial

20 mg/10 mL (2 mg/mL)
INTRAVENOUS USE ONLY
Usual Dosage: See insert.

Discard unused portion.
NDC 12345-678-90   **Rx only**

Contraindications: Known sensitivity. Use in pregnancy only if the potential benefits justify the potential risk to the fetus. Do not use during labor and avoid in nursing mothers.

Dosage:
- **Adult:** 0.2 to 0.6 mg/kg slow IV, IO (over 30 to 60 seconds); 0.3 mg/kg is used in many protocols/references. A typical adult intubating dose of etomidate is 20 mg slow IV. Consider less (e.g., 10 mg) in older adults or patients with cardiac conditions.
- **Pediatric:**
  - **Older than 10 years:** Same as adult dosing.
  - **Younger than 10 years:** Safety has not been established.

Special Considerations:
Etomidate is used to prepare a patient for orotracheal intubation. Both personnel and equipment must be present to manage the patient's airway before administration.
Pregnancy class C.

KETAMINE (KETALAR)

Classification: General anesthetic, analgesic, sedative.

Action: Produces a state of anesthesia while maintaining airway reflexes, heart rate, and blood pressure.

Indications: Pain and as anesthesia for procedures of short duration.

Adverse Effects: Emergence phenomena, hypertension and sinus tachycardia, hypotension and sinus bradycardia, other cardiac arrhythmias (rare), respiratory depression, apnea, laryngospasms and other forms of airway obstruction (rare), tonic-clonic movements, vomiting.

Contraindications: Patients in whom a significant elevation in blood pressure would be hazardous (hypertension, stroke, head trauma, increased intracranial mass or bleeding, myocardial infarction). Use with caution in patients with increased ICP or increased intraocular pressure (glaucoma) and patients with hypovolemia, dehydration, or cardiac disease (especially angina and heart failure).

© Julia Hiebaum/Alamy Stock Photo.

Dosage: Administer slowly over a period of 60 seconds.

IV, IO:
- **Adult:** 1 to 4.5 mg/kg IV, IO. 1 to 2 mg/kg produces anesthesia usually within 30 seconds that typically lasts 5 to 10 minutes.
- **Pediatric:** 0.5 to 2 mg IV, IO over a 1-minute period.

IM:
- **Adult:** 6.5 to 13 mg/kg IM. 10 mg/kg IM is capable of producing anesthesia within 3 to 4 minutes with an effect typically lasting 12 to 25 minutes. In adults, concomitant administration of 5 to 15 mg of diazepam reduces the incidence of emergence phenomena.
- **Pediatric:** 4 to 5 mg/kg IM.

Special Considerations:
Pregnancy class C.

RAPID SEQUENCE INTUBATION

The procedure for RSI can be characterized by following the seven Ps (**FIGURE 20-2**):

1. **P**reparations (Time ≥ t – 5 minutes)

Patient is attached to pulse oximeter, electrocardiogram monitor, and end-tidal CO_2 monitor (if available). Medications are chosen after considering underlying patient condition and potential contraindications. Intubation and suction equipment are readied, including rescue devices such as an LMA or King Airway. Ensure that oxygen is connected and flowing at the maximal rate. Remember personal protective gear because blood and body fluids often erupt from the airways. Move the patient into the optimal position for intubation (if possible). This position may be supine, low Fowler, or reverse Trendelenburg, depending on the situation.

2. **P**reoxygenation (Time = t – 5 minutes)

Patient is placed on tight-fitting 100% nonrebreather face mask for 5 minutes. Attempt to wash out excess nitrogen from the pulmonary alveoli, providing a reservoir of oxygen to enable tolerance of an apneic period. As much as possible, avoid ventilating the patient with positive pressure unless oxygen saturation falls below 90%. If positive pressure ventilation is required, apply downward pressure over the cricothyroid membrane (Sellick maneuver) to limit passage of air into the stomach, which would otherwise increase the risk of emesis and aspiration. Consult local protocols regarding use of the Sellick maneuver as it is no longer recommended by certain sources.[16,17] If the patient is alert, coach him or her to take 8 maximal (i.e., as deep as possible) breaths, a technique that also eliminates space-wasting nitrogen.

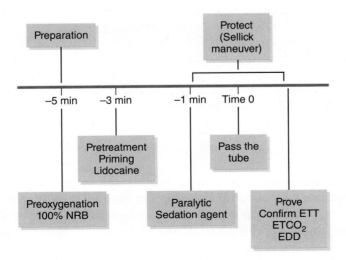

FIGURE 20-2 RSI technique. *Abbreviations:* EDD, esophageal detector device; $ETCO_2$, end-tidal CO_2; ETT, endotracheal tube; NRB, nonrebreather mask.

3. *P*retreatment/priming (Time = t – 3 minutes)

If using succinylcholine, administer one-tenth of the paralyzing dose. Be sure equipment is ready in the event of premature paralysis. Consider pretreatment with lidocaine, although quality supportive evidence is lacking.[12] Manipulation of the larynx causes both reflex elevation of ICP and secretion of catecholamines such as epinephrine. These can cause decreased blood flow to the brain and put increased stress on cardiac oxygen consumption. Lidocaine may blunt these effects. Whether any additive protection is applied to deep sedation is unclear, but no downside exists in trying to maximize cerebral and cardiac protection. If a patient does not have a head injury, intracranial process, or cardiac problems, lidocaine can be omitted.

4. *P*aralytic/sedation (Time = t – 1 minute)

Administer a sedation agent followed immediately by a paralytic agent. Allow for adequate relaxation before attempting to intubate; the use of a watch is best. Some cases allow you to administer sedation, maintain spontaneous breathing, and assess the ability to visualize the laryngeal opening, following with full paralysis and intubation. Administering sedation before the paralytic is generally better in case IV access is lost.

5. *P*ass the tube (Time = 0)

6. *P*rove it! (Time = t+)

Confirm tube position. Although determining ET position is especially difficult in the prehospital environment, several studies have demonstrated unacceptable rates of undetected ET malposition in field intubations.[18] Confirmatory methods must be used, such as end-tidal CO_2 detectors and esophageal detector devices, in addition to clinical assessment of ET tube position. Waveform capnography should be considered the gold standard for ETT placement confirmation. Other methods, including colorimetric end-tidal CO_2 devices, have significant clinical limitations.

7. *P*ost-intubation management

Provide additional doses of sedative and analgesic medications as appropriate. Consider subsequent doses of a chemical paralytic medication. Continue monitoring airway patency. Monitor end-tidal CO_2 waveforms for changes in ventilation, perfusion, or ETT compromise. Provide additional supportive measures such as IV fluids while continuing to monitor the patient's vital signs.

CASE STUDY

You and your partner respond to a call for a gunshot wound to the face. After the scene is secured by police, you find a 46-year-old man who attempted suicide by placing a shotgun under his chin and firing. He is awake and sitting forward. Although he cannot speak beyond mumbles, he is able to follow commands and communicate. Blood is draining at a moderate rate out of what is left of his mouth. His blood pressure is 150/85 mm Hg, heart rate is 110 beats/min, and respiratory rate is 30 breaths/min and unlabored. Oxygen saturation is 92%. You have concerns about his airway and consider intubating him, using your knowledge of the RSI technique.

In this common scenario, the paramedic is faced with several decisions. First, does the patient need immediate intubation (question 6 from the earlier list of questions that should be asked to determine barriers to RSI)? As long as he leans forward, he should be able to maintain his airway until he goes into shock. The decision really depends on how much he is bleeding and how far away you are from the destination hospital (or helicopter). If you decide to intubate, maintain him in a position of comfort (sitting up) for as long as possible and consider intubating him while he is sitting up. The patient's risk of cervical spine injury with this mechanism of injury is low. He is at a higher risk for losing his airway.

If his blood loss, ability to control his airway, and time to the trauma center are too great, a modified intubation plan may be warranted. Following the previously outlined steps, proceed through the seven Ps. During preparation, ask yourself the five remaining questions:

1. *Can I intubate?*

Surprisingly, patients who sustain a gunshot wound to their mandible and teeth/tongue are often easy to intubate because of little resistance to laryngoscopy. Bleeding can obscure the view, however, so suction should be optimized. The patient should remain leaning forward throughout the procedure if possible.

2. *Can I ventilate?*

It would not be appropriate to ventilate with a bag-mask device.

3. *Do I have other options?*

Plan on an alternate airway. The LMA and King Airway devices have been shown to be a valuable adjunct and may also provide some tamponade of pharyngeal bleeding.[19]

4. *Is the equipment assembled?*

5. *Are any contraindications to medications or technique present?*

The major problem may be visualization. Because the patient is currently breathing, you could choose a technique that maintains his breathing, at least until confirmation that the laryngeal opening can be visualized. Consider using ketamine (if part of approved protocols) or etomidate at a reduced dose (0.15 to 0.2 mg/kg). If you can visualize the laryngeal opening, proceed with full paralysis. If not, defer to the receiving hospital unless the patient deteriorates further. This plan should be established in advance, with alternatives considered at that time, as well.

▶ Review Questions

1. What are six questions to ask yourself when preparing to perform rapid sequence intubation?
2. What is the neurotransmitter used to make muscles contract?
3. What is the chemical that normally breaks down acetylcholine?
4. What are the two classes of paralytics?
5. How quickly does succinylcholine induce paralysis?
6. What electrolyte is released into the bloodstream after the administration of succinylcholine?
7. In what medical conditions should a patient *not* be given succinylcholine?
8. What is malignant hyperthermia?
9. In children younger than 8 years, what medication should be administered before succinylcholine? Why?
10. What are the effects of rocuronium on the cardiovascular system?
11. What is the unique relation between the deep sedation medications midazolam and flumazenil?
12. Explain why etomidate is the preferred drug for deep sedation in intubation.
13. List the seven Ps of RSI and the time frame required for each step of the procedure.

References

1. Wallace C, McGuire B. Rapid sequence induction: its place in modern anaesthesia. *Contin Educ Anaesthes Crit Care Pain.* 2013;14(3):130–135.
2. Nason KS. Acute intraoperative pulmonary aspiration. *Thorac Surg Clin.* 2015;25(3):301–307.
3. Pepe PE, Roppolo LP, Fowler RL. Prehospital endotracheal intubation: elemental or detrimental? *Crit Care.* 2015;19(1):121.
4. Nickson C. Rapid sequence airway (RSA) and PALM. Life in the Fast Lane. https://lifeinthefastlane.com/ccc/rapid-sequence-airway-rsa. Updated March 7, 2015. Accessed September 12, 2018.
5. Rubenson Wahlin R, Nelson DW, Bellander B-M, Svensson M, Helmy A, Thelin EP. Prehospital intubation and outcome in traumatic brain injury—assessing intervention efficacy in a modern trauma cohort. *Frontiers Neurol.* 2018;9:194. doi:10.3389/fneur.2018.00194.
6. Raghavendra T. Neuromuscular blocking drugs: discovery and development. *J Royal Soc Med.* 2002;95(7):363–367.

7. Pavlov I, Medrano S, Weingart, S. Apneic oxygenation reduces the incidence of hypoxemia during emergency intubation: a systematic review and meta-analysis. *Am J Emerg Med.* 2017;35(8):1184–1189.

8. Okubo M, Gibo K, Hagiwara Y, Nakayama Y, Hasegawa K, Japanese Emergency Medicine Network Investigators. The effectiveness of rapid sequence intubation (RSI) versus non-RSI in emergency department: an analysis of multicenter prospective observational study. *Int J Emerg Med.* 2017;10:1. doi:10.1186/s12245-017-0129-8.

9. Kotsovolis G, Komninos G. Awareness during anesthesia: how sure can we be that the patient is sleeping indeed? *Hippokratia.* 2009;13(2):83–89.

10. Chung HS. Awareness and recall during general anesthesia. *Korean J Anesthesiol.* 2014;66(5):339–345.

11. Simon B. Pharmacologic aids in airway management. In: Dailey R, ed. *The Airway: Emergency Management.* St. Louis, MO: Mosby; 1992:145–170.

12. Caro D. Induction agents for rapid sequence intubation in adults outside the operating room. UpToDate. https://www.uptodate.com/contents/induction-agents-for-rapid-sequence-intubation-in-adults-outside-the-operating-room. Updated March 29, 2017. Accessed September 12, 2018.

13. Mosier JM, Sakles JC, Stolz U, et al. Neuromuscular blockade improves first-attempt success for intubation in the intensive care unit. A propensity matched analysis. *Ann Am Thorac Soc.* 2015;12(5):734–741.

14. Goyal S, Agrawal A. Ketamine in status asthmaticus: a review. *Indian J Crit Care Med.* 2013;17(3):154–161.

15. Driver BE, Reardon RF. Apnea after low-dose ketamine sedation during attempted delayed sequence intubation. *Ann Emerg Med.* 2017;69(1):34–35.

16. Stronczek MJ. Airway management changes—2015–2020 ACLS Guidelines. OMS Guardian. https://www.dds4dds.com/Documents/Public%20Resources/Social/AirwayManagementChanges.pdf. Accessed September 12, 2018.

17. Brown CA, Sakles JC. Rapid sequence intubation for adults outside the operating room. UpToDate. https://www.uptodate.com/contents/rapid-sequence-intubation-for-adults-outside-the-operating-room. Updated November 16, 2017. Accessed September 13, 2018.

18. Bernhard M, Becker TK, Böttiger BW. Prehospital airway management for out-of-hospital cardiac arrest. *JAMA.* 2013;309(18):1888. doi:10.1001/jama.2013.3098.

19. Davis DP, Valentine C, Ochs M, Voke GM, Hoyt DB. The Combitube as a salvage airway device for paramedic rapid sequence intubation. *Ann Emerg Med.* 2003;42:697.

Appendix A

Medications, Classifications, and Body Systems Affected

Medication	Classification	Body System Affected	Chapter	Page Number(s)
Abciximab (ReoPro)	GP IIb/IIIa inhibitor	Cardiovascular	6: Acute Coronary Syndromes	145
Activated charcoal	Antidote, adsorbent	Gastrointestinal	13: Poisonings, Overdoses, and Intoxications	250
Adenosine (Adenocard)	Antiarrhythmic	Cardiovascular	9: Cardiac Arrhythmias 19: Special Considerations	192 379
Albumin	Volume expander, colloid	Cardiovascular	5: Intravenous Fluids and Administration	107
Albuterol (Proventil, Ventolin)	Bronchodilator, beta agonist	Respiratory	8: Anaphylaxis 14: Respiratory Emergencies 19: Special Considerations	180–181 282 364–365
Albuterol/ipratropium (Combivent)	Combination bronchodilator	Respiratory	14: Respiratory Emergencies	284
Amiodarone (Cordarone)	Antiarrhythmic, Class III	Cardiovascular	9: Cardiac Arrhythmias 18: Critical Care Transport 19: Special Considerations	198–199 343–344 380
Angiotensin-converting enzyme (ACE) inhibitors: Captopril (Capoten), Enalapril (Vasotec), Lisinopril (Prinivil, Zestril), Ramipril (Altace)	ACE inhibitor	Cardiovascular	6: Acute Coronary Syndromes 10: Congestive Heart Failure	147 212
Aspirin, ASA	Antiplatelet, nonnarcotic analgesic, antipyretic	Cardiovascular, central nervous	6: Acute Coronary Syndromes 12: Hypertensive Emergencies 13: Poisonings, Overdoses, and Intoxications	135 239 263

(continues)

Medication	Classification	Body System Affected	Chapter	Page Number(s)
Atenolol (Tenormin)	Beta-adrenergic antagonist, antianginal, antihypertensive, Class II antiarrhythmic	Cardiovascular	6: Acute Coronary Syndromes	140
Atracurium (Tracrium)	Nondepolarizing neuromuscular blocker	Musculoskeletal	20: Pharmacology-Assisted Intubation	397
Atropine sulfate	Anticholinergic (antimuscarinic)	Cardiovascular, parasympathetic nervous	1: Principles of Pharmacology 9: Cardiac Arrhythmias 13: Poisonings, Overdoses, and Intoxications 19: Special Considerations 20: Pharmacology-Assisted Intubation	27 188 256–257 377–378 395
Bivalirudin (Angiomax)	Anticoagulant	Hematologic, cardiovascular	6: Acute Coronary Syndromes	144
Calcium gluconate	Electrolyte solution	Cardiovascular, renal	5: Intravenous Fluids and Administration 18: Critical Care Transport	110 341
Carbamazepine (Tegretol)	Anticonvulsant	Central nervous	15: Seizures	295
Clopidogrel (Plavix)	Antiplatelet	Hematologic, cardiovascular	6: Acute Coronary Syndromes	142–143
Dexamethasone (Decadron)	Corticosteroid	Endocrine, respiratory, immune	14: Respiratory Emergencies	285
Dextrose (50%, 25%, 10%)	Antihypoglycemic	Endocrine	5: Intravenous Fluids and Administration 11: Endocrine Emergencies	111 220
Diazepam (Valium)	Benzodiazepine, Schedule C-IV	Central nervous	7: Analgesia and Sedation 12: Hypertensive Emergencies 13: Poisonings, Overdoses, and Intoxications 15: Seizures	164–165 243–244 254 291–292
Digoxin (Lanoxin)	Cardiac glycoside	Cardiovascular	10: Congestive Heart Failure	211
Diltiazem (Cardizem)	Calcium channel blocker, Class IV antiarrhythmic	Cardiovascular	9: Cardiac Arrhythmias	193

Medication	Classification	Body System Affected	Chapter	Page Number(s)
Diphenhydramine hydrochloride (Benadryl)	Antihistamine	Immune system, cardiovascular, respiratory	8: Anaphylaxis 19: Special Considerations	181 363
Dobutamine (Dobutrex)	Adrenergic agent	Cardiovascular	1: Principles of Pharmacology 16: Shock	23 312
Dolasetron (Anzemet)	Antiemetic	Central nervous	7: Analgesia and Sedation	169
Dopamine (Intropin)	Adrenergic agonist, inotropic, vasopressor	Cardiovascular	1: Principles of Pharmacology 9: Cardiac Arrhythmias 16: Shock	22 190 312
Enoxaparin (Lovenox)	Anticoagulant	Hematologic, cardiovascular	6: Acute Coronary Syndromes	144
Epinephrine	Adrenergic agent, inotropic	Cardiovascular, respiratory	1: Principles of Pharmacology 8: Anaphylaxis 9: Cardiac Arrhythmias 19: Special Considerations	22 178 189 377
Epinephrine autoinjectors (EpiPen, EpiPen Jr)	Adrenergic agonist inotropic	Cardiovascular, respiratory	8: Anaphylaxis	179
Eptifibatide (Integrilin)	GP IIb/IIIa inhibitor	Hematologic, cardiovascular	6: Acute Coronary Syndromes 18: Critical Care Transport	146 344
Esmolol (Brevibloc)	Beta-adrenergic antagonist, Class II antiarrhythmic	Cardiovascular	6: Acute Coronary Syndromes 9: Cardiac Arrhythmias 11: Endocrine Emergencies 12: Hypertensive Emergencies	141 196 227–228 235
Etomidate (Amidate)	Hypnotic, anesthesia induction agent	Central nervous	7: Analgesia and Sedation 20: Pharmacology-Assisted Intubation	162 402
Felbamate (Felbatol)	Anticonvulsant	Central nervous	15: Seizures	294
Fentanyl citrate (Sublimaze)	Narcotic analgesic, Schedule C-II	Central nervous	7: Analgesia and Sedation 18: Critical Care Transport	157 351
Fibrinolytic: tissue plasminogen activator (tPA)	Thrombolytic agents	Hematologic, cardiovascular	6: Acute Coronary Syndromes	150

(continues)

Medication	Classification	Body System Affected	Chapter	Page Number(s)
Flumazenil (Romazicon)	Benzodiazepine receptor antagonist, antidote	Central nervous	7: Analgesia and Sedation 20: Pharmacology-Assisted Intubation	167–168 401
Fosphenytoin (Cerebyx)	Anticonvulsant	Central nervous	13: Poisonings, Overdoses, and Intoxications 15: Seizures 18: Critical Care Transport	255 295 339
Furosemide (Lasix)	Loop diuretic	Renal	10: Congestive Heart Failure 12: Hypertensive Emergencies	208 236
Gabapentin (Neurontin)	Anticonvulsant	Central nervous	15: Seizures	297
Glucagon	Hormone	Endocrine	8: Anaphylaxis 11: Endocrine Emergencies 13: Poisonings, Overdoses, and Intoxications	182–183 221 257
Haloperidol (Haldol)	Antipsychotic agent	Central nervous	13: Poisonings, Overdoses, and Intoxications	260–261
Heparin (unfractionated heparin)	Anticoagulant	Hematologic, cardiovascular	6: Acute Coronary Syndromes	143–144
HMG-CoA Reductase Inhibitors (Statins): Atorvastatin (Lipitor), Fluvastatin (Lescol), Lovastatin (Mevacor), Pravastatin (Pravachol), Rosuvastatin (Crestor), Simvastatin (Zocor)	HMG-CoA Reductase Inhibitors (Statins)	Cardiovascular	6: Acute Coronary Syndromes	147–148
Hydralazine (Apresoline)	Antihypertensive agent, vasodilator	Cardiovascular	12: Hypertensive Emergencies 18: Critical Care Transport 19: Special Considerations	242 339 370
Hydrocortisone sodium succinate (Cortef, Solu-Cortef)	Corticosteroid	Endocrine, respiratory, immune	8: Anaphylaxis 11: Endocrine Emergencies 19: Special Considerations	181–182 226 368
Hypertonic saline (3% saline)	Volume expander, electrolyte solution	Central nervous, cardiovascular	5: Intravenous Fluids and Administration 17: Traumatic Brain Injury	108 323
Ibuprofen	NSAID	Cardiovascular, central nervous	7: Analgesia and Sedation	158

Medication	Classification	Body System Affected	Chapter	Page Number(s)
Insulin, regular (Humulin R, Novolin R)	Hormone	Endocrine, renal	5: Intravenous Fluids and Administration 11: Endocrine Emergencies 18: Critical Care Transport 19: Special Considerations	111 224 347–348 372–373
Ipratropium bromide (Atrovent)	Bronchodilator, anticholinergic	Respiratory	14: Respiratory Emergencies 19: Special Considerations	283–284 366
Ketamine (Ketalar)	General anesthetic	Central nervous	7: Analgesia and Sedation 20: Pharmacology-Assisted Intubation	161–162 402–403
Ketorolac (Toradol)	NSAID	Central nervous, peripheral tissue	7: Analgesia and Sedation	159
Labetalol (Normodyne, Trandate)	Beta-adrenergic antagonist, antianginal, antihypertensive	Cardiovascular	1: Principles of Pharmacology 6: Acute Coronary Syndromes 11: Endocrine Emergencies 12: Hypertensive Emergencies 18: Critical Care Transport 19: Special Considerations	26 141–142 228 237 340 369–370
Lamotrigine (Lamictal)	Anticonvulsant, antimanic agent	Central nervous	15: Seizures	298
Levalbuterol (Xopenex)	Beta agonist	Respiratory	14: Respiratory Emergencies	283
Levetiracetam (Keppra)	Anticonvulsant	Central nervous	15: Seizures	296
Lidocaine (Xylocaine)	Antiarrhythmic, Class IB	Cardiovascular	9: Cardiac Arrhythmias 19: Special Considerations	199 381
Lorazepam (Ativan)	Benzodiazepine, Schedule C-IV	Central nervous	7: Analgesia and Sedation 13: Poisonings, Overdoses, and Intoxications 15: Seizures	166 260 293
Magnesium sulfate	Electrolyte, tocolytic, mineral	Cardiovascular	9: Cardiac Arrhythmias 12: Hypertensive Emergencies 13: Poisonings, Overdoses, and Intoxications 14: Respiratory Emergencies 18: Critical Care Transport 19: Special Considerations	201 241–242 252 286 337–338 371

(continues)

Medication	Classification	Body System Affected	Chapter	Page Number(s)
Mannitol (Osmitrol)	Osmotic diuretic	Central nervous, cardiovascular, renal	17: Traumatic Brain Injury 18: Critical Care Transport	322–323 351
Methylprednisolone sodium succinate (Solu-Medrol)	Corticosteroid	Central nervous, endocrine, respiratory, immune	8: Anaphylaxis 14: Respiratory Emergencies 19: Special Considerations	182 286 367
Metoprolol (Lopressor, Toprol XL)	Beta-adrenergic antagonist, antianginal, antihypertensive, Class II antiarrhythmic	Cardiovascular	1: Principles of Pharmacology 6: Acute Coronary Syndromes 9: Cardiac Arrhythmias 10: Congestive Heart Failure 11: Endocrine Emergencies	26 140 195 212 229
Midazolam (Versed)	Benzodiazepine, Schedule C-IV	Central nervous	7: Analgesia and Sedation 13: Poisonings, Overdoses, and Intoxications 18: Critical Care Transport 20: Pharmacology-Assisted Intubation	165–166 259–260 342–343 400–401
Milrinone (Primacor)	Inotropic	Cardiovascular	16: Shock	313
Morphine sulfate	Opiate agonist, Schedule C-II	Cardiovascular, central nervous	6: Acute Coronary Syndromes 7: Analgesia and Sedation 10: Congestive Heart Failure 13: Poisonings, Overdoses, and Intoxications	139 156–157 208–209 264
Naloxone (Narcan)	Opioid antagonist	Central nervous	7: Analgesia and Sedation 13: Poisonings, Overdoses, and Intoxications	168 266
Nicardipine (Cardene)	Calcium channel blocker	Cardiovascular	12: Hypertensive Emergencies	235
Nitroglycerin (Nitro-lingual, NitroQuick, Nitro-Dur)	Antianginal agent	Cardiovascular	6: Acute Coronary Syndromes 10: Congestive Heart Failure 12: Hypertensive Emergencies 13: Poisonings, Overdoses, and Intoxications	138–139 209–210 239–240 261
Nitrous oxide	Inorganic gas, inhaled anesthetic	Central nervous	7: Analgesia and Sedation	160

Medication	Classification	Body System Affected	Chapter	Page Number(s)
Norepinephrine (Levophed)	Adrenergic agonist, inotropic, vasopressor	Cardiovascular	1: Principles of Pharmacology 13: Poisonings, Overdoses, and Intoxications 16: Shock	22 253 313
Ondansetron (Zofran)	Antiemetic	Gastrointestinal	7: Analgesia and Sedation	170
Oxygen	Elemental gas	Respiratory, cardiovascular	6: Acute Coronary Syndromes 14: Respiratory Emergencies	135 276
Pancuronium (Pavulon)	Nondepolarizing neuromuscular blocker	Musculoskeletal	20: Pharmacology-Assisted Intubation	398
Phenobarbital (Luminal)	Anticonvulsant, barbiturate, Schedule C-IV	Central nervous	15: Seizures	296
Phentolamine (Regitine)	Alpha antagonist, antihypertensive	Cardiovascular	12: Hypertensive Emergencies 13: Poisonings, Overdoses, and Intoxications	244 264
Phenylephrine (Neo-Synephrine)	Adrenergic agonist	Cardiovascular	1: Principles of Pharmacology 13: Poisonings, Overdoses, and Intoxications 16: Shock	23 252–253 315
Phenytoin (Dilantin)	Anticonvulsant	Central nervous	13: Poisonings, Overdoses, and Intoxications 15: Seizures 18: Critical Care Transport	255 294–295 338
Potassium chloride	Electrolyte replacement	Cardiovascular, central nervous, renal	5: Intravenous Fluids and Administration	112
Pralidoxime (2-PAM, Protopam)	Cholinergic agonist, antidote	Parasympathetic nervous	13: Poisonings, Overdoses, and Intoxications	268
Prednisone	Corticosteroid	Endocrine, respiratory, immune	19: Special Considerations	367
Procainamide (Pronestyl)	Antiarrhythmic, Class IA	Cardiovascular	9: Cardiac Arrhythmias 19: Special Considerations	200 380
Promethazine (Phenergan)	Antiemetic, antihistamine	Central nervous	7: Analgesia and Sedation	169
Propofol (Diprivan)	Anesthetic	Central nervous	18: Critical Care Transport	349–350

(continues)

Medication	Classification	Body System Affected	Chapter	Page Number(s)
Propranolol (Inderal)	Beta-adrenergic antagonist, antianginal, antihypertensive, antiarrhythmic Class II	Cardiovascular	1: Principles of Pharmacology 9: Cardiac Arrhythmias	25 195
Racemic epinephrine/racepinephrine (microNefrin, S_2)	Bronchodilator, adrenergic agent	Respiratory	14: Respiratory Emergencies	287
Rocuronium (Zemuron)	Neuromuscular blocker, nondepolarizing	Musculoskeletal	20: Pharmacology-Assisted Intubation	397
Scopolamine (Transderm Scop)	Neurologic antivertigo, antimuscarinic	Cardiovascular, parasympathetic nervous	1: Principles of Pharmacology	28
Sodium bicarbonate	Electrolyte replacement	Cardiovascular, pulmonary, renal	5: Intravenous Fluids and Administration 13: Poisonings, Overdoses, and Intoxications	110 251
Sodium nitroprusside (Nitropress)	Antihypertensive agent	Cardiovascular	12: Hypertensive Emergencies	236–237
Succinylcholine (Anectine)	Neuromuscular blocker, depolarizing	Musculoskeletal	20: Pharmacology-Assisted Intubation	394
Terbutaline (Brethine)	Adrenergic agonist	Respiratory	19: Special Considerations	365
Thiamine (vitamin B_1)	vitamin B_1	Central nervous	11: Endocrine Emergencies	221
Tirofiban (Aggrastat)	GP IIb/IIIa inhibitor	Cardiovascular	6: Acute Coronary Syndromes	146
Tranexamic Acid (Cyklokapron, TXA)	Antifibrinolytic, hemostatic agent	Hematologic	16: Shock	309
Valproic acid (Depakote)	Anticonvulsant, antimanic	Central nervous	15: Seizures	297
Vecuronium (Norcuron)	Neuromuscular blocker, nondepolarizing	Musculoskeletal	18: Critical Care Transport 20: Pharmacology-Assisted Intubation	344–345 397
Verapamil (Isoptin)	Calcium channel blocker, Class IV antiarrhythmic	Cardiovascular	9: Cardiac Arrhythmias	194

Appendix B

Compilation of Drug Profiles

ABCIXIMAB (REOPRO)

Classification: GP IIb/IIIa inhibitor.

Action: Prevents the aggregation of platelets by inhibiting the integrin GP IIb/IIIa receptor.

Indications: UA/NSTEMI patients undergoing planned or emergent percutaneous coronary intervention.

Adverse Effects: Bleeding from the GI tract, internal bleeding, intracranial hemorrhage, hypotension, stroke, anaphylactic shock.

Contraindications: Bleeding from any source, severe uncontrolled hypertension, surgery or trauma within the previous 6 weeks, stroke within the previous 30 days, renal failure, thrombocytopenia, intracranial mass.

© Bob London/Alamy Stock Photo.

Dosage:

UA/NSTEMI with Planned PCI Within 24 Hours:

- 0.25 mg/kg IV, IO (10 to 60 minutes before procedure), then 0.125 mcg/kg per minute IV, IO infusion for 12 to 24 hours.

Percutaneous Coronary Intervention Only:

- 0.25 mg/kg IV, IO, then 10 mcg/min IV, IO infusion.

Special Considerations:
Pregnancy class C.

ACTIVATED CHARCOAL

Classification: Antidote, adsorbent.

Action: When certain chemicals and toxins are in proximity to the activated charcoal, the chemical will attach to the surface of the charcoal and become trapped.

Indications: Toxic ingestion.

Adverse Effects: Nausea/vomiting, constipation, or diarrhea. If aspirated into the lungs, charcoal can induce a potentially fatal form of pneumonitis.

Contraindications: Ingestion of acids, alkalis, ethanol, methanol, cyanide, ferrous sulfate or other iron salts, lithium; coma; GI obstruction, known minimally toxic ingestion.

Dosage:

- **Adult:** 50 to 100 g/dose.
- **Pediatric:** 1 to 2 g/kg.

Special Considerations:
Pregnancy class C.

ADENOSINE (ADENOCARD)

Classification: Antiarrhythmic.
Action: Slows the conduction of electrical impulses at the AV node.
Indications: Stable reentry SVT. Does not convert AF, atrial flutter, or VT.
Adverse Effects: Common adverse reactions are generally mild and short-lived: sense of impending doom, complaints of flushing, chest pressure, throat tightness, numbness. Patients will have a brief episode of asystole after administration.
Contraindications: Sick sinus syndrome, second- or third-degree heart block, poison-/drug-induced tachycardia, asthma, or bronchospasm.

© Jones & Bartlett Learning.

Dosage: Note: Adenosine should be delivered only by rapid IV bolus with a peripheral IV or directly into a vein, in a location as close to the heart as possible, preferably in the antecubital fossa. Administration of adenosine must be immediately followed by a saline flush, and then the extremity should be elevated.

- **Adult:** Initial dose 6 mg rapid IV, IO (over a 1- to 3-second period) immediately followed by a 20-mL rapid saline flush. If the first dose does not eliminate the rhythm in 1 to 2 minutes, administer a second dose of 12 mg rapid IV, IO.
- **Pediatric:**
  - **Children >110 pounds (50 kg):** Same as adult dosing.
  - **Children <110 pounds (50 kg):** Initial dose 0.1 mg/kg IV, IO (max dose: 6 mg) immediately followed by a ≥5-mL rapid saline flush; may repeat at 0.2 mg/kg (max dose: 12 mg).

Special Considerations:
Use with caution in patients with preexisting bronchospasm and those with a history of AF.
Older adults with no history of paroxysmal SVT should be carefully evaluated for dehydration and rapid sinus tachycardia requiring volume fluid replacement rather than simply treated with adenosine.
Pregnancy class C.

ALBUMIN

Classification: Volume expander, colloid.
Action: Increases oncotic pressure in intravascular space.
Indications: Expand intravascular volume.
Adverse Effects: Allergic reaction in some patients; an excessive volume of fluid can result in and pulmonary edema in susceptible patients.
Contraindications: Severe anemia or cardiac failure in the presence of normal or increased intravascular volume, solution appears turbid or after 4 hours since opening the container, known sensitivity.
Dosage: Two preparations: 500 mL of a 5% solution (250 mL of a 5% solution also available) and 100 mL of a 25% solution (50 mL of a 25% solution also available).

- **Adult:**
  - **5% albumin:** 500 to 1,000 mL IV, IO.
  - **25% albumin:** 50 to 200 mL IV, IO.

ALBUMIN   *(continued)*

- **Pediatric:**
  - **5% albumin:** 0.5 to 1 g/kg IV; the initial dose may be repeated in 15 to 30 minutes if the clinical response is inadequate.
  - **25% albumin:** 1 g/kg IV, IO.

Special Considerations:

Patients with a history of CHF, cardiac disease, hypertension, and pulmonary edema should be given 5% albumin, or the 25% albumin should be diluted. Because 25% of albumin increases intravascular volume greater than the volume administered, slowly administer 25% albumin in normovolemic patients to prevent complications such as pulmonary edema.

Pregnancy class C.

ALBUTEROL (PROVENTIL, VENTOLIN)

Classification: Bronchodilator, beta agonist.

Action: Binds and stimulates beta$_2$ receptors, resulting in relaxation of bronchial smooth muscle.

Indications: Asthma, bronchitis with bronchospasm, and COPD.

Adverse Effects: Hyperglycemia, hypokalemia, palpitations, sinus tachycardia, anxiety, tremor, nausea/vomiting, throat irritation, dry mouth, hypertension, dyspepsia, insomnia, headache, epistaxis, paradoxical bronchospasm.

Contraindications: Angioedema, sensitivity to albuterol or levalbuterol. Use with caution in lactating patients, cardiovascular disorders, cardiac arrhythmias.

© Joseph Gaul/Alamy Stock Photo.

Dosage:

Acute Bronchospasm:

- **Adult:**
  - **MDI:** 4 to 8 puffs every 1 to 4 hours may be required.
  - **Nebulizer:** 2.5 to 5 mg every 20 minutes for a maximum of three doses. After the initial three doses, escalate the dose or start a continuous nebulization at 10 to 15 mg/hr.
- **Pediatric:**
  - **MDI:**
    - **4 years and older:** 2 inhalations every 4 to 6 hours; however, in some patients, 1 inhalation every 4 hours is sufficient. More frequent administration or more inhalations are not recommended.
    - **Younger than 4 years:** Administer by nebulization.
  - **Nebulizer:**
    - **Older than 12 years:** The dose for a continuous nebulization is 0.5 mg/kg per hour.
    - **Younger than 12 years:** 0.63 to 2.5 mg every 20 minutes for a maximum of three doses. Alternatively, continuous nebulization at 0.5 mg/kg per hour can be delivered to children younger than 12 years.

Asthma in Pregnancy:

- **MDI:** Two inhalations every 4 hours. In acute exacerbation, start with 2 to 4 puffs every 20 minutes.

(continues)

ALBUTEROL (PROVENTIL, VENTOLIN)   *(continued)*

- **Nebulizer:** 2.5 mg (0.5 mL) by 0.5% nebulization solution. Place 0.5 mL of the albuterol solution in 2.5 mL of sterile normal saline. Flow is regulated to deliver the therapy over a 5- to 20-minute period. In refractory cases, some physicians order 10 mg nebulized over a 60-minute period.

Special Considerations:
Pregnancy class C.

ALBUTEROL/IPRATROPIUM (COMBIVENT; DUONEB)

Classification: Combination bronchodilator.
Action: Binds and stimulates beta$_2$ receptors, resulting in relaxation of bronchial smooth muscle, and antagonizes the acetylcholine receptor, producing bronchodilation.
Indications: Second-line treatment (if bronchodilator is ineffective) in COPD or severe acute asthma exacerbations during medical transport.
Adverse Effects: Headache, cough, nausea, arrhythmias, paradoxical acute bronchospasm.
Contraindications: Allergy to soybeans or peanuts; known sensitivity to atropine, albuterol, or their respective derivatives. Used with caution in patients with asthma, hypertension, angina, cardiac arrhythmias, tachycardia, cardiovascular disease, congenital long QT syndrome, closed-angle glaucoma.
Dosage:
MDI:

- **Adult:** 8 inhalations every 20 minutes for up to 3 hours.

Nebulization:

- **Adult:** 3 mL every 20 minutes for 3 doses, then as needed.

Special Considerations:
Pregnancy class C.

AMIODARONE (CORDARONE)

Classification: Antiarrhythmic, Class III.
Action: Acts directly on the myocardium to delay repolarization and increase the duration of the action potential.
Indications: Ventricular arrhythmias; second-line agent for atrial arrhythmias.
Adverse Effects: Burning at the IV site, hypotension, bradycardia.
Contraindications: Sick sinus syndrome, second- and third-degree heart block, cardiogenic shock, when episodes of bradycardia have caused syncope, sensitivity to benzyl alcohol and iodine.

© Jones & Bartlett Learning.

Dosage:
Ventricular Fibrillation and Pulseless Ventricular Tachycardia:

- **Adult:** 300 mg IV, IO. May be followed by one dose of 150 mg in 3 to 5 minutes.
- **Pediatric:** 5 mg/kg (max dose: 300 mg); may repeat 5 mg/kg IV, IO up to 15 mg/kg.

AMIODARONE (CORDARONE) *(continued)*

Relatively Stable Patients with Arrhythmias Such as Premature Ventricular Contractions or Wide-Complex Tachycardias with a Strong Pulse:
- **Adult:** 150 mg in 100 mL D_5W IV, IO over a 10-minute period; once return of spontaneous circulation is accomplished, begin an infusion of 1 mg/min for 6 hours, then decrease to 0.5 mg/min; may repeat in 10 minutes up to a maximum dose of 2.2 g over 24 hours.
- **Pediatric:** 5 mg/kg very slow IV, IO (over 20 to 60 minutes); may repeat in 5-mg/kg doses up to 15 mg/kg (max dose: 300 mg).

Special Considerations:
Pregnancy class D.

ANGIOTENSIN-CONVERTING ENZYME (ACE) INHIBITORS: CAPTOPRIL (CAPOTEN), ENALAPRIL (VASOTEC), LISINOPRIL (PRINIVIL, ZESTRIL), RAMIPRIL (ALTACE)

Classification: ACE inhibitors.
Action: Blocks the enzyme responsible for the production of angiotensin II, resulting in a decrease in blood pressure.
Indications: CHF, hypertension, post-MI.
Adverse Effects: Headache, dizziness, fatigue, depression, chest pain, hypotension, palpitations, cough, dyspnea, upper respiratory infection, nausea/vomiting, rash, pruritus, angioedema, renal failure.
Contraindications: Angioedema related to previous treatment with an ACE inhibitor, known sensitivity. Use with caution in aortic stenosis, bilateral renal artery stenosis, hypertrophic obstructive cardiomyopathy, pericardial tamponade, elevated serum potassium levels, acute kidney failure.
Dosage:
- **Adult:** Medication is administered PO. Dosage is individualized.
- **Pediatric:** Medication is administered PO. Dosage is individualized.

Special Considerations:
Pregnancy class D.

ASPIRIN, ASA

Classification: Antiplatelet, nonnarcotic analgesic, antipyretic.
Action: Prevents the formation of a chemical known as thromboxane A2, which causes platelets to clump together, or aggregate, and form plugs that cause obstruction or constriction of small coronary arteries.
Indications: Fever, inflammation, angina, AMI, and patients complaining of pain, pressure, squeezing, or crushing in the chest that may be cardiac in origin.
Adverse Effects: Anaphylaxis, angioedema, bronchospasm, bleeding, stomach irritation, nausea/vomiting.

© ClassicStock/S. FELD/Medical Images.

Contraindications: GI bleeding, active ulcer disease, hemorrhagic stroke, bleeding disorders, children with chickenpox or flulike symptoms, known sensitivity.
Dosage: Note: "Baby aspirin" 81 mg, standard adult aspirin dose 325 mg.

(continues)

ASPIRIN, ASA (continued)

Myocardial Infarction:
- **Adult:** 160 to 325 mg PO (alternatively, four 81-mg baby aspirin are often given), 300-mg rectal suppository.
- **Pediatric:** 3 to 5 mg/kg per day to 5 to 10 mg/kg per day given as a single dose.

Pain or Fever:
- **Adult:** 325 to 650 mg PO (1 to 2 adult tablets) every 4 to 6 hours.
- **Pediatric:** 60 to 90 mg/kg per day in divided doses every 4 to 6 hours.

Special Considerations:
Pregnancy class C except the last 3 months of pregnancy, when aspirin is considered pregnancy class D.

ATENOLOL (TENORMIN)

Classification: Beta adrenergic antagonist, antianginal, antihypertensive, Class II antiarrhythmic.

Action: Inhibits the strength of the heart's contractions and heart rate, resulting in a decrease in cardiac oxygen consumption. Also saturates the beta receptors and inhibits dilation of bronchial smooth muscle (beta$_2$ receptor).

Indications: ACS, hypertension, SVT, atrial flutter, AF.

Adverse Effects: Bradycardia, bronchospasm, hypotension.

Contraindications: Cardiogenic shock, AV block, bradycardia, known sensitivity. Use with caution in hypotension, chronic lung disease (asthma and COPD).

Dosage:

ACS:
- **Adult:** Oral dosing only, not administered acutely for ACS.
- **Pediatric:** Not recommended for pediatric patients.

Special Considerations:
Pregnancy class D.

ATRACURIUM (TRACRIUM)

Classification: Nondepolarizing neuromuscular blocker.

Action: Antagonizes acetylcholine receptors at the motor end plate, producing muscle paralysis.

Indications: Neuromuscular blockade to facilitate ET intubation.

Adverse Effects: Flushing, edema, urticaria, pruritus, bronchospasm and/or wheezing, alterations in heart rate, decrease in blood pressure.

Contraindications: Cardiac disease, electrolyte abnormalities, dehydration, known sensitivity.

Dosage:
- **Adult:** 0.4 to 0.5 mg/kg IV, IO; repeat with 0.08 to 0.1 mg/kg every 20 to 45 minutes as needed for prolonged paralysis.
- **Pediatric:**
  - **Older than 2 years:** Same as adult dosing.
  - **Younger than 2 years:** 0.3 to 0.4 mg/kg IV, IO.

Special Considerations:
Do not give by IM injection.
Pregnancy class C.

ATROPINE SULFATE

Classification: Anticholinergic (antimuscarinic).

Action: Competes reversibly with acetylcholine at the site of the muscarinic receptor. Receptors affected, in order from the most sensitive to the least sensitive, include salivary, bronchial, sweat glands, eye, heart, and GI tract.

Indications: Symptomatic bradycardia, asystole or pulseless electrical activity, nerve agent exposure, organophosphate poisoning.

© Jones & Bartlett Learning.

Adverse Effects: Decreased secretions resulting in dry mouth and hot skin temperature, intense facial flushing, blurred vision or dilation of the pupils with subsequent photophobia, tachycardia, and restlessness. Atropine may cause paradoxical bradycardia if the dose administered is too low or if the drug is administered too slowly.

Contraindications: Acute MI; myasthenia gravis; GI obstruction; closed-angle glaucoma; known sensitivity to atropine, belladonna alkaloids, or sulfites. Will not be effective for infranodal (type II) AV block and new third-degree block with wide QRS complex.

Dosage:

Symptomatic Bradycardia:

- **Adult:** 0.5 mg IV, IO every 3 to 5 minutes to a maximum dose of 3 mg.
- **Adolescent:** 0.02 mg/kg (minimum 0.1 mg/dose; maximum 1 mg/dose) IV, IO up to a total dose of 2 mg.
- **Pediatric:** 0.02 mg/kg (minimum 0.1 mg/dose; maximum 0.5 mg/dose) IV, IO, to a total dose of 1 mg.

Nerve Agent or Organophosphate Poisoning:

- **Adult:** 1 to 6 mg IV, IM; repeat if needed every 5 minutes until symptoms dissipate.
- **Pediatric:** 0.05 mg/kg IV, IM every 10 to 30 minutes as needed until symptoms dissipate.
- **Infants <15 pounds:** 0.05 mg/kg IV, IM every 5 to 20 minutes as needed until symptoms dissipate.

Special Considerations:

Severe organophosphate exposures may require *massive* amounts of atropine, well beyond what is carried in most EMS vehicles.

Half-life is 2.5 hours.

Pregnancy class C; possibly unsafe in lactating mothers.

BIVALIRUDIN (ANGIOMAX)

Classification: Anticoagulant; direct thrombin inhibitor.

Action: Binds with thrombin to inhibit various clotting pathways

Indications: ACS, cardiac surgery.

Adverse Effects: Bleeding, hypotension, hypertension, allergic reactions.

Contraindications: Predisposition to bleeding, aortic aneurysm, peptic ulceration; intracranial hemorrhage.

Dosage:

Cardiac Indications:

- **Adult:** 0.75 mg/kg bolus followed by IV infusion 1.75 mg/kg per hour

Special Considerations:

Rapid onset. Anticoagulant effects subside approximately 1 hour after discontinuing.

Pregnancy class B.

CALCIUM GLUCONATE

Classification: Electrolyte solution.
Action: Counteracts the toxicity of hyperkalemia by stabilizing the membranes of the cardiac cells, reducing the likelihood of fibrillation.
Indications: Hyperkalemia, hypocalcemia, hypermagnesemia.
Adverse Effects: Soft-tissue necrosis, hypotension, bradycardia (if administered too rapidly).
Contraindications: VF, digitalis toxicity, hypercalcemia.
Dosage: Supplied as 10% solution; therefore, each milliliter contains 100 mg of calcium gluconate.

- **Adult:** 500 to 1,000 mg IV, IO administered slowly at a rate of approximately 1 to 1.5 mL/min; maximum dose 3 g IV, IO. It may also be ordered as 60 mg/kg per dose.
- **Pediatric:** 60 to 100 mg/kg IV, IO slowly over a 5- to 10-minute period; maximum dose 3 g IV, IO.

Special Considerations:
Do not administer by IM or subcutaneous routes, which causes significant tissue necrosis.
Pregnancy class C.

CARBAMAZEPINE (TEGRETOL)

Classification: Anticonvulsant, also possesses antidepressant, antimanic, anticholinergic, antiarrhythmic and muscle relaxant properties. It may be prescribed for a wide variety of indications not related to a seizure disorder.

Action: Decreases the spread of the seizure.
Indications: Partial and generalized tonic-clonic seizures.
Adverse Effects: Dizziness, drowsiness, ataxia, nausea/vomiting, blurred vision, confusion, headache, transient diplopia, visual hallucinations, life-threatening rashes.
Contraindications: AV block, bundle branch block, agranulocytosis, bone marrow suppression, monoamine oxidase inhibitor therapy, hypersensitivity to carbamazepine or tricyclic antidepressants. Use with caution in petit mal, atonic, or myoclonic seizures; liver disease; patients with blood dyscrasia caused by drug therapies or blood disorders; patients with a history of cardiac disease; or patients with a history of alcoholism.
Dosage:
- **Adult:** 200 mg PO every 12 hours.
- **Pediatric:**
  - **6 to 12 years:** 100 mg PO twice daily.
  - **Younger than 6 years:** 10 to 20 mg/kg per day PO 2 or 3 times per day.

Special Considerations:
Pregnancy class D.

CLOPIDOGREL (PLAVIX)

© Dr P. Marazzi/Science Source.

Classification: Antiplatelet.
Action: Blocks platelet aggregation by antagonizing the GP IIb/IIIa receptors.
Indications: ACS, chronic coronary and vascular disease, ischemic stroke.
Adverse Effects: Nausea, abdominal pain, and hemorrhage.
Contraindications: History of intracranial hemorrhage, GI bleed or trauma, known sensitivity.
Dosage:
Unstable Angina Pectoris or
Non-Q-Wave AMI:
- **Adult:** Single loading dose of 300 to 600 mg PO followed by a daily dose of 75 mg PO.
- **Pediatric:** Not recommended for pediatric patients.

Special Considerations:
Pregnancy class B.

DEXAMETHASONE (DECADRON)

Classification: Corticosteroid.
Action: Reduces inflammation by multiple mechanisms.
Indications: Anti-inflammatory agent for a wide variety of medical conditions, including asthma, airway edema, acute mountain sickness, cerebral edema, etc.
Adverse Effects: Depression, euphoria, headache, restlessness, hypertension, bradycardia, nausea/vomiting, swelling, diarrhea, weakness, fluid retention, paresthesias.
Contraindications: Fungal infection, known sensitivity (including sulfites). Use with caution in active infections, renal disease, penetrating spinal cord injury.

Dosage:
Numerous dosing options for a wide variety of adult and pediatric indications, including asthma

Special Considerations:
Parenteral formulation may also be administered PO if needed.
Pregnancy class C.

DEXTROSE (50%, 25%, 10%)

Classification: Antihypoglycemic.
Action: Increases blood glucose concentrations.
Indications: Hypoglycemia
Adverse Effects: Hyperglycemia, warmth, burning from IV infusion. Concentrated solutions may cause pain and thrombosis of the peripheral veins.
Contraindications: Intracranial and intraspinal hemorrhage, delirium tremens, solution is not clear, seals are not intact.
Dosage:
Hyperkalemia:
- **Adult:** 25 g of dextrose 50% IV, IO.
- **Pediatric:** 0.5 to 1 g/kg IV, IO.

Hypoglycemia:
- **Adult:** 10 to 25 g of dextrose 50% IV (20 to 50 mL of dextrose solution).
- **Pediatric:**
  - **Older than 2 years:** 2 mL/kg of dextrose 50%.
  - **Younger than 2 years:** 2 to 4 mL/kg of dextrose 10%.

Special Considerations:
Pregnancy class C

DIAZEPAM (VALIUM)

Classification: Benzodiazepine, Schedule C-IV.
Action: Binds to the benzodiazepine receptor and enhances the effects of GABA. Benzodiazepines act at the level of the limbic, thalamic, and hypothalamic regions of the CNS and can produce any level of CNS depression required (including sedation, skeletal muscle relaxation, and anticonvulsant activity).
Indications: Anxiety, skeletal muscle relaxation, alcohol withdrawal, seizures.
Adverse Effects: Respiratory depression, drowsiness, fatigue, headache, pain at the injection site, confusion, nausea, hypotension, oversedation.
Contraindications: Children younger than 6 months, acute-angle glaucoma, CNS depression, alcohol intoxication, known sensitivity.
Dosage:
Anxiety:
- **Adult:**
  - **Moderate:** 2 to 5 mg slow IV, IM.
  - **Severe:** 5 to 10 mg slow IV, IM (administer no faster than 5 mg/min).
  - **Low:** Low dosages are often required for older adults or debilitated patients.
- **Pediatric:** 0.2 to 0.3 mg/kg per dose IV, IM every 4 hours to a maximum dose of 0.6 mg/kg.

Delirium Tremens from Acute Alcohol Withdrawal:
- **Adult:** 10 mg IV

Seizure:
- **Adult:** 5 to 10 mg slow IV, IO every 10 to 15 minutes; maximum total dose 30 mg.
- **Pediatric:**
  - **IV, IO:**
    - **5 years and older:** 1 mg over a 3-minute period every 2 to 5 minutes to a maximum total dose of 10 mg.

DIAZEPAM (VALIUM) *(continued)*

- **Older than 30 days to younger than 5 years:** 0.2 to 0.5 mg over a 3-minute period; may repeat every 2 to 5 minutes to a maximum total dose of 5 mg.
- **Neonate:** 0.1 to 0.3 mg/kg per dose given over a 3- to 5-minute period; may repeat every 15 to 30 minutes to a maximum total dose of 2 mg. (Not a first-line agent due to sodium benzoic acid in the injection.)
- **Rectal administration:** If vascular access is not obtained, diazepam may be administered rectally to children.
  - **12 years and older:** 0.2 mg/kg.
  - **6 to 11 years:** 0.3 mg/kg.
  - **2 to 5 years:** 0.5 mg/kg.
  - **Younger than 2 years:** Not recommended.

Special Considerations:

Make sure that IV, IO lines are well secured. Extravasation of diazepam causes tissue necrosis. Diazepam is insoluble in water and must be dissolved in propylene glycol. This produces a viscous solution; give slowly to prevent pain on injection.

Pregnancy class D.

DIGOXIN (LANOXIN)

Classification: Cardiac glycoside.

Action: Inhibits sodium-potassium-adenosine triphosphatase membrane pump, resulting in an increase in calcium inside the heart muscle cell, which causes an increase in the force of the heart's contraction.

Indications: CHF, to control the ventricular rate in chronic AF and atrial flutter, narrow-complex paroxysmal SVT.

Adverse Effects: Headache, weakness, GI disturbances, arrhythmias, nausea/vomiting, diarrhea, vision disturbances.

Contraindications: Digitalis allergy, VT and VF, heart block, sick sinus syndrome, tachycardia without heart failure, pulse lower than 50 to 60 beats/min, MI, ischemic heart disease, patients with preexcitation AF or atrial flutter (i.e., a delta wave, characteristic of Wolff-Parkinson-White syndrome, visible during normal sinus rhythm).

Dosage: Dosage is individualized.

Special Considerations:

Low levels of serum potassium can lead to digoxin toxicity and bradycardia. Conditions such as administration of steroids or diuretics or vomiting and diarrhea can produce low levels of potassium and subsequent digoxin toxicity.

Pregnancy class C.

DILTIAZEM (CARDIZEM)

Classification: Calcium channel blocker, Class IV antiarrhythmic.
Action: Blocks calcium from moving into the heart muscle cell, which prolongs the conduction of electrical impulses through the AV node.
Indications: Ventricular rate control in rapid AF.
Adverse Effects: Flushing; headache; bradycardia; hypotension; heart block; myocardial depression; severe AV block; and, at high doses, cardiac arrest.
Contraindications: Hypotension, heart block, heart failure.
Dosage:
- **Adult:** Optimum dose is 0.25 mg/kg IV, IO over a 2-minute period to control rapid AF; 20 mg is a reasonable dose for the average adult patient. A second, higher dose of 0.35 mg/kg IV, IO (25 mg is a typical second dose) may be administered over a 2-minute period if rate control is not obtained with the lower dose. For continued reduction in heart rate, a continuous infusion can be started at a dose range of 5 to 15 mg/hr.
- **Pediatric:** Not recommended for pediatric patients.

© Allik Camazine/Alamy Stock Photo.

Special Considerations:
Use with extreme caution in patients who are taking beta blockers because these two drug classes potentiate each other's effects and toxicities.
Patients with a history of heart failure and heart block are at a higher risk for toxicity.
Pregnancy class C.

DIPHENHYDRAMINE HYDROCHLORIDE (BENADRYL)

Classification: Antihistamine.
Action: Binds and blocks H_1 histamine receptors.
Indications: Anaphylactic reactions.
Adverse Effects: Drowsiness, dizziness, headache, excitable state (children), wheezing, thickening of bronchial secretions, chest tightness, palpitations, hypotension, blurred vision, dry mouth, nausea/vomiting, diarrhea.
Contraindications: Acute asthma, which thickens secretions; patients with cardiac histories; known sensitivity.
Dosage:
- **Adult:** 25 to 50 mg IV, IO, IM.
- **Pediatric: 2 to 12 years:** 1 to 1.25 mg/kg IV, IO, IM.

Special Considerations:
Pregnancy class B.

DOBUTAMINE (DOBUTREX)

Classification: Adrenergic agent, inotropic.
Action: Acts primarily as an agonist at $beta_1$ adrenergic receptors with minor $beta_2$ and $alpha_1$ effects. Consequently, dobutamine increases myocardial contractility and stroke volume with minor chronotropic effects, resulting in increased cardiac output.
Indications: CHF, cardiogenic shock.
Adverse Effects: Tachycardia, premature ventricular contractions, hypertension, hypotension, palpitations, arrhythmias.
Contraindications: Suspected or known poisoning/drug-induced shock, systolic blood pressure < 100 mm Hg with signs of shock, idiopathic hypertrophic subaortic stenosis, known sensitivity (including sulfites). Use with caution in hypertension, recent MI, arrhythmias, hypovolemia.

DOBUTAMINE (DOBUTREX) *(continued)*

Dosage:
- **Adult:** Initial 0.5 to 1 mcg/kg per minute IV, IO. Maintenance infusions are typically 2 to 20 mcg/kg per minute. At doses > 20 mcg/kg per minute, increases of heart rate of > 10% may induce or exacerbate myocardial ischemia.
- **Pediatric:** Same as adult dosing.

Special Considerations:
Half-life 2 minutes
Pregnancy class C

DOLASETRON (ANZEMET)

Classification: Antiemetic.
Action: Prevents/reduces nausea/vomiting by binding and blocking a receptor for the brain chemical serotonin.
Indications: Prevent and treat nausea/vomiting.
Adverse Effects: Headache, fatigue, diarrhea, dizziness, abdominal pain, hypotension, hypertension, ECG changes (prolonged PR and QT intervals, widened QRS), bradycardia, tachycardia, syncope.
Contraindications: Known sensitivity. Use with caution in hypokalemia, hypomagnesemia, cardiac arrhythmias.
Dosage:
- **Adult:** 12.5 mg IV, IO.
- **Pediatric: 2 to 16 years:** 0.35 mg/kg IV, IO (max dose: 12.5 mg).

Special Considerations:
Pregnancy class B.

DOPAMINE (INTROPIN)

Classification: Adrenergic agonist, inotropic, vasopressor.
Action: Stimulates alpha and beta adrenergic receptors. At moderate doses (2 to 10 mcg/kg per minute), dopamine stimulates beta$_1$ receptors, resulting in inotropy and increased cardiac output while maintaining dopaminergic-induced vasodilatory effects. At high doses (> 10 mcg/kg per minute), alpha adrenergic agonism predominates, and increased peripheral vascular resistance and vasoconstriction result.
Indications: Hypotension and decreased cardiac output associated with cardiogenic shock and septic shock, hypotension after return of spontaneous circulation following cardiac arrest, symptomatic bradycardia unresponsive to atropine.
Adverse Effects: Tachycardia, arrhythmias, skin and soft tissue necrosis, severe hypertension from excessive vasoconstriction, angina, dyspnea, headache, nausea/vomiting.
Contraindications: Pheochromocytoma, VF, VT, or other ventricular arrhythmias, known sensitivity (including sulfites). Correct any hypovolemia with volume fluid replacement before administering dopamine.

© Jones & Bartlett Learning.

(continues)

DOPAMINE (INTROPIN) *(continued)*

Dosage:
- **Adult:** 2 to 20 mcg/kg per minute IV, IO infusion. Starting dose 5 mcg/kg per minute; may gradually increase the infusion by 5 to 10 mcg/kg per minute to desired effect. Cardiac dose is usually 5 to 10 mcg/kg per minute; vasopressor dose is usually 10 to 20 mcg/kg per minute. Little benefit is gained beyond 20 mcg/kg per minute.
- **Pediatric:** Same as adult dosing.

Special Considerations:
Half-life 2 minutes
Pregnancy class C

ENOXAPARIN (LOVENOX)

Classification: Anticoagulant.
Action: Acts on antithrombin III to reduce the ability of the blood to form clots, thus preventing clot deposition in the coronary arteries; inhibits factor Xa.
Indications: ACS, acute pulmonary embolism, deep venous thrombosis.
Adverse Effects: Bleeding, thrombocytopenia, allergic reactions.
Contraindications: Predisposition to bleeding, aortic aneurysm, peptic ulceration; known sensitivity or history of heparin-induced thrombocytopenia, severe thrombocytopenia, sulfite sensitivity.

Dosage:
Cardiac Indications:
- **Adult:** 30 mg IV × 1, then 1 mg/kg every two hours subcutaneously.
- **Pediatric:** 0.5 to 1.5 mg subcutaneously every 12 hours.

Deep Vein Thrombosis:
- **Adult:** 1 mg/kg every 12 hours.
- **Pediatric:** 0.5 to 1.5 mg subcutaneously every 12 hours.

Special Considerations:
Onset is approximately 3 to 5 hours; duration is approximately 12 hours.
Pregnancy class B.

EPINEPHRINE

Classification: Adrenergic agent, inotropic.
Action: Binds strongly with both alpha and beta receptors, producing increased blood pressure, increased heart rate, bronchodilation.
Indications: Bronchospasm, allergic and anaphylactic reactions, restoration of cardiac activity in cardiac arrest.
Adverse Effects: Anxiety, headache, cardiac arrhythmias, hypertension, nervousness, tremors, chest pain, nausea/vomiting.
Contraindications: Arrhythmias other than VF, asystole, pulseless electrical activity; cardiovascular disease; hypertension; cerebrovascular disease; shock secondary to causes other than anaphylactic shock; closed-angle glaucoma; diabetes; pregnant women in active labor; known sensitivity to epinephrine or sulfites.

© Jones & Bartlett Learning.

Dosage:
Cardiac Arrest:
- **Adult:** 1 mg (1:10,000 solution) IV, IO; may repeat every 3 to 5 minutes.
- **Pediatric:** 0.01 mg/kg (1:10,000 solution) IV, IO; repeat every 3 to 5 minutes as needed (max dose: 1 mg).

EPINEPHRINE   *(continued)*

Symptomatic Bradycardia:
- **Adult:** 2 to 10 mcg per minute (1:10,000 solution) as a continuous IV infusion; usual dosage range: 2 to 10 mcg per minute IV; titrate to effect.
- **Pediatric:** 0.01 mg/kg (1:10,000 solution) IV, IO; may repeat every 3 to 5 minutes (max dose: 1 mg). If giving epinephrine by ET tube, administer 0.1 mg/kg.

Asthma Attacks and Certain Allergic Reactions:
- **Adult:** 0.3 to 0.5 mg (1:1,000 solution) IM or subcutaneous; may repeat every 10 to 15 minutes (max dose: 1 mg).
- **Pediatric:** 0.01 mg/kg (1:1,000 solution) IM or subcutaneous (max dose: 0.5 mg).

Anaphylactic Shock:
- **Adult:** 0.5 mg (1:1,000 solution) IM repeated as needed every 5 to 15 minutes, or transition to IV infusion of 1 to 4 mcg per minute, titrated to effect.
- **Pediatric:** 0.01 mg/kg IM, repeated as needed every 5 to 15 minutes, or transitioned to continuous IV infusion rate of 0.1 to 1 mcg/kg per minute (1:10,000 solution); titrate to response.

Special Considerations:
Half-life 1 minute
Pregnancy class C

© Jones & Bartlett Learning.

EPINEPHRINE AUTOINJECTORS (EPIPEN, EPIPEN JR)

Classification: Adrenergic agonist, inotropic.
Action: Binds strongly with both alpha and beta receptors, producing increased blood pressure, increased heart rate, bronchodilation.
Indications: Anaphylactic shock, certain allergic reactions, asthma attacks.
Adverse Effects: Headaches, nervousness, tremors, arrhythmias, hypertension, chest pain, nausea/vomiting.
Contraindications: Arrhythmias other than VF, asystole, pulseless electrical activity; cardiovascular disease; hypertension; cerebrovascular disease; shock secondary to causes other than anaphylactic shock; closed-angle glaucoma; diabetes; pregnant women in active labor; known sensitivity to epinephrine or sulfites.

© smartstock/iStock Editorial/Getty Images Plus/Getty Images.

Dosage:
- **Adult:** An EpiPen contains 0.3 to 0.5 mg epinephrine to be administered IM into the anterolateral thigh area.
- **Pediatric:** For children weighing <66 pounds (30 kg), an EpiPen Jr delivers 0.15 mg IM.

Special Considerations:
Half-life 1 minute
Pregnancy class C.

EPTIFIBATIDE (INTEGRILIN)

Classification: GP IIb/IIIa inhibitor.
Action: Prevents the aggregation of platelets by binding to the GP IIb/IIIa receptor.
Indications: UA/NSTEMI—to manage medically and for those undergoing percutaneous coronary intervention.
Adverse Effects: Bleeding from the GI tract, internal bleeding, intracranial hemorrhage, hypotension, stroke, anaphylactic shock.
Contraindications: Bleeding from any source, severe uncontrolled hypertension, surgery or trauma within the previous 6 weeks, stroke within the previous 30 days, renal failure, thrombocytopenia.

Dosage:
- **Adult:** Loading dose: 180 mcg/kg IV, IO (max dose: 22.6 mg) over 1 to 2 minutes, then 2 mcg/kg per minute IV, IO infusion (max dose: 15 mg/hr).
- **Pediatric:** No current dosing recommendations exist for pediatric patients.

Special Considerations:
Half-life approximately 90 to 150 minutes
Pregnancy class B.

ESMOLOL (BREVIBLOC)

Classification: Beta adrenergic antagonist, Class II antiarrhythmic.
Action: Inhibits the strength of the heart's contractions, as well as heart rate, resulting in a decrease in cardiac oxygen consumption.
Indications: ACS, MI, acute hypertension, supraventricular tachyarrhythmias, thyrotoxicosis.
Adverse Effects: Hypotension, sinus bradycardia, AV block, cardiac arrest, nausea/vomiting, hypoglycemia, injection site reaction.
Contraindications: Acute bronchospasm, COPD, second- or third-degree heart block, bradycardia, cardiogenic shock, pulmonary edema, sick sinus syndrome, known sensitivity. Use with caution in patients with pheochromocytoma, Prinzmetal's angina, cerebrovascular disease, stroke, poorly controlled diabetes mellitus, hyperthyroidism, thyrotoxicosis, renal disease.

Dosage:
- **Adult:** 500 mcg/kg (0.5 mg/kg) IV, IO over a 1-minute period, followed by a 50-mcg/kg per minute (0.05 mg/kg) infusion over a 4-minute period (maximum total: 200 mcg/kg). If patient response is inadequate, administer a second bolus 500 mcg/kg (0.5 mg/kg) over a 1-minute period, and then increase infusion to 100 mcg/kg per minute. Maximum infusion rate: 300 mcg/kg per minute.
- **Pediatric:** 500 mcg/kg (0.5 mg/kg) IV, IO over a 1-minute period, followed by an infusion at 25 to 200 mcg/kg per minute.

Special Considerations:
Half-life 5 to 9 minutes
Any adverse effects caused by administration of esmolol are brief because of the drug's short half-life.
Resolution of effects usually within 10 to 20 minutes.
Pregnancy class C.

ETOMIDATE (AMIDATE)

Classification: Hypnotic, anesthesia induction agent.

Action: Although the exact mechanism is unknown, etomidate appears to have GABA-like effects.

Indications: Induction for rapid sequence intubation and pharmacologic-assisted intubation, induction of anesthesia.

Adverse Effects: Hypotension, respiratory depression, pain at the site of injection, temporary involuntary muscle movements, frequent nausea/vomiting on emergence, adrenal insufficiency, hyperventilation, hypoventilation, apnea of short duration, hiccups, laryngospasm, snoring, tachypnea, hypertension, cardiac arrhythmias.

Contraindications: Known sensitivity. Use in pregnancy only if the potential benefits justify the potential risk to the fetus. Do not use during labor and avoid in nursing mothers.

Dosage:

- **Adult:** 0.2 to 0.6 mg/kg slow IV, IO (over 30 to 60 seconds); 0.3 mg/kg is used in many protocols/references. A typical adult intubating dose of etomidate is 20 mg slow IV. Consider less (e.g., 10 mg) in older adults or patients with cardiac conditions.
- **Pediatric:**
  - **Older than 10 years:** Same as adult dosing.
  - **Younger than 10 years:** Safety has not been established.

Special Considerations:

Etomidate is used to prepare a patient for orotracheal intubation. Both personnel and equipment must be present to manage the patient's airway before administration.

Pregnancy class C.

FELBAMATE (FELBATOL)

Classification: Anticonvulsant.

Action: Although the mechanism of action is not known, it increases the seizure threshold in absence seizures, and prevents the spread of generalized tonic-clonic and partial seizures. It appears to affect both N-methyl-D-aspartate and GABA function.

Indications: Partial seizures with and without generalization in epileptic adults; partial and generalized seizures associated with Lennox-Gastaut syndrome in children.

Adverse Effects: Nausea/vomiting, suicidal ideation and behavior, depression, insomnia, dyspepsia, upper respiratory tract infection, fatigue, headache, constipation, diarrhea, rhinitis, anxiety, (occasionally fatal) aplastic anemia, photosensitivity.

Contraindications: Blood dyscrasias, hepatic disease, known sensitivity to carbamates.

Dosage: Should be individualized based on condition.

Special Considerations:

Use should be limited to very particular situations. The manufacturer recommends written informed consent prior to initiating therapy.

Pregnancy class C.

FENTANYL CITRATE (SUBLIMAZE)

Classification: Narcotic analgesic, Schedule C-II.
Action: Binds to opiate receptors, producing analgesia and euphoria.
Indications: Pain.
Adverse Effects: Respiratory depression, apnea, hypotension, nausea/vomiting, dizziness, sedation, euphoria, sinus bradycardia, sinus tachycardia, palpitations, hypertension, diaphoresis, syncope, pain at injection site.
Contraindications: Known sensitivity. Use with caution in traumatic brain injury, respiratory depression.

© Joe Amon/Contributor/Denver Post/Getty Images.

Dosage: Note: Dosage should be individualized.
- **Adult:** 50 to 100 mcg/dose (0.05 to 0.1 mg) IM or slow IV, IO (administered over 1 to 2 minutes).
- **Pediatric:** 1 to 2 mcg/kg IM or slow IV, IO (administered over 1 to 2 minutes).

Special Considerations:
Pregnancy class B.

FIBRINOLYTIC: TISSUE PLASMINOGEN ACTIVATOR (TPA)

Classification: Thrombolytic agent.
Action: Dissolves thrombi plugs in the coronary arteries and reestablishes blood flow.
Indications: ST-segment elevation ($\geq$1 mm in two or more contiguous leads), new or presumed-new left bundle branch block.
Adverse Effects: Bleeding, intracranial hemorrhage, stroke, cardiac arrhythmias, hypotension, bruising.
Contraindications: ST-segment depression, cardiogenic shock, recent (within 10 days) major surgery, cerebrovascular disease, recent (within 10 days) GI bleeding, recent trauma, severe hypertension (systolic blood pressure $\geq$180 mm Hg or diastolic blood pressure $\geq$110 mm Hg), high likelihood of left heart thrombus, acute pericarditis, subacute bacterial endocarditis, severe renal or liver failure with bleeding complications, significant liver dysfunction, diabetic hemorrhagic retinopathy, septic thrombophlebitis, advanced age (older than 75 years), patients taking warfarin (Coumadin).
Dosage: Dosing per medical direction.
Special Considerations:
Pregnancy class C.

FLUMAZENIL (ROMAZICON)

Classification: Benzodiazepine receptor antagonist, antidote.
Action: Competes with benzodiazepines for binding at the benzodiazepine receptor, reverses the sedative effects of benzodiazepines.
Indication: Benzodiazepine oversedation.
Adverse Effects: Resedation, seizures, dizziness, pain at injection site, nausea/vomiting, diaphoresis, headache, visual impairment.
Contraindications: Cyclic antidepressant overdose; life-threatening conditions that require treatment with benzodiazepines, such as status epilepticus and intracranial hypertension; known sensitivity to flumazenil or benzodiazepines. Use with caution where there is the possibility of unrecognized benzodiazepine dependence and in patients who have a history of substance abuse, who are known substance abusers, or have a history of seizures.

FLUMAZENIL (ROMAZICON)   *(continued)*

Dosage:
- **Adult:** Initial dose is 0.2 mg IV, IO over a 15-second period. If the desired effect is not observed after 45 seconds, administer a second 0.2-mg dose, again over a 15-second period. Doses can be repeated a total of four times until a total dose of 1 mg has been administered.
- **Pediatric:** Children older than 1 year, 0.01 mg/kg IV, IO given over a 15-second period. May repeat in 45 seconds and then every minute to a maximum cumulative dose of 0.05 mg/kg or 1 mg, whichever is the lower dose.

Special Considerations:
Monitor for signs of hypoventilation and hypoxia for approximately 2 hours.
If the half-life of the benzodiazepine is longer than flumazenil, an additional dose may be needed.
May precipitate withdrawal symptoms in patients dependent on benzodiazepines.
Flumazenil has not been shown to benefit patients who have overdosed on multiple drugs.
Pregnancy class C.

FOSPHENYTOIN (CEREBYX)

Classification: Anticonvulsant.
Action: Depresses seizures by affecting the movement of sodium and calcium into neural tissue.
Indications: Generalized tonic-clonic seizures.
Adverse Effects: Depression of cardiac conduction, sedation, nystagmus, delirium, tremors, ataxia, dysarthria, hypertension, hypotension, pain or irritation at injection site.
Contraindications: Sinus bradycardia, sinoatrial block, second- and third-degree heart block, Adams-Stokes syndrome, known sensitivity to hydantoins.
Dosage:

- **Adult and Pediatric:** Dosing is ordered in *milligram phenytoin equivalents* (PE) rather than in milligrams. Administer 15 to 20 mg PE/kg IV, IO, administered at a rate of <150 PE/min.

Special Considerations:
Continuously monitor the ECG and blood pressure during administration. Monitor IV site for signs of infiltration.
Pregnancy class D.

FUROSEMIDE (LASIX)

Classification: Loop diuretic.
Action: Inhibits the absorption of the sodium and chloride ions and water in the loop of Henle, as well as the convoluted tubule of the nephron. This results in decreased absorption of water and increased production of urine.
Indications: Pulmonary edema, CHF, hypertensive emergency.
Adverse Effects: Vertigo, dizziness, weakness, orthostatic hypotension, hypokalemia, thrombophlebitis. Patients with anuria, severe renal failure, untreated hepatic coma, increasing azotemia, and electrolyte depletion can develop life-threatening consequences.
Contraindications: Known sensitivity to sulfonamides or furosemide.

(continues)

FUROSEMIDE (LASIX) (continued)

Dosage:
Congestive Heart Failure and Pulmonary Edema:
- **Adult:** 20 to 40 mg IV, IO administered slowly over a 1- to 2-minute period. Begin with 40 mg in emergent situations. If a satisfactory response is not achieved within 1 hour, an additional dose of 80 mg can be given. A maximum single IV dose is 160 to 200 mg.
- **Pediatric:** 1 mg/kg IV, IO, or IM. If the response is not satisfactory, an additional dose of 2 mg/kg may be administered no sooner than 2 hours after the first dose.

Hypertensive Emergency:
- **Adult:** 40 mg IV, IO.
- **Pediatric:** 1 mg/kg IV or IM.

Special Considerations:
Onset of action for IV, IO administration occurs within 5 minutes and will peak within 30 minutes. Furosemide is a diuretic, so the patient will likely have urinary urgency. Be prepared to help the patient void.
Pregnancy class C.

GABAPENTIN (NEURONTIN)

Classification: Anticonvulsant.
Action: The exact mechanism of action has not been determined.
Indications: Seizures, neuropathic pain syndromes.
Adverse Effects: Dizziness, ataxia, sleepiness, gait disturbances, upset stomach, peripheral edema.
Contraindications: Known sensitivity. Use with caution in elderly patients, renal impairment.

© Christine Whitehead/Alamy Stock Photo.

Dosage:
- **Adult:** 300 to 1,800 mg PO daily.
- **Pediatric:**
  - **5 to 12 years:** Up to 35 mg/kg per day PO divided in three divided doses daily.
  - **3 to 4 years:** 10 to 15 mg/kg per day PO divided in three divided doses daily.

Special Considerations:
Pregnancy class C.

GLUCAGON

Classification: Hormone.
Action: Converts glycogen to glucose.
Indications: Hypoglycemia, beta blocker overdose.
Adverse Effects: Nausea/vomiting, rebound hyperglycemia, hypotension, sinus tachycardia.
Contraindications: Pheochromocytoma, insulinoma, known sensitivity.

Dosage:
Hypoglycemia:
- **Adult:** 1 mg IM, IV, IO, or subcutaneous.
- **Pediatric (<44 pounds [20 kg]):** 0.5 mg IM, IV, IO, or subcutaneous.

Beta Blocker Overdose:
- **Adult:** 3 to 10 mg IV, IO over a 1-minute period, followed by a second dose of 10 mg IV
  (or IV infusion 3 to 5 mg/hr) if the symptoms of bradycardia and

GLUCAGON   *(continued)*

hypotension recur. (Note that this dose is much higher than the dose required to treat hypoglycemia; avoid using the supplied glycerin-based reconstitution solution when larger doses of glucagon are being administered.)

- **Pediatric:** For patients weighing <44 pounds (20 kg), the dose is 0.5 mg.

Special Considerations:
Pregnancy class B.

HALOPERIDOL (HALDOL)

Classification: Antipsychotic agent.
Action: Selectively blocks postsynaptic dopamine receptors.
Indications: Psychotic disorders, agitation.
Adverse Effects: Extrapyramidal symptoms, drowsiness, tardive dyskinesia, hypotension, hypertension, VT, sinus tachycardia, QT prolongation, torsades de pointes.
Contraindications: Depressed mental status, Parkinson disease.
Dosage:

- **Adult:**
  - **Mild agitation:** 0.5 to 2 mg PO or IM.
  - **Moderate agitation:** 5 to 10 mg PO or IM.
  - **Severe agitation:** 10 mg PO or IM.
- **Pediatric:** 1 to 5 mg IM or PO for acute psychosis or agitation.

Special Considerations:
IV use is considered "off-label" although it is used routinely in many settings. Consult department protocols or state/regional guidelines prior to administering. Monitor ECG if administered IV.
Pregnancy class C.

HEPARIN (UNFRACTIONATED HEPARIN)

Classification: Anticoagulant.
Action: Acts on antithrombin III to reduce the ability of the blood to form clots, thus preventing clot deposition in the coronary arteries.
Indications: ACS, acute pulmonary embolism, deep venous thrombosis.
Adverse Effects: Bleeding, thrombocytopenia, allergic reactions.
Contraindications: Predisposition to bleeding, aortic aneurysm, peptic ulceration; known sensitivity or history of heparin-induced thrombocytopenia, severe thrombocytopenia, sulfite sensitivity.
Dosage:
Cardiac Indications:

- **Adult:** 60 units/kg IV (max 4,000 units), followed by 12 units/kg per hour (max 1,000 units). Once in the hospital, additional dosing is determined based on laboratory blood tests.
- **Pediatric:** 75 units/kg followed by 20 units/kg per hour.

Pulmonary Embolism and Deep Vein Thrombosis:

- **Adult:** 80 units/kg IV, followed by 18 units/kg per hour.
- **Pediatric:** 75 units/kg IV followed by 20 units/kg per hour.

Special Considerations:
Half-life approximately 90 minutes
Pregnancy class C.

HMG COENZYME A STATINS: ATORVASTATIN (LIPITOR), FLUVASTATIN (LESCOL), LOVASTATIN (MEVACOR), PRAVASTATIN (PRAVACHOL), ROSUVASTATIN (CRESTOR), SIMVASTATIN (ZOCOR))

Classification: HMG-CoA reductase inhibitors (statins).

Action: Reduces the level of circulating total cholesterol, low-density lipoprotein cholesterol, and serum triglycerides; reduces the incidence of reinfarction, recurrent angina, rehospitalization, and stroke when initiated within a few days after onset of ACS.

Indications: ACS/AMI prophylaxis, hypercholesterolemia, hyperlipoproteinemia, hypertriglyceridemia, stroke prophylaxis.

Adverse Effects: Constipation, flatulence, dyspepsia, abdominal pain, infection, headache, flu-like symptoms, back pain, allergic reaction, asthenia, diarrhea, sinusitis, pharyngitis, rash, arthralgia, nausea/vomiting, myopathy, myasthenia, renal failure, rhabdomyolysis, chest pain, bronchitis, rhinitis, insomnia.

Contraindications: Active hepatic disease, pregnancy, breastfeeding, rhabdomyolysis.

Dosage:
- **Adult:** Medication is administered PO. Dosage is individualized.
- **Pediatric:** Safe use has not been established.

Special Considerations:
Pregnancy class X.

HYDRALAZINE (APRESOLINE)

Classification: Antihypertensive agent, vasodilator.

Action: Directly dilates the peripheral blood vessels.

Indications: Hypertension associated with preeclampsia and eclampsia, hypertensive crisis.

Adverse Effects: Headache, angina, flushing, palpitations, reflex tachycardia, anorexia, nausea/vomiting, diarrhea, hypotension, syncope, peripheral vasodilation, peripheral edema, fluid retention, paresthesias.

Contraindications: Patients taking diazoxide or MAOIs, coronary artery disease, stroke, angina, dissecting aortic aneurysm, mitral valve and rheumatic heart diseases.

Dosage:

Preeclampsia and Eclampsia:
- **Adult:** 5 to 10 mg IV. Repeat every 20 to 30 minutes until systolic blood pressure of 90 to 105 mm Hg is attained.

Acute Hypertension Not Associated with Preeclampsia:
- **Adult:** 10 to 20 mg IV, or IM.
- **Pediatric:**
  - **1 month to 12 years:** 0.1 to 0.2 mg/kg IV or IM every 4 to 6 hours as needed (max: 20 mg/dose).

Special Considerations:
Pregnancy class C.

HYDROCORTISONE SODIUM SUCCINATE (CORTEF, SOLU-CORTEF)

Classification: Corticosteroid.
Action: Reduces inflammation by multiple mechanisms. As a steroid, it replaces the steroids that are lacking in adrenal insufficiency.
Indications: Adrenal insufficiency, allergic reactions, anaphylaxis, asthma, COPD.
Adverse Effects: Leukocytosis, hyperglycemia, increased infection, decreased wound healing, increased rate of death from sepsis.
Contraindications: Cushing syndrome, known sensitivity to benzyl alcohol. Use with caution in diabetes, hypertension, CHF, known systemic fungal infection, renal disease, idiopathic thrombocytopenia, psychosis, seizure disorder, GI disease, glaucoma, known sensitivity.
Dosage:
Anaphylactic Shock:
- **Adult:** 100 to 500 mg IV, IO, or IM.
- **Pediatric:** 2 to 10 mg/kg per day IV, IO, or IM (max: 500 mg).
Special Considerations:
Pregnancy class C.

HYPERTONIC SALINE (3% SALINE)

Classification: Volume expander, electrolyte solution.
Action: The hypertonic nature of this fluid pulls extravascular fluid into the vascular space. Hypertonic saline may therefore be used as a volume expander in cases of hypovolemia or to reduce the edema of the swollen brain. Three percent saline has an electrolyte concentration of 514 mEq/L sodium.
Indications: Reduction of increased ICP resulting from traumatic brain injury, hypovolemic shock.
Adverse Effects: Increased rate of bleeding, alteration of blood-clotting ability, osmotic demyelination syndrome.
Contraindications: Pulmonary congestion, pulmonary edema, known sensitivity. Hypertonic saline should not be administered by the IO route.
Dosage: Note: Hypertonic saline is available in several concentrations from 3% to 5%.
- **Adult:** 100 to 200 mL/hr
- **Pediatric:** 0.1 to 1 mL/kg per hour (off-label for most pediatric indications; consult with online medical control)
Special Considerations:
Hypertonic saline can cause damage to the vein in which it is administered.
Pregnancy class C.

IBUPROFEN

Classification: NSAID.
Action: Inhibits prostaglandin synthesis by inhibiting cyclooxygenase isoenzymes, resulting in analgesic, antipyretic, and anti-inflammatory effects.
Indications: Mild to moderate pain, fever, osteoarthritis, rheumatoid arthritis.
Adverse Effects: Anorexia, nausea/vomiting, epigastric/abdominal pain, dyspepsia, constipation, diarrhea, gastritis, melena, flatulence, headache, dizziness.

(continues)

IBUPROFEN

(continued)

Contraindications: Sensitivity to NSAID or salicylate. Use with caution in asthma, hepatic disease, renal disease, CHF, hypertension, cardiac disease, cardiomyopathy, cardiac arrhythmias, significant coronary artery disease, peripheral vascular disease, cerebrovascular disease, fluid retention, or edema.

Dosage:

Mild to Moderate Pain:

- **Adult:** 400 mg PO every 4 hours as needed, not to exceed 1,200 mg/day.
- **Pediatric: 6 months to 12 years:** 5 to 10 mg/kg PO every 6 to 8 hours as needed, not to exceed 40 mg/kg per day.

Fever:

- **Adult:** 200 to 400 mg PO every 4 to 6 hours as needed, not to exceed 1,200 mg/day.
- **Pediatric: 6 months to 12 years:** 5 mg/kg PO if baseline temperature is less than 102.5°F (39°C), or 10 mg/kg PO if baseline temperature is greater than 102.5°F (39°C) (max dose: 40 mg/kg per day).

Osteoarthritis or Rheumatoid Arthritis:

- **Adult:** 400 to 800 mg PO 3 to 4 times per day, not to exceed 3,200 mg/day.
- **Pediatric: 1 to 12 years:** 30 to 40 mg/kg per day PO in 3 to 4 divided doses, not to exceed 50 mg/kg per day.

Special Considerations:
Pregnancy class B.

© digitalreflections/Shutterstock.

INSULIN, REGULAR (HUMULIN R, NOVOLIN R)

Classification: Hormone.

Action: Binds to a receptor on the membrane of cells and facilitates the transport of glucose into cells.

Indications: Hyperglycemia, insulin-dependent diabetes mellitus, hyperkalemia.

Adverse Effects: Hypoglycemia, tachycardia, palpitations, diaphoresis, anxiety, confusion, blurred vision, weakness, depression, seizures, coma, insulin shock, hypokalemia.

Contraindications: Hypoglycemia, known sensitivity.

Dosage:

Diabetic Ketoacidosis:

- **Adult:** 0.1 U/kg IV, IO, or subcutaneous.
  Because of poor perfusion of the peripheral tissues, subcutaneous administration is much less effective than the IV, IO route. IV, IO insulin has a very short half-life; therefore, IV, IO insulin without an infusion is not that effective. The rate for an insulin infusion is 0.05 to 0.1 U/kg per hour IV, IO. When dosing insulin, use a U-100 insulin syringe to measure and deliver the insulin. The time from administration to action, as well as the duration of action, varies greatly among different people, as well as at different times in the same person.

Hyperkalemia:

- **Adult:** 10 U IV, IO of regular insulin (Insulin R), coadministered with 50 mL of $D_{50}W$ over 5 minutes.
- **Pediatric:** 0.1 U/kg Insulin R IV, IO.

Special Considerations:
Only regular insulin can be given IV, IO.
Pregnancy class B.

IPRATROPIUM BROMIDE (ATROVENT)

Classification: Bronchodilator, anticholinergic.
Action: Antagonizes the acetylcholine receptor on bronchial smooth muscle, producing bronchodilation.
Indications: Asthma, bronchospasm associated with COPD.
Adverse Effects: Paradoxical acute bronchospasm, cough, throat irritation, headache, dizziness, dry mouth, palpitations.
Contraindications: Closed-angle glaucoma, bladder neck obstruction, prostatic hypertrophy, known sensitivity including peanuts or soybeans and atropine or atropine derivatives.
Dosage:
MDI:

- **Adult:** 8 inhalations every 20 minutes for up to 3 hours.
- · **Pediatric: <12 years:** 4 to 8 inhalations every 20 minutes for up to 3 hours.

Nebulization:

- **Adult:** 0.5 mg every 20 minutes for 3 doses, then as needed.
- **Pediatric: 5 to 14 years:** 0.25 to 0.5 mg every 20 minutes for 3 doses as needed.

Special Considerations:
Ipratropium bromide is not typically used as a sole medication in the treatment of acute exacerbation of asthma. Ipratropium bromide is commonly administered after a beta agonist.
Care should be taken to not allow the aerosol spray (especially in the MDI) to come into contact with the eyes. This can cause temporary blurring of vision that resolves without intervention within 4 hours.
Pregnancy class B.

Image label: NDC 12345-678-90 — Ipratropium Inhalation Aerosol — Rx only — (Ipratropium bromide HFA) — Each actuation delivers 17 mcg ipratropium bromide from the mouthpiece. — 12.9 grams — 200 metered actuations — with Dose indicator — LOT — EXP

KETAMINE (KETALAR)

Classification: General anesthetic, analgesic, sedative.
Action: Produces a state of anesthesia while maintaining airway reflexes, heart rate, and blood pressure.
Indications: Pain and as anesthesia for procedures of short duration.
Adverse Effects: Emergence phenomena, hypertension and sinus tachycardia, hypotension and sinus bradycardia, other cardiac arrhythmias (rare), respiratory depression, apnea, laryngospasms and other forms of airway obstruction (rare), tonic-clonic movements, vomiting.
Contraindications: Patients in whom a significant elevation in blood pressure would be hazardous (hypertension, stroke, head trauma, increased intracranial mass or bleeding, MI). Use with caution in patients with increased ICP or increased intraocular pressure (glaucoma) and patients with hypovolemia, dehydration, or cardiac disease (especially angina and CHF).

© Julia Hiebaum/Alamy Stock Photo.

Dosage: Administer slowly over a period of 60 seconds.
IV, IO:

- **Adult:** 1 to 4.5 mg/kg IV, IO. 1 to 2 mg/kg produces anesthesia usually within 30 seconds that typically lasts 5 to 10 minutes.
- **Pediatric:** 0.5 to 2 mg IV, IO over a 1-minute period.

IM:

- **Adult:** 6.5 to 13 mg/kg IM. 10 mg/kg IM is capable of producing anesthesia within 3 to 4 minutes with an effect typically lasting 12 to 25 minutes. In adults, concomitant administration of 5 to 15 mg of diazepam reduces the incidence of emergence phenomena.
- **Pediatric:** 4 to 5 mg/kg IM.

Special Considerations:
Pregnancy class C.

KETOROLAC (TORADOL)

Classification: NSAID.
Action: Inhibits the production of prostaglandins in inflamed tissue, which decreases the responsiveness of pain receptors.
Indications: Moderately severe acute pain.
Adverse Effects: Headache, drowsiness, dizziness, abdominal pain, dyspepsia, nausea/vomiting, diarrhea.
Contraindications: Patients with a history of peptic ulcer disease or GI bleed, patients with renal insufficiency, hypovolemic patients, pregnancy (third trimester), nursing mothers, allergy to aspirin or other NSAIDs, stroke or suspected stroke or head trauma, need for major surgery in the immediate or near future (i.e., within 7 days).
Dosage: For patients weighing <110 pounds (50 kg) and/or aged ≥65 years refer to older adult dosing.

© Allik Camazine/Alamy Stock Photo.

- **Adult:**
  - **IV:** 30 mg a single dose or 30 mg every 6 hours not to exceed a maximal total daily dose of 120 mg.
  - **IM:** 60 mg as a single dose or 30 mg every 6 hours not to exceed a maximal total daily dose of 120 mg.
- **Older adult (age ≥65 years or weight <110 pounds [50 kg]):**
  - **IV:** 15 mg as a single dose or 15 mg every 6 hours not to exceed a maximal total daily dose of 60 mg.
  - **IM:** 30 mg as a single dose or 15 mg every 6 hours not to exceed a maximal dose of 60 mg.

For patients with moderate renal impairment, administer half the recommended doses, not to exceed a total daily dose of 60 mg/day IV or IM.
Special Considerations:
Pregnancy class C; class D in third trimester.

LABETALOL (NORMODYNE, TRANDATE)

Classification: Beta adrenergic antagonist, antianginal, antihypertensive.
Action: Binds with both the beta$_1$ and beta$_2$ receptors and alpha$_1$ receptors in vascular smooth muscle. Inhibits the strength of the heart's contractions, as well as heart rate. This results in a decrease in cardiac oxygen consumption.
Indications: ACS, SVT, severe hypertension.
Adverse Effects: Usually mild and transient; hypotensive symptoms, nausea/vomiting, bronchospasm, arrhythmia, bradycardia, AV block.

Labetalol Hydrochloride

Injection, USP

20 mL Multi-Dose vial

100 mg/20 mL (5 mg/mL)
For Intravenous Injection Only
Sterile   NDC 12345-678-90

Rx only

Contraindications: Hypotension, cardiogenic shock, acute pulmonary edema, heart failure, severe bradycardia, sick sinus syndrome, second- or third-degree heart block, asthma or acute bronchospasm, cocaine-induced ACS, known sensitivity. Use caution in pheochromocytoma, cerebrovascular disease or stroke, poorly controlled diabetes, with hepatic disease. Use with caution at lowest effective dose in chronic lung disease.
Dosage:
Cardiac Indications: Note: Monitor blood pressure and heart rate closely during administration.
- **Adult:** 10 mg IV, IO over a 1- to 2-minute period. May repeat every 10 minutes to a maximum dose of 150 mg or give initial bolus and then follow with infusion at 2 to 8 mg per minute.
- **Pediatric:** 0.4 to 1 mg/kg per hour to a maximum dosage of 3 mg/kg per hour.

LABETALOL (NORMODYNE, TRANDATE)

(continued)

Severe Hypertension:

- **Adult:** Initial dose is 20 mg IV, IO slow infusion over a 2-minute period. After the initial dose, blood pressure should be checked every 5 minutes. Repeat doses can be given at 10-minute intervals. The second dose should be 40 mg IV, IO, and subsequent doses should be 80 mg IV, IO, to a maximum total dose of 300 mg. The effect on blood pressure typically will occur within 5 minutes from the time of administration. Alternatively, may be administered via IV infusion at 2 mg per minute to a total maximum dose of 300 mg.
- **Pediatric:** 0.4 to 1 mg/kg per hour IV, IO infusion with a maximum dose of 3 mg/kg per hour.

Special Considerations:
Pregnancy class C

LAMOTRIGINE (LAMICTAL)

Classification: Anticonvulsant, antimanic agent.
Action: The exact mechanism of action has not been determined. Studies suggest lamotrigine stabilizes neuronal membranes by acting at voltage-sensitive sodium channels, thereby decreasing presynaptic release of glutamate and aspartate, resulting in decreased seizure activity.

Lamotrigine Tablets USP	NDC 12345-678-90 Rx only **100 mg**
Each uncoated tablet contains: Lamotrigine USP 100 mg Dispense in a tight container as defined in the USP. Store at 20°–25°C (68°–77°F); excursion permitted to 15°–30°C (59°–86°F) [see USP Controlled Room Temperature]. PHARMACIST: Dispense the accompanying Medication Guide to each patient.	**30 Tablets**
LOT EXP	See package outsert for Dosage & Administration.

Indications: Seizures, bipolar disorders.
Adverse Effects: Headache, dizziness, nausea/vomiting, ataxia, diplopia, severe skin rash, amnesia, abnormal thoughts, speech and depression.
Contraindications: Known sensitivity.
Dosage:

- **Adult:** Medication is administered PO. Dosage is individualized.
- **Pediatric:** Medication is administered PO. Dosage is individualized.

Special Considerations:
Pregnancy class C.

LEVALBUTEROL (XOPENEX)

Classification: Beta agonist.
Action: Stimulates beta$_2$ receptors, resulting in relaxation of the smooth muscle in the lungs, uterus, and vasculature that supply skeletal muscle.
Indications: Acute bronchospasm or bronchospasm prophylaxis in patient with asthma.

Levalbuterol tartrate HFA Inhalation Aerosol **45 mcg/actuation**	NDC 12345-678-90 Net Contents 15g
Contents: Each actuation delivers from the mouthpiece a suspension of 59 mcg of micronized levalbuterol tartrate equivalent to 45 mcg levelbuterol in propellant (HFA-134a) dehydrated alcohol USP, and oleic acid NF.	
FOR ORAL INHALATION WITH *Xopenex HFA* ACTUATOR ONLY	**200** metered inhalations
LOT EXP	

Adverse Effects: Hyperglycemia, hypokalemia, palpitations, sinus tachycardia, anxiety, tremor, nausea/vomiting, throat irritation, hypertension, dyspepsia, insomnia, headache.
Contraindications: Angioedema, sensitivity to albuterol or levalbuterol. Use with caution in lactating patients, cardiovascular disorders, cardiac arrhythmias. Do not use in patients taking phenothiazines because this may cause prolonged QT interval and cardiac arrhythmias. Also avoid use in patients getting sotalol or other beta blockers because they may decrease bronchodilating effects and cause bronchospasm, prolonged QT interval, and cardiac arrhythmias.

(continues)

LEVALBUTEROL (XOPENEX)

(continued)

Dosage:

MDI:

- **Adult:** 2 inhalations every 4 to 6 hours. In some patients, 1 inhalation may be sufficient. For acute exacerbations, 4 to 8 inhalations every 20 minutes up to 4 hours, then every 1 to 4 hours as needed (off label).
- **Pediatric:**
  - **4 to 12 years:** 2 inhalations every 4 to 6 hours. In some patients, 1 inhalation may be sufficient. For acute exacerbations, 4 to 8 inhalations every 20 minutes for 3 doses, then 2 to 4 inhalations every 1 to 4 hours as needed.
  - **Younger than 4 years:** Safe and effective use has not been established. For acute exacerbations, 2 to 4 inhalations using a valved holding chamber and face mask every 20 minutes for 3 doses, then 2 to 4 inhalations every 1 to 4 hours as needed.

Nebulizer:

- **Adult:** Usually, 0.63 mg 3 times/day. For acute exacerbations, 1.25 to 2.5 mg every 20 minutes for 3 doses, then 1.25 to 5 mg every 1 to 4 hours as needed.
- **Pediatric:**
  - **6 to 11 years:** Usually, 0.31 mg 3 times/day. For acute exacerbations, 0.075 mg/kg (1.25 mg minimum) every 20 minutes for 3 doses, then 0.075 to 0.15 mg/kg (5 mg maximum) every 1 to 4 hours as needed.
  - **Younger than 6 years:** Safe and effective use has not been established. For acute exacerbations, 1.25 to 2.5 mg every 20 minutes for 3 doses, then 1.25 to 5 mg every 1 to 4 hours as needed.

Special Considerations:

Pregnancy class C.

LEVETIRACETAM (KEPPRA)

Classification: Anticonvulsant.

Action: Unknown mechanism, appears to regulate GABA transmission.

Indications: Partial and generalized tonic-clonic seizures.

Adverse Effects: Behavior changes (frequent reason for discontinuation), ataxia, confusion, drowsiness, anorexia, constipation, diarrhea

Contraindications: Hypersensitivity; use in caution in patients prone to emotional or behavioral disorders.

Dosage:

- **Adult:**
  - Status epilepticus: 1,000 to 3,000 mg IV, IO administered over 15 minutes.
  - Oral maintenance: Up to 3,000 mg/day in divided doses.
- **Pediatric:**
  - Status epilepticus: 20 to 60 mg/kg IV/IO, infused at 2 to 5 mg/kg per minute.
  - Oral maintenance: 7 to 10 mg/kg per dose.

Special Considerations:

Pregnancy class C. Monitor emotional and behavioral changes while patients are receiving levetiracetam. Known to cause toxic epidermal necrosis and Stevens-Johnson syndrome.

LIDOCAINE (XYLOCAINE)

Classification: Antiarrhythmic, Class IB.
Action: Blocks sodium channels, increasing the recovery period after repolarization; suppresses automaticity in the His-Purkinje system and depolarization in the ventricles.
Indications: Ventricular arrhythmias, when amiodarone is not available: cardiac arrest from VF/VT, stable monomorphic VT with preserved ventricular function, stable polymorphic VT with normal baseline QT interval and preserved left ventricular function (when ischemia and electrolyte imbalance are treated), stable polymorphic VT with baseline QT prolongation suggestive of torsades de pointes.

> **2%** **Lidocaine**
> HCl Injection, USP
> 1,000 mg per 50 mL
> For Infiltration and Nerve Block.
> Methylparaben as preservative
> Not for Caudal or Epidural Use.
> 25 × 50 mL.
> Multiple-Dose Vials
> **(20 mg/mL)** **Rx only**

Adverse Effects: Toxicity (signs may include anxiety, apprehension, euphoria, nervousness, disorientation, dizziness, blurred vision, facial paresthesias, tremors, hearing disturbances, slurred speech, seizures, sinus bradycardia), seizures without warning, cardiac arrhythmias, hypotension, cardiac arrest, pain at injection site.
Contraindications: AV block; bleeding; thrombocytopenia; known sensitivity to lidocaine, sulfite, or paraben. Use with caution in bradycardia, hypovolemia, cardiogenic shock, Adams-Stokes syndrome, Wolff-Parkinson-White syndrome.
Dosage:
Pulseless Ventricular Tachycardia and Ventricular Fibrillation:
- **Adult IV, IO:** 1 to 1.5 mg/kg IV, IO; may repeat at half the original dose (0.5 to 0.75 mg/kg) every 5 to 10 minutes to a maximum dose of 3 mg/kg. If a maintenance infusion is warranted, the rate is 1 to 4 mg/min.
- **Pediatric IV, IO:** 1 mg/kg IV, IO (maximum: 100 mg). If a maintenance infusion is warranted, the rate is 20 to 50 mcg/kg per minute.

Perfusing Ventricular Rhythms:
- **Adult:** 0.5 to 0.75 mg/kg IV, IO (up to 1 to 1.5 mg/kg may be used). Repeat 0.5 to 0.75 mg/kg every 5 to 10 minutes to a maximum total dose of 3 mg/kg. A maintenance infusion of 1 to 4 mg/min (30 to 50 mcg/kg per minute) is acceptable.
- **Pediatric:** 1 mg/kg IV, IO. May repeat every 5 to 10 minutes to a maximum dose of 3 mg/kg. Maintenance infusion rate is 20 to 50 mcg/kg per minute.

Special Considerations:
Half-life approximately 90 minutes.
Pregnancy class B.

LORAZEPAM (ATIVAN)

Classification: Benzodiazepine, Schedule C-IV.
Action: Binds to the benzodiazepine receptor and enhances the effects of the brain chemical GABA, an inhibitory transmitter, and may result in a state of sedation, hypnosis, skeletal muscle relaxation, anticonvulsant activity, coma.
Indications: Preprocedure sedation induction, anxiety, status epilepticus.
Adverse Effects: Headache, drowsiness, ataxia, dizziness, amnesia, depression, dysarthria, euphoria, syncope, fatigue, tremor, vertigo, respiratory depression, paradoxical CNS stimulation.
Contraindications: Known sensitivity to lorazepam, benzodiazepines, polyethylene glycol, propylene glycol, or benzyl alcohol; COPD; sleep apnea (except while being mechanically ventilated); shock; coma; acute closed-angle glaucoma.

© Scott Camazine/Science Source.

(continues)

LORAZEPAM (ATIVAN)

(continued)

Dosage: Note: IV, IO lorazepam needs to be administered slowly.
Analgesia and Sedation:
- **Adult:** 2 mg or 0.44 mg/kg IV, IO, whichever is smaller. This dosage will provide adequate sedation in most patients and should not be exceeded in patients older than 50 years.
- **Pediatric:** 0.05 mg/kg IV, IO. Each dose should not exceed 2 mg IV, IO.

Seizures:
- **Adult:** 2 mg to 4 mg IV, IO given over 2 to 5 minutes; may repeat in 10 to 15 minutes (max total dose: 8 mg in a 12-hour period).
- **Pediatric:** 0.1 mg/kg slow IV, IO given over 2 to 5 minutes (max single dose: 4 mg). May repeat at half the original dose in 10 to 15 minutes if seizure activity resumes.

Special Considerations:
Be prepared to support the patient's airway and ventilation.
Pregnancy class D.

MAGNESIUM SULFATE

Classification: Electrolyte, tocolytic, mineral.
Action: Required for normal physiologic functioning. Magnesium is a cofactor in neurochemical transmission and muscular excitability. Magnesium sulfate controls seizures by blocking peripheral neuromuscular transmission. Magnesium is also a peripheral vasodilator and an inhibitor of platelet function.
Indications: Torsades de pointes, cardiac arrhythmias associated with hypomagnesemia, eclampsia and seizure prophylaxis in preeclampsia, status asthmaticus.

Adverse Effects: Magnesium toxicity (signs include flushing, diaphoresis, hypotension, muscle paralysis, weakness, hypothermia, and cardiac, CNS, or respiratory depression).
Contraindications: AV block, GI obstruction. Use with caution in renal impairment.
Dosage:
Pulseless Ventricular Fibrillation/Ventricular Tachycardia with Torsades de Pointes or Hypomagnesemia:
- **Adult:** 1 to 2 g in 10 mL D$_5$W IV, IO administered over 15 minutes or faster with cardiac arrest.
- **Pediatric:** 25 to 50 mg/kg IV, IO over 10 to 20 minutes; may administer faster for torsades de pointes (max single dose: 2 g).

Torsades de Pointes with a Pulse or Cardiac Arrhythmias with Hypomagnesemia:
- **Adult:** 1 to 2 g in 50 to 100 mL D$_5$W IV, IO administered over 5 to 60 minutes. Follow with 0.5 to 1 g/hr IV, IO titrated to control torsades de pointes.
- **Pediatric:** 25 to 50 mg/kg IV, IO over 10 to 20 minutes (max single dose: 2 g).

Eclampsia and Seizure Prophylaxis in Preeclampsia:
- **Adult:** 4 to 6 g IV, IO over 20 to 30 minutes, followed by an infusion of 1 to 2 g/hr.

Status Asthmaticus:
- **Adult:** 1.2 to 2 g slow IV, IO (over 20 minutes).
- **Pediatric:** 25 to 50 mg/kg (diluted in D$_5$W) slow IV, IO (over 10 to 20 minutes).

Special Considerations:
Pregnancy class A.

MANNITOL (OSMITROL)

Classification: Osmotic diuretic.

Action: Facilitates the flow of fluid out of tissues (including the brain) and into interstitial fluid and blood, thereby dehydrating the brain and reducing swelling. Reabsorption by the kidney is minimal, consequently increasing urine output.

Indications: Increased ICP.

Adverse Effects: Pulmonary edema, headache, blurred vision, dizziness, seizures, hypovolemia, nausea/vomiting, diarrhea, electrolyte imbalances, hypotension, hypertension, sinus tachycardia, premature ventricular contractions, angina, phlebitis.

Contraindications: Active intracranial bleeding, heart failure, pulmonary edema, severe dehydration. Use with caution in hypovolemia, renal failure.

Dosage:

- **Adult:** 0.25 to 1 g/kg IV, IO followed by 0.25 to 1 g/kg infused over 20 to 30 minutes, administered every 4 hours.
- **Pediatric:** 0.25 to 1 g/kg IV, IO followed by 0.25 to 0.5 g/kg infused over 20 to 30 minutes every 4 hours.

Special Considerations:

Mannitol should not be given in the same IV, IO line as blood.

Pregnancy class C.

METHYLPREDNISOLONE SODIUM SUCCINATE (SOLU-MEDROL)

Classification: Corticosteroid.

Action: Reduces inflammation by multiple mechanisms.

Indications: Anaphylaxis, asthma, COPD.

Adverse Effects: Depression, euphoria, headache, restlessness, hypertension, bradycardia, nausea/vomiting, swelling, diarrhea, weakness, fluid retention, paresthesias.

Contraindications: Cushing syndrome, fungal infection, measles, varicella, known sensitivity (including sulfites). Use with caution in active infections, renal disease, penetrating spinal cord injury, hypertension, seizures, CHF.

Dosage:

Asthma and COPD:

- **Adult:** 40 to 80 mg/day IV in divided doses.
- **Pediatric:** 1 mg/kg (up to 60 mg) IV, IO per day in two divided doses.

Anaphylactic Shock:

- **Adult:** 0.5 to 1 mg/kg IV every 12 hours.
- **Pediatric:** Same as adult dosing.

Special Considerations:

May mask signs and symptoms of infection.

Pregnancy class C.

METOPROLOL (LOPRESSOR, TOPROL XL)

Classification: Beta adrenergic antagonist, antianginal, antihypertensive, class II antiarrhythmic.

Action: Inhibits the strength of the heart's contractions, as well as heart rate. This results in a decrease in cardiac oxygen consumption.

Indications: ACS, hypertension, SVT, atrial flutter, AF, thyrotoxicosis.

Adverse Effects: Tiredness, dizziness, diarrhea, heart block, bradycardia, bronchospasm, drop in blood pressure.

Contraindications: Cardiogenic shock, AV block, bradycardia, known sensitivity. Use with caution in hypotension, chronic lung disease (asthma and COPD).

Dosage:

Cardiac Indications:

- **Adult:** 5 mg slow IV, IO over a 2-minute period; repeat at 5-minute intervals up to a total of three infusions totaling 15 mg IV, IO.
- **Pediatric:** Oral dosing only.

Special Considerations:

Blood pressure, heart rate, and ECG activity should be monitored carefully. Use with caution in patients with asthma.

Pregnancy class C.

MIDAZOLAM (VERSED)

Classification: Benzodiazepine, Schedule C-IV.

Action: Binds to the benzodiazepine receptor and enhances the effects of the brain chemical (neurotransmitter) GABA. Benzodiazepines act at the level of the limbic, thalamic, and hypothalamic regions of the CNS to produce short-acting CNS depression (including sedation, skeletal muscle relaxation, and anticonvulsant activity).

Indications: Sedation, anxiety, skeletal muscle relaxation.

Adverse Effects: Respiratory

© Dr P. Marazzi/Science Source.

depression, respiratory arrest, hypotension, nausea/vomiting, headache, hiccups, cardiac arrest.

Contraindications: Acute-angle glaucoma, pregnant women, known sensitivity.

Dosage:

Sedation:

Note: The dose of midazolam needs to be individualized. Every dose should be administered slowly over a period of 2 minutes. Allow 2 minutes to evaluate the clinical effect of the dose given.

- **Adult:**
  - **Healthy and younger than 60 years:** *Some patients require as little as 1 mg IV, IO. No more than 2.5 mg should be given over a 2-minute interval.* If additional sedation is required, continue to administer small increments over 2-minute periods (max dose: 5 mg). If the patient also has received a narcotic, he or she will typically require 30% less midazolam than the same patient not given the narcotic.

MIDAZOLAM (VERSED) *(continued)*

- ○ **60 years and older and debilitated or chronically ill patients:** This group of patients has a higher risk of hypoventilation, airway obstruction, and apnea. The peak clinical effect can take longer in these patients; therefore, dose increments should be smaller, and the rate of injection should be slower. *Some patients require a dose as small as 1 mg IV, IO, and no more than 1.5 mg should be given over a 2-minute period.* If additional sedation is required, additional midazolam should be given at a rate of no more than 1 mg over a 2-minute period (max dose: 3.5 mg). If the patient also has received a narcotic, he or she will typically require 50% less midazolam than the same patient not given the narcotic.
- ○ **Continuous infusion:** Continuous infusions can be required for prolonged transport of intubated, critically ill, and injured patients. After an initial bolus dose, the adult patient will require a maintenance infusion dose of 0.02 to 0.1 mg/kg per hour (1–7 mg/hr).
- **Pediatric (weight-based):** Pediatric patients typically require higher doses of midazolam than do adults on the basis of weight (in mg/kg). Younger pediatric patients (younger than 6 years) require higher doses (in mg/kg) than older pediatric patients. Midazolam takes approximately 3 minutes to reach peak effect; therefore, wait at least 2 minutes to determine the effectiveness of the drug and the need for additional dosing.
  - ○ **12 to 16 years:** Same as adult dosing. Some patients in this age group require a higher dose than that used in adults, but rarely does a patient require more than 10 mg.
  - ○ **6 to 12 years:** 0.025 to 0.05 mg/kg IV, IO up to a total dose of 0.4 mg/kg. Exceeding 10 mg as total dose usually is not necessary.
  - ○ **6 months to 5 years:** 0.05 to 0.1 mg/kg IV, IO up to a total dose of 0.6 mg/kg. Exceeding 6 mg as total dose usually is not necessary.
  - ○ **Younger than 6 months:** Dosing recommendations for this age group is unclear. Because this age group is especially vulnerable to airway obstruction and hypoventilation, use small increments with frequent clinical evaluation. Dose: 0.05 to 0.1 mg/kg IV, IO.

Special Considerations:
Patients receiving midazolam require frequent monitoring of vital signs and pulse oximetry. Be prepared to support the patient's airway and ventilation.
Pregnancy class D.

MILRINONE (PRIMACOR)

Classification: Inotropic.
Action: Milrinone is a positive inotropic drug and vasodilator with minimal chronotropic effect. Milrinone inhibits an enzyme, cAMP phosphodiesterase, which results in an increase in the concentration of calcium inside the cardiac cell. The result is improvement in diastolic function and myocardial contractility.
Indications: Cardiogenic shock, heart failure.
Adverse Effects: Cardiac arrhythmias, nausea/vomiting, hypotension.
Contraindications: Valvular heart disease, known sensitivity.
Dosage:

- **Adult:** 50 mcg/kg IV, IO over a period of 10 minutes, followed by an infusion of 0.375 to 0.5 mcg/kg per minute (max dose: 0.75 mcg/kg per minute).
- **Pediatric:** Same as adult dosing.

Special Considerations:
Pregnancy class C.

MORPHINE SULFATE

Classification: Opiate agonist, Schedule C-II.
Action: Binds with opioid receptors. Morphine is capable of inducing hypotension by depression of the vasomotor centers of the brain, as well as release of the chemical histamine. In the management of angina, morphine reduces stimulation of the sympathetic nervous system caused by pain and anxiety. Reduction of sympathetic stimulation reduces heart rate, cardiac work, and myocardial oxygen consumption.
Indications: Moderate to severe pain, including chest pain associated with ACS, CHF, pulmonary edema.
Adverse Effects: Respiratory depression, hypotension, nausea/vomiting, dizziness, lightheadedness, sedation, diaphoresis, euphoria, dysphoria, worsening of bradycardia and heart block in some patients with acute inferior wall MI, seizures, cardiac arrest, anaphylactoid reactions.
Contraindications: Respiratory depression, shock, known sensitivity. Use with caution in hypotension, acute bronchial asthma, respiratory insufficiency, head trauma.
Dosage:
- **Adult:** 2 to 10 mg IV, IO, IM, or subcutaneous administered slowly over a period of several minutes. The dose is the same whether administered IV, IO, IM, or subcutaneous.
- **Pediatric <110 pounds (50 kg):** 0.025 to 0.2 mg/kg IV, IO, IM, or subcutaneous.

Special Considerations:
Monitor vital signs and pulse oximetry closely. Be prepared to support patient's airway and ventilations.
Patients may report a "flushed" or hot feeling immediately following administration. Assess for signs of allergic reaction; however, this is typically a histamine release.
Overdose should be treated with naloxone.
Pregnancy class C.

NALOXONE (NARCAN)

Classification: Opioid antagonist.
Action: Binds the opioid receptor and blocks the effect of narcotics.
Indications: Narcotic overdoses, reversal of narcotics used for procedure-related anesthesia.
Adverse Effects: Nausea/vomiting, restlessness, diaphoresis, tachycardia, hypertension, tremulousness, seizures, cardiac arrest, narcotic withdrawal. Patients who have gone from a state of somnolence from a narcotic overdose to wide awake may become combative.
Contraindications: Known sensitivity to naloxone, nalmefene, or naltrexone. Use with caution in patients with supraventricular arrhythmias or other cardiac disease, head trauma, brain tumor.

© Tomas Nevesely/Shutterstock.

Dosage:
- **Adult:** 0.4 to 2 mg IV, IO, ET, IM, or subcutaneous. Alternatively, administer 2 mg intranasally. Higher doses (10–20 mg) may be required for overdoses of synthetic narcotics. A repeat dose of one third to two thirds the original dose is often necessary.
- **Pediatric:**
  - **5 years or older or weight >20 kg:** 2 mg IV, IO, ET, IM, or subcutaneous.
  - **Younger than 5 years or weight <20 kg:** 0.1 mg/kg IV, IO, ET, IM, or subcutaneous; may repeat every 2 to 3 minutes.

Special Considerations:
Pregnancy class C.

NICARDIPINE (CARDENE)

Classification: Calcium channel blocker.
Action: Blocks calcium movement into the smooth muscle of the blood vessel walls, causing vasodilation.
Indications: Hypertension, angina
Adverse Effects: Edema, headaches, flushing, sinus tachycardia, hypotension.
Contraindications: Aortic stenosis, hypotension, known sensitivity. Use with caution in heart failure, cardiac conduction abnormalities, cerebrovascular disease, depressed AV node conduction.

Dosage:
- **Adult:** 5 mg/hr IV, IO; may increase by 2.5 mg/hr every 5 to 15 minutes (max dose: 15 mg/hr). Once the patient has achieved the desired blood pressure, decrease infusion to a maintenance dose of 3 mg/hr.
- **Pediatric:** 0.5 to 5 mcg/kg per minute IV, IO infusion.

Special Considerations:
Pregnancy class C.

NITROGLYCERIN (NITROLINGUAL, NITROQUICK, NITRO-DUR)

Classification: Antianginal agent.
Action: Relaxes vascular smooth muscle, thereby dilating peripheral arteries and veins. This causes pooling of venous blood and decreased venous return to the heart, which decreases preload. Nitroglycerin also reduces left ventricular systolic wall tension, which decreases afterload.
Indications: Angina, ongoing ischemic chest discomfort, hypertension, myocardial ischemia associated with cocaine intoxication.

© Sue Heaton/Alamy Stock Photo.

© Allik Camazine/Alamy Stock Photo.

Adverse Effects: Headache, hypotension, bradycardia, lightheadedness, flushing, cardiovascular collapse, methemoglobinemia.
Contraindications: Hypotension, severe bradycardia or tachycardia, right-sided MI, increased ICP, intracranial bleeding, patients taking any medications for erectile dysfunction (such as sildenafil [Viagra], tadalafil [Cialis], or vardenafil [Levitra]), known sensitivity to nitrates. Use with caution in anemia, closed-angle glaucoma, hypotension, postural hypotension, uncorrected hypovolemia.
Dosage:
- **Adult:**
  - **Sublingual tablets:** 1 tablet (0.3–0.4 mg) at 5-minute intervals to a maximum of 3 doses.
  - **Translingual spray:** 1 (0.4 mg) spray at 5-minute intervals to a maximum of 3 sprays.
  - **Ointment:** 2% topical (Nitro-Bid ointment): Apply 1 to 2 inches of paste over the chest wall, cover with transparent wrap, and secure with tape.
  - **IV infusion:** 5 mcg/min; may increase rate by 5 to 10 mcg/min every 5 to 10 minutes as needed. End points of dose titration for nitroglycerin include a drop in the blood pressure of 10%, relief of chest pain, and return of ST segment to normal on a 12-lead ECG.
- **Pediatric IV infusion:** The initial pediatric infusion is 0.25 to 0.5 mcg/kg per minute IV, IO titrated by 0.5 to 1 mcg/kg/min. Usual required dose is 1 to 3 mcg/kg per minute to a maximum dose of 5 mcg/kg per minute.

Special Considerations:
Administration of nitroglycerin to a patient with right ventricular MI can result in hypotension. Pregnancy class C.

NITROUS OXIDE

Classification: Inorganic gas, inhaled anesthetic.
Action: Exact mechanism is not known.
Indications: Mild to severe pain.
Adverse Effects: Delirium, hypoxia, respiratory depression, nausea/vomiting.
Contraindications: Use with caution in head trauma, increased ICP, pneumothorax, bowel obstruction, patients with COPD who require a hypoxic respiratory drive.
Dosage: Inhaled: 20% to 50% concentration mixed with oxygen.
Special Considerations:
Ensure the safety of healthcare professionals. Use only with a scavenger gas system to ensure that unused gas is collected, or scavenged, and that providers are not exposed to significant levels of the agent.
Pregnancy class not noted.

NOREPINEPHRINE (LEVOPHED)

Classification: Adrenergic agonist, inotropic, vasopressor.
Action: Norepinephrine is an alpha$_1$, alpha$_2$, and beta$_1$ agonist. Alpha-mediated peripheral vasoconstriction is the predominant clinical result of administration, resulting in increasing blood pressure and coronary blood flow. Beta adrenergic action produces inotropic stimulation of the heart and dilates the coronary arteries.
Indications: Cardiogenic shock, septic shock, severe hypotension.
Adverse Effects: Dizziness, anxiety, cardiac arrhythmias, dyspnea, exacerbation of asthma.
Contraindications: Patients taking MAOIs, known sensitivity. Use with caution in hypovolemia.
Dosage:
- **Adult:** Add 4 mg to 250 mL of D$_5$W or D$_5$NS, but not normal saline alone. 0.1 to 0.5 mcg/kg per minute as IV, IO, titrated to maintain blood pressure > 80 mm Hg. Many settings still use non-weight-based dosing of 2 to 4 mcg per minute titrated upward for the desired clinical effect. Refractory shock may require doses as high as 30 mcg per minute.
- **Pediatric:** 0.05 to 2 mcg/kg per minute IV, IO infusion, to a maximum dose of 2 mcg/kg per minute.

Special Considerations:
Do not administer in same IV line as alkaline solutions.
Half-life 1 minute
Pregnancy class C

ONDANSETRON (ZOFRAN)

Classification: Antiemetic.
Action: Prevents/reduces nausea/vomiting by binding and blocking a receptor for the brain chemical serotonin.
Indications: Prevent and treat nausea/vomiting.
Adverse Effects: Headache, fatigue, diarrhea, dizziness, abdominal pain, hypotension, hypertension, ECG changes (prolonged PR and QT intervals, widened QRS), bradycardia, tachycardia, syncope.

© Margaret M Stewart/Shutterstock.

ONDANSETRON (ZOFRAN)   *(continued)*

Contraindications: Known sensitivity. Use with caution in hypokalemia, hypomagnesemia, cardiac arrhythmias.
Dosage:
- **Adult:** 4 to 8 mg IV, IO, PO.
- **Pediatric: 2 to 16 years:** 0.15 mg/kg IV, IO (max dose: 16 mg).

Special Considerations:
Pregnancy class B.

OXYGEN

Classification: Elemental gas.
Action: Facilitates cellular energy metabolism.
Indications: Hypoxia, ischemic chest pain, respiratory distress, suspected carbon monoxide poisoning, traumatic injuries, shock.
Adverse Effects: High concentrations can cause a decreased level of consciousness and respiratory depression in patients with chronic carbon dioxide retention or chronic lung disease. Oxygen causes systemic and coronary vasoconstriction, possibly coronary artery perfusion.
Contraindications: Known paraquat poisoning.
Dosage:
Low-Concentration Oxygen:
- A dose of 1 to 4 L/min by a nasal cannula is appropriate.

High-Concentration Oxygen:
- A dose of 10 to 15 L/min via nonrebreather mask is appropriate.

Special Considerations:
Pregnancy class A.

© Jones & Bartlett Learning.

PANCURONIUM (PAVULON)

Classification: Nondepolarizing neuromuscular blocker.
Action: Antagonizes acetylcholine at the motor end plate, producing skeletal muscle paralysis.
Indications: To induce neuromuscular blockade for the facilitation of ET intubation.
Adverse Effects: Muscle paralysis, apnea, dyspnea, respiratory depression, cutaneous flushing, sinus tachycardia.
Contraindications: Known sensitivity to bromides. Use with caution in heart disease, renal disease.
Dosage:
- **Adult:** 0.06 to 0.1 mg/kg IV, IO; repeat dosing is 0.01 mg/kg every 25 to 60 minutes.
- **Pediatric:** Same as adult dosing.

Special Considerations:
Pregnancy class C.

PHENOBARBITAL (LUMINAL)

Classification: Anticonvulsant, barbiturate, Schedule C-IV.
Action: Depresses seizure activity in the cortex, thalamus, and limbic system; increases threshold for electrical stimulation of motor cortex; produces state of sedation.
Indications: Seizures, may also be used for severe alcohol withdrawal or withdrawal from sedative hypnotic medications (off-label).
Adverse Effects: Depression, agitation, respiratory depression, accelerated metabolism of several other medications.
Contraindications: Liver dysfunction, porphyria, agranulocytosis, known sensitivity to barbiturates. Use with caution with respiratory dysfunction.
Dosage:
- **Adult:** 20 mg/kg IV, IO; infuse at a rate not faster than 50 to 100 mg/min.
- **Pediatric:** 20 mg/kg IV, IO; infuse over 10 minutes.

Special Considerations:
Be prepared to manage the patient's airway.
Pregnancy class D.

PHENTOLAMINE (REGITINE)

Classification: Alpha antagonist, antihypertensive.
Action: Blocks alpha adrenergic receptors, causing vasodilation.
Indications: Hypertensive emergencies and hypertension caused by pheochromocytoma, cocaine-induced vasospasm of the coronary arteries.
Adverse Effects: Sinus tachycardia, angina, dizziness, orthostatic hypotension, prolonged hypotensive episodes, nausea/vomiting, diarrhea, weakness, flushing, nasal congestion.
Contraindications: Known sensitivity. Use with caution in AMI, angina, coronary insufficiency, evidence suggestive of coronary artery disease, peptic ulcer disease.
Dosage:
Hypertensive Crisis:
- **Adult:** 5 to 15 mg IV, IO, or IM.
- **Pediatric:** 0.05 to 0.1 mg/kg IV, IO; or 1 mg/dose

Cocaine-Induced Vasospasm:
- **Adult:** 5 mg IV, IO or IM.
- **Pediatric:** 0.05 to 0.1 mg/kg IV, IO; or 1 mg/dose

Special Considerations:
Pregnancy class C.

PHENYLEPHRINE (NEO-SYNEPHRINE)

Classification: Adrenergic agonist.

Action: Stimulates the alpha receptors, causing vasoconstriction, which results in increased blood pressure.

Indications: Neurogenic shock, spinal shock, cases of shock in which the patient's heart rate does not need to be increased, drug-induced hypotension.

Adverse Effects: Hypertension, VT, headache, excitability, tremor, MI, exacerbation of asthma, cardiac arrhythmias, reflex bradycardia, soft tissue necrosis.

Contraindications: Acute MI, angina, cardiac arrhythmias, severe hypertension, coronary artery disease, pheochromocytoma, narrow-angle glaucoma, cardiomyopathy, MAOI therapy, known sensitivity to phenylephrine or sulfites.

Dosage:

- **Adult:** 100 to 180 mcg per minute IV, IO. Once the blood pressure has been stabilized, the dose can be reduced to 40 to 60 mcg per minute.
- **Pediatric (2 to 12 years):** 5 to 20 mcg/kg IV, IO followed by 0.1 to 0.5 mcg/kg per minute IV, IO (max dose: 3 mcg/kg per minute IV, IO).

Special Considerations:

Pregnancy class C

PHENYTOIN (DILANTIN)

Classification: Anticonvulsant.

Action: Depresses seizures by affecting the movement of sodium and calcium into neural tissue.

Indications: Generalized tonic-clonic seizures.

Adverse Effects: Nausea/vomiting, depression of cardiac conduction, sedation, nystagmus, tremors, ataxia, dysarthria, gingival hypertrophy, hirsutism, facial coarsening, hypotension.

Contraindications: Sinus bradycardia, sinoatrial block, second- and third-degree heart block, Adams-Stokes syndrome, known sensitivity to hydantoins.

Dosage:

- **Adult:** 15 to 20 mg/kg IV, IO should be administered slowly at a rate not exceeding 50 mg/min. (This requires approximately 20 minutes in a 70-kg patient.)
- **Pediatric:** 15 to 20 mg/kg IV, IO, administered at a rate of 1 to 3 mg/kg per minute.

Special Considerations:

Continuously monitor the ECG and blood pressure during administration. Monitor IV site for signs of infiltration.

Pregnancy class D.

POTASSIUM CHLORIDE

Classification: Electrolyte replacement.
Action: Replaces potassium. Slight alterations in extracellular potassium levels can cause serious alterations in both cardiac and nervous function.
Indications: Hypokalemia.
Adverse Effects: Hyperkalemia; AV block; cardiac arrest; GI bleeding, obstruction, or perforation; tissue necrosis if the infusion infiltrates into the soft tissues.
Contraindications: Use with caution in patients with cardiac arrhythmias, renal failure, muscle cramps, severe tissue trauma.
Dosage:

- **Adult:** Dosage must be individualized according to patient serum potassium concentration.
- **Pediatric:** Dosage must be individualized according to patient serum potassium concentration.

Special Considerations:
Pregnancy class C

PRALIDOXIME (2-PAM, PROTOPAM)

Classification: Cholinergic agonist, antidote.
Action: Reactivates cholinesterase.
Indications: Toxicity from nerve agents (organophosphates) having cholinesterase activity.
Adverse Effects: Dizziness, blurred vision, hypertension, diplopia, hyperventilation, laryngospasm, nausea/vomiting, sinus tachycardia.
Contraindications: Myasthenia gravis, renal failure, inability to control the airway.
Dosage:

- **Adult:** 1 to 2 g (dilute in 100 mL normal saline) over a 15- to 30-minute period. If this is not practical or if pulmonary edema is present, the dose should be given slowly ($\geq$5 min) by IV as a 5% solution in water. Consider IM or subcutaneous administration if IV administration is not possible.
  - **Autoinjector:** Pralidoxime is also available as an autoinjector that delivers 600 mg IM. Repeat doses can be given every 15 minutes to a total of three doses (1,800 mg). Pralidoxime autoinjector is not recommended for pediatric patients.
- **Pediatric:** 15 to 50 mg/kg IV, IO, depending on severity. Consider IM or subcutaneous administration if IV administration is not possible.

Special Considerations:
Pregnancy class C

PREDNISONE

Classification: Corticosteroid.
Action: Reduces inflammation.
Indications: Inflammatory conditions, such as asthma with bronchospasm.
Adverse Effects: Many adverse effects of steroid use are not related to short-term use but typically are seen with long-term use and during withdrawal.
Contraindications: Cushing's syndrome, fungal infections, measles, varicella, known sensitivity.
Dosage:
- **Adult:** Dosage must be individualized.
- **Pediatric:** Dosage must be individualized.

Special Considerations:
Pregnancy class C.

PROCAINAMIDE (PRONESTYL)

Classification: Antiarrhythmic, Class IA.
Action: Blocks influx of sodium through membrane pores, consequently suppresses atrial and ventricular arrhythmias by slowing conduction in myocardial tissue.
Indications: Alternative to amiodarone for stable monomorphic VT with normal QT interval and preserved ventricular function, reentry SVT if uncontrolled by adenosine and vagal maneuvers if blood pressure stable, AF with rapid rate in Wolff-Parkinson-White syndrome.

Adverse Effects: Asystole, VF, flushing, hypotension, PR prolongation, QRS widening, QT prolongation.
Contraindications: AV block, QT prolongation, torsades de pointes. Use with caution in hypotension, heart failure.
Dosage:
- **Adult:** 500 to 600 mg over 25 to 3 minutes IV, or 20 to 50 mg/min slow IV, IO (max total dose: 17 mg/kg until one of the following occurs: arrhythmia resolves, hypotension, QRS widens by >50% of original width).
- **Maintenance:** Infusion (after resuscitation from cardiac arrest): mix 1 g in 250 mL solution (4 mg/mL), infuse at 1 to 4 mg/min.
- **Pediatric:** 10 to 15 mg/kg slow IV, IO over 30 to 60 minutes.

Special Considerations:
Pregnancy class C.

PROMETHAZINE (PHENERGAN)

Classification: Antiemetic, antihistamine.
Action: Decreases nausea and vomiting by antagonizing H_1 receptors.
Indications: Nausea/vomiting.
Adverse Effects: Paradoxic excitation in children and older adults.
Contraindications: Altered level of consciousness, jaundice, bone marrow suppression, known sensitivity. Use with caution in seizure disorder.
Dosage:
- **Adult:** 12.5 to 25 mg IV, IO or IM.
- **Pediatric: 2 years and older:** 0.25 to 1 mg/kg IV, IO, IM (maximum rate of IV, IO administration is 25 mg/min).

Special Considerations:
Must dilute to at least 10 mL before IV administration.
Monitor IV site for signs of infiltration.
Use caution in older adults.
Pregnancy class C.

© Allik Camazine/Alamy Stock Photo.

PROPOFOL (DIPRIVAN)

Classification: Anesthetic.
Action: Produces rapid and brief state of general anesthesia.
Indications: Anesthesia induction.
Adverse Effects: Apnea, cardiac arrhythmias, asystole, hypotension, hypertension, pain at injection site.
Contraindications: Hypovolemia, known sensitivity (including soybean oil, eggs).
Dosage: A general induction dose used to produce a state of unconsciousness rapidly is 1.5 to 3 mg/kg IV, IO.

After the induction bolus, the patient must be given intermittent boluses or a maintenance infusion. For an average adult, an intermittent dose is 20 to 50 mg as needed. Alternatively, a propofol infusion may

© Julia Hiebaum/Alamy Stock Photo.

Patient Group	Dosage	Rate of Administration (10 mg/mL)
Healthy adults younger than 55 years	2 to 2.5 mg/kg IV, IO	40 mg every 10 seconds
Older or debilitated patients	1 to 1.5 mg/kg IV, IO	20 mg every 10 seconds
Cardiac patients	0.5 to 1.5 mg/kg IV, IO	20 mg every 10 seconds
Patients with head injuries	1 to 2 mg/kg IV, IO	20 mg every 10 seconds
Pediatric (3 to 16 years)	2.5 to 3.5 mg/kg IV, IO	20 mg every 10 seconds

PROPOFOL (DIPRIVAN)   *(continued)*

be ordered. Maintenance of anesthesia with a propofol infusion can be achieved by following the following protocols:

- **Adult patients:** 25 to 75 mcg/kg per minute IV, IO. Prolonged infusions begin at 5 mcg/kg per minute and are titrated up to a maximum dose of 50 mcg/kg per minute.
- **Older adult, debilitated, or head-injured patients:** Use approximately 80% of the normal adult dose.
- **Pediatric:** 30 to 300 mcg/kg per minute IV, IO.

Special Considerations:

Propofol should be administered only by personnel trained and equipped to manage the patient's airway and provide mechanical ventilation. Propofol bolus administration may be restricted to only be administered by physicians and licensed-independent providers—consult your state EMS regulations and local protocols. In older adults and debilitated patients, avoid rapid administration to prevent hypotension, apnea, airway obstruction, and/or oxygen desaturation. Continue to monitor the patient's oxygenation and vital signs and try to limit use of propofol to patients who are intubated. Propofol should not be administered through the same IV catheter as blood or plasma. Pain can occur at the site of injection, which can be minimized by the use of larger veins, slower rates of administration, and administration of 1 mL 1% lidocaine before propofol administration.

Propofol is listed as a pregnancy class B; however, propofol should be avoided in pregnant women because it crosses the placenta and can cause neonatal depression.

PROPRANOLOL (INDERAL)

Classification: Beta adrenergic antagonist, antianginal, antihypertensive, antiarrhythmic class II.

Action: Nonselective beta antagonist that binds with both the beta$_1$ and beta$_2$ receptors. Propranolol inhibits the strength of the heart's contractions, as well as heart rate. This results in a decrease in cardiac oxygen consumption.

Indications: Angina; narrow-complex tachycardias that originate from either a *reentry mechanism* (reentry SVT) or an *automatic focus* (junctional, ectopic, or multifocal tachycardia) uncontrolled by vagal maneuvers and adenosine in patients with preserved ventricular function; AF and atrial flutter in patients with preserved ventricular function; hypertension; migraine headaches.

Adverse Effects: Bradycardia, AV block, bronchospasm, hypotension.

Contraindications: Cardiogenic shock, heart failure, AV block, bradycardia, pulmonary edema, sick sinus syndrome, known sensitivity. Use with caution in chronic lung disease (asthma and COPD).

Dosage:

- **Adult:** 1 to 3 mg IV, IO at a rate of 1 mg per minute; may repeat the dose 2 minutes later.
- **Pediatric:** 0.01 to 0.1 mg/kg slow IV, IO over a 10-minute period.

Special Considerations:

Monitor blood pressure and heart rate closely during administration.

Pregnancy class C

RACEMIC EPINEPHRINE/RACEPINEPHRINE (MICRONEFRIN, S₂)

© Jones & Bartlett Learning.

Classification: Bronchodilator, adrenergic agent.
Action: Stimulates both alpha and beta receptors, causing vasoconstriction, reduced mucosal edema, and bronchodilation.
Indications: Bronchial asthma, croup.
Adverse Effects: Anxiety, dizziness, headache, tremor, palpitations, tachycardia, cardiac arrhythmias, hypertension, nausea/vomiting.
Contraindications: Glaucoma, elderly, cardiac disease, hypertension, thyroid disease, diabetes, known sensitivity to sulfites.
Dosage:

- **Adult:** Add 0.5 mL to nebulizer; for hand-bulb nebulizer, administer 1 to 3 inhalations; for jet nebulizer, add 3 mL of diluent, swirl the nebulizer and administer for 15 minutes.
- **Pediatric:**
  - **Older than 4 years:** Same as adult dosing.
  - **Younger than 4 years:** Safe and effective use has not been demonstrated.

Special Considerations:
Monitor blood pressure, heart rate, and cardiac rhythm for changes.
Onset of action is 1 to 5 minutes.
Pregnancy class C.

ROCURONIUM (ZEMURON)

© Dr P. Marazzi/Science Source.

Classification: Neuromuscular blocker, nondepolarizing.
Action: Antagonizes acetylcholine at the motor end plate, producing skeletal muscle paralysis.
Indications: To induce neuromuscular blockade for the facilitation of ET intubation.
Adverse Effects: Muscle paralysis, apnea, dyspnea, respiratory depression, sinus tachycardia, urticaria.
Contraindications: Known sensitivity to bromides. Use with caution in heart disease, liver disease.
Dosage:

- **Adult:** 0.6 to 1.2 mg/kg IV, IO (using ideal body weight).
- **Pediatric (older than 3 months):** 0.9 to 1.2 mg/kg IV, IO (off-label).

Special Considerations:
Onset of action is 30 seconds to 2 minutes.
Duration of action is approximately 30 minutes.
Pregnancy class B.

SCOPOLAMINE (TRANSDERM SCOP)

Classification: Neurologic antivertigo, antimuscarinic.
Action: Antagonizes acetylcholine at muscarinic receptors.
Indications: Motion sickness.
Adverse Effects: Dry mouth, drowsiness, dilated pupils and blurred vision, hallucinations, confusion.
Contraindications: Glaucoma, cardiac arrhythmias, coronary artery disease, known sensitivity.
Dosage:

- **Adult and children older than 12 years:** 1 disc applied to skin behind the ear.

Special Considerations:
Half-life 8 hours
Pregnancy class C

Scopolamine
Transdermal system
1 mg/3 days
Formulated delivery of approximately 1 mg over three days
Motion Sickness and Post-operative Nausea & Vomiting Prevention Patches
NDC 12345-678-90   **Rx only**

SODIUM BICARBONATE

Classification: Electrolyte replacement.
Action: Counteracts existing acidosis.
Indications: Acidosis, drug intoxications (e.g., barbiturates, salicylates, methyl alcohol).
Adverse Effects: Metabolic alkalosis, hypernatremia, injection site reaction, sodium and fluid retention, peripheral edema.
Contraindications: Metabolic alkalosis, hypocalcemia.
Dosage:
Metabolic Acidosis During Cardiac Arrest:

- **Adult:** 1 mEq/kg slow IV, IO; may repeat at 0.5 mEq/kg in 10 minutes.
- **Pediatric:** Same as adult dosing.

Metabolic Acidosis Not Associated with Cardiac Arrest:

- **Adult:** Dosage should be individualized.
- **Pediatric:** Dosage should be individualized.

Special Considerations:
Do not administer into an IV, IO line in which another medication is being given.
Because of the high concentration of sodium within each ampule of sodium bicarbonate, use with caution in patients with CHF and renal disease.
Pregnancy class C.

SODIUM NITROPRUSSIDE (NIPRIDE, NITROPRESS)

WARNING

PROTECT FROM LIGHT

Monitor blood pressure before and during administration.

2 mL   Single-Dose Fliptop Vial   NDC 0409-3024-01

Sodium Nitroprusside

50 mg/mL Vial

(25 mg/mL)   Rx only
FOR IV INFUSION ONLY

RL-2267 (8/07)

Classification: Antihypertensive agent.
Action: Causes direct relaxation of both arteries and veins.
Indications: Hypertensive emergencies.
Adverse Effects: Cyanide or thiocyanate toxicity, nausea/vomiting, dizziness, headache, restlessness, abdominal pain, methemoglobinemia.
Contraindications: Hypotension, increased ICP, cerebrovascular disease, coronary artery disease, hepatic disease, renal disease, pulmonary disease.
Dosage:
- **Adult:** 0.3 to 10 mcg/kg per minute IV, IO. Titrate to desired blood pressure.
- **Pediatric:** 0.5 to 10 mcg/kg per minute IV, IO. Titrate to desired blood pressure.

Special Considerations:

Nitroprusside will break down when exposed to ultraviolet light. Therefore, the infusion should be shielded from light by wrapping the bag with aluminum foil. Doses less than 2 mcg/kg per minute are less likely to cause toxicity.
Pregnancy class C.

SUCCINYLCHOLINE (ANECTINE)

Classification: Neuromuscular blocker, depolarizing.
Action: Competes with the acetylcholine receptor of the motor end plate on the muscle cell, resulting in muscle paralysis.
Indications: To induce neuromuscular blockade for the facilitation of ET intubation.
Adverse Effects: Anaphylactoid reactions, respiratory depression, apnea, bronchospasm, cardiac arrhythmias, malignant hyperthermia, hypertension, hypotension, muscle fasciculation, post-procedure muscle pain, hypersalivation, rash.
Contraindications: Malignant hyperthermia, burns, trauma. Use with caution in children, cardiac disease, hepatic disease, renal disease, peptic ulcer disease, cholinesterase-inhibitor toxicity, pseudocholinesterase deficiency, digitalis toxicity, glaucoma, hyperkalemia, hypothermia, rhabdomyolysis, myasthenia gravis.
Dosage:
- **Adult:**
  - **IV:** 0.6 mg/kg IV, IO (range 0.3 to 1.1 mg/kg). (Off-label 1 to 1.5 mg/kg for RSI.)
  - **IM:** 3 to 4 mg/kg (max dose: 150 mg).
- **Pediatric:**
  - **IV:**
    - **Adolescents and older children:** 1 mg/kg IV, IO.
    - **Small children and infants:** 2 mg/kg IV, IO.
  - **IM:** 3 to 4 mg/kg (max dose: 150 mg).

SUCCINYLCHOLINE (ANECTINE)   *(continued)*

Special Considerations:
IV administration results in neuromuscular blockade in 0.5 to 1 minute. IM administration results in neuromuscular blockade in 2 to 3 minutes.
IV administration in infants and children can potentially result in profound bradycardia and, in some cases, asystole. The incidence of bradycardia is greater after the second dose. The occurrence of bradycardia can be reduced with the pretreatment of atropine.
Succinylcholine can have a significantly prolonged effect in the setting of poisoning with nerve gas agents and organophosphate pesticides.
Pregnancy class C.

TERBUTALINE (BRETHINE, BRETHAIRE)

Classification: Adrenergic agonist.
Action: Stimulates the beta$_2$ receptor, producing relaxation of bronchial smooth muscle and bronchodilation.
Indications: Prevention and reversal of bronchospasm.
Adverse Effects: Cardiac arrhythmias, arrhythmia exacerbation, angina, anxiety, headache, tremor, palpitations, dizziness.
Contraindications: Known sensitivity to sympathomimetics. Use with caution in hypertension, cardiac disease, cardiac arrhythmias, diabetes, older adults, MAOI therapy, pheochromocytoma, thyrotoxicosis, seizure disorder.
Dosage:
- **Adult:** 0.25 mg subcutaneous every 20 minutes for 3 doses. The usual site for the subcutaneous injection is the lateral deltoid.
- **Pediatric:** 0.005 to 0.01 mg/kg subcutaneous every 20 minutes for 3 doses.

Special Considerations:
Pregnancy class B.

THIAMINE (VITAMIN B$_1$)

Classification: Vitamin B$_1$.
Action: Thiamine combines with adenosine triphosphate to produce thiamine diphosphate, which acts as a coenzyme in carbohydrate metabolism.
Indications: Wernicke-Korsakoff syndrome, beriberi, nutritional supplementation.
Adverse Effects: Itching, rash, pain at injection site.
Contraindications: Known sensitivity.
Dosage:
Wernicke-Korsakoff Syndrome:
- **Adult:** 100 mg IV, IO.
- **Pediatric:** Not recommended for pediatric patients.

Special Considerations:
Pregnancy class A.

TIROFIBAN (AGGRASTAT)

Classification: GP IIb/IIIa inhibitor.
Action: Prevents the aggregation of platelets by binding to the GP IIb/IIIa receptor.
Indications: UA/NSTEMI—to manage medically and for those undergoing percutaneous coronary intervention.
Adverse Effects: Bleeding from the GI tract, internal bleeding, intracranial hemorrhage, hypotension, stroke, anaphylactic shock.
Contraindications: Bleeding from any source, severe uncontrolled hypertension, surgery or trauma within the previous 6 weeks, stroke within the previous 30 days, renal failure, thrombocytopenia.
Dosage: 25 mcg/kg IV given over 5 minutes; 0.15 mcg/kg/min IV, IO infusion for 48 hours.
Special Considerations:
Half-life approximately 2 hours
Pregnancy class B.

Tirofiban
(hydrochloride)
Injection   NDC 12345-678-90
250 mL   Single-Dose Container
Sterile Nonpyrogenic
Iso-osmotic
12.5 mg per 250 mL
(50 mcg per mL)
Rx only

TRANEXAMIC ACID (TXA; CYKLOKAPRON)

Classification: Antifibrinolytic agent; hemostatic agent.
Action: Inhibits intrinsic fibrinolysis, promoting blood clot formation.
Indications: Severe traumatic hemorrhage (off-label); surgical hemorrhage; hyphema (off-label), severe menstrual bleeding, dental bleeding.
Adverse Effects: Visual changes, anxiety, tachycardia, rash, hives.
Contraindications: Hypersensitivity, subarachnoid hemorrhage, thromboembolism.
Dosage:
Acute Traumatic Hemorrhage:
- **Adult:** 1,000 mg IV over 10 minutes, followed by 1,000 mg IV over 8 hours.

Special Considerations:
Pregnancy class B.

NDC 12345-678-90
TRANEXAMIC ACID
INJECTION 10 X 10 mL
1000 mg/10 mL (100 mg/mL)
FOR INTRAVENOUS USE ONLY
Single-Dose Vials   **Rx only**

VALPROIC ACID (DEPAKOTE)

Classification: Anticonvulsant, antimanic.
Action: It is suggested that valproic acid increases brain concentrations of GABA.
Indications: Seizures, mood disorders.
Adverse Effects: Tremor, confusion, sedation, hypotension, hypertension, tachycardia, transient hair loss, weight gain, weight loss, fatal hepatic failure.
Contraindications: Liver disease.
Dosage: Dosing is individualized.
Special Considerations:
Although generally well tolerated, valproic acid does require regular monitoring of blood levels to ensure maintenance of therapeutic levels while minimizing adverse drug reactions.
Pregnancy class D.

NDC 12345-678-90
Valproic Acid
Oral Solution USP
250 mg/5 mL*
16 fl oz (473 mL)
Rx only

VECURONIUM (NORCURON)

Classification: Neuromuscular blocker, nondepolarizing.
Action: Antagonizes acetylcholine at the motor end plate, producing skeletal muscle paralysis.
Indications: To induce neuromuscular blockade for the facilitation of ET intubation.
Adverse Effects: Muscle paralysis, apnea, dyspnea, respiratory depression, sinus tachycardia, urticaria.
Contraindications: Known sensitivity to bromides. Use with caution in heart disease, liver disease.
Dosage:
- **Adult:** 0.08 to 0.1 mg/kg IV, IO. Use an infusion of 0.8 to 1.2 mcg/kg per minute for ongoing chemical paralysis.
- **Pediatric:** 0.1 to 0.15 mg/kg. Use an infusion of 1 to 2.5 mcg/kg per minute for ongoing chemical paralysis.

Special Considerations:
Pregnancy class C.
Carefully monitor and provide adequate sedation and analgesia for patients who are chemically paralyzed with vecuronium. This medication has no sedative or analgesic effects. Patients may appear to be unconscious while having completely intact awareness, hearing, and sensation of pain.

© Food Collection/Alamy Stock Photo.

VERAPAMIL (ISOPTIN)

Classification: Calcium channel blocker; Class IV antiarrhythmic.
Action: Blocks calcium from moving into the heart muscle cell, which prolongs the conduction of electrical impulses through the AV node. Also dilates arteries.
Indications: AF, hypertension, paroxysmal SVT, paroxysmal SVT prophylaxis.
Adverse Effects: Sinus bradycardia; first-, second-, or third-degree AV block; CHF; reflex sinus tachycardia; transient asystole; AV block; hypotension.
Contraindications: Second- or third-degree AV block (except in patients with a functioning artificial pacemaker); hypotension (systolic pressure <90 mm Hg) or cardiogenic shock; sick sinus syndrome (except in patients with a functioning artificial pacemaker); Wolff-Parkinson-White syndrome; Lown-Ganong-Levine syndrome; severe left ventricular dysfunction; known sensitivity to verapamil or any component of the formulation; atrial flutter or fibrillation and an accessory bypass tract (Wolff-Parkinson-White, Lown-Ganong-Levine syndrome); in infants <1 year.
Dosage:
- **Adult:** 2.5 to 10 mg IV, IO over 2 minutes (3 minutes in older adults). May repeat at 5 to 10 mg every 15 to 30 minutes to a maximum dose of 30 mg.
- **Pediatric:**
  - **Children 1 to 16 years:** 0.1 mg/kg IV, IO (maximum 5 mg/dose) over 2 minutes. May repeat in 30 minutes to a maximum dose of 10 mg.
  - **Infants <1 year:** Not recommended.

Special Considerations:
Do not administer to patients with heart failure or impaired ventricular function.
Pregnancy class C.

Appendix C

Commonly Prescribed and Over-the-Counter Medications

Generic Name	Trade Names	Classifications	Indications
acetaminophen	Tylenol	Analgesic/antipyretic	Pain, fever
acyclovir	Acyclo-V, Zovirax, others	Antiviral	Herpes
adalimumab	Humira	Immunosuppressant	Crohn disease, arthritis
adapalene	Differin	Dermatologic	Acne
albuterol	Proventil, Proventil HFA, Ventolin, others	Bronchodilator/adrenergic agonist	Asthma, bronchospasm
alendronate	Fosamax	Bisphosphonate	Osteoporosis, Paget disease
allopurinol	Zyloprim	Antigout	Gout
alprazolam	Xanax, others	Anxiolytic/ benzodiazepine/ sedative-hypnotic	Anxiety, panic disorder
amitriptyline HCl	Elavil, others	Tricyclic antidepressant	Depression
amlodipine besylate	Norvasc	Calcium channel blocker	Angina, hypertension
amlodipine besylate/ benazepril HCl	Lotrel	ACE inhibitor/calcium channel blocker	Hypertension
amoxicillin	Amoxil, Trimox	Antibiotic, penicillin	Infection
amoxicillin/clavulanate	Augmentin, Augmentin ES-600	Antibiotic, penicillin	Infection
amphetamine mixed salts	Adderall, Adderall XR	Adrenergic agent/ amphetamine/central nervous system stimulant	ADHD, narcolepsy
apixaban	Eliquis	Anticoagulant	Blood clots
aripiprazole	Abilify	Antipsychotic	Bipolar disorder, schizophrenia, depression

(continues)

Generic Name	Trade Names	Classifications	Indications
aspirin	Zorprin, others	Analgesic/antipyretic/ salicylate	Arthritis, pain
atenolol	Tenormin, others	Antiadrenergic/beta blocker	Angina, hypertension, myocardial infarction
atomoxetine	Strattera	Norepinephrine reuptake inhibitor	ADHD
atorvastatin	Lipitor	Antihyperlipidemic	High cholesterol
azelastine	Astelin	Antihistamine	Allergy
azithromycin	Zithromax	Antibiotic	Infection
benazepril HCl	Lotensin	ACE inhibitor	Hypertension
benazepril HCl/ hydrochlorothiazide	Lotensin HCT	ACE inhibitor/diuretic	Hypertension
benzonatate	Tessalon Perles	Antitussive	Cough
benzoyl peroxide/ clindamycin	BenzaClin	Antibiotic/dermatologic	Acne
benztropine mesylate	Cogentin, others	Anticholinergic (antiparkinson)	Parkinson disease, extrapyramidal disorder
bimatoprost	Lumigan	Ophthalmologic	Glaucoma
bisoprolol/HCTZ	Ziac	Beta blocker/diuretic	Hypertension
brimonidine	Alphagan P	Adrenergic agonist; ophthalmologic	Glaucoma
budesonide	Pulmicort, Rhinocort, others	Inhaled corticosteroid	Asthma, Crohn disease, inflammatory bowel disease, rhinitis
budesonide	Rhinocort Aqua	Corticosteroid	Rhinitis
budesonide and formoterol	Symbicort	Corticosteroid and beta agonist	Asthma, COPD
buprenorphine and naloxone	Suboxone	Partial opioid agonist	Opioid addiction and withdrawal
bupropion HCl	Wellbutrin, Zyban	Antidepressant	Depression, smoking cessation
buspirone HCl	BuSpar	Anxiolytic	Anxiety
butalbital/APAP/ caffeine	Fioricet with codeine	Analgesic/barbiturate/ xanthine	Pain

Generic Name	Trade Names	Classifications	Indications
calcitonin	Miacalcin	Hormone	High calcium levels, Paget disease
candesartan	Atacand	Angiotensin II receptor antagonist	Hypertension
captopril	Capoten	ACE inhibitor	Congestive heart failure, hypertension, myocardial infarction, diabetic neuropathy
carisoprodol	Soma, others	Skeletal muscle relaxant	Musculoskeletal pain
carvedilol	Coreg	Antiadrenergic/beta blocker	Hypertension, myocardial infarction
cefdinir	Omnicef	Antibiotic/cephalosporin	Infection
cefprozil	Cefzil	Antibiotic	Infection
cefuroxime axetil	Ceftin	Antibiotic	Infection
celecoxib	Celebrex	Analgesic/NSAID	Arthritis
cephalexin	Keflex	Antibiotic/cephalosporin	Infection
cetirizine HCl	Zyrtec	Antihistamine	Allergy
cetirizine/ pseudoephedrine	Zyrtec-D	Antihistamine/ decongestant	Allergy
cimetidine HCl	Tagamet, others	Antihistamine, H_2/ gastrointestinal	Gastroesophageal reflux disease, ulcer
ciprofloxacin HCl	Ciloxan, Cipro, others	Antibiotic	Infection (e.g., bone, respiratory, urinary), anthrax
Citalopram hydrobromide	Celexa	SSRI antidepressant	Depression
clarithromycin	Biaxin	Antibiotic	Infection
clindamycin HCl	Cleocin	Antibiotic	Infection
clonazepam	Klonopin	Anxiolytic/benzodiazepine	Epilepsy
clonidine HCl	Catapres, Catapres-TTS, others	Antiadrenergic (central)	Pain, hypertension
clopidogrel bisulfate	Plavix	Platelet inhibitor	Myocardial infarction and stroke prevention
clotrimazole	Lotrimin	Antifungal	Fungal infection

(continues)

Generic Name	Trade Names	Classifications	Indications
clotrimazole/ betamethasone	Lotrisone	Antifungal	Fungal infection
codeine phosphate	Codeine Phosphate	Narcotic analgesic	Pain
conjugated estrogens	Premarin	Hormone (estrogen)	Cancer, menopause
conjugated estrogens/ medroxyprogesterone	Prempro	Hormone	Menopause
cyclobenzaprine HCl	Flexeril	Skeletal muscle relaxant	Muscle spasm
dabigatran	Pradaxa	Anticoagulant	Blood clots
desloratadine	Clarinex	Antihistamine	Allergy
desogestrel/ethinyl estradiol	Apri, Desogen, Kariva, Mircette	Contraceptive	Contraception
desvenlafaxine	Pristiq	Antidepressant	Depression
dexamethasone/ tobramycin	TobraDex	Anti-infective/corticosteroid; ophthalmologic	Eye injury, infection
dexlansoprazole	Dexilant	Proton-pump inhibitor	GERD, gastritis
dexmethylphenidate	Focalin	Central nervous system stimulant	ADHD
diazepam	Valium	Anxiolytic/benzodiazepine/muscle relaxant	Ethyl alcohol withdrawal, epilepsy, muscle spasm
diclofenac	Voltaren	Analgesic/NSAID	Pain, arthritis
digoxin	Digitek, Lanoxin	Antiarrhythmic/cardiac glycoside/inotropic	Atrial fibrillation, congestive heart failure
diltiazem/diltiazem HCl	Tiazac	Calcium channel blocker	Angina, hypertension, atrial fibrillation or flutter, paroxysmal supraventricular tachycardia
diphenhydramine	Benadryl	Antihistamine	Allergic reaction
divalproex	Depakote	Anticonvulsant	Epilepsy
docetaxel	Taxotere	Antineoplastic	Breast cancer
donepezil HCl	Aricept	Cholinesterase inhibitor	Dementia, Alzheimer disease
dorzolamide HCl/ timolol maleate	Cosopt	Antiadrenergic/beta blocker/ophthalmologic	Glaucoma

Generic Name	Trade Names	Classifications	Indications
doxazosin mesylate	Cardura	Alpha$_1$ blocker	Benign prostatic hypertrophy, hypertension
doxepin HCl	Sinequan	Tricyclic antidepressant	Anxiety, depression
doxycycline	Vibramycin, others	Antibiotic/tetracycline	Infection
drospirenone/ethinyl estradiol	Yasmin 28	Contraceptive	Contraception
duloxetine	Cymbalta	SSRI antidepressant	Depression
dutasteride	Avodart	Alpha blocker	Prostatic hypertrophy
enalapril maleate	Vasotec	ACE inhibitor	Congestive heart failure, hypertension, left ventricular dysfunction
epoetin alfa	Epogen, Procrit	Hematopoietic/hormone	Anemia
erythromycin	Ilotycin	Antibiotic	Infection
escitalopram	Lexapro	SSRI antidepressant	Depression
esomeprazole	Nexium	Gastrointestinal/PPI	Ulcer, gastroesophageal reflux disease, esophagitis
estradiol	Climara, Estraderm, Vivelle-DOT, others	Estrogen hormone	Menopause, cancer, vaginal atrophy
estradiol/norethindrone acetate	Activella	Hormone	Menopause
eszopiclone	Lunesta	Sedative	Difficulty sleeping
etanercept	Enbrel	Antirheumatic	Rheumatoid arthritis
ethinyl estradiol/ norethindrone	Ovcon-35	Contraceptive	Contraception
ethinyl estradiol/ ethynodiol diacetate	Zovia 1/35	Contraceptive	Contraception
ethinyl estradiol/ferrous fumarate/hormone nore-thindrone acetate	Estrostep Fe	Contraceptive	Contraception
ethinyl estradiol/ levonorgestrel	Levora, Triphasil, Trivora-28	Contraceptive	Contraception
ethinyl estradiol/ norethindrone	Necon	Contraceptive	Contraception

(continues)

Generic Name	Trade Names	Classifications	Indications
ethinyl estradiol/ norgestimate	Ortho-Cyclen, Ortho Tri-Cyclen	Contraceptive	Contraception
ethinyl estradiol/ norelgestromin	Ortho Evra	Contraceptive	Contraception
etonogestrel/ethinyl estradiol	NuvaRing	Contraceptive	Contraception
ezetimibe	Zetia	Antihyperlipidemic	High cholesterol
ezetimibe/simvastatin	Vytorin	Antihyperlipidemic	High cholesterol
famotidine	Pepcid	Antihistamine, H_2 blocker/ gastrointestinal	Adenoma, gastroesopha- geal reflux disease, ulcer
felodipine	Plendil	Calcium channel blocker	Hypertension
fenofibrate	Lipidil, TriCor	Antihyperlipidemic	High triglyceride level
fentanyl citrate	Duragesic	Narcotic analgesic	Pain
fexofenadine HCl	Allegra	Antihistamine	Rhinitis, seasonal allergy
fexofenadine HCl/pseudo- ephedrine HCl	Allegra-D	Antihistamine/ decongestant	Rhinitis, seasonal allergy
finasteride	Proscar	Antiandrogen/hormone	Hair loss, benign prostatic hypertrophy
fluconazole	Diflucan	Antifungal	Candidiasis, meningitis, bone marrow transplant adjunct
fluoxetine HCl	Prozac	SSRI antidepressant	Depression, bulimia, obsessive-compulsive disorder
fluticasone propionate	Flonase, Flovent	Inhaled corticosteroid	Allergic rhinitis, dermatosis
fluticasone propionate, salmeterol xinafoate	Advair Diskus	Adrenergic agonist/ bronchodilator/ inhaled corticosteroid	Asthma
fluvastatin	Lescol XL	Antihyperlipidemic	High cholesterol
folic acid	Folvite	Hematinic/vitamin	Anemia
fosinopril	Monopril	ACE inhibitor	Hypertension, congestive heart failure
flunisolide inhaled	AeroBid	Inhaled corticosteroid	Asthma prophylaxis

Generic Name	Trade Names	Classifications	Indications
furosemide	Lasix	Loop diuretic	Edema, pulmonary conditions, congestive heart failure, hypertension
gabapentin	Neurontin	Anticonvulsant	Epilepsy
gatifloxacin	Tequin	Antibiotic	Infection
gemfibrozil	Lopid	Antihyperlipidemic	High cholesterol
glimepiride	Amaryl	Antidiabetic agent	Diabetes mellitus
glipizide	Glucotrol, Glucotrol XL	Antidiabetic agent	Diabetes mellitus
glyburide	DiaBeta, others	Antidiabetic agent	Diabetes mellitus
glyburide/metformin	Glucovance	Antidiabetic agent	Diabetes mellitus
human insulin 70/30	Humulin 70/30	Antidiabetic agent/insulin	Diabetes mellitus
human insulin NPH	Humulin N	Antidiabetic agent/insulin	Diabetes mellitus
hydrochlorothiazide	Esidrix	Diuretic	Edema, hypertension
hydrochlorothiazide/ losartan	Hyzaar	Angiotensin II receptor antagonist/diuretic	Hypertension
hydrocodone/ibuprofen	Vicoprofen	Narcotic analgesic/NSAID	Pain
hydroxyzine	Atarax	Antiemetic/antihistamine/ anxiolytic/sedative	Ethyl alcohol withdrawal, anxiety, nausea and vomiting
hyoscyamine sulfate	Levsin, others	Anticholinergic/ gastrointestinal	Bladder, bowel, pancreatic problems; Parkinson disease
ibuprofen	Advil, Motrin, others	Analgesic/ anti-inflammatory/ antipyretic/NSAID	Rheumatoid arthritis and osteoarthritis, mild to moderate pain, primary dysmenorrhea, fever, pain
infliximab	Remicade	Antirheumatic/ gastrointestinal/ immunomodulator	Rheumatoid arthritis, Crohn disease
insulin aspart	NovoLog	Antidiabetic agent/insulin	Diabetes mellitus
insulin detemir	Levemir	Antidiabetic agent/insulin	Diabetes mellitus
insulin glargine	Lantus	Antidiabetic agent/insulin	Diabetes mellitus
insulin lispro	Humalog	Antidiabetic agent/insulin	Diabetes mellitus

(continues)

Generic Name	Trade Names	Classifications	Indications
ipratropium	Atrovent	Anticholinergic bronchodilator	Bronchospasm associated with chronic obstructive pulmonary disease
ipratropium/albuterol	Combivent	Adrenergic agonist/ anticholinergic/ bronchodilator	Bronchitis, chronic obstructive pulmonary disease
irbesartan	Avapro	Angiotensin II receptor antagonist	Hypertension
irbesartan/HCTZ	Avalide	Angiotensin II receptor antagonist/diuretic	Hypertension
isosorbide mononitrate	Isomer, others	Nitrate/vasodilator	Angina
isotretinoin	Accutane	Acne	Acne
ketoconazole	Nizoral shampoo	Antifungal	Skin infection
lamivudine/zidovudine	Combivir	Antiviral	HIV
lamotrigine	Lamictal	Anticonvulsant	Epilepsy
lansoprazole	Prevacid	Gastrointestinal/PPI	Esophagitis, gastroesophageal reflux disease, ulcer
latanoprost	Xalatan	Ophthalmologic	Glaucoma
leuprolide acetate	Lupron Depot	Antineoplastic/hormone	Cancer, endometriosis
levalbuterol HCl	Xopenex	Adrenergic agonist/ bronchodilator	Asthma
levofloxacin	Levaquin	Antibiotic	Infection
levonorgestrel/ethinyl estradiol	Alesse, Aviane	Contraceptive/hormone	Contraception
levothyroxine	Levothroid, Levoxyl, Synthroid, others	Hormone (thyroid)	Goiter, hypothyroidism
lisdexamfetamine	Vyvanse	Central nervous system stimulant	ADHD
lisinopril	Prinivil, Zestril, others	ACE inhibitor	Congestive heart failure, hypertension
lisinopril/HCTZ	Zestoretic	ACE inhibitor/diuretic	Congestive heart failure, hypertension
loratadine	Claritin	Antihistamine	Allergy

Generic Name	Trade Names	Classifications	Indications
losartan	Cozaar	Angiotensin II receptor antagonist	Hypertension
lovastatin/niacin	Advicor	Cholesterol lowering	Elevated cholesterol
meclizine	Antivert, others	Antiemetic/antivertigo	Motion sickness, vertigo
memantine	Namenda	NDMA receptor antagonist	Alzheimer disease
medroxyprogesterone acetate	Depo-Provera	Hormone/antineoplastic/contraceptive	Amenorrhea, cancer, contraception, uterine bleeding
mesalamine	Asacol, Rowasa, others	Gastrointestinal/salicylate	Colitis, proctitis
metaxalone	Skelaxin	Musculoskeletal relaxant	Pain
metformin HCl	Glucophage	Antidiabetic	Diabetes mellitus
metformin/sitagliptin	Janumet	Antidiabetic	Diabetes mellitus
methotrexate	Folex, Rheumatrex, others	Antineoplastic/antirheumatic	Arthritis, cancer
methylphenidate XR	Concerta	Central nervous system stimulant	ADHD
methylprednisolone	Medrol	Corticosteroid	Adrenocortical insufficiency, anemia, arthritis, allergy, gastrointestinal conditions, inflammatory conditions
metoclopramide	Reglan	Antiemetic/gastrointestinal stimulant	Gastrointestinal conditions
metolazone	Zaroxolyn	Diuretic	Edema, hypertension
metoprolol succinate	Toprol XL	Antiadrenergic/beta blocker	Angina, hypertension, myocardial infarction, congestive heart failure
metoprolol tartrate	Lopressor	Antiadrenergic/beta blocker	Angina, hypertension, myocardial infarction, congestive heart failure
metronidazole	Flagyl	Antibiotic	Infection
minocycline HCl	Minocin	Antibiotic/tetracycline	Infection
mirtazapine	Remeron, others	Tricyclic antidepressant	Depression

(continues)

Generic Name	Trade Names	Classifications	Indications
mometasone	Elocon, Nasonex	Inhaled corticosteroid	Dermatosis, rhinitis
montelukast	Singulair	Leukotriene blocker/inhibitor	Asthma
mupirocin	Bactroban	Anti-infective/dermatologic	Skin infection
nabumetone	Relafen	Analgesic/NSAID	Arthritis
naproxen	Naprosyn	Analgesic/NSAID	Arthritis, pain
nebivolol	Bystolic	Beta blocker	Hypertension
nefazodone HCl	Serzone	Antidepressant	Depression
niacin	Niaspan	Antihyperlipidemic/vitamin	High cholesterol, high triglyceride level
Nifedipine	Adalat, Nifediac CC, Nifedipine ER, Procardia XL	Calcium channel blocker	Angina, hypertension
nitrofurantoin	Macrobid	Antibiotic	Urinary tract infection
nitroglycerin	NitroQuick, Transderm, others	Vasodilator	Angina, congestive heart failure, hypertension
norethindrone/ethinyl estradiol	Microgestin Fe, Ortho-Novum, Ortho-Novum 7/7/7, Loestrin Fe 1/20, Lo-Ovral, Low-Ogestrel	Hormone/contraceptive	Contraception
nortriptyline HCl	Pamelor	Tricyclic antidepressant	Depression
ofloxacin	Floxin, Ocuflox	Antibiotic/antifungal	Infection
olanzapine	Zyprexa	Antipsychotic	Schizophrenia, bipolar disorder
olmesartan medoxomil	Benicar	Angiotensin II receptor blocker	Hypertension
olopatadine HCl	Patanol	Antihistamine	Conjunctivitis
omeprazole	Prilosec, others	Gastrointestinal/PPI	Esophagitis, gastroesophageal reflux disease, ulcer
oseltamivir	Tamiflu	Antiviral	Influenza
oxybutynin	Ditropan XL	Anticholinergic	Incontinence, bladder dysfunction
oxycodone HCl	OxyContin	Narcotic analgesic	Pain

Generic Name	Trade Names	Classifications	Indications
oxycodone/ acetaminophen	Percocet, Roxicet, Endocet	Narcotic analgesic	Pain
pantoprazole	Protonix	Gastrointestinal/PPI	gastroesophageal reflux disease
paroxetine HCl	Paxil	SSRI antidepressant	Anxiety, panic disorder, depression, obsessive-compulsive disorder
penicillin VK	Penicillin VK, Veetids	Antibiotic	Infection
phenazopyridine HCl	Pyridium	Analgesic	Dysuria
phenobarbital	Luminal, Phenobarbital, others	Anticonvulsant/ barbiturate/sedative	Epilepsy, insomnia
phenytoin	Dilantin	Anticonvulsant	Epilepsy
pimecrolimus	Elidel	Dermatologic	Dermatitis
pioglitazone	Actos	Antidiabetic	Diabetes mellitus
potassium chloride	K-Dur, Klor-Con, Klor-Con M20	Electrolyte	Hypokalemia
pravastatin	Pravachol	Antihyperlipidemic	High cholesterol
prednisone	Deltasone	Corticosteroid	Adrenal insufficiency, inflammatory conditions
pregabalin	Lyrica	Anticonvulsant	Chronic pain, neuropathy, seizures
progesterone	Prometrium, Progestasert, others	Antiemetic/antihistamine/ phenothiazine	Amenorrhea, uterine bleeding
promethazine HCl	Phenergan, Promethegan, others	Antiemetic/antihistamine/ phenothiazine	Allergy, motion sickness
propranolol	Inderal, Inderal LA, others	Antiadrenergic/beta blocker/antiarrhythmic	Angina, atrial arrhythmia, migraine, hypertension, myocardial infarction
quetiapine fumarate	Seroquel	Antipsychotic	Schizophrenia
quinapril	Accupril	ACE inhibitor	Congestive heart failure, hypertension
rabeprazole	Aciphex	PPI	Gastroesophageal reflux disease, ulcers
raloxifene HCl	Evista	Hormone (estrogen)	Osteoporosis

(continues)

Generic Name	Trade Names	Classifications	Indications
ramipril	Altace	ACE inhibitor	Myocardial infarction and stroke prevention, congestive heart failure, hypertension
ranitidine HCl	Zantac	Antihistamine, H_2/ gastrointestinal	Esophagitis, gastroesophageal reflux disease, ulcer
risedronate	Actonel	Bisphosphonate	Paget disease
risperidone	Risperdal	Antipsychotic	Psychosis, schizophrenia
rivaroxaban	Xarelto	Anticoagulant	Blood clots
rivastigmine tartrate	Exelon	Cholinesterase inhibitor	Dementia, Alzheimer disease
rosuvastatin	Crestor	Antihyperlipidemic	High cholesterol
salmeterol	Serevent	Adrenergic agonist/ bronchodilator	Asthma, bronchospasm
sertraline HCl	Zoloft	SSRI antidepressant	Depression, obsessive-compulsive disorder, panic disorder, premenstrual syndrome, post-traumatic stress disorder
sildenafil citrate	Viagra	Impotence agent	Erectile dysfunction
simvastatin	Zocor	Antihyperlipidemic	Congestive heart failure and myocardial infarction prevention, high cholesterol
sitagliptin	Januvia	Antidiabetic agent	Diabetes mellitus
solifenacin	Vesicare	Anticholinergic agent	Overactive bladder
spironolactone	Aldactone	Diuretic	Adenoma, edema, hypertension
sulfamethoxazole/ trimethoprim	Bactrim, Cotrim, SMX-TMP, others	Antibiotic/sulfonamide	Infection
sumatriptan	Imitrex	Serotonin receptor agonist	Migraine headache
tadalafil	Cialis	Impotence agent	Erectile dysfunction
tamoxifen citrate	Nolvadex	Antineoplastic/hormone	Breast cancer
tamsulosin	Flomax	Antiadrenergic/alpha blocker	Benign prostatic hypertrophy

Generic Name	Trade Names	Classifications	Indications
temazepam	Restoril	Benzodiazepine/sedative	Insomnia
terazosin HCl	Hytrin	Alpha$_1$ blocker	Benign prostatic hypertrophy
terbinafine HCl	Lamisil Oral	Antifungal	Fungal infection
theophylline	Theophylline SR	Methylxanthine bronchodilator	Asthma, bronchospasm
timolol	Timoptic	Beta blocker, ophthalmologic	Glaucoma
tiotropium	Spiriva	Bronchodilator	Asthma, COPD
tolterodine tartrate	Detrol, Detrol LA	Anticholinergic/urinary tract relaxant	Incontinence
topiramate	Topamax	Anticonvulsant	Epilepsy
tramadol HCl	Ultram	Narcotic-like analgesic	Pain
tramadol/acetaminophen	Ultracet	Narcotic-like analgesic	Pain
trandolapril	Mavik	ACE inhibitor	Hypertension, congestive heart failure
travoprost	Travatan Z	Ophthalmic agent	Glaucoma
trazodone HCl	Desyrel	Antidepressant	Depression
triamcinolone	Aristocort	Corticosteroid	Anemia, inflammatory conditions
Triamcinolone acetonide	Nasacort AQ	Corticosteroid	Anemia, inflammatory conditions
triamterene	Dyrenium	Diuretic	Edema, congestive heart failure
valacyclovir	Valtrex	Antiviral	Herpes
valdecoxib	Bextra	Analgesic/NSAID	Arthritis, dysmenorrhea
valsartan	Diovan	Angiotensin II receptor blocker	Hypertension, congestive heart failure
valsartan/HCTZ	Diovan HCT	Angiotensin II antagonist/ diuretic	Hypotension, congestive heart failure
vardenafil HCl	Levitra	Impotence agent	Erectile dysfunction
varenicline	Chantix	Nicotine agonist	Smoking cessation

(continues)

Generic Name	Trade Names	Classifications	Indications
venlafaxine HCl	Effexor, Effexor XR	Antidepressant	Depression, anxiety
verapamil	Calan	Calcium channel blocker	Angina, arrhythmia, hypertension
warfarin	Coumadin	Anticoagulant	Arrhythmia, pulmonary embolism, deep vein thrombosis
zolpidem tartrate	Ambien	Sedative-hypnotic	Insomnia

ACE, Angiotensin-converting enzyme; *ADHD,* attention deficit–hyperactivity disorder; *APAP,* acetaminophen; *HCl,* hydrochloride; *HCTZ,* hydrochlorothiazide; *NSAID,* nonsteroidal anti-inflammatory drug; *PPI,* proton pump inhibitor; *SSRI,* selective serotonin reuptake inhibitor.

Appendix D

Common Herbal Supplements

Herbal Product	Uses	Important Facts
Acai	Decreasing fasting glucose and improving total cholesterol; other uses include erectile dysfunction, weight loss, and improving overall health	Has not been shown to improve low-density lipoprotein, high-density lipoprotein, or blood pressure
Alfalfa	Digestive disorders, arthritis, to increase blood clotting, as a diuretic, cystitis; may also improve cholesterol and reduce blood glucose levels	Should not be used during pregnancy or in patients with lupus erythematosus; seeds should not be eaten; may increase prothrombin time and prolong bleeding when taken with anticoagulants; may contain vitamin K, which may decrease the effect of oral anticoagulants; potentiate hypoglycemic action; avoid concurrent use with estrogen and oral contraceptives; may cause hypotension, photosensitivity
Aloe	Minor burns, sunburns, cuts, abrasions, bed sores, diabetic ulcers, acne, stomatitis, weight loss	Should not be used internally during pregnancy; should not be given to children younger than 12 years; should not be used by persons with kidney disease, cardiac disease, or bowel obstruction; should not be used topically by persons hypersensitive to aloe, garlic, onions, or tulips; may cause gastrointestinal spasms, intestinal mucosa damage, hemorrhagic diarrhea, red-colored urine, nephrotoxicity, contact dermatitis, delayed healing of deep wounds, hypokalemia, uterine contractions causing spontaneous abortion, premature labor; aloe products taken internally may increase the effects of antiarrhythmics, cardiac glycosides, antidiabetics, loop diuretics, potassium-wasting drugs, systemic steroids, and thiazides; if taken internally, avoid concurrent use with licorice, which may cause hypokalemia; aloe may lower serum potassium levels with long-term use; *avoid prolonged use or higher doses*
Arginine	Congestive heart failure, erectile dysfunction, peripheral vascular disease, angina, interstitial cystitis, chronic renal failure, sexual dysfunction	Safety in pregnancy and children not established; should not be used by persons with severe hepatic disease; may cause nausea, vomiting, anorexia, increased blood urea nitrogen level, hyperkalemia; angiotensin-converting enzyme inhibitors taken with arginine IV may lead to fatal hypokalemia; concurrent use of alcohol, NSAIDs, platelet inhibitors, and salicylates may cause an increased risk of bleeding

(continues)

Herbal Product	Uses	Important Facts
Astragalus	Bronchitis, chronic obstructive pulmonary disease, colds, flu, gastrointestinal conditions, weakness, fatigue, chronic hepatitis, ulcers, hypertension, viral myocarditis, numerous other indications	Should not be used during pregnancy and lactation; may cause allergic reactions; may decrease or increase action of antihypertensives, avoid concurrent use
Belladonna	Irritable bowel syndrome, nervous system disorders, headache, asthma, menopausal symptoms, premenstrual syndrome, radiation burns, muscle and bone aches	Should not be used during pregnancy and lactation; should not be used in children; may cause dilated pupils, flushed skin, dry mouth, tachycardia, confusion, nervousness, hallucinations, allergic rashes; should not be used in persons sensitive to anticholinergic drugs or who are allergic to members of the nightshade family such as bell peppers, potatoes, and eggplant; atropine is an ingredient in belladonna, therefore, drugs that interact with atropine will interact with belladonna
Betel nut	CNS stimulation, schizophrenia, anemia	Should not be used during pregnancy and lactation; should not be used in children; may cause skin color changes, dilated pupils, blurred vision, difficulty breathing, increased salivation, incontinence, diaphoresis, fever, confusion, psychosis, amnesia, feeling of euphoria; may cause tremors, stiffness in persons also taking antipsychotic medications; chewing betel nuts may cause nausea, vomiting, stomach cramps, diarrhea, chest pain, arrhythmias; do not use concurrently with alcohol, antiglaucoma agents, monoamine oxidase inhibitors, neuroleptics
Bilberry	To improve night vision; prevent cataracts, macular degeneration, and glaucoma; treat varicose veins and hemorrhoids; prevent hemorrhage after surgery; prevent and treat diabetic retinopathy and myopia; decrease diarrhea and dyspepsia; control insulin levels	Safety in pregnancy not established; may cause constipation; use caution if taking concurrently with anticoagulants, antiplatelets, aspirin, insulin, NSAIDs, oral antidiabetics
Black cohosh	Menopausal symptoms, arthritis	Use during pregnancy may cause uterine stimulation; should not be used during lactation; should be given to children only under supervision of a qualified herbalist; should not be used in patients with a history of estrogen receptor–positive breast cancer; may cause bradycardia, uterine stimulation, spontaneous abortion, nausea, vomiting, anorexia; oral contraceptives, use cautiously with hormone replacement therapy
Blessed thistle	Anorexia, gastrointestinal discomfort, and dyspepsia	Should not be used during pregnancy; may cause nausea, vomiting, anorexia, contact dermatitis. Has been known to increase gastric acid secretion

Herbal Product	Uses	Important Facts
Burdock	Arthritis, diabetes, some skin disorders (e.g., psoriasis, eczema, poison ivy), hypertension, inflammatory disorders	May cause hypotension, hypoglycemia; use with caution in persons with diabetes or cardiac disorders; avoid concurrent use with antidiabetics, antihypertensives, calcium channel blockers
Capsicum	Diarrhea, cramps, osteoarthritis, neuralgia, neuropathy, back pain, muscle spasms, migraines	Generally recognized as safe when used in typical food preparations. Avoid high doses or long-term use. May cause hypertensive crisis in higher doses. May cause abdominal discomfort and skin/eye irritation. Inhalation may cause dyspnea, congestion; when used as a "pepper spray" respiratory arrest and death has occurred
Chamomile	Wide variety of uses, including restlessness, anxiety, gastrointestinal distress, fibromyalgia attention deficit hyperactivity disorder	Generally recognized as safe when used in foods; medicinal doses may not be safe when taken long-term; unclear if safe during pregnancy and lactation; has mild sedative effects, use caution when taking other medications with sedative properties; may interfere with contraceptive medications; may increase bleeding risks when taken with warfarin (Coumadin); interacts with certain cytochrome P450 substrates
Chondroitin	Joint conditions (in combination with glucosamine), coronary artery disease, interstitial cystitis, hyperlipidemia	Safety in pregnancy and children not established; should not be used in persons with bleeding disorders; may cause headache, restlessness, euphoria, nausea, vomiting, anorexia
Coenzyme Q10	Ischemic heart disease, congestive heart failure, angina pectoris, hypertension, arrhythmias, diabetes mellitus, breast cancer, deafness, Bell's palsy, decreased immunity, mitral valve prolapse, periodontal disease, infertility	Should not be used at excessive levels during pregnancy and lactation; safety in children not established; may cause nausea, vomiting, anorexia, diarrhea, epigastric pain; avoid concurrent use with anticoagulants, beta blockers, HMG-CoA reductase inhibitors
Cranberry	Urinary tract disorders, susceptibility to kidney stones	Should not be used by persons with oliguria, anuria; may cause diarrhea (large doses), hypersensitivity reactions
Creatine	Enhanced athletic performance, prevention of age-related muscle loss	Safety in pregnancy and children not established; may cause nausea, vomiting, anorexia, bloating, weight gain, diarrhea, dehydration, cramping (high doses)
Dandelion	As a laxative, antihypertensive, diuretic	Safety in children not established; several notable medication interactions, including anticoagulants, antidiabetic agents, potassium-sparing diuretics, and certain antibiotics; generally recognized as safe in typical food quantities
Devil's claw	Anorexia, joint pain and inflammation, allergies, headache, heartburn, dysmenorrhea, gastrointestinal upset	Should not be used during pregnancy and lactation; should not be given to children; may cause nausea, vomiting, anorexia; use cautiously with antiarrhythmics; many significant medication interactions

(continues)

Herbal Product	Uses	Important Facts
DHEA	Atherosclerosis, hyperglycemia, cancer, to improve memory and cognitive functioning	Safety in pregnancy and children not established; avoid use in persons with estrogen-sensitive tumors, prostate cancer, or benign prostatic hypertrophy; may cause arrhythmias (high doses), insomnia, restlessness, irritability, anxiety, increased mood, aggressiveness, acne; avoid concurrent use with hormone replacement therapy
Dong quai	Menopausal symptoms, menstrual irregularities (e.g., dysmenorrhea, premenstrual syndrome, menorrhagia), headache, neuralgia, herpes infections, malaria	Safety in pregnancy and children not established; avoid use in persons with bleeding disorders, excessive menstrual flow, or acute illness; may cause nausea, vomiting, diarrhea, anorexia, increased menstrual flow, hypersensitivity reactions, photosensitivity, fever, bleeding; do not combine with antiplatelets and oral anticoagulants; may exacerbate estrogen-sensitive cancers and conditions
Echinacea	Prevention and treatment of infection (especially a cold or the flu), impaired immune status	Should not be used during pregnancy and lactation; should not be given to children younger than 2 years; avoid use in persons with autoimmune diseases; may cause hepatotoxicity, hypersensitivity reactions, acute asthma attack, angioedema: numerous medication interactions
Evening primrose oil	Premenstrual syndrome, hot flashes, inflammatory disorders, migraine headache, Alzheimer disease, schizophrenia, liver cancer, chronic fatigue syndrome	May cause uterine contraction in pregnant women; may lower seizure threshold in seizure disorders or individuals taking phenothiazines; do not use concurrently with phenothiazines; may prolong bleeding time
Feverfew	Fever, migraine headache prophylaxis, arthritis, asthma, nausea, vomiting, allergies	Do not use in pregnancy; may cause nausea, heartburn, diarrhea, constipation, abdominal pain, and other gastrointestinal issues; many notable medication interactions
Fish oil	Wide variety of uses including hyperlipidemia, hypertension, coronary artery disease, depression, ventricular arrhythmias	Generally recognized as safe with typical food doses. Dietary sources may contain other toxins with serious harmful effects; >3 g/day may inhibit platelet aggregation; may lower blood pressure, particularly in combination with other antihypertensive agents
Flaxseed oil	Wide variety of uses including constipation, rheumatoid arthritis, weight loss, cardiovascular disease, hypertension, elevated cholesterol	Avoid use in pregnancy, may increase risk of premature birth, otherwise considered safe for short-term use; may decrease platelet aggregation; use caution when combining with antihypertensive medications; may cause loose stools and diarrhea
Garlic	Improve circulation, lower blood lipid levels, hypertension, inflammatory/menstrual disorders, earaches, diarrhea, cold and flu symptoms	May increase bleeding time; should not be used before or immediately after surgery or with drugs or herbs that affect clotting; may cause hypersensitivity reactions, contact dermatitis, diaphoresis, garlic odor, irritation of the oral cavities; do not use concurrently with anticoagulants; may increase effects of antihypertensive medications; avoid concurrent use with isoniazid

Herbal Product	Uses	Important Facts
Ginger	Nausea, indigestion, sore throat, motion and morning sickness, inflammation, migraine headaches	Safety in pregnancy not established; may cause nausea, vomiting, anorexia, hypersensitivity reactions; may increase the risk of bleeding when used concurrently with anticoagulants or antiplatelets
Ginkgo	Decrease disturbances of cerebral functioning and peripheral vascular insufficiency in persons with Alzheimer disease or other types of age-related dementia, as an antioxidant, to improve peripheral artery disease, enhance circulation throughout the body, depressive mood disorders, sexual dysfunction, asthma, glaucoma, menopausal symptoms, multiple sclerosis, headaches, tinnitus, dizziness, arthritis, altitude sickness, intermittent claudication	Safety in pregnancy and children not established; should not be used in persons with coagulation or platelet disorders, hemophilia; may cause transient headache, anxiety, restlessness, nausea, vomiting, anorexia, diarrhea, hypersensitivity reactions, rash; avoid concurrent use with anticonvulsants or in patients prone to seizures; avoid concurrent use with anticoagulants, monoamine oxidase inhibitors, platelet inhibitors
Ginseng	Physical/mental exhaustion, stress, viral infection, diabetes, headache	Safety in pregnancy and children not established; may cause increased QT interval, chest pain, palpitations, insomnia, restlessness (high doses), headache, nausea, vomiting, anorexia, diarrhea (high doses), hypersensitivity reactions, rash; avoid concurrent use with immunosuppressants, insulin, monoamine oxidase inhibitors, oral antidiabetics, stimulants, and many other common medications
Glucosamine	Joint conditions (in combination with chondroitin)	Should not be used during pregnancy and lactation; may cause drowsiness, headache, nausea, vomiting, anorexia, constipation or diarrhea, heartburn, epigastric pain, cramps, indigestion, hypersensitivity reactions, rash (rare); may increase the effects of antidiabetics; do not use concurrently with warfarin (Coumadin)
Goldenseal	Gastritis, gastrointestinal ulceration, peptic ulcer disease, mouth ulcer, bladder infection, sore throat, postpartum hemorrhage, skin disorders (e.g., pruritus, boils, hemorrhoids, anal fissures, eczema), cancer, tuberculosis, may promote wound healing and reduce inflammation	Uterine stimulant—should not be used during pregnancy; safety during lactation and in children not established; *numerous significant medication interactions*
Gotu kola	Improves venous and arterial blood flow, fatigue, anxiety, wound healing, common cold, influenza, Alzheimer disease, epilepsy, striae gravidarum (stretch marks)	Safety in pregnancy and children not established; may cause hepatotoxicity; use with caution with other medications known to cause liver injury; may cause increased sedation when taken concurrently with other sedative medications
Grapeseed	Antioxidant, disease prevention, leg cramps, inflammation, vision problems	Safety in pregnancy and children not established; may cause dizziness, nausea, anorexia, hepatotoxicity, rash

(continues)

Herbal Product	Uses	Important Facts
Green tea	Used as a general antioxidant, anticancer agent, diuretic, antibacterial, antilipidemic, antiatherosclerotic, cognitive performance	Caffeine content may cause hypertension, palpitations, arrhythmia (high doses), anxiety, nervousness, insomnia (high doses), nausea, heartburn, increased stomach acid (high doses), hypersensitivity reactions; antacids may decrease the therapeutic effects of green tea; large amounts may increase the action of some bronchodilators
Hawthorn	Cardiovascular disorders (e.g., hypertension, arrhythmias, arteriosclerosis, congestive heart disease, stable angina pectoris)	Safety in pregnancy and children not established; may cause hypotension, arrhythmias, fatigue, sedation, nausea; avoid concurrent use with antihypertensives (especially nitrates and phosphodiesterase inhibitors), CNS depressants; carefully monitor concurrent use with cardiac glycosides
Horse chestnut	Fever, phlebitis, hemorrhoids, prostate enlargement, edema, inflammation, diarrhea, varicose veins	Do not consume raw bark, seeds, flower, or leaves; safety in pregnancy and children not established; may cause nephrotoxicity, hepatotoxicity, severe bleeding, shock, nausea, vomiting, anorexia, pruritus, hypersensitivity, rash, urticaria, muscle spasms; do not use concurrently with anticoagulants, aspirin, and other salicylates; may increase the hypoglycemic effects of diabetic medications
Horsetail	**Internally:** Oral diuretic for treatment of edema, osteoporosis **Externally:** To promote wound healing	Safety in pregnancy and children not established; certain preparations may lead to thiamine deficiency; may cause nausea or mild gastrointestinal distress; interacts with many diuretic and antidiabetic agents
Kava	Anxiety, depression, insomnia, stress, to promote wound healing	Unsafe in pregnancy and lactation; has been implicated in numerous cases of liver failure, prompting market withdrawals in certain countries; monitor liver function tests during use; may produce a wide variety of CNS, hematologic, hepatic, and other adverse effects; do not use concurrently with antiparkinsonian, benzodiazepines, CNS depressants; antipsychotics taken with kava may result in neuroleptic movement disorders; concurrent use with barbiturates may result in increased sedation
Lavender	Anxiety, insomnia, depression, anorexia, nausea, vomiting, migraine headaches	Safety in pregnancy and children not established; may cause headache, drowsiness, nausea, vomiting, increased appetite, hypersensitivity reactions, contact dermatitis; avoid concurrent use with alcohol, antihistamines, opioids, sedatives/hypnotics
Licorice	Constipation, asthma, malaria, hepatitis, abdominal pain, gastrointestinal disorders, infections, eczema, chronic fatigue syndrome, insomnia	Unsafe in pregnancy; should not be used by persons with renal disease, hypokalemia, hypertension, arrhythmias, congestive heart failure; may cause hypokalemia, hypertension, edema, headache, weakness, nausea, vomiting, anorexia, hypersensitivity reactions; do not use concurrently with antiarrhythmics, antihypertensives, coumadin, or many other medications metabolized by certain cytochrome P450 substrates

Herbal Product	Uses	Important Facts
Lycopene	Cancer prevention, atherosclerosis, cardiovascular disease, Parkinson disease, asthma, hypertension	Considered safe when taken in foods; higher doses may be harmful during pregnancy; may cause nausea, vomiting, anorexia, abdominal discomfort
Marshmallow	Cough, sore throat, gastric disorders (e.g., irritable bowel syndrome, gastritis, constipation), minor skin disorders	Safety in pregnancy and children not established; may cause nausea, vomiting, anorexia, hypersensitivity reactions; may reduce the absorption of oral medications, do not use concurrently; may increase effects of hypoglycemic and anticoagulant agents
Melatonin	Insomnia, to inhibit cataract formation, increase longevity, treat jet lag, circadian rhythm disruption, prevent weight loss in cancer patients	Safety in pregnancy not established; may cause tachycardia, headache, change in sleep patterns, confusion, sedation; nausea, vomiting, anorexia; hypersensitivity reactions (rash, pruritus); use cautiously with benzodiazepines; avoid concurrent use with cerebral stimulants, DHEA, magnesium, succinylcholine, zinc
Milk thistle	Hepatotoxicity caused by poisonous mushrooms, cirrhosis of the liver, chronic candidiasis, hepatitis C, exposure to toxic chemicals, liver transplantation, anorexia	Safety in pregnancy and children not established; may cause nausea, vomiting, anorexia, diarrhea, menstrual changes, hypersensitivity reactions; should not be used with drugs metabolized by certain cytochrome P-450 enzyme
Passion flower	Anxiety, sleep disorders, neuralgia, nervous tachycardia, restlessness, opiate withdrawal	Safety in pregnancy not established; may cause CNS depression (usually at high doses), severe nausea, vomiting, drowsiness, prolonged QT interval, nonsustained ventricular tachycardia, liver toxicity, hypersensitivity reactions, anorexia; avoid concurrent use with CNS depressants
Propolis	Inflammation, to promote wound healing, bacterial and fungal infections, canker sores, warts	Safety in pregnancy and children not established; may cause nausea, anorexia, oral mucositis, stomatitis, hypersensitivity reactions, dermatitis, eczema
Pycnogenol	Wound healing, inflammation, elevated cholesterol, menopause, neuroprotective effects, also used as an antioxidant and an antitumor	Safety in pregnancy and children not established; may cause reduced blood platelet aggregation; use with caution with autoimmune conditions or bleeding disorders
Pygeum	Urinary tract infections, benign prostatic hypertrophy, to increase prostatic secretions that may cause sterility	Safety in pregnancy and children not established; may cause nausea, vomiting, anorexia, gastrointestinal irritation; minimal interaction with other medications, herbs and foods
Saw palmetto	Benign prostatic hypertrophy; urinary problems; chronic and subacute cystitis; to increase breast size, sperm count, and sexual potency	Should not be used during pregnancy; safety during lactation and in children not established; may cause hypertension, headache, nausea, vomiting, anorexia, constipation or diarrhea, abdominal pain and cramping, dysuria, urine retention, impotence, hypersensitivity reactions, back pain

(continues)

Herbal Product	Uses	Important Facts
Slippery elm	Cough, gastrointestinal conditions; topically, for smoothing skin and as a poultice to treat skin inflammation, wounds, burns	May cause spontaneous abortion if used during pregnancy; safety during lactation and in children not established; may cause nausea, vomiting, anorexia
Soy	To lower cholesterol, treat hyperactivity, fever, headache, anorexia, chronic hepatitis, menopausal symptoms, osteoporosis, various cancers	Considered generally safe for pregnancy, lactation, and use in children; no absolute contraindications are known; may cause hypersensitivity reactions, nausea, bloating, diarrhea, abdominal pain; avoid concurrent use with thyroid agents; several other notable interactions with various medication categories
Spirulina (blue-green algae)	Malnutrition, promote weight loss, decrease cholesterol, treat fibromyalgia, stress, fatigue, anxiety, depression	Safety in pregnancy not established; contaminants, including heavy metals, may make certain preparations unsafe for children; may cause nausea, vomiting, anorexia, hypersensitivity reactions (including anaphylaxis); may interact with anticoagulant and immunosuppressant medications
St. John's wort	Anxiety, depression, sleep disorders, viral infection, hemorrhoids, fibromyalgia, burns, premenstrual syndrome, chronic fatigue syndrome	Appears unsafe in pregnancy and lactation; may cause dizziness, insomnia, restlessness, fatigue, constipation, abdominal cramps, photosensitivity, rash, hypersensitivity reactions, hypoglycemia, headache, insomnia; *numerous significant medication interactions*; avoid concurrent use with angiotensin-converting enzyme inhibitors, loop diuretics, thiazide diuretics, alcohol (inconclusive research), immunosuppressants, monoamine oxidase inhibitors (inconclusive research), NSAIDs, oral contraceptives, selective serotonin reuptake inhibitors, sulfonamides, sulfonylureas, tetracyclines; concurrent use of amphetamines, antidepressants, trazodone may cause serotonin syndrome; taken orally in combination with indinavir may decrease the antiretroviral action of this drug
Valerian root	Anxiety, stress, depression, insomnia, muscle and joint pain	Safety in pregnancy and children not established; may cause insomnia, headache, restlessness, nausea, vomiting, anorexia, hepatotoxicity (overdose), hypersensitivity reactions, vision changes, palpitations; may enhance effects of alcohol or sedating substances; avoid if taking antidepressants, pain medications, tranquilizers, antihistamines, anticholinergic drugs, or kava; may increase effects of anesthetic; avoid before surgery; avoid concurrent use with CNS depressants

CNS, central nervous system; *DHEA*, dehydroepiandrosterone; *HMG-CoA*, 3-hydroxy-3-methylglutaryl coenzyme A; *NSAIDs*, nonsteroidal anti-inflammatory drugs.
Data from Skidmore-Roth L. *Mosby's Handbook of Herbs and Natural Supplements*. 3rd ed. St. Louis, MO: Mosby; 2006; and Therapeutic Research Center. Natural medicines. https://naturalmedicines.therapeuticresearch.com. Accessed December 29, 2018.

Appendix E

Answers to Chapter Review Questions

▶ Part I

Chapter 1

1. The generic name is usually an abbreviated form of the drug's chemical name. These names often describe the chemical structure or properties of the drug molecule. Generic names are often long and difficult to remember and are registered with the U.S. Food and Drug Administration. Generic drug names are written in lower case. Trade names are names created by the drug companies, often created to help providers remember the action or properties of the drug. Trade names always begin with a capital letter.

2. The properties of medications include mechanism of action, absorption, distribution, metabolism, elimination, and toxicity.

3. Typically, the higher the dosage, the higher the concentration of the medication at the site of action. The greater the amount of drug at the site of action, the greater the physiologic effect. Typically, as the dosage of a medication is increased, the physiologic effect manifested by the drug is increased. This effect continues with increasing doses of the medication up to a point at which increasing the medication no longer produces an increase in the desired physiologic effect.

4. A patient having an asthmatic attack requires a medication that has nearly immediate delivery and action. Once swallowed, the oral medication needs to be absorbed and delivered to the site of action, which may take more than half an hour. Additionally, a patient having difficulty breathing may not be able to swallow an oral medication or any water to help swallow the pill.

5. Medications absorbed through the gastrointestinal tract must first pass through the liver before being distributed throughout the body. While passing through the liver, the drug is often partially metabolized, reducing the amount of medication available for distribution to the body.

6. Factors include the patient's age, route of drug administration, dosage of the medication, patient's genetic predisposition, diet or starvation, and preexisting disease.

7. Both active transport and carrier-mediated diffusion require a macromolecule to assist in transport. Both processes require specific binding of the drug molecule to the macromolecule, and both are capable of reaching a point of saturation.

8. A half-life is the period of time required to eliminate half of an administered medication from the body.

9. The two factors required to calculate the therapeutic index are the effective dose 50 (ED50) and lethal dose 50 (LD50). The lethal dose is fatal in 50% of the laboratory animals tested. The ED50 produces a therapeutic effect in 50% of the animals tested. Once these two values are determined, the therapeutic index is calculated as LD50/ED50. The closer the therapeutic index is to 1, the more dangerous the drug. In contrast, the closer this number is to 0, the safer the drug.

10. An agonist is a drug that produces the desired physiologic effect upon binding with a drug receptor. Agonists turn things on. In contrast, an antagonist is a drug that either diminishes or eradicates the physiologic effect of the agonist. Antagonists turn things off.

11. A drug interaction occurs when the actions of one drug modify or interfere with the actions of a second drug.

12. The two types of drug interactions alter the plasma level of a medication or alter the effects of a medication.

13. Epinephrine binds to both the alpha and beta receptors. This results in an increase in blood pressure, heart rate, and cardiac contractility. Epinephrine is quite arrhythmogenic; that is, it is prone to causing cardiac arrhythmias.

14. Stimulation of beta$_1$ receptors increases the heart rate (chronotropism) and the force of cardiac contraction (inotropism).

15. Stimulation of beta$_2$ receptors causes relaxation of bronchial smooth muscle.

16. In a dose smaller than recommended, atropine causes a paradoxic slowing of the heart rate.

Chapter 2

1. Ordinary negligence is the failure to exercise the degree of care that another reasonable person would exercise in the same or a similar situation in which harm to another person results.

2. The basic principle of Good Samaritan laws is to encourage others to assist an ill or injured person to the best of their ability without the fear of a lawsuit for potential mistakes they may make.

3. To prove that a paramedic was negligent after a medication error, it must be proven that the paramedic breached his or her duty to the patient and the paramedic deviated from the standard of care. There must be actual harm to the patient, and the actions of the paramedic must be responsible for causing that harm. Under these conditions, proving negligence is difficult.

4. Standing orders and protocols are advance orders from a medical director and are to be followed in the event that certain medical conditions are determined by the paramedic. When protocols and standing orders are used, online medical direction is not necessary. They tend to be rigid and do not allow for unique patient conditions or situations. Standing orders are usually part of a larger treatment protocol.

5. Schedule I drugs are the most dangerous and have the highest abuse potential. Drugs in this class have no recognized medical use and include agents such as heroin, LSD, and methaqualone.

6. Shelf life is the period that a medication may be stored and remain suitable for administration to patients. Drugs that have exceeded the expiration date have expired.

Expired medications may not produce the intended beneficial effects when administered to patients.

7. The Ryan White Law provides safeguards for EMS personnel in the event of a needlestick. If a patient tests positive for HIV, EMS personnel will be advised of the necessary precautions and other steps to take.

8. The EMS system medical director ultimately approves which medications will be used by a local EMS system.

9. The paramedic must ensure that the patient is competent to make that refusal. All refusals of care must be carefully documented to prevent the risk of a claim of abandonment or negligence. Failure to assess the patient's ability to give consent properly and improper documentation of a refusal of care are significant areas of liability risk.

10. A partial refusal occurs when a patient agrees to some, but not all, of the treatment offered. If a patient refuses a portion of treatment, such as the administration of a specific medication, the paramedic can still provide other treatment that the patient does consent to receive. A complete refusal occurs in situations in which the patient refuses all aspects of treatment.

11. Minors are usually permitted by most state laws to be able to consent to treatment, but they usually are not considered legally competent to refuse treatment.

12. Under advanced directives, the healthcare provider is allowed to treat the patient with palliative or comfort measures and restrict the use of resuscitative measures such as cardiopulmonary resuscitation, endotracheal intubation, and medication administration.

13. (1) Do not scribble or write illegibly. (2) Do not misspell words or medication names. (3) Do not forget to check the patient's response to the medication. (4) Do not create abbreviations or use inappropriate acronyms in documentation. Use only approved abbreviations. (5) Do not assume that other crew members will take care of your documentation. (6) Do not prepare your report late if you can avoid it.

14. Once an incident report is completed, submit it to your immediate supervisor. In many cases, attaching the incident report to the patient care record is not wise because anything attached to it can become part of the medical record.

Chapter 3

1. Standing orders are instructions for treatment that are usually specific to a particular patient presentation and may or may not require consultation with medical control. Standing orders are most appropriate for life-threatening conditions that require immediate intervention.

2. As-needed orders can be obtained from medical control to treat a condition if it develops.

3. The nine patient rights of drug administration are right patient, right drug and indication, right dose, right route, right time, right education, right to refuse, right response and evaluation, and right documentation.

4. Parenteral drug administration is a more effective route for drug administration in the prehospital environment because medications given intravenously produce blood levels that are reliable and almost immediately available. Enteral medications enter the bloodstream by absorption through the gastrointestinal tract.

5. Oral medications have several disadvantages for use in emergencies. A patient with an altered or depressed level of consciousness will not be able to take an oral medication safely. Oral medication must be transported through the gastrointestinal tract and then absorbed into the bloodstream, which delays transport and absorption. Thus a medication that is administered orally is not rapidly available for treatment of a potentially life-threatening condition.

6. A provider should never attempt to recap or bend a needle. Immediately after using a needle or sharp, place it in an approved, puncture-resistant, leak-proof needle box.

7. Some medications used in IM injections are irritating to the soft tissues and can result in permanent staining of the skin. The Z-track technique allows delivery of medications deep into muscle tissue and prevents the medication from leaking into the surrounding soft tissue and skin.

8. Medications that can be delivered by endotracheal tube include lidocaine, epinephrine, atropine, and naloxone. These medications can be remembered by the mnemonic LEAN. This route is still an option; however, medication uptake is unreliable. Consider an alternate method such as intraosseous if intravenous access cannot be established.

9. When administering a medication by endotracheal tube, the paramedic needs to give 2 to 2.5 times the standard IV dose. In addition to this increased dose, the medication should be diluted in 10 mL of normal saline. This exposes the medication to the large surface area of the lung and facilitates greater absorption.

Chapter 4

Answers to Practical Application Problems

1. 10 mL
2. 2 mL
3. 6 mL
4. 3 mL
5. 250 gtt/min
6. 4 gtt/sec
7. 5 mL
8. 2 tablets
9. 50 kg; 200 mcg/min
10. 1,600 mcg/mL
11. 7 to 8 gtt/min
12. 1 gtt/7 to 8 sec
13. 4 mcg/mL
14. 30 gtt/min
15. 1 gtt/sec
16. 4 mL
17. 0.5 mL
18. 75 mL
19. 5 mL
20. 2 mL

Chapter 5

1. Intracellular fluid is found inside the cells. Intracellular fluid composes two thirds of the total body water.

2. Extracellular fluid is composed of the fluid between the cells (the interstitial fluid) and the fluid inside the blood vessels.

3. Osmosis is the movement of water across a semipermeable membrane.

4. 83 mL

5. 250 mL

6. Crystalloid solutions are IV fluids in which sodium is the primary particle that controls volume distribution. The most common types of crystalloid fluids used by prehospital providers are Ringer's lactate and normal saline. Colloid solutions use complex molecules such as proteins and complex sugars

to provide osmotic pressure. Crystalloid solutions use electrolytes for osmotic pressure. Isotonic fluids contain sodium and other electrolyte concentrations that closely mimic the concentration of the extracellular fluid.

7. Hyperkalemia may be caused by kidney failure, burns, crush injuries, diabetic ketoacidosis, and severe infections.

8. A fluid bolus in a pediatric patient is 10 to 20 mL/kg.

9. Drop factor is the number of drops into the chamber required to administer 1 mL.

10. Microdrip chambers have 60 gtt/mL.

11. 60 mL/hr

12. Factors affecting the drip rate include the height of the IV bag, position of the extremity with the IV, caliber of the IV catheter, and coiling of the IV tubing.

13. The size of the IV catheter is the principal determinant of the maximal rate of fluid administration.

14. Infiltration occurs when the tip of the catheter dislodges from the lumen of the vein and the fluid or medication is delivered to soft tissues around the vein.

15. The paramedic should suspect IV infiltration when the IV no longer drips freely and when a patient has pain or swelling at the IV site.

16. The way to prevent catheter shear is to never try to resheath an angiocatheter back over the needle while the needle is still inside the patient.

▶ Part II

Chapter 6

1. The American Heart Association has identified the following risk factors for the development of acute myocardial ischemia: cigarette smoking, high blood pressure, high blood cholesterol, lack of exercise, obesity, and heart disease.

2. Stable angina pectoris occurs when the oxygen demands of the heart exceed the body's ability to deliver oxygen to the heart muscle. Providing the patient with oxygen increases oxygen delivery to the heart.

3. Erectile dysfunction. Administration of nitroglycerin to a patient taking a medication for erectile dysfunction, such as sildenafil (Viagra), tadalafil (Cialis), and vardenafil (Levitra), can result in profound hypotension.

4. Morphine helps relieve the pain from myocardial ischemia and causes vasodilation, which increases blood flow to the heart.

5. Beta blockers are widely prescribed to patients with heart disease. Beta blockers decrease the heart rate, which decreases the amount of oxygen consumed by the heart. Also, blood flows through the heart during the diastolic portion of the cardiac cycle; therefore, slowing the heart rate increases the blood through the coronary arteries.

6. Contraindications for the use of beta blockers include current cocaine use, signs of heart failure, evidence of low output state, cardiogenic shock or increased risk for cardiogenic shock, PR interval greater than 0.24 second, second- or third-degree heart block, and active asthma or reactive airway disease.

7. Drugs that block or antagonize the glycoprotein IIb/IIIa receptors prevent platelet aggregation and reduce platelet plugs within the coronary arteries.

8. Contraindications to the administration of fibrinolytic drugs include age greater than 75 years, ST-segment depression, cardiogenic shock, surgery within the previous 10 days, cerebrovascular disease, gastrointestinal bleeding within the previous 10 days, recent trauma, systolic blood pressure greater than 180 mm Hg or diastolic blood pressure greater than 110 mm Hg, recent trauma, high likelihood of left heart thrombus, acute pericarditis, subacute bacterial endocarditis, severe kidney or liver failure with bleeding complications, diabetic hemorrhagic retinopathy, septic thrombophlebitis, and warfarin (Coumadin) administration.

Chapter 7

1. Pain

2. Patients in pain may not be given narcotics because of concerns of respiratory depression and hypotension. Other concerns that prevent narcotic use include the masking of symptoms in patients with head injuries or acute abdominal pain.

3. Morphine can produce hypotension by the release of histamine, which produces vasodilation and subsequently hypotension. This hypotension can be especially profound in patients who are hypovolemic.

4. Fentanyl administration does not release histamine and is less likely to cause hypotension after administration.

5. Administration of narcotics to a patient with abdominal pain can mask the progression of an intra-abdominal disease process (e.g., appendicitis), which typically manifests as an increase in the intensity of pain. The patient can subjectively feel better, but in reality the condition is worsening.

6. Ketorolac (Toradol) is a powerful nonsteroidal anti-inflammatory analgesic that can be given parenterally.

7. Nitrous oxide is self-administered, and once the patient has received an adequate dose the mask falls away from the patient's face. Nitrous oxide provides mild analgesia while allowing the patient to maintain and protect the airway.

8. Benzodiazepines

9. Antegrade amnesia is the inability to remember events from a point in time forward. Antegrade amnesia is an effect of benzodiazepine administration. Therefore, before an unpleasant procedure or situation, administer a benzodiazepine and the patient will be unable to recall the event.

10. Nausea and vomiting are common adverse effects of narcotic administration.

Chapter 8

1. The symptoms of anaphylactic shock are shortness of breath, syncope, itching, swelling of the throat, and a sudden fall in blood pressure.

2. The antigen triggers the body's allergic response. An antigen provokes the body to produce an allergic response, which in turn stimulates cells within the body to release the chemicals histamine, serotonin, bradykinin, and slow-reacting substance of anaphylaxis. These chemicals, when released, cause vasodilation, increased capillary permeability, and smooth muscle spasm.

3. Histamine is the chemical released by the body that is responsible for many of the symptoms associated with anaphylaxis.

4. The most common cause of death in patients with anaphylaxis is airway obstruction.

5. Allergy to shellfish is a common food allergy, and the patient reports a history of such reactions to seafood in the past.

6. Epinephrine is the first-line drug therapy for patients having an anaphylactic reaction. The concentration and dose of epinephrine depend on the route of administration.

7. Epinephrine causes the relaxation of bronchial smooth muscle and constriction of blood vessels.

8. EpiPen and EpiPen Jr

Chapter 9

1. Electrical defibrillation is the single best method of treatment for the patient with VF. The likelihood that a patient will survive an arrest from VF will significantly diminish the longer this rhythm is not converted using electrical therapy. When defibrillation is applied within 1 minute of the development of VF, the survival rate can be greater than 90%. This rate of successful defibrillation drops by 7% to 10% for each minute defibrillation is delayed.

2. Atropine is used to treat sinus bradycardia because it inhibits the effects of the vagus nerve. The vagus nerve, when stimulated, causes slowing of the heart rate, much like applying the brakes when driving a vehicle. Therefore, a drug that inhibits the vagus nerve will increase the heart rate, as if you took your foot off the brake pedal in the vehicle.

3. The half-life of adenosine is 5 to 20 seconds.

4. Class I antiarrhythmics are sodium channel blockers. These agents are further divided into subclasses based on what effect they have on the sodium channel. Class IA agents block the fast sodium channels and depress depolarization. Class IB sodium channel blockers shorten the action potential duration. Class IC sodium channel blockers depress depolarization and conductivity. This subclass is the most potent sodium channel blocker. Class II agents are beta blockers. Class III agents block potassium channels. Class IV agents block calcium channels.

5. Calcium channel blockers are Class IV agents. The overall effect is that the rapid electrical impulses traveling down from the atria to the ventricles through the atrioventricular (AV) node are slowed, and the ventricular rate is slowed.

6. Beta blockers exert their pharmacologic effects on both $beta_1$ and $beta_2$ receptors. $Beta_1$ receptors are located in the heart and act as

the main mediator of rate and contractility. Beta blockers are negative inotropic drugs that decrease the force and velocity of myocardial contractility, thus lowering blood pressure and oxygen consumption. The negative chronotropic effects of beta blockers result in a lower heart rate, automaticity, and conduction. Thus, beta blockers can dramatically decrease cardiac output.

7. The drug of choice for ventricular arrhythmias is amiodarone.

8. Magnesium sulfate should be used for the treatment of torsades de pointes.

9. Pulseless electrical activity is characterized by detectable electrical activity on the monitor but no mechanical cardiac activity as detected by the presence of a pulse or audible heart tones. In asystole, the patient has neither electrical nor mechanical cardiac activity.

Chapter 10

1. Heart failure may be the result of ischemic heart disease, diabetes mellitus, hypertension, or disease of the heart valves. The onset of heart failure may be rather acute after a myocardial infarction or may take years to develop in conditions such as valvular heart disease, hypertension, or diabetes mellitus.

2. Diuretics increase urine output and decrease the intravascular volume. Diuretics are commonly used in the treatment of congestive heart failure in patients with pulmonary edema. The decrease in the intravascular volume offloads the weakened and failing heart and reduces the congestion, or the backing up, of fluids in the lung.

3. In the treatment of congestive heart failure, morphine is beneficial by causing venodilation, which reduces patient anxiety and lowers myocardial oxygen demand.

4. Diastole is the portion of the cardiac cycle at which the heart is relaxed and blood is flowing through the coronary arteries. Systole is the portion of the cardiac cycle when the heart squeezes and ejects blood out of the ventricles. During systole, when the heart is contracting, blood cannot flow through the coronary arteries. With an elevated heart rate, the time in systole remains constant, but the diastolic time decreases. Because blood flows through the coronary

arteries during diastole, an elevated heart rate causes decrease coronary blood flow and decreased myocardial oxygen delivery. Therefore, decreasing the heart rate improves oxygen delivery to the diseased heart.

5. Digoxin is used in patients with congestive heart failure to increase myocardial contractility and often to slow the heart rate. Digoxin helps the heart beat stronger and more slowly.

6. Angiotensin-converting enzyme (ACE) inhibitors inhibit the production of the most powerful vasoconstrictor in the body (angiotensinogen). As a result, the patient has a decrease in blood pressure and mild diuresis. ACE inhibitors also reduce cardiac ischemic events, mortality rate, and hospital admissions for individuals with congestive heart failure.

7. After a beta blocker is administered, the blood pressure, heart rate, and ECG should be carefully monitored.

Chapter 11

1. Patients with type 1 diabetes do not produce insulin. In type 2 diabetes, patients are capable of making insulin; however, the insulin is not used properly by the body, a condition known as *insulin resistance*. Most people with diabetes have type 2.

2. The use of beta blockers in patients with diabetes can render the patient unaware of low blood sugar and create a condition known as *hypoglycemic unawareness*. Beta blockers mask the common symptoms of hypoglycemia: increased heart rate, hypertension, sweating, and a sense of anxiety.

3. After glucagon is administered, the patient may have nausea and vomiting.

4. Too-aggressive fluid resuscitation can lead to cerebral edema. A patient with diabetic ketoacidosis will be dehydrated; note that the dehydration developed over a protracted period. Therefore, do not replace all the patient's fluid losses in the first hour or two of treatment.

5. Diabetic ketoacidosis can be treated by prehospital providers without insulin. Patients with this condition have blood sugar levels that are alarming, but correcting the blood sugar levels too rapidly can be more harmful

than no immediate treatment at all. Often the initiation of IV fluids is sufficient initial therapy for treatment of the hyperglycemia and metabolic acidosis until the patient can be treated at the hospital.

6. In times of stress, cortisol prepares the body by increasing the blood pressure, heart rate, and blood sugar level.

7. Patients with thyrotoxicosis commonly have tachycardia, tremor, diaphoresis, weight loss, and intolerance for warm rooms and environments.

Chapter 12

1. Specific hypertensive emergencies include hypertensive encephalopathy, hypertensive intracranial hemorrhage, pulmonary edema with hypertension, myocardial ischemia with hypertension, and preeclampsia and eclampsia (hypertension with proteinuria in pregnancy).

2. When treating a patient with a hypertensive emergency, do not reduce the diastolic blood pressure by more than 10% to 15%. An overzealous reduction of blood pressure can result in cerebral ischemia.

3. Contraindications to the use of nitroprusside include coronary ischemia or infarction, pregnancy, and conditions associated with elevated intracranial pressure.

4. Nitroprusside should be protected from light by wrapping the IV bag with aluminum foil. Nitroprusside will break down when exposed to ultraviolet light.

5. Labetalol decreases blood pressure by blocking beta-mediated contraction of vascular smooth muscle.

6. Labetalol should not be used in patients who are hypertensive as a result of cocaine intoxication. A patient whose blood pressure is elevated as a result of cocaine intoxication will have an increase in blood pressure after the administration of labetalol.

7. Nitroglycerin is the drug of choice for treating elevated blood pressure in a patient having a myocardial infarction.

8. Magnesium sulfate

9. Administration of hydralazine will cause a drop in blood pressure but a reflexive increase in heart rate.

10. Contraindications to the use of beta blockers include asthma, heart failure, pheochromocytoma, cocaine toxicity, and heart block.

Chapter 13

1. Administration of activated charcoal commonly induces vomiting; if aspirated into the lungs, the charcoal can induce a sometimes fatal pneumonitis.

2. Do not give activated charcoal to someone who has overdosed on acetaminophen (Tylenol) because activated charcoal interferes with the absorption of medications that are administered at the hospital to treat the poisoning.

3. If the patient is having wide-complex QRS rhythms, treatment with sodium bicarbonate is appropriate.

4. Too-rapid administration results in hypotension.

5. Glucagon

6. Methamphetamines increase the body's levels of norepinephrine and epinephrine, resulting in tachycardia, hypertension, hyperthermia, agitation, and mydriasis.

7. Neither gastric lavage nor activated charcoal has a role in methamphetamine intoxication because the majority of the drug has been absorbed by the time the patient is seen by a prehospital provider.

8. The initial treatment for cocaine-related agitation is diazepam (Valium).

9. The most dangerous clinical manifestations of organophosphate poisoning are excessive respiratory secretions (bronchorrhea), bronchospasm, and respiratory insufficiency.

10. Succinylcholine should not be used because it cannot be broken down, resulting in prolonged paralysis of the patient.

Chapter 14

1. Increasing the concentration of inspired oxygen increases the content of oxygen in the blood and subsequently the amount of oxygen delivered to the heart and peripheral tissues.

2. Rebreather face masks, or partial rebreathing face masks, have a face mask and a reservoir bag. Oxygen accumulates in the reservoir bag. During inhalation, the patient inhales the oxygen in the reservoir, as well as some room air through the side ports. When the patient exhales, some of the exhaled breath goes back into the reservoir bag, where it is then rebreathed. Partial rebreather masks are capable of delivering 60% oxygen. Nonrebreather

face masks are similar to rebreather masks in appearance and function, with the exception of having one-way exhalation valves on the sides of the mask and on the reservoir bag. The valves on the sides of the mask prevent inhalation of room air during inhalation. The valve on the reservoir prevents any of the exhaled breath from entering the oxygen-rich reservoir. Nonrebreather face masks require a higher flow rate of 12 to 15 L/min and are capable of delivering oxygen concentrations close to 100%.

3. The class of drugs commonly used to treat bronchospasm are beta$_2$-specific agonists. These drugs cause dilation of bronchial smooth muscle by stimulating the beta$_2$ receptor.

4. The two methods of delivering medications directly to the bronchioles are the pneumatically powered nebulizer and metered-dose inhaler.

5. The objective of delivering inhaled medications is to deliver the medications to the lung. Particles that are too large will not make it to their intended site of action, the lung. Particles that are too small will be inhaled and then exhaled without binding to their receptors inside the lung.

6. The purpose of using the spacer is to slow the velocity of the medication particles so that they do not collide with the soft tissues of the oropharynx and the medication particles can reach their intended site in the lung.

7. The principal goal in the management of the asthmatic patient is the reversal of the acute bronchospasm.

8. Patients with a long-standing history of chronic obstructive pulmonary disease require a mild degree of hypoxia to continue breathing. This need for mild hypoxia to continue a respiratory drive is known as *hypoxic respiratory drive*. If the patient is given too much oxygen, the hypoxic respiratory drive is removed, as well as the patient's stimulus for spontaneous respirations.

Chapter 15

1. Status epilepticus is defined as continuous seizure activity for more than 30 minutes or a series of seizures without full recovery of consciousness between seizures.

2. Rectal medication administration may be required in a patient who is actively having a seizure and in whom IV access is not obtainable.

3. The most common class of agents used in the initial management of seizure activity, particularly in the prehospital setting, are the benzodiazepines.

4. Acute-angle glaucoma is a contraindication to benzodiazepine administration because the drug relaxes the ciliary muscle of the pupil and can cause an acute increase in intraocular pressure.

5. A prodrug is a medication administered in an inactive form and then converted to the active form after administration. Fosphenytoin (Cerebyx) is an example of a prodrug.

Chapter 16

1. The early clinical signs of shock in patients include delayed capillary refill, cold and clammy skin, and an increased respiratory rate.

2. The five types of shock are hypovolemic, cardiogenic, neurogenic, septic, and anaphylactic shock.

3. A common therapy for any patient in shock is the expansion of the intravascular volume with IV fluids.

4. An initial therapy for the treatment of hypovolemic shock is to stop the bleeding. This may be difficult for someone in shock from a gastrointestinal bleed. Control of hemorrhage from traumatic blood loss can be achieved by direct pressure or tourniquets.

5. The preferred IV fluid for use in trauma patients who are likely to require blood products is normal saline. The principal reason for this choice is that saline is compatible with the administration of blood products in the same IV line. The optimal IV fluid in patients with hypovolemic shock remains controversial. There is supporting evidence for both normal saline and lactated Ringer's solution, depending on the study or source.

6. Patients who demonstrate improved perfusion, heart rate, or blood pressure with crystalloid infusion can be categorized as rapid responders, transient responders, or nonresponders. Rapid responders do not need further aggressive resuscitation. They have no ongoing hemorrhage; the source of bleeding has been controlled with pressure or the patient's normal hemostatic mechanisms. Transient responders improve as their

intravascular volume is replenished. However, with ongoing manifestations of poor perfusion return, transient responders require blood transfusion and control of hemorrhage. Nonresponders have uncontrolled hemorrhage and require blood transfusion and control of bleeding.

7. Standard blood banking practices involve separating donated whole blood into components. Red blood cells, platelets, and plasma are all separated. In this manner, a single unit of blood can provide therapy for many patients.

8. Rh⁻ patients who receive Rh⁺ blood develop antibodies against the Rh factor in approximately 80% of cases. The seroconversion that occurs can complicate a subsequent pregnancy if the Rh⁻ mother becomes pregnant with an Rh⁺ fetus. The fetus can have chronic hemolytic disease of the newborn.

9. Milrinone, a drug classified as a phosphodiesterase inhibitor, is a good drug to use in a patient in cardiogenic shock but not responding to an adrenergic agonist such as dobutamine. Milrinone works by a different mechanism than dobutamine.

10. Fluid infusion to improve preload is the initial therapy for neurogenic shock. Neurogenic shock mainly involves managing a bigger vascular container, and fluid administration simply refills that vascular container. Fluids, not vasopressors, are the initial treatment for neurogenic shock.

11. In septic shock, the patient has a source of infection that initiates a complex sequence of events in the body known as a *systemic inflammatory response*. The inflammatory reaction produces toxins within the body that result in dilation of the blood vessels. Another effect of the produced toxins is that the blood vessels become "leaky," and the patient can become hypovolemic as he or she loses intravascular fluid to the extravascular space. Therefore, these patients have vasodilation such as that seen in neurogenic shock and decreased intravascular volume as seen in hypovolemic shock.

Chapter 17

1. Two types of trauma can occur to the brain: primary brain injury occurs directly to the brain from mechanical forces at the time of the initial insult. Secondary brain injury occurs hours after the time of the injury. In a significant number of patients, secondary brain injury leads to delayed death and disability in head-injured patients.

2. Hypotension and hypoxia result in a significant increase in mortality rate from traumatic brain injury. Therefore, the paramedic should strive to prevent or treat these conditions rapidly.

3. The treatment of severe traumatic brain injury has two goals: to identify an intracranial injury that may require surgery rapidly and to prevent conditions that result in secondary brain injury (hypoxia and hypotension).

4. Mannitol is an osmotic diuretic that decreases brain swelling by dehydrating the brain.

5. Hypertonic saline must be administered slowly to avoid an increase in the rate of bleeding and an alteration of the ability to clot blood. Too-rapid infusion can result in osmotic demyelination syndrome.

▶ Part III

Chapter 18

1. Types of infusion sets include macrodrip infusion sets, microdrip infusion sets, blood tubing sets, volume-control chamber sets, vented and nonvented infusion sets, and multiple-drip infusion sets.

2. The drip rate is 30 gtt/min.

3. The treatment for magnesium toxicity includes the administration of IV calcium gluconate.

4. Amiodarone prevents the patient from experiencing additional arrhythmias.

5. Blood glucose level should not be decreased at a rate faster than 10% per hour. Dextrose in the form of D_5 should be added to the IV fluids once the blood glucose is less than 250 mg/dL.

6. Cerebral perfusion pressure is calculated from the mean arterial pressure and intracranial pressure. A goal for the cerebral perfusion pressure of 70 mm Hg is needed to ensure adequate cerebral perfusion. Therefore, increases in intracranial pressure and decreases in mean arterial pressure can result in an insufficient blood flow to the brain.

7. Fluid replacement is essential in preventing hypovolemia in critically ill burn patients. Major fluid shifts and losses occur during the first 24 hours of a burn injury. Large amounts of fluids leak from the vascular space to the extravascular space. Additionally, with large areas of burned skin, the body also loses large amounts of fluids from evaporation from the burns. Large amounts of crystalloid must be administered to replace the intravascular fluid loss that results from shifts to the interstitial space.

8. The rule of nines divides the patient's body surface area into units that are divisible by nine. This calculation is accurate for use in adult patients but is not adequate for calculating total body surface area of children because of the disproportion of their body surface area.

9. If a transfusion reaction is suspected, stop the transfusion, disconnect any blood tubing (to keep extra blood from entering the body), and flush the primary IV line with saline.

Chapter 19

1. Pregnant women have a delay in gastric emptying that results in a delay from the time a patient takes an oral medication to the time the drug is delivered to the intestine, where oral medications are absorbed. Pregnant women have higher minute ventilation than nonpregnant women, so inhaled medications result in more rapid systemic effects than in nonpregnant women. Pregnancy increases the percentage of body fat, which creates a larger volume of distribution for fat-soluble drugs. Pregnancy also induces a decrease in liver function and an increase in renal function. As a result, the breakdown of a drug by the liver can be slowed, but the excretion of that drug's by-products can be increased by an improvement in kidney function.

2. Teratogenic drugs are medications that result in a characteristic set of malformations in the fetus.

3. Drugs are categorized as A, B, C, D, or X. A is the safest, with B, C, and D progressively more dangerous. Category X drugs are the most dangerous to use in pregnancy and should be avoided. The Pregnancy Safety Category system is limited in its usefulness because most research studies conducted to determine the safety of drugs have used animals. This system is being phased out as the Food and Drug Administration implements a more elaborate system to describe medication risks to fertility, pregnancy, and lactation.

4. Peanut or soy allergy is a contraindication to ipratropium bromide.

5. When the initial peak expiratory flow rate is less than 50% of predicted, corticosteroids should be administered after ipratropium bromide. Corticosteroids should also be considered when the peak expiratory flow rate does not improve by at least 10% after bronchodilator therapy or is less than 70% after 1 hour of therapy.

6. Chronic hypertension occurs when the pregnant woman has a history of hypertension that precedes the pregnancy. Gestational hypertension is elevated blood pressure that first occurs during pregnancy but does not meet the diagnostic criteria of eclampsia.

7. The threshold for treatment that has been suggested is a diastolic blood pressure greater than 110 mm Hg or a systolic blood pressure in excess of 160 mm Hg.

8. Diabetic ketoacidosis is a state of insulin deficiency that produces a condition of hyperglycemia, dehydration, and metabolic acidosis. Diabetic ketoacidosis in pregnancy can be fatal for the fetus, with fetal mortality rates approaching 50%.

9. A decrease in blood pressure is a late sign of shock in both adults and children. Tachycardia is a more reliable sign than hypotension.

10. Stroke volume is the amount of blood ejected by the heart with each heartbeat. An adult has some variability of stroke volume; however, the stroke volume is held relatively stable in children.

11. Complications of intraosseous infusions include osteomyelitis, cellulitis, infiltration of fluid, anterior compartment syndrome, tibial fractures, and fat embolus.

12. Information on pediatric drug dosing is usually given based on age, weight, or body surface area. In most cases, drugs recommended for pediatric use usually propose a particular dose in milligrams per kilogram or pound. For many drugs, the recommended weight-based dose (or weight-normalized dose) is presented for children of different ages or weight groups. For many drugs, the

weight-normalized dose increases as the weight of the child decreases. These changes in weight-based doses are attributable to changes in the child's body composition and metabolism. The percentage of total body water of an infant is approximately 80%, and this proportion decreases to approximately 60% by adulthood. In the first year of life, the percentage of fat nearly doubles in infants. Infants have a much smaller percentage of muscle mass than do adults, but they have much larger brains and livers in relation to their total body weight. Infants and children also have large volumes of distribution and rapid metabolic rates. Because of differences in a child's metabolism during the various stages of development, a simple linear reduction of an adult drug dose is not appropriate.

13. Hypoxia
14. Adenosine administration can cause transient atrioventricular block, which can appear to be asystole for the first 10 seconds.
15. Too-aggressive fluid administration in a child with diabetic ketoacidosis can result in cerebral edema.
16. Polypharmacy occurs when an individual patient is taking multiple medications for the treatment of several medical disorders. The danger of polypharmacy is the increased likelihood of an adverse effect or serious drug interaction.
17. The causes of renal failure include trauma, pregnancy, hemorrhage, and complications of drug therapy.
18. Hypertension and diabetes mellitus
19. Medications that have the potential of becoming toxic in kidney disease include digoxin, antibiotics, antihypertensives, and antiarrhythmics.
20. Hemodialysis is the removal of toxic substances from the bloodstream by filtering the patient's blood through a machine and then passing the blood back to the patient.

Chapter 20

1. If I give these drugs and if/when this patient stops breathing, will I be able to intubate? If I am unable to intubate the patient, will I be able to ventilate? If I am unable to either intubate or ventilate this patient, do I have other options? Do I have the right equipment on hand? Is the equipment assembled? Does the patient have any medical problems or conditions for which these drugs and techniques are contraindicated? If I do not act, will this patient die or have permanent brain damage?
2. Acetylcholine
3. Acetylcholinesterase
4. Depolarizing and nondepolarizing
5. Succinylcholine is able to induce paralysis in approximately 45 seconds.
6. Potassium
7. Patients who should not be given succinylcholine are those with major burns, neuromuscular conditions, myopathic diseases, or hyperkalemia. Succinylcholine should be used with caution in patients with renal failure because these patients often have elevated potassium levels.
8. Malignant hyperthermia is a genetic abnormality in which a patient has exaggerated, sustained muscle contractions in response to certain inhaled general anesthetics and succinylcholine. The increased muscle activity can lead to fatal hyperthermia.
9. To avoid bradycardia after administration of succinylcholine, the paramedic should administer atropine to children younger than 8 years.
10. Rocuronium has no negative effects on cardiovascular function and does not lower blood pressure or raise or lower heart rate. For these reasons it is a safe drug to use in a potentially hypovolemic patient.
11. Flumazenil can completely reverse the effects of midazolam.
12. Etomidate has favorable properties for rapid sequence intubation sedation; it has a rapid onset (30 seconds), short duration of action (3 to 5 minutes), and minimal effects on the heart and blood vessels.
13. (1) Preparations (Time = t – 5 minutes or greater); (2) preoxygenation (Time = t – 5 minutes); (3) pretreatment/priming (Time = t – 3 minutes); (4) paralytic/sedation (Time = t – 1 minute); (5) pass the tube (Time = 0); (6) prove it! (Time = t+); (7) Post-intubation management (Time = t+).

Glossary

5-HT₃ receptor antagonist receptor for the neurotransmitter and peripheral signal mediator serotonin, also known as *5-hydroxytryptamine* or *5-HT*. 5-HT receptors are located on the cell membrane of nerve cells and other cell types, including smooth muscle in animals, and mediate the effects of serotonin as the endogenous ligand and of a broad range of pharmaceutical and hallucinogenic drugs. 5-HT receptors affect the release and activity of other neurotransmitters such as glutamate, dopamine, and GABA. 5-HT_{2A} receptors increase the activity of glutamate in many areas of the brain, whereas some other serotonin receptors have the effect of suppressing glutamate.

A

$A^3E^3P^3$ ("A three, E three, P three") refusal guidelines a method of remembering and documenting the critical considerations when a patient refuses treatment. $A^3E^3P^3$ stands for *a*ssess, *a*dvise, *a*void; *e*nsure, *e*xploit, *e*xplain; *p*ersist, *p*rotocols, *p*rotect.

absorption the incorporation of matter by other matter through chemical, molecular, or physical action, such as the dissolving of a gas in a liquid or the taking up of a liquid by a porous solid.

acetylcholine a direct-acting cholinergic neurotransmitter agent widely distributed in body tissues, with a primary function of mediating synaptic activity of the nervous system and skeletal muscles.

acetylcholine receptor a receptor that specifically binds the neurotransmitter acetylcholine and results in contraction of a muscle fiber.

acetylcholinesterase an enzyme present at endings of voluntary nerves, parasympathetic involuntary nerves, and autonomic nerve ganglia. It inactivates and prevents accumulation of the neurotransmitter acetylcholine released during nerve impulse transmission by hydrolyzing the substance to choline and acetate.

activated charcoal a general-purpose emergency antidote and a powerful pharmaceutical adsorbent prescribed in the treatment of acute poisoning.

active transport the movement of materials across the membranes and epithelial layers of a cell by chemical activity that allows the cell to admit otherwise impermeable molecules against a concentration gradient.

acute adrenal insufficiency a life-threatening emergency caused by inadequate amounts of cortisol and stress hormones at times of stress, such as injury and illness.

acute coronary syndrome (ACS) a classification encompassing clinical presentations ranging from unstable angina through myocardial infarction not characterized by alterations in Q waves. The classification sometimes also includes myocardial infarction characterized by altered Q waves.

adrenal medulla the inner portion of the adrenal gland. Adrenal medulla cells secrete epinephrine and norepinephrine when stimulated by the sympathetic division of the autonomic nervous system.

adrenergic agonist medication that acts on the adrenergic receptor to stimulate the sympathetic nervous system.

adrenergic receptor a site in a sympathetic effector cell that reacts to adrenergic stimulation. Two types of adrenergic receptors are recognized: alpha adrenergic, which act in response to sympathomimetic stimuli, and beta adrenergic, which block sympathomimetic activity.

adrenocorticotropin (ACTH) the adrenocorticotropic hormone secreted by the anterior pituitary gland that stimulates secretion of corticosteroid hormones by the adrenal cortex.

advance directive an advance declaration by a person of treatment preferences if he or she is unable to communicate his or her wishes.

adverse effect an undesirable or harmful effect from a medication.

affinity the measure of the binding strength of the antibody-antigen reaction.

agonist a drug that produces a desired physiologic effect on binding with the receptor. Agonists turn things on.

albumin a water-soluble, heat-coagulable protein containing carbon, hydrogen, oxygen, nitrogen, and sulfur.

allergen an environmental substance that can produce a hypersensitive allergic reaction in the body but may not be intrinsically harmful. Common allergens include pollen, animal dander, house dust, feathers, and various foods.

allergic response an exaggerated hypersensitivity reaction to a previously encountered antigen; a potentially life-threatening series of events that affects multiple body systems. Also called an *anaphylactic response.*

alpha₁ receptor receptor in the sympathetic nervous system located on the peripheral blood vessels that, when stimulated with an alpha agonist, typically produces constriction of blood vessels and an increase in blood pressure.

alpha₂ receptor receptor located on nerve endings that provides negative feedback to nerves in the sympathetic nervous system.

alveolus a small outpouching of walls of alveolar space through which gas exchange between alveolar air and pulmonary capillary blood takes place. The term is often used interchangeably with *acinus*.

ampule a small, sterile glass or plastic container that usually contains a single dose of a solution.

analgesic a drug that relieves pain. The opioid analgesics act on the central nervous system and alter the patient's perception; they are more often used for severe pain.

anaphylactic reaction acute allergic response involving immunoglobulin E–mediated, antigen-stimulated mast cell activation resulting in histamine release. Exposure to the antigen may result in dyspnea, airway obstruction, shock, urticaria and, in some cases, death.

anaphylactic shock a severe and sometimes fatal systemic allergic reaction to a sensitizing substance, such as a drug, vaccine, specific food, serum, allergen extract, insect venom, or chemical.

anaphylaxis an exaggerated, life-threatening hypersensitivity reaction to a previously encountered antigen.

anemia a decrease in hemoglobin in the blood to levels below the normal range of 12 to 16 g/dL for women and 13.5 to 18 g/dL for men. Anemia may be caused by a decrease in red cell production, an increase in red cell destruction, or a loss of blood.

angina pectoris a paroxysmal thoracic pain most often caused by myocardial anoxia as a result of atherosclerosis or spasm of the coronary arteries.

angioedema swelling of the mucous membranes of the airway.

angiotensin-converting enzyme (ACE) inhibitor protease inhibitor found in serum that promotes vasodilation by blocking the formation of angiotensin II and slowing the degradation of bradykinin and other kinins. It decreases sodium retention, water retention, blood pressure, and heart size and increases cardiac output.

angiotensin II a potent vasoconstrictor that also acts to stimulate the secretion of the antidiuretic hormone.

angiotensinogen a serum glycoprotein produced in the liver that is the precursor of angiotensin.

antagonist a drug that diminishes or eradicates the physiologic effect of an agonist. Antagonists turn things off.

anterograde amnesia the inability to recall events that occur after the onset of amnesia.

antibody an immunoglobulin produced by lymphocytes in response to bacteria, viruses, or other antigenic substances. An antibody is specific to an antigen. Each class of antibody is named for its action.

anticonvulsant a substance or procedure that prevents or reduces the severity of epileptic or other convulsive seizures.

antigen a substance, usually a protein, that the body recognizes as foreign and that can evoke an immune response.

antiplatelet any agent that destroys platelets or inhibits their function.

antisialagogue a substance or medication that reduces or prevents the production of saliva or secretions.

apothecary system an obsolete unit of measure used in pharmaceutical preparations. The basic unit of weight is the grain (gr), and the basic unit of volume is the minim (m).

arrhythmia any deviation from the normal pattern of the heartbeat.

arterial line an arterial blood monitoring system consisting of a catheter inserted into an artery and connected to pressure tubing, a transducer, and a monitor. The device permits continuous direct blood pressure readings, as well as access to the arterial blood supply when samples are needed for analysis.

as-needed order order that applies as necessary for a certain and specified condition; often referred to as a prn order (*prn* is an abbreviation for the Latin phrase *pro re nata*, which means "as the situation demands").

assisted medication administration the act of assisting a patient in self-administering medications previously prescribed by a personal physician for preexisting or chronic medical conditions.

asthma a respiratory disorder characterized by recurring episodes of paroxysmal dyspnea, wheezing on expiration, and/or inspiration caused by constriction of the bronchi, coughing, and viscous mucoid bronchial secretions.

atrial fibrillation (AF) a cardiac arrhythmia characterized by disorganized electrical activity in the atria accompanied by an irregular ventricular response that is usually rapid.

atrial flutter a type of atrial tachycardia characterized by contraction rates between 230 and 380 per minute. Two kinds, typical and atypical, have been identified and are distinguished from each other by their rates and ECG patterns.

atrioventricular (AV) node an area of specialized cardiac muscle that receives the cardiac impulse from the sinoatrial (SA) node and conducts it to the AV bundle and then to the Purkinje fibers and walls of the ventricles. The AV node is located in the septal wall between the left and right atria.

autonomic nervous system the part of the nervous system that regulates involuntary body functions, including the activity of the cardiac muscle, smooth muscles, and glands. It has two divisions, the sympathetic nervous system and the parasympathetic nervous system.

autoresuscitate the shift of fluid from extravascular fluid spaces (intracellular and interstitial spaces) to the intravascular space in an attempt to compensate for a state of hypovolemia.

B

baroreceptor one of the pressure-sensitive nerve endings in the walls of the atria of the heart, the aortic arch, and the carotid sinuses. Baroreceptors stimulate central reflex mechanisms that allow physiologic adjustment and adaptation to changes in blood pressure by changes in heart rate, vasodilation, or vasoconstriction.

barrel the portion of the syringe that contains the medication.

belladonna alkaloids a group of anticholinergic alkaloids occurring in belladonna (*Atropa belladonna*).

benzodiazepine a class of medications that reduces anxiety (anxiolysis), relaxes muscles, and treats seizures. Benzodiazepines induce a state of anterograde amnesia.

beta agonist medication that exerts a positive effect by binding to the beta receptor. Beta agonists increase heart rate, increase the cardiac force of contraction, and produce bronchodilation.

beta blocker a popular term for beta agonist, a medication that binds and blocks the receptor. Beta blockers mediate a negative effect on the beta receptor. Such medications bind the beta receptor and have the potential to decrease heart rate, decrease force of contraction, and even produce bronchospasm.

beta1 receptor a type of beta receptor found on the heart and blood vessels. When stimulated with an agonist, $beta_1$ receptors increase heart rate, increase the force of cardiac contraction, and produce vasodilation.

beta2 receptor a type of beta receptor found on bronchial smooth muscle. When stimulated with an agonist, $beta_2$ receptors produce bronchodilation.

bevel the angled tip of a hypodermic needle.

bioavailability the degree of activity or amount of an administered drug or other substance that becomes available for activity in the target tissue.

biotransformation the chemical changes a substance undergoes in the body, such as by the action of enzymes.

blood tubing set tubing specific for the administration of blood and blood products.

bradykinin a peptide containing nine amino acid residues produced from $alpha_2$-globulin by the enzyme kallikrein. Bradykinin is a potent vasodilator.

breach of duty to act failure to provide a level of care dictated by the local EMS policies or protocols.

bronchodilator a substance, especially a drug, that relaxes contractions of the smooth muscle of the bronchioles to improve ventilation to the lungs. Pharmacologic bronchodilators are prescribed to improve aeration in asthma, bronchiectasis, bronchitis, and emphysema.

bronchospasm an excessive and prolonged contraction of the smooth muscle of the bronchi and bronchioles, resulting in an acute narrowing and obstruction of the respiratory airway.

buccal administration (of medication) oral administration of a drug, usually in the form of a tablet, by placing it between the cheek and the teeth or gum until it dissolves.

buccal area the vestibule of the mouth, specifically the area lying between the teeth and cheeks.

BURP maneuver a mnemonic for a series of manual techniques to improve visualization during endotracheal intubation. BURP stands for *b*ackward-*u*pward (toward the head), *r*ightward (toward the patient's right), and *p*ressure.

butterfly needle a short needle attached to plastic stabilizers at 90 degrees. It is used for IV access of small veins of adults and children. Usual gauge is 22 to 25.

C

calcium channel blocker a drug that inhibits the flow of calcium ions across the membranes of smooth muscle cells. By reduction of the calcium flow, smooth muscle tone is relaxed and the risk of muscle spasms is diminished.

cardiac output (CO) the volume of blood expelled by the ventricles of the heart with each beat (the stroke volume) multiplied by the heart rate.

cardiogenic shock an abnormal condition often characterized by a low cardiac output associated with acute myocardial infarction and congestive heart failure.

cardioselective beta blocker the common name for a $beta_1$ antagonist.

carrier-mediated facilitated diffusion transportation of a drug into a particular cell by using a second molecule to carry the drug molecule.

catheter shear the cutting, separating, and perhaps embolization of an IV catheter by the reinsertion of a needle while the catheter is still in the patient.

causation the existence of a reasonable connection between the misfeasance, malfeasance, or nonfeasance of the defendant and the injury or damage suffered by the plaintiff.

centi combining form meaning "one hundred" or "one hundredth."

central nervous system (CNS) one of the two main divisions of the nervous system, consisting of the brain and the spinal cord.

central venous catheter a catheter that is threaded through the internal jugular, antecubital, or subclavian vein, usually with the tip resting in the superior vena cava or the right atrium of the heart. It is used to administer fluids or medications for hemodynamic monitoring and to measure central venous pressure.

chelating agents medications administered to bind with heavy metals in the body.

cholinergic agonist a class of drugs that act on the parasympathetic nervous system by binding and stimulating cholinergic receptors.

cholinergic receptor a specialized sensory nerve ending that responds to the stimulation of acetylcholine.

chronic hypertension a long-standing condition of elevated blood pressure.

chronic obstructive pulmonary disease (COPD) a progressive and irreversible condition characterized by diminished inspiratory and expiratory capacity of the lungs.

chronotropic drug a medication that increases heart rate.

chronotropism the act or process of affecting the regularity of a periodic function, especially interference with the rate of heartbeat.

colloid solution a solution in which small particles, such as large polymeric molecules, are homogenously dispersed through a liquid medium.

coma cocktail a combination of medications used to treat a patient with an altered mental status and no history of trauma.

compensated shock a shock condition in which blood volume is low but the body can maintain blood pressure and organ perfusion by increasing the heart rate and constricting the blood vessels.

competitive antagonist a substance that interferes with usual metabolic activity by competing for binding sites on a substrate (the substance on which an enzyme acts in a chemical reaction) or on an enzyme that ordinarily attacks the substrate. The antagonist is usually an analog of the substrate.

complete refusal the right of a patient to refuse treatment after the provider has informed the patient of the diagnosis, prognosis, available alternative interventions, risks and benefits of those options, and risks and probable outcomes of no intervention.

congenital adrenal hyperplasia (CAH) a group of disorders that have in common an enzyme defect resulting in low levels of cortisol and increased secretion of adrenocorticotrophic hormone. The net effects are adrenal gland hyperplasia and increased production of cortisol precursors and androgens.

congestive heart failure (CHF) an abnormal condition that reflects impaired cardiac pumping. Its causes include myocardial infarction, ischemic heart disease, and cardiomyopathy.

consent to give approval, assent, or permission.

cortisol a steroid hormone produced naturally by the adrenal gland, identical to chemically synthesized hydrocortisone.

crystalloid a substance in a solution that can diffuse through a semipermeable membrane.

cyclic adenosine monophosphate (cAMP) a cyclic nucleotide formed from adenosine triphosphate by the action of adenylyl cyclase. This cyclic compound, known as the "second messenger," participates in the action of catecholamines, vasopressin, adrenocorticotropic hormone, and many other hormones.

cytochrome P-450 a protein involved with extramitochondrial electron transport in the liver and during drug detoxification.

D

decompensated shock loss of physiologic adaptation to a condition that predisposes and eventually leads to a shock condition characterized by tachycardia, hypotension, and tachypnea.

dehydration excessive loss of water from body tissues. Dehydration is accompanied by a disturbance in the balance of essential electrolytes, particularly sodium, potassium, and chloride. It may follow prolonged fever, diarrhea, vomiting, acidosis, and any condition in which rapid depletion of body fluids occurs.

deltoid muscle a large, thick, triangular muscle that covers the shoulder joint.

depolarization the reduction of a membrane potential caused by the influx of cations, such as sodium and calcium, through ion channels in the membrane.

diabetic ketoacidosis (DKA) diabetic coma, an acute, life-threatening complication of uncontrolled diabetes mellitus. In this condition, urinary loss of water, potassium, ammonium, and sodium results in hypovolemia, electrolyte imbalance, extremely high blood glucose levels, and the breakdown of free fatty acids, causing acidosis, often with coma.

distribution the location of medications in various organs and tissues after administration.

diuresis increased formation and secretion of urine.

diuretic a drug or other substance that tends to promote the formation and excretion of urine.

dorsogluteal injection injection of a medication into a region of the upper outer quadrant of the buttocks where intramuscular injections can safely be administered.

dosage the regimen governing the size, amount, frequency, and number of doses of a therapeutic agent to be administered to a patient.

dose the amount of a drug or other substance to be administered at one time.

dose-response curve a range of doses over which response occurs. Doses lower than the threshold produce no response, whereas those in excess of the threshold exert no additional response.

dose-response relationship a mathematic relationship between the dose of a drug or radiation and the body's reaction to it.

drip chamber the compartment immediately below the IV bag where the IV fluid drips at a predetermined volume.

drop factor the number of drops into the chamber required to administer 1 mL of fluid.

drug interaction an occurrence in which the effects of one drug are modified by or interfere with the effects of a second drug administered concurrently.

duration of action the period from which the drug initially exhibits its desired action to the point in time when the effect is no longer perceptible. Duration of action is different than biologic half-life.

duty to act a duty to respond to the patient and provide the level of care that reasonable paramedics are expected to provide.

E

eclampsia the gravest form of pregnancy-induced hypertension. It is characterized by grand mal seizure, coma, hypertension, proteinuria, and edema.

ectopy a condition in which an organ or substance is not in its natural or proper place, such as an ectopic pregnancy that develops outside the uterus or an ectopic heartbeat.

effective dose 50 (ED50) the dose needed to cause the desired response in 50% of the people to whom it is given.

efficacy (of a drug or treatment) the ability of a drug or treatment to produce a specific result, regardless of dosage.

electrical therapy the restoration of the heart's normal sinus rhythm through an electrical shock delivered by a defibrillator. Application of the shock is synchronized to the QRS complex.

electrocardiogram (ECG) a graphic record produced by an electrocardiograph, a device for recording electrical conduction through the heart.

electrolytes salts that have been dissolved in water and have the potential to conduct electricity.

emergence phenomena a condition often experienced by patients awakening from ketamine-induced anesthesia; characterized by frightening and vivid nightmares.

endocytosis uptake by a cell of material from the environment by invagination of its plasma membrane, which may be either phagocytosis or pinocytosis.

endotracheal (ET) tube a large-bore catheter inserted through the mouth or nose and into the trachea to a point above the bifurcation of the trachea. It is used for delivering oxygen under pressure when ventilation must be totally controlled and in general anesthetic procedures.

end-stage renal disease (ESRD) a point at which the kidney is so badly damaged or scarred that dialysis or transplantation is required for patient survival.

enteral administration (of medication) the provision of nutrients through the gastrointestinal tract when the patient cannot ingest, chew, or swallow food but can digest and absorb nutrients.

enzyme a complex produced by living cells that catalyzes chemical reactions in organic matter.

epidural hematoma accumulation of blood in the epidural space, caused by damage to and leakage of blood from the middle meningeal artery, producing compression of the dura mater and thus of the brain.

erythropoietin a glycoprotein hormone synthesized mainly in the kidneys and released into the bloodstream in response to anoxia. The hormone acts to stimulate and regulate the production of erythrocytes and thus increases the oxygen-carrying capacity of the blood.

essential hypertension an elevated systemic arterial pressure for which no cause can be found.

excretion the process of eliminating, shedding, or getting rid of substances by body organs or tissues as part of a natural metabolic activity. Excretion usually begins at the cellular level, where water, carbon dioxide, and other waste products of cellular life are emptied into the capillaries.

exponential kinetics of absorption another name for *first-order kinetics of absorption*. A constant fraction of the medication is absorbed into the bloodstream over a defined period.

extracellular fluid (ECF) the portion of the body fluid composing the interstitial fluid and blood plasma.

extrinsic pertaining to anything external or originating outside a structure or organism, including parts of an organ that are not wholly contained within it, such as an extrinsic muscle.

F

fight-or-flight response the reaction of the body to stress in which the sympathetic nervous system and the adrenal medulla act to increase the cardiac output; dilate the pupils of the eyes; increase the rate of the heartbeat; constrict the blood vessels of the skin; increase the levels of glucose and fatty acids in the circulation; and induce an alert, aroused mental state.

first-order kinetics a chemical reaction in which the rate of decrease in the number of molecules of a substrate is proportional to the concentration of substrate molecules remaining.

first-pass metabolism medications absorbed through the gastrointestinal tract pass through the liver and are partially metabolized before distribution to the rest of the body. This metabolism reduces the amount of medication available for distribution.

flow controller a device used to regulate the flow of an IV fluid or medication though IV tubing.

fluid bolus the rapid administration of a volume of IV fluid.

fluid warmer an instrument that warms administered IV fluids or blood to a safe temperature and helps prevent hypothermia.

fraction of inspired oxygen (FiO$_2$) the proportion of oxygen in the air that is inspired.

G

gamma-aminobutyric acid (GABA) an amino acid that functions as an inhibitory neurotransmitter in the brain and spinal cord. It is also found in the heart, lungs, and kidneys.

gastrointestinal (GI) pertaining to the organs of the gastrointestinal tract, from mouth to anus.

generic name the official established nonproprietary name assigned to a drug.

gestational hypertension elevated blood pressure that first occurs during pregnancy but does not meet the diagnostic criteria of eclampsia.

glucagon a polypeptide hormone, produced by alpha cells in the islets of Langerhans, that stimulates the conversion of glycogen to glucose in the liver.

glucocorticoid an adrenocortical steroid hormone that increases gluconeogenesis, exerts an anti-inflammatory effect, and influences many body functions.

glucose a primary source of energy used by body tissues.

glycogen a polysaccharide that is the major carbohydrate stored in animal cells. It is formed from repeating units of glucose and stored chiefly in the liver and, to a lesser extent, in muscle cells.

glycoprotein (GP) any of the large group of conjugated proteins in which the nonprotein substance is a carbohydrate. These include the mucins, the mucoids, and the chondroproteins.

Good Samaritan legislation laws enacted in some states to protect health professionals from liability in rendering emergency medical or dental aid, unless willful wrong or gross negligence is proven.

gram (g) a unit of mass in the metric system equal to 1/1,000 kilogram.

gross negligence the commission of an act that a prudent person would not have done or the omission of a duty that a prudent person would have fulfilled, resulting in injury or harm to another person.

H

half-life the time required for a radioactive substance to lose 50% of its activity through decay. Each radionuclide has a unique half-life.

harm to the patient physical or emotional injury that causes damage to the patient as a result of negligence by the provider.

HELLP syndrome mnemonic for a form of severe pre-eclampsia, a hypertensive complication of late pregnancy. The abbreviation stands for *h*emolysis, *e*levated *l*iver function, and *l*ow *p*latelet level.

hemodialysis a procedure in which impurities or wastes are removed from the blood. It is used in treating patients with renal failure and various toxic conditions.

heparin a naturally occurring substance that prevents intravascular clotting. The substance is produced by basophils and mast cells, which are found in large numbers in the connective tissue surrounding capillaries, particularly in the lungs and liver.

histamine a compound found in all cells that is produced by the breakdown of histidine. It is released in allergic inflammatory reactions and causes dilation of capillaries, a decrease in blood pressure, an increase in the secretion of gastric juice, and constriction of smooth muscles of the bronchi and uterus.

hub the part of a syringe where the needle attaches.

Huber needle a special needle used to access implantable medical ports. The Huber needle has a hole on the side rather than on the tip. This design slices through the membrane of the implantable medication port and does not core out a segment of the membrane. This reduces the chance of leaking through the opening of the port.

hyperkalemia greater than normal amounts of potassium in the blood.

hypersensitivity reaction an inappropriate and excessive response of the immune system to a sensitizing antigen called an allergen.

hypertension a common disorder that is a known cardiovascular disease risk factor. Hypertension is characterized by elevated blood pressure over the normal values of 120/80 mm Hg in an adult older than 18 years.

hypertensive emergency a severe elevation in blood pressure complicated by evidence of end-organ damage. End-organ damage can occur in the kidneys (kidney failure), heart (heart failure), and brain (intracranial bleed or altered level of consciousness). Also known as *malignant hypertension*.

hypertensive urgency a severe elevation of blood pressure without evidence of end-organ damage.

hypertonic pertaining to a solution that causes cells to shrink. Hypertonic solution increases the degree of osmotic pressure on a semipermeable membrane.

hypertonic saline solution a saline solution that contains 1 to 23.4% sodium chloride (compared with normal saline solution at 0.9%).

hypoglycemia a less than normal amount of glucose in the blood, usually caused by administration of too much insulin, excessive secretion of insulin by the islet cells of the pancreas, or dietary deficiency.

hypoglycemic unawareness the inability to recognize impending hypoglycemic episodes; often considered an adverse effect of beta blockers.

hypokalemia a condition in which an inadequate amount of potassium, the major intracellular cation, is found in the circulating bloodstream.

hypotension an abnormal condition in which the blood pressure is not adequate for normal perfusion and oxygenation of the tissues.

hypotensive resuscitation a resuscitation strategy to provide fluids to a trauma patient in which the goal is not to return the vital signs to normal, but to maintain physiologic functioning until the source of hemorrhage can be controlled.

hypothyroidism a condition in which thyroid hormone levels are low.

hypotonic a solution having a lower concentration of solute than another solution and thus exerting less osmotic pressure than that solution.

hypovolemic shock a state of physical collapse and prostration caused by massive blood loss, approximately one fifth or more of total blood volume.

hypoxia inadequate oxygen tension at the cellular level.

hypoxic respiratory drive a condition in which patients require a mild degree of hypoxia to continue breathing as a result of chronic respiratory disease.

I

idiosyncratic response a rare and unpredicted response to a drug that is unique to the patient experiencing the response. Such a response is not allergic in nature.

IM injection administration of a drug into the musculature.

immune system an elaborate system of the human body that is designed to mitigate the effects of harmful substances that might enter the body and compromise essential body functions.

immunities exemption from a duty or an obligation generally required by law, such as an exemption from taxation or penalty for wrongdoing, or protection against liability.

immunoglobulin see *antibody*.

infiltration the process in which a fluid passes into the tissues, such as when a local anesthetic is administered or an IV infusion infiltrates.

infusion pump an apparatus designed to deliver measured amounts of a drug or IV solution through injection over time.

infusion set another term to describe IV administration sets, or setups. Includes a bag of IV fluids, drip chamber, roller clamp, administration port, and IV catheter.

inhalation administration (of medication) the administration of a drug by inspiration of the vapor released from a fragile ampule packed in a fine mesh that is crushed for immediate administration.

inhaled medication medication that can be administered parenterally to bronchi and lungs by having the patient breathe or inhale the medication. In the prehospital setting, inhaled medications can be administered in two basic ways: the metered-dose inhaler and the pneumatically powered nebulizer.

inhaler a device for administering medications to be inhaled, such as vapors, fine powders, or volatile substances.

injectable medication parenteral delivery of a medication by using either IV, intramuscular, or subcutaneous routes of administration.

injection port area placed along the IV tubing where the provider can inject the contents of a syringe into the IV line.

inotropic drug a drug or substance that increases the force of cardiac contractions.

inotropism the force of cardiac contraction.

insulin a naturally occurring polypeptide hormone secreted by the beta cells of the islets of Langerhans in the pancreas in response to increased levels of glucose in the blood, as well as the parasympathetic nervous system and other stimuli.

insulin syringe a specially designed and labeled syringe in which the barrel is calibrated and labeled with the units of insulin and not volume, as most syringes are labeled. Most insulin syringes are calibrated and labeled for use with U-100 insulin.

interstitial fluid an extracellular fluid that fills the spaces between most of the cells of the body and provides a substantial portion of the liquid environment of the body.

intracellular fluid (ICF) an extracellular fluid that fills the spaces between most of the cells of the body and provides a substantial portion of the liquid environment of the body.

intracranial pressure (ICP) following injury to the brain, the brain will swell within the confines of the rigid skull, increasing the pressure within the skull and on the brain.

intramedullary space the highly vascular, central cavity of the bone in which an intraosseous needle can be placed to allow the administration of IV fluids, blood, and medications.

intramuscular (IM) the introduction of a hypodermic needle into a muscle to administer a medication.

intraosseous (IO) infusion the injection of blood, medications, or fluids into bone marrow rather than into a vein.

intranasal a route of medication administration that occurs within the nose; includes nasal spray for congestion or solutions to moisten the nasal mucosa.

intraparenchymal hematoma typically refers to bleeding within the brain caused by trauma or hemorrhagic stroke. Also can be used to refer to bleeding within the substance of other organs such as the liver or spleen.

intravascular fluid a form of extracellular fluid; principally, the blood.

intravascular space pertaining to the inside of a blood vessel.

intravenous (IV) pertaining to the inside of a vein, or a route of administration of an injection, an infusion, or a catheter.

intravenous infusion a solution administered into a vein through an infusion set that includes a plastic or glass vacuum bottle or bag containing the solution and tubing connecting the bottle to a catheter or a needle in the patient's vein.

intravenous pump a pump designed to regulate the rate of flow of a fluid administered through an IV catheter.

intrinsic originating from or situated within an organ or tissue.

intubation the insertion of a breathing tube through the mouth or nose into the trachea to ensure a patent airway for the delivery of anesthetic gases, oxygen, or both.

irreversible binding a condition in which a drug permanently binds to a receptor.

ischemia a decreased supply of oxygenated blood to a body part.

ischemic heart disease a pathologic condition caused by lack of oxygen in cells of the myocardium.

isotonic fluids pertaining to a solution that causes no change in cell volume.

IV piggyback (IVPB) a special coupling in the primary tubing that allows a supplementary, or piggyback, solution to run into the IV system.

IV push (IVP) a rapid form of a bolus typically used in life-threatening conditions in which a syringe containing a medication is connected to the injection port of IV tubing and then injected slowly into the IV line.

K

ketoacidosis acidosis accompanied by an accumulation of ketones in the body, resulting from the extensive breakdown of fats because of faulty carbohydrate metabolism.

ketone bodies products of lipid pyruvate metabolism, beta-hydroxybutyric acid, and aminoacetic acid, from which acetone may spontaneously arise. Excessive production leads to their excretion in urine, such as in diabetes mellitus.

ketonemia the presence of ketones, mainly acetone, in the blood. It is characterized by the fruity breath odor of ketoacidosis.

kilo combining form meaning "one thousand."

KVO a common abbreviation meaning "keep vein open."

L

lactic acidosis a disorder characterized by an accumulation of lactic acid in the blood, resulting in a lowered pH in muscle and serum.

laryngoedema swelling of the vocal cords.

latent period the interval between the time of exposure to an injurious dose of radiation and the adverse response. The term is also used to refer to the interval from administration of a drug to the desired effect. When speaking of medications, another name for latent period is "onset of action."

lethal dose (LD50) the amount of toxin that produces death in all members of a species population within a specified period of time.

lipophilic a drug or substance that dissolves in lipids (fat). Medications that are lipophilic are able to be dissolved in body fat and easily cross the membranes that separate the various body compartments.

lipophobic a drug or substance that does not dissolve in lipids (fat). Medications that are lipophobic are not able to dissolve in body fat and cannot cross the membranes that separate the various body compartments.

loading dose a rapidly administered and often larger dose of a medication used to elevate serum drug concentration to a therapeutic concentration.

loop of Henle the U-shaped part of a renal tubule, consisting of a thin descending limb and a thick ascending limb.

low-molecular-weight heparin a class of drugs used to prevent potentially fatal blood clots in patients undergoing surgery or other patients at risk for blood clots.

Luer-lock syringes a syringe fitted with a threaded tip, allowing a needle to be screwed into the tip. The Luer-lock allows the needle to be attached to the barrel with greater security. This type of syringe is required for use in needleless IV systems.

M

macrodrip chamber the drip compartment immediately below the IV bag where the IV fluid drips at a predetermined volume. Macrodrip chambers drip at 10, 12, 15, and 20 drops/mL.

macrodrip infusion set an IV tubing set that contains a macrodrip chamber.

malignant hypertension the most lethal form of hypertension, characterized by severely elevated blood pressure that commonly damages the intima of small vessels, the brain, the retina, the heart, and the kidneys.

malignant hyperthermia a rare genetic hypermetabolic condition characterized by severe hyperthermia and rigidity of the skeletal muscles occurring in affected people exposed to inhalation anesthetics and succinylcholine, a nondepolarizing muscle relaxant.

mechanism of action the chemical or physiologic method of how a medication affects the target tissue.

medical direction the process by which physicians direct and monitor the care given in the prehospital environment within an EMS system.

Medical Order for Life-Sustaining Treatment (MOLST) a form designed to convert patient wishes into actionable medical orders that are then followed by various medical professionals, including EMS providers, as patients move throughout the healthcare system. Also called *Physician Order for Life-Sustaining Treatment (POLST)*.

metabolism the aggregate of all chemical processes that take place in living organisms, resulting in growth, generation of energy, elimination of wastes, and other body functions as they relate to the distribution of nutrients in the blood after digestion.

medication administration record (MAR) a document in which healthcare settings typically document patient medication orders, schedules, and time of administration.

metered-dose inhaler (MDI) a device designed to deliver a measured dose of an inhaled drug.

methemoglobin a poisonous form of hemoglobin that does not release oxygen as well as normal hemoglobin.

metric system a decimal system of measurement based on the meter (39.37 inches) as the unit of length, or the gram (15.432 grains) as the unit of weight or mass, and—as a derived unit—on the liter (0.908 U.S. dry quart or 1.0567 U.S. liquid quart) as the unit of volume.

micro prefix meaning "one millionth."

microdrip chamber the compartment immediately below the IV bag where the IV fluid drips at a predetermined volume. Microdrip chambers administer 60 gtt/mL. The number of drops per minute equals the rate of infusion in milliliters per hour. Therefore, if 30 drops occur per minute, the infusion rate is 30 mL/hr.

microdrip infusion set an apparatus for delivering relatively small amounts of IV solution at specific flow rates. The size of the drop is controlled by the fixed diameter of the plastic delivery tube. With a microdrip set, 60 drops deliver 1 mL of solution. Microdrip sets deliver small amounts of solution over time, such as when it is necessary to keep a vein open.

microgram (mcg) a unit of measurement of mass equal to one millionth of a gram.

milli combining form meaning "one thousandth."

milligram (mg) a metric unit of weight equal to one thousandth of a gram.

milliliter (mL) a metric unit of volume that is one thousandth (10^{-3}) of a liter, or 1 cm.

mineralocorticoid a hormone secreted by the adrenal cortex that maintains normal blood volume, promotes sodium and water retention, and increases urinary excretion of potassium and hydrogen ions.

monoamine oxidase inhibitor (MAOI) any of a chemically heterogeneous group of drugs used primarily in the treatment of depression.

motor end plate a large special synaptic contact between motor axons and each skeletal muscle fiber. Each muscle fiber forms one end plate.

MTWHF a mnemonic for remembering the effects of nicotinic receptor blockage. The abbreviation stands for *M*ydriasis (dilation of pupils), *T*achycardia, *W*eakness, *H*ypertension and hyperglycemia, and *F*asciculations (involuntary contractions, twitching).

multidrip infusion set an infusion set that allows the paramedic to alternate among a 10-, 15-, and 60-drop set in one system.

muscarinic receptor a type of cholinergic receptor in the parasympathetic nervous system. Muscarinic receptors are found in the cardiac and smooth muscle, exocrine glands, and brain.

myocardial infarction (MI) necrosis of a portion of cardiac muscle caused by an obstruction in a coronary artery from atherosclerosis, a thrombus, or a spasm.

myxedema coma a severe form of hypothyroidism that is a life-threatening medical emergency with a high mortality rate.

N

narcotic a drug that acts by binding to opiate receptors in the central nervous system and alters the perception of pain; induces euphoria, mood changes, mental clouding, and deep sleep; depresses respirations and the cough reflex; constricts the pupils; and causes smooth muscle spasm, decreased peristalsis, emesis, and nausea.

narcotic antagonist a drug that binds to the opiate or narcotic receptor to prevent the opiate from exerting its effects of altered mental status, hypotension, and respiratory depression. Also known as *opiate antagonist*.

nasal cannula a device for delivering oxygen by way of two small tubes inserted into the nares.

nasogastric (NG) pertaining to the nose and stomach, as in (nasogastric) aspiration of the stomach's contents.

nebulization a method of administering a drug by spraying it into the respiratory passages of the patient.

nebulize to vaporize or disperse a liquid in a fine spray.

nebulizer a device for producing a fine spray of medication.

nephrolithiasis a disorder characterized by the presence of calculi in the kidney.

neurogenic shock a form of shock that results from peripheral vascular dilation due to loss of neural input maintaining vascular tone.

neuromuscular junction the area of contact between the ends of a large myelinated nerve fiber and a fiber of skeletal muscle. Neurotransmitters communicate with the muscle tissue in this area.

neurotransmitter any one of numerous chemicals that modify or result in the transmission of nerve impulses between synapses.

nicotinic receptor a type of cholinergic receptor in the parasympathetic nervous system. Nicotinic receptors are found in the central nervous system, autonomic ganglia, and striated muscle.

nine patient rights of drug administration a checklist that should be performed before administering a medication to a patient to improve patient safety in drug administration. The nine patient rights are right patient, right drug and right indication, right dose, right route, right time, right education, right to refuse, right response and evaluation, and right documentation.

noncompetitive antagonist an antagonist that irreversibly binds to a receptor. Regardless of how much of the agonist is given, the effect of the noncompetitive antagonists on the receptor cannot be overcome.

nondepolarizing muscle relaxant medication that produces relaxation of skeletal muscles by preferentially binding to the acetylcholine receptor site, preventing binding of acetylcholine and thereby preventing muscle contraction.

nondepolarizing paralytic another name for a nondepolarizing muscle relaxant.

non-Luer-lock syringe a syringe in which the needle fits tightly on the tip, which is not threaded.

nonrebreather face mask oxygen face mask with one-way exhalation valves on the sides of the mask and the reservoir bag. Nonrebreather face masks require a higher flow rate of 12 to 15 L/min and are capable of delivering oxygen concentrations close to 100%.

nonselective beta blocker beta blockers that bind at both the beta$_1$ and the beta$_2$ receptor.

nonsteroidal anti-inflammatory drug (NSAID) any of a group of drugs having antipyretic, analgesic, and anti-inflammatory effects.

nonvented infusion set infusion set that does not have a port for air to flow into the closed fluid container. Nonvented sets are used for fluids not packaged in glass containers, such as crystalloid solutions.

O

offline medical direction medical control in which the physician is not available for real-time interactions.

one-time order when a prehospital provider consults medical direction and receives an order for immediate drug intervention.

online medical direction medical direction in which the prehospital provider is able to consult and obtain direction and orders in real time by radio or telephone communication.

onset of action the time required after administration of a drug for a response to be observed.

Opiate an opioid drug that contains opium, derivatives of opium, or any of several semisynthetic or synthetic drugs with opium-like activity. A substance that causes sleep or relief of pain.

opioid a medication that acts upon opioid receptors in the body. Most true narcotics administered by EMS providers are opioids.

opioid receptor transmembrane protein that binds to endogenous opioid neuropeptides and exogenous morphine and similar natural or synthetic compounds.

ordinary negligence the failure to exercise the degree of care that another reasonable person would exercise in the same or similar situation in which harm to another person results. Also known as *basic negligence*.

organophosphate a class of anticholinesterase chemicals used in certain pesticides and war gases. They act by causing irreversible inhibition of cholinesterase.

osmosis the movement of a pure solvent, such as water, through a differentially permeable membrane, from a solution that has a lower solute concentration to one that has a higher solute concentration.

osmotic demyelination syndrome (ODS) a neurologic condition associated with the too-rapid correction of hyponatremia. Symptoms include headache, alterations in behavior, obtundation, coma, and death.

osmotic diuretic a medication that when excreted by the kidneys cannot be reabsorbed by the kidneys and prevents the reabsorption of excreted water. This produces the rate of urine production.

P

packed red blood cells (PRBCs) a preparation of blood cells separated from liquid plasma, often administered in severe anemia to restore adequate levels of hemoglobin and red cells without overloading the vascular system with excess fluids.

parasympathetic nervous system the division of the autonomic nervous system that slows heart rate, increases intestinal peristalsis and gland activity, and relaxes sphincters.

parenteral administration route that bypasses the GI tract.

parenteral route pertaining to a medication administered by a route other than the gastrointestinal tract, such as a drug given by injection.

paroxysmal supraventricular tachycardia (PSVT) an ectopic heart rhythm with a rate of 170 to 250 beats/min. It begins abruptly with a premature atrial or ventricular beat and is supported by an atrioventricular nodal reentry mechanism or by an atrioventricular reentry mechanism involving an accessory pathway.

partial agonist a medication that binds to a receptor site and initiates a reduced amount of cellular activity compared to other chemicals or medications that may also be present at the cells, reducing the efficacy of other agonist chemicals.

partial rebreather face mask see *rebreather face mask*.

partial refusal when a patient agrees to some, but not all, of the treatment offered.

passive diffusion when medications penetrate cells by diffusion through the cell membrane.

passive transport the movement of small molecules across the membrane of a cell by diffusion. Passive transport occurs when the chemicals outside a cell become concentrated and start moving into the cell, changing the intracellular equilibrium.

peak expiratory flow rate (PEFR) the greatest rate of airflow that can be achieved during forced expiration beginning with the lungs fully inflated.

percutaneous coronary intervention (PCI) the management of coronary artery occlusion by any of various catheter-based techniques, such as percutaneous transluminal coronary angioplasty, atherectomy, angioplasty using the excimer laser, and implementation of coronary stents and related devices.

percutaneous transluminal coronary angioplasty (PTCA) a technique in the treatment of atherosclerotic coronary heart disease and angina pectoris in which some plaques in the arteries of the heart are flattened against the arterial walls, resulting in improved circulation.

pericardial tamponade compression of the heart produced by the accumulation of blood or other fluid in the pericardial sac.

peripheral line a term that applies to an IV catheter inserted in a peripheral vein.

peripherally inserted central catheter (PICC line) a long catheter introduced through a vein in the arm, then through the subclavian vein into the superior vena cava or right atrium to administer parenteral fluids or medications or to measure central venous pressure.

peritoneal dialysis a dialysis procedure performed to correct an imbalance of fluid or electrolytes in the blood or to remove toxins, drugs, or other wastes normally excreted by the kidney. The peritoneum is used as a diffusible membrane.

permissive hypotension a hypotensive state that is permitted with the goal of maintaining physiologic functioning until the source of hemorrhage can be controlled.

pharmacodynamics the study of how a drug acts on a living organism, including the pharmacologic response and the duration and magnitude of response observed relative to the concentration of the drug at an active site in the organism.

pharmacokinetics the study of the action of drugs within the body, including studies of the mechanisms of drug absorption, distribution, metabolism, and excretion; onset of action; duration of effect; biotransformation; and effects and routes of excretion of the metabolites of the drug.

pharmacologic antagonism occurs when a drug binds to a receptor and prevents the biologic effect of that receptor.

pharmacology the study of the preparation, properties, uses, and actions of drugs.

phenytoin equivalent (PE) to avoid the need to perform dose conversions between phenytoin and fosphenytoin, the dosage for fosphenytoin is prescribed in phenytoin equivalents (PE).

pheochromocytoma a vascular tumor of chromaffin tissue of the adrenal medulla or sympathetic paraganglia, characterized by hypersecretion of epinephrine and norepinephrine, causing persistent or intermittent hypertension.

phlebitis inflammation of a vein accompanied by the formation of a clot.

phosphodiesterase inhibitor a class of drugs that increase inotropism by increasing the concentration of calcium inside the cardiac cell.

photophobia abnormal sensitivity to light, especially by the eyes. The condition is prevalent in albinism and various diseases of the conjunctiva and cornea and may be a symptom of such disorders as measles, psittacosis, encephalitis, Rocky Mountain spotted fever, and Reiter's syndrome.

piggyback infusion see *IV piggyback.*

placenta a highly vascular fetal organ that exchanges with the maternal circulation, mainly by diffusion of oxygen, carbon dioxide, and other substances.

plunger the inner portion of the syringe that pushes the liquid medication to the tip of the syringe and out the needle.

pneumothorax the presence of air or gas in the pleural space, causing a lung or collapse. Pneumothorax may be the result of an open chest wound that permits the entrance of air, the rupture of an emphysematous vesicle on the surface of the lung, or without apparent cause.

Poiseuille's law the law of physics that governs the movement of an incompressible fluid through a circular tube.

polypharmacy the use of a number of different drugs, possibly prescribed by different doctors and filled in different pharmacies, by a patient who may have one or several health problems.

potency a term used to compare the different doses of two medications in producing the same effect.

potentiation when a drug lacking a particular effect of its own increases the effect of a second drug.

precursor a prognostic characteristic or feature of a patient's health data, such as a radiographic or laboratory finding, that is associated with a higher or lower risk of death than average.

preeclampsia an abnormal condition of pregnancy characterized by the onset of acute hypertension after the twenty-fourth week of gestation.

prefilled tube a medication-filled cylinder to assist in medication administration.

preloaded syringe a two-piece kit with a medication-filled cylinder that rapidly screws to an included syringe to allow rapid drug administration.

premature ventricular complex (PVC) a ventricular depolarization that occurs earlier than expected.

pressure bag a sleeve placed around a bag of IV fluids to increase the pressure of the IV fluids and increase the flow rate of the IV fluid. Pressure bags may be applied to arterial lines to prevent backflow of blood into the tubing.

primary brain injury an injury that occurs directly to the brain from mechanical forces at the time of the initial insult.

Prinzmetal's angina chest pain caused by reversible, severe coronary artery spasm. It is associated with ST-segment elevation that reverts to normal within minutes. The ST-segment elevation indicates total occlusion of the epicardial coronary artery.

prn order abbreviation for *pro re nata,* a Latin phrase meaning "as needed," referring to administration times that are determined by the patient's needs.

prodrug an inactive or partially active drug that is metabolically changed in the body to an active drug.

protocol a written plan specifying the procedures to be followed in giving a particular examination, conducting research, or providing care for a particular condition.

proximate cause a legal concept of cause-and-effect relations in determining, for example, whether an injury would have resulted from a particular cause.

pseudocholinesterase an enzyme that acts as a catalyst in the hydrolysis of acetylcholine to choline and acetate; provides the "off" mechanism during cholinergic neurotransmission.

pulmonary edema the accumulation of extravascular fluid in lung tissues and alveoli, caused most commonly by congestive heart failure.

pulseless electrical activity (PEA) continued electrical rhythmicity of the heart in the absence of effective mechanical function.

pulseless ventricular tachycardia a rapid heart rate that originates in the ventricles and is not associated with a pulse.

Q

qualified immunity immunity that has qualification; the caregiver may not act in a reckless, wanton manner in total disregard to the patient.

R

rapid sequence induction a series of techniques to start general anesthesia with a lower risk of aspiration.

rapid sequence intubation adoption of the techniques of rapid sequence induction for the use of emergency intubation.

rebreather face mask breathing device with a face mask and a reservoir bag. Oxygen accumulates in the reservoir bag. During inhalation, the patient inhales oxygen in the reservoir, as well as some room air through the side ports. When the patient exhales, some of the exhaled breath goes back into the reservoir bag, where it is then rebreathed.

receptor a chemical structure, usually of protein/carbohydrate, on the surface of a cell that combines with an antigen to produce a discrete immunologic component.

rectal administration (of a medication) the instillation of a medicated suppository, cream, or gel into the rectum.

refractory period a period during the action potential in which the nerve or muscle tissue will not produce a response if stimulated.

reperfusion therapy administration of a medication that dissolves clots within an artery and reestablishes blood flow.

reversible binding a condition in which a drug is able to separate from the cell's receptor, as in removing a key from a lock. When the drug is removed from the receptor, the effect of the drug stops.

Reye's syndrome a combination of acute encephalopathy and fatty infiltration of the internal organs that may follow acute viral infections. The cause is unknown; however, the administration of aspirin seems to be an association.

roller clamp a device, usually made of plastic, equipped with a small roller that may be rolled counterclockwise to close off primary IV tubing or clockwise to open it.

S

sarin a nerve agent used in chemical warfare.

saturable process when referring to movement of drugs across membranes, a process in which the external concentrations of the drug can reach a point at which increasing the concentration does not result in an increase in the rate of transportation into the cell.

Schedule I a category of drugs not considered legitimate for medical use. Special licensing procedures must be followed to use these substances.

Schedule II a category of drugs considered to have a strong potential for abuse or addiction but that have legitimate medical use.

Schedule III a category of drugs that have less potential for abuse or addiction than Schedule II or I drugs.

Schedule IV a category of drugs that have less potential for abuse or addiction than those of Schedules I to III.

Schedule V a category of drugs that have a small potential for abuse or addiction. The specific drugs in Schedule V vary greatly from state to state.

scope of practice the legally approved skills or practices that may be performed by a provider and the medications authorized to administer as defined in state law.

secondary brain injury a delayed injury to the brain that occurs from swelling of the brain within the rigid confines of the skull, resulting in a decrease in blood flow and oxygen delivery.

sedative an agent that decreases functional activity, diminishes irritability, and allays excitement. Some sedatives have a general effect on all organs; others principally affect the activities of the heart, stomach, intestines, nerve trunks, respiratory system, or vasomotor system.

selective beta blocker a beta blocker that binds with either the beta$_1$ or the beta$_2$ receptor but not both.

Sellick maneuver a technique to reduce the risk of aspiration of stomach contents during induction of general anesthesia; applied before intubation, immediately after injection of anesthetic drugs, and as a part of rapid sequence intubation.

septic shock a form of shock that occurs in septicemia when endotoxins or exotoxins are released from certain bacteria in the bloodstream.

serotonin a naturally occurring derivative of tryptophan found in platelets and cells of the brain and the intestine. Serotonin is released from platelets when damage occurs to the blood vessel walls.

shaft the long portion of the needle that attaches to the hub.

shelf life the period of time a medication can be stored and remain suitable for use.

side effect any reaction to or consequence of a medication or therapy, usually undesirable.

single dose administration of one dose of a medication without the need for repeat administration to be therapeutic.

sinus rhythm a cardiac rhythm stimulated by the sinus node. A rate of 60 to 100 beats/min is normal.

slow-reacting substance of anaphylaxis (SRS-A) a group of active substances, including histamine and leukotrienes, that are released during an anaphylactic reaction. They cause the smooth muscle contraction and vascular dilation that result in the signs and symptoms of anaphylaxis.

somatic nervous system the division of the nervous system that controls skeletal muscles and movement.

spacer device on a metered-dose inhaler, a chamber between the inhaler canister and the patient's mouth where droplets of medication can slow and evaporate so that there is less direct impact on the oropharynx.

stable angina pectoris transient episode of chest pain resulting from myocardial ischemia that predictably occurs with exercise, exertion, and stressful situations.

standard of care a written statement describing the rules, actions, or conditions that direct patient care. Standards of care guide practice and can be used to evaluate performance.

standing orders instructions for treatment that are usually specific to a particular patient presentation and may or may not require consultation with medical direction. Standing orders are most appropriate for life-threatening conditions that require immediate intervention.

status epilepticus a medical emergency characterized by continuous seizures occurring without interruptions and lasting more than 30 minutes.

sternum the elongated flattened bone forming the middle part of the thorax.

steroid hormones any of the ductless gland secretions that contain the basic steroid nucleus in their chemical formulas. The natural steroid hormones include the androgens, estrogens, and adrenal cortex secretions.

stroke volume the amount of blood ejected by a ventricle during contraction.

subcutaneous the introduction of a hypodermic needle into the subcutaneous tissue beneath the skin, usually on the upper arm, thigh, or abdomen.

subcutaneous administration injection of a drug under the skin.

subcutaneous space a continuous layer of connective tissue over the entire body between the skin and the deep fascial investment of the specialized structures of the body, such as the muscles.

subdural hematoma an accumulation of blood in the subdural space, usually caused by an injury.

sublingual (SL) administration (of a medication) the administration of a drug, usually in tablet form, by placing it beneath the tongue until the tablet dissolves.

substrate a chemical acted on and changed by an enzyme in a chemical reaction.

summation the concentration of a neurotransmitter at a synapse, either by increasing the frequency of nerve impulses in each fiber or by increasing the number of fibers stimulated, so that the threshold of the postsynaptic neuron is overcome and an impulse is transmitted.

suppurative thrombophlebitis an infection of a vein that can be complicated by septic thrombosis, bacteremia, metastatic abscesses, and even death.

supraventricular tachycardia (SVT) any cardiac rhythm with a rate exceeding 100 beats/min that originates above the branching part of the atrioventricular bundle.

sympathetic nervous system the division of the autonomic nervous system that accelerates heart rate, constricts blood vessels, and raises blood pressure.

sympathomimetic drug a pharmacologic agent that mimics the effects of stimulation of organs and structures by the sympathetic nervous system. It functions by occupying adrenergic receptor sites and acting as an agonist or by increasing the release of the neurotransmitter norepinephrine at postganglionic nerve endings.

synapse the region surrounding the point of contact between two neurons or between a neuron and an effector organ, across which nerve impulses are transmitted through the action of a neurotransmitter.

synaptic cleft the microscopic extracellular space at the synapse that separates the membrane of the terminal nerve endings of a presynaptic neuron and the membrane of a postsynaptic cell.

synergism the observed effect of two medications, when given at the same time, being greater than the effects of the medications when given individually.

syringe a device for withdrawing, injecting, or instilling fluids. A syringe for the injection of medication usually consists of a calibrated glass or plastic cylindric barrel that has a close-fitting plunger at one end and a small opening at the other to which the head of a hollow-bore needle is fitted.

syrup of ipecac an emetic preparation of ipecac fluid extract, glycerin, and syrup used to treat certain types of poisonings and drug overdoses.

T

tall man lettering a convention for writing drug names so that similar-sounding drug names are not confused with one another. Uppercase letters are set against lowercase letters to highlight the key letters that distinguish a particular drug name. For example, "DOBUTamine" and "DOPamine."

tardive dyskinesia an abnormal condition characterized by involuntary repetitious movements of the muscles of the face, limbs, and trunk. This disorder most commonly affects older people who have been treated for extended periods with phenothiazine.

teratogenic any substance, agent, or process that interferes with normal prenatal development, causing the formation of one or more developmental abnormalities in the fetus.

therapeutic index (TI) the difference between the minimal therapeutic and minimal toxic concentrations of a drug.

thionamide agent oral antithyroid medications commonly used for the long-term management of hyperthyroidism.

thrombolytic a drug or other agent that dissolves thrombi.

thrombophlebitis inflammation of a vein accompanied by the formation of a clot.

thyroid storm a life-threatening manifestation of thyrotoxicosis.

thyrotoxicosis a multisystemic autoimmune disorder characterized by pronounced hyperthyroidism, usually associated with an enlarged thyroid gland and exophthalmos (abnormal protrusion of the eyeball).

tibial tuberosity a characteristic elevation on the anterior and proximal portion of the tibia that can be palpated as a small bony bump on the lower leg immediately below the knee.

tip the portion of a syringe where the needle attaches.

TKO an abbreviation for "to keep open," referring to a minimal IV infusion rate to keep the catheter from clotting.

tonic-clonic seizure an epileptic seizure characterized by a generalized involuntary muscular contraction and cessation of respiration followed by tonic and clonic spasms of the muscles.

torsades de pointes a type of ventricular tachycardia with a spiral-like appearance ("twisting of the points") and complexes that at first appear to be positive and then negative on an electrocardiogram.

total body water (TBW) all the water within the body, including intracellular and extracellular water plus the water in the gastrointestinal and urinary tracts.

trade name a name for a drug created by pharmaceutical companies; also known as a *proprietary* or *brand name*. Trade names always begin with a capital letter.

transdermal/topical administration (of a medication) a method of applying a drug to unbroken skin. The drug is continuously absorbed through the skin and enters the systemic system.

traumatic brain injury (TBI) a broad term applied to mechanical injury to the brain, including such injuries as concussion, subarachnoid hemorrhage, subdural hematoma, and epidural hematoma.

triple-lumen catheter (TLC) any catheter with three separate passages.

type 1 diabetes an autoimmune disease characterized by the inability to metabolize fuels, carbohydrates, protein, and fat because of absolute insulin deficiency; can occur at any age, but its incidence is more common in children.

type 2 diabetes a type of diabetes mellitus characterized by insulin resistance in appropriate hepatic glucose production and impaired insulin secretion; onset is usually after 40 years of age but can occur at any age, including during childhood and adolescence.

U

United States Pharmacopeia-National Formulary (USP-NF) a compendium recognized officially by the Federal Food, Drug, and Cosmetic Act that contains descriptions, uses, strengths, and standards of purity for selected drugs and for all their forms of dosage.

unstable angina pectoris (UA) angina pectoris, commonly known as angina, is chest pain due to ischemia (a lack of blood and hence oxygen supply) of the heart muscle, generally due to obstruction or spasm of the coronary arteries (the heart's blood vessels). Coronary artery disease, the main cause of angina, is due to atherosclerosis of the cardiac arteries. The term derives from the Greek *ankhon* (strangling) and the Latin *pectus* (chest), and can, therefore, be translated as "a strangling feeling in the chest."

V

variant angina see *Prinzmetal's angina*.

vastus lateralis the largest of the four muscles of the quadriceps femoris group, situated on the lateral side of the thigh.

vented infusion set infusion set necessary for the administration of fluids. Vented sets have a side port at the drip chamber that can be opened to allow air to flow into the closed fluid container.

ventricular fibrillation (VF) a cardiac arrhythmia marked by rapid depolarizations of the ventricular myocardium.

ventricular tachycardia (VT) tachycardia of at least three consecutive ventricular complexes with a rate greater than 100 per minute. It originates in a focus within the ventricle.

ventrogluteal injection a region of the hip where injections can be safely administered in children.

Venturi mask a respiratory therapy face mask designed to allow inspired air to mix with oxygen, which is supplied through a jet at a fixed concentration.

vial a glass container with a metal-enclosed rubber seal.

volume the amount of space occupied by a body, expressed in cubic units.

volume-control chamber any one of several types of transparent plastic reservoirs with graduated volumetric markings used to regulate the flow of IV solutions. These devices are components of IV volume control sets and accommodate the injection and mixing of medications by special built-in ports.

volume of distribution a measure of how rapidly and to what extent a drug can move throughout the body. A drug with a high volume of distribution is fat soluble and can easily pass through membranes and into the various body compartments.

VX a thin, amber-colored, odorless liquid that resembles motor oil and may be used as a nerve agent.

W

Wernicke-Korsakoff syndrome the coexistence of Wernicke's encephalopathy and Korsakoff's syndrome.

Wolff-Parkinson-White (WPW) syndrome a disorder of atrioventricular conduction involving an accessory pathway; often identified by a characteristic delta wave seen on an electrocardiogram at the beginning of the QRS complex.

Z

Z-track technique a technique for injecting irritating preparations into a muscle without tracking residual medication through sensitive tissues.

zero-order kinetics a state at which the rate of an enzyme reaction is independent of the concentration of the substrate.

Index

Note: Page numbers followed by *f* indicate figures; *t*, tables; *b*, boxes